Chronic Liver Disease

Chronic Liver Disease

Edited by Heidi Hamlin

hayle medical
New York

Hayle Medical,
750 Third Avenue, 9th Floor,
New York, NY 10017, USA

Visit us on the World Wide Web at:
www.haylemedical.com

ISBN: 978-1-63241-635-3

Printed in China.

Cataloging-in-Publication Data

Chronic liver disease / edited by Heidi Hamlin.
p. cm.
Includes bibliographical references and index.
ISBN 978-1-63241-635-3
1. Liver--Diseases. 2. Liver--Diseases--Diagnosis. 3. Liver--Diseases--Treatment.
4. Hepatology. I. Hamlin, Heidi.
RC845 .C47 2019
616.362--dc23

Preface

Chronic liver disease refers to a series of stages in the liver condition that involves progressive destruction and regeneration of the liver parenchyma, thereby leading to cirrhosis and fibrosis. This progression usually lasts over a period of six months. Chronic liver disease may be caused by viral agents such as Hepatitis B and C, right heart failure, drugs and toxins such as alcohol, paracetamol, methotrexate, nitrofurantoin, amiodarone, etc. Metabolic conditions such as haemochromatosis, non-alcoholic fatty liver disease, Wilson's disease, and autoimmune response such as primary sclerosing cholangitis and primary biliary cholangitis are also associated with chronic liver disease. Some of the factors that may enhance the risks of developing chronic liver disease are obesity, certain prescription medications, excessive alcohol use, metabolic syndrome such as raised blood lipids, etc. Liver biopsy, ultrasonography and liver function tests may help diagnose the liver condition. This book covers in detail some existing theories and innovative concepts revolving around chronic liver disease. The objective of this book is to give a general view of the different clinical aspects along with the medical and surgical treatment strategies of chronic liver disease. It will help the readers in keeping pace with the rapid changes in the treatment of chronic liver disease.

This book is a result of research of several months to collate the most relevant data in the field.

When I was approached with the idea of this book and the proposal to edit it, I was overwhelmed. It gave me an opportunity to reach out to all those who share a common interest with me in this field. I had 3 main parameters for editing this text:

1. Accuracy - The data and information provided in this book should be up-to-date and valuable to the readers.

2. Structure - The data must be presented in a structured format for easy understanding and better grasping of the readers.

3. Universal Approach - This book not only targets students but also experts and innovators in the field, thus my aim was to present topics which are of use to all.

Thus, it took me a couple of months to finish the editing of this book.

I would like to make a special mention of my publisher who considered me worthy of this opportunity and also supported me throughout the editing process. I would also like to thank the editing team at the back-end who extended their help whenever required.

Editor

1

A New Child-Turcotte-Pugh Class 0 for Patients with Hepatocellular Carcinoma: Determinants, Prognostic Impact and Ability to Improve the Current Staging Systems

Yun-Hsuan Lee[1,7], Chia-Yang Hsu[1,4,8], Chen-Wei Chu[1,7], Po-Hong Liu[1,4], Cheng-Yuan Hsia[1,5], Yi-Hsiang Huang[2,4], Chien-Wei Su[1,4], Yi-You Chiou[1,6], Han-Chieh Lin[1,4], Teh-Ia Huo[1,3,4]*

1 Faculty of Medicine, National Yang-Ming University School of Medicine, Taipei, Taiwan, **2** Institute of Clinical Medicine, National Yang-Ming University School of Medicine, Taipei, Taiwan, **3** Institute of Pharmacology, National Yang-Ming University School of Medicine, Taipei, Taiwan, **4** Department of Medicine, Taipei Veterans General Hospital, Taipei, Taiwan, **5** Department of Surgery, Taipei Veterans General Hospital, Taipei, Taiwan, **6** Department of Radiology, Taipei Veterans General Hospital, Taipei, Taiwan, **7** Department of Medicine, Yuanshan Branch of Taipei Veterans General Hospital, Taipei, Taiwan, **8** Department of Biostatistics, University of California Los Angeles, Los Angeles, California, United States of America

Abstract

Background/Aim: Majority of patients with hepatocellular carcinoma (HCC) belonged to Child-Turcotte-Pugh (CTP) class A. We aimed to identify a new class of patients with very well-preserved liver function and analyze its impact on outcome prediction, tumor staging and treatment allocation.

Methods: A total of 2654 HCC patients were retrospectively analyzed. The prognostic ability was compared by the Akaike information criterion (AIC).

Results: The CTP class 0 was defined by fulfilling all criteria of albumin $\geqq 4$ g/dL, bilirubin $\leqq 0.8$ mg/dL, prothrombin time prolongation <0 seconds, no ascites and encephalopathy. A total of 23% of patients of CTP class A were reclassified as CTP class 0. Patients with CTP class 0 had a higher serum sodium level, lower serum creatinine, alanine aminotransferase, α-fetoprotein levels, shorter prothrombin time, better general well-being, smaller tumor burden with more solitary nodules, lower rates of vascular invasion, ascites formation, hepatic encephalopathy, more frequently treated with curative interventions and better Barcelona Clinic Liver Cancer (BCLC) stages (all $p<0.001$). In the Cox proportional hazards model, the adjusted hazard ratios for CTP class A, B and C were 1.739, 3.120 and 5.107, respectively, compared to class 0 (all $p<0.001$). Reassigning patients with CTP class 0, A, B, B and C to stage 0, A, B, C and D, respectively, provided the lowest AIC score among all BCLC-based models.

Conclusions: The proposal of CTP class 0 independently predicted better survival in HCC patients. Modification of tumor staging systems according to the modified CTP classification further enhances their prognostic ability.

Editor: Yujin Hoshida, Icahn School of Medicine at Mount Sinai, United States of America

Funding: This study was supported by grants from the Center of Excellence for Cancer Research at Taipei Veterans General Hospital (DOH102-TD-C-111-007), Taiwan, from Taipei Veterans General Hospital (V102C-012), Taipei, Taiwan. The funders had no role in study design, data collection and analysis, decision to publish, or preparation of the manuscript.

Competing Interests: The authors have declared that no competing interests exist.

* E-mail: tihuo@vghtpe.gov.tw

Introduction

Hepatocellular carcinoma (HCC) is a common malignancy accounting for 500,000 deaths per year [1]. Chronic inflammation of liver parenchyma, mainly arising from viral hepatitis or alcoholism, may subsequently result in HCC. Notably, majority of patients with HCC have a coexisting liver cirrhosis or chronic liver disease. The Child-Turcotte-Pugh (CTP) classification was originally created to predict mortality in patients receiving surgery for portal hypertension [2,3], and is currently used to determine the survival of patients with chronic liver disease and cirrhosis. Among the commonly used cancer staging systems, CTP classification is an important outcome indicator in the Barcelona Clinic Liver Cancer (BCLC), Cancer of the Liver Italian Program (CLIP) and Taipei Integrated Scoring (TIS) staging systems [4–7]. CTP classification is also included as an important index for treatment suggestion, according to the BCLC staging system [7,8].

The current CTP classification is determined by serum albumin, bilirubin and international normalized ratio (INR) of prothrombin time (PT) levels, ascites formation and encephalopathy. Interestingly, even though CTP class A comprises only patients with total scores of 5 and 6, it represents a majority of patients with HCC [9]. Furthermore, the composition of HCC

Table 1. Definitions for the original and modified CTP classifications.

	Child-Turcotte-Pugh Scoring				
	Albumin (g/dL)	**Bilirubin (mg/dL)**	**Prothrombin time prolong (seconds)**	**Ascites**	**Encephalopathy**
1	>3.5	<2	<4	None	None
2	2.8–3.5	2–3	4–6	Mild	Grade 1–2
3	<2.8	>3	>6	Moderate to severe	Grade 3–4

Modified CTP class 0: Fulfill all criteria of albumin ≧4.0 g/dL, bilirubin ≦0.8 mg/dL, prothromin time prolongation <0 seconds, no ascites and no encephalopathy. Modified CTP class A: total scores of 5–6 and not fulfilling criteria for class 0; class B: total scores of 7–9; class C: total scores of 10–15.
Abbreviations: CTP, Child-Turcotte-Pugh.

patients with CTP score of 5 encompasses different strata of clinical scenarios, including patients with no chronic liver disease, patients with only chronic inflammation and patients with well-compensated cirrhosis. The long-term outcomes of these patients are considered to be different [10,11] and the current CTP classification may not be capable of distinguishing these patients in estimating liver function and survival prediction. Moreover, the current cancer staging system, based on the original CTP classification, may not be informative enough [12–14]. A new definition for an earlier stage of CTP classification is considered for better discrimination of liver functional reserve. No study to date has specifically aimed to explore the rationale of using the CTP classification with an attempt to identify the early stage of these patients. In this study, we proposed a new CTP class 0 and validated its ability in predicting outcome for HCC. Moreover, modified models of the BCLC, CLIP and TIS staging systems were proposed according to the modified CTP classification, and the prognostic ability of these models were investigated.

Patients and Methods

Patients

Between 2002 and 2012, patients who were newly diagnosed with HCC in Taipei Veterans General Hospital were consecutively enrolled and retrospectively analyzed. The baseline information was comprehensively collected at the time of diagnosis. This study has been approved by the institutional review board of Taipei Veterans General Hospital and complies with the standards of the Declaration of Helsinki and current ethical guidelines. Waiver of consent was obtained, and patient records/information was anonymized and de-identified prior to analysis. Part of our patients had been enrolled in our previous studies [9,15].

Diagnosis and Definitions

The inclusion criteria were: (1) patients with newly diagnosed HCC; (2) aged above 18 years; (3) did not receive management for HCC before enrollment. Patients who were diagnosed with malignant tumor other than HCC were excluded from the study. The diagnosis of HCC was established by histology or based on the findings of typical radiological features in a 4-phase multi-detector computed tomography scan or dynamic contrast-enhanced magnetic resonance imaging [8,16,17]. Vascular invasion was defined by the presence of adjacent thrombus to the tumor in portal vein with blurring boundary confirmed by at least one imaging modality. Alcoholism was diagnosed in subjects with a documented history of alcohol excess of at least 40 g alcohol daily for 5 years or more [18]. The performance status was assessed by using the Eastern Cooperative Oncology Group (ECOG) performance scale: 0 (asymptomatic) to 4 (confined to bed). The original CTP classification and the model for end-stage liver disease (MELD) score were defined as reported [2,3,19]. Total tumor volume (TTV) was calculated as the sum of all tumor nodule volume, and each tumor nodule volume is calculated as $4/3 \times 3.14 \times (\text{maximum radius of the tumor nodule in cm})^3$ as previously described [6]. The BCLC, CLIP and TIS systems were used to define clinical staging [4–6].

Treatment

Treatment for each individual patient was suggested by a multidisciplinary HCC team of our hospital. Curative treatment was defined as patients undergoing surgical resection, local ablation therapy or liver transplantation. Other treatment modalities were mostly palliative and collectively defined as non-curative treatment. Patients with HCC selected for surgical resection (SR) were (a) patients with tumor involving no more than 3 Healey's segments, (b) patients with preserved liver function and had less than 25% retention of indocyanine green 15 minutes

Table 2. The distribution of HCC patients after modification of the CTP classifications.

		Modified Child-Turcotte-Pugh Classification				
		0	**A**	**B**	**C**	**No. (%)**
Original Child-Turcotte-Pugh Classification	A	441	1483	-	-	1924 (72)
	B	-	-	583	-	583 (22)
	C	-	-	-	147	147 (6)
	No. (%)	441 (17)	1483 (56)	583 (22)	147 (6)	

Abbreviations: CTP, Child-Turcotte-Pugh; HCC, hepatocellular carcinoma; No., number.

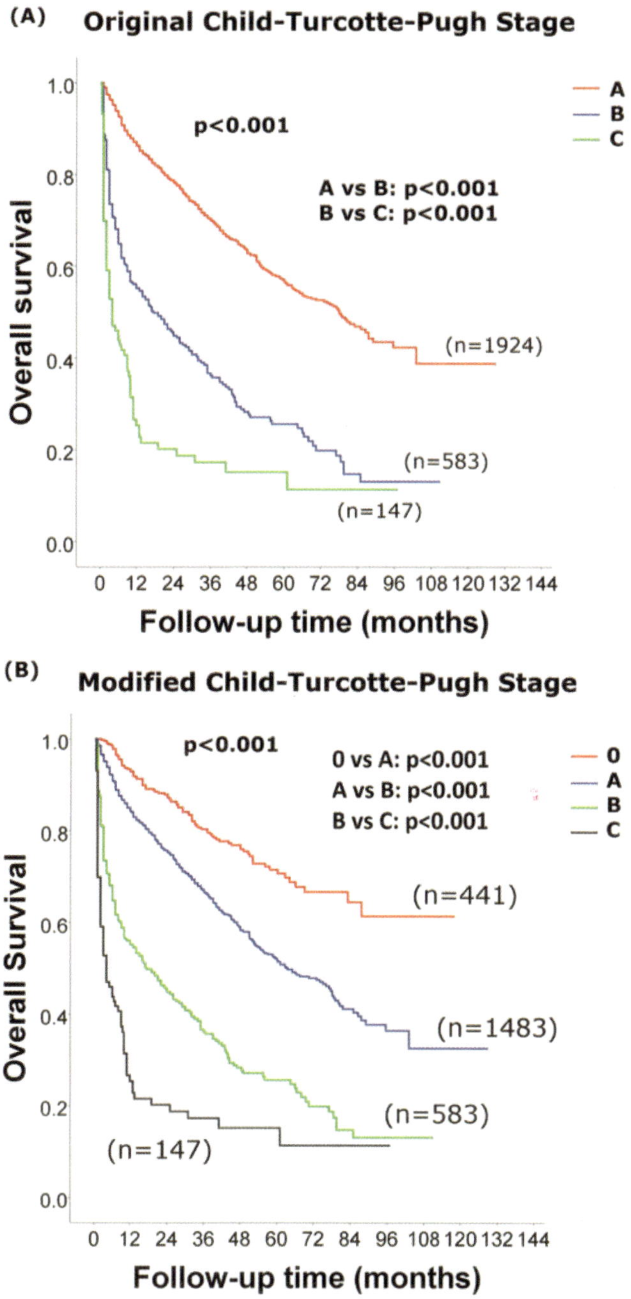

Figure 1. Comparison of survival distributions between patients of different CTP classifications. Patients with the new CTP class 0 were associated with a better long-term survival (panel B; $p<0.001$). Pairwise comparison between each CTP and modified CTP classes showed significant survival differences (panel A $p<0.001$).

(ICG15) after injection [20], and (c) patients who had no main portal vein trunk involvement or distant metastasis [8,17]. The ICG15 of each patient was then individually evaluated for the feasibility of SR according to their tumor size and the extent of hepatic resection. Radiofrequency ablation (RFA) was considered in patients with solitary tumor nodule ≤5 cm or up to 3 tumor nodules with sizes ≤3 cm and not suitable or unwilling to receive surgery [8,17]. RFA was also considered as the alternative first-line treatment in patients with single solitary tumor nodule ≤2 cm [21].

Proposal of a New CTP Class 0 and Modified BCLC, CLIP and TIS Models

In order to select new cutoff values for serum albumin, bilirubin and INR of PT for patients with very well-preserved liver function, the distribution of the study patients and clinical feasibility were taken into consideration. The cutoff values were set more strictly with a higher standard than the normal range of our center laboratory to identify patients without overt liver dysfunction. Modified models for tumor staging were proposed by re-defining the CTP class for each stage of the original BCLC, CLIP and TIS staging systems.

Statistical Methods

The chi-squared test and the Kruskal-Wallis test were used to compare categorical and continuous data of more than 2 groups. The Kaplan-Meier method with a log-rank test was applied to compare the survival. For continuous variables, the median of each variable was used as the cutoff to dichotimize patients in the survival analysis. Factors which were significant ($p<0.05$) in the univariate analysis were introduced into multivariate Cox proportional hazards model. For all comparisons, a p value<0.05 was considered statistically significant.

The overall predictive accuracy of the survival between different tumor staging models was compared to determine which system possessed the most accurate prediction of survival (monotonicity of the score). Homogeneity (small difference in survival among patients in the same score category within each model) was determined by likelihood ratio χ^2 which was generated by the Cox proportional hazards model [22,23]. The consequences of the Cox regression were expressed with the Akaike information criterion (AIC), which revealed how the scoring systems affected the patient survival. The lower the AIC, the more explanatory and informative the model is [24].

Results

Definitions for the New CTP Class 0

The new CTP class 0 were defined by fulfilling all the criteria of serum albumin ≧4.0 g/dL, bilirubin ≤0.8 mg/dL, PT prolongation <0 second, no ascites and no encephalopathy (Table 1). A total of 917 patients (48% of original CTP class A) had a serum albumin level ≧4.0 g/dL, 1110 patients (58% of original CTP class A) had a serum bilirubin ≤0.8 mg/dL, 1454 patients (76% of original CTP class A) had a PT prolongation <0 second, and 1798 patients (94% of original CTP class A) did not have ascites. When combining these criteria together, 441 patients (23% of original CTP class A) fulfilled all the above mentioned criteria and were redefined as CTP class 0. Patients with CTP score of 5–6 and not fulfilling the criteria for CTP class 0 were classified as modified CTP class A; the definitions for CTP class B and C remained the same.

Distribution of Patients after Modifying CTP Classification

A total of 2654 HCC patients were consecutively enrolled and analyzed in this study. There were a total of 1924 (72%), 583 (22%) and 147 (6%) patients in the original CTP class A, B and C, respectively (Table 2). After modifying the CTP classification, 441 (23%) patients in the original CTP class A were reassigned to the modified CTP class 0. A total of 441 (17%), 1483 (56%), 583 (22%) and 147 (6%) patients were in the modified CTP class 0, A, B and C, respectively.

Table 3. Baseline demographics of all HCC patients and HCC patients with modified CTP class 0, A, B and C.

	All	Modified CTP class				p
		0	A	B	C	
Number of patients	2654	441	1483	583	147	
Age (years, mean±SD)	64±13	63±13	65±13	64±14	60±13	<0.001
Male/female (%)	77/23	81/19	76/24	77/23	80/20	0.22
Etiology of chronicliver disease (%)						<0.001
HBV only	1103(42)	213(48)	619(42)	209(36)	62(42)	
HCV only	609(23)	79(18)	384(26)	124(21)	22(15)	
HBV+HCV only	90(3)	15(3)	54(4)	17(3)	4(3)	
Alcohol only	121(5)	13(3)	59(4)	38(7)	11(8)	
Multiple etiologies and others	731(28)	121(27)	367(25)	195(33)	48(33)	
Serum biochemistry (mean±SD)						
Albumin (g/dL)	3.7±0.6	4.3±0.2	3.8±0.4	3.1±0.5	2.6±0.5	<0.001
Bilirubin (mg/dL)	1.5±2.7	0.6±0.2	0.9±0.4	2.4±3.3	6.8±7.0	<0.001
BUN (mg/dL)	19±12	18±10	18±10	21±16	24±17	<0.001
Creatinine (mg/dL)	1.2±1.0	1.2±1.2	1.1±0.9	1.3±1.2	1.5±1.4	<0.001
INR of PT	1.09±0.18	0.99±0.07	1.05±0.09	1.17±0.20	1.46±0.34	<0.001
ALT (U/L)	73±92	54±47	71±87	81±92	110±187	<0.001
Sodium (mmol/L)	138±4	140±3	139±3	137±4	133±6	<0.001
AFP [ng/mL, mean±SD (median; IQR)]	26,155±241,302 (49; 849)	5,852±37,162 (21; 186)	20,628±288,840 (43; 483)	46,144±198,882 (111; 4768)	63,551±211,663 (186; 4392)	<0.001
Performance status 0/1/2/3/4 (%)	58/18/12/8/4	82/10/6/2/0	68/18/10/3/1	28/25/20/17/11	4/13/20/42/22	<0.001
Mean CTP score [mean±SD (median; IQR)]	6.1±1.6 (5; 2)	5.0±0 (5; 0)	5.4±0.5 (5; 1)	7.7±0.8 (7; 1)	10.9±1.0 (11; 1)	<0.001
MELD score						
<8/8–12/12–16/>16 (%)	44/36/11/8	72/23/3/2	53/39/6/3	13/45/28/14	0/6/29/65	<0.001
Score [mean±SD (median; IQR)]	9.8±4.2 (8.3; 3.8)	7.8±2.4 (7.1; 1.7)	8.6±2.6 (7.9; 2.3)	12.0±4.0 (11.2; 4.8)	19.0±6.0 (17.3; 6.1)	<0.001
No. and size of tumor (%)						
Single/multiple	60/40	69/31	61/39	56/44	44/56	<0.001
≤5 cm/>5 cm	56/44	66/34	59/41	41/59	46/54	<0.001
TTV [cm^3, mean±SD (median; IQR)]	374±729 (51; 392)	201±458 (29; 139)	332±708 (39; 291)	584±890 (183; 773)	491±688 (166; 679)	<0.001
Vascular invasion (%)	928(35)	106(24)	429(29)	307(53)	86(59)	<0.001
Ascites (%)	646(24)	0(0)	126(9)	380(65)	140(95)	<0.001
Encephalopathy (%)	83(3)	0(0)	0(0)	42(7)	41(28)	<0.001
Treatment modality (%)						<0.001
Resection	705(27)	198(45)	459(31)	46(8)	2(1)	
Transplantation	8(0.3)	1(0.2)	1(0.1)	1(0.2)	5(3)	
Local ablation	529(20)	97(22)	323(22)	91(16)	18(12)	
TACE	769(29)	117(27)	489(33)	144(25)	19(13)	
Sorafenib	169(6)	5(1)	62(4)	87(15)	15(10)	
Others	474(18)	23(5)	149(10)	214(37)	88(60)	
BCLC stage 0/A/B/C/D (%)	9/22/14/42/14	13/31/19/35/2	11/24/17/43/5	0/13/7/54/27	0/0/0/0/100	<0.001

Table 3. Cont.

	All	Modified CTP class				p
		0	A	B	C	
CLIP score 0/1/2/3/4/5/6 (%)	27/26/16/12/12/6/2	46/27/14/8/5/0/0	34/30/15/11/10/0.1/0	0/21/21/14/20/24/0	0/0/14/20/18/20/27	<0.001
TIS score 0/1/2/3/4/5/6 (%)	35/22/12/12/11/6/1	53/23/10/9/5/0/0	46/21/9/13/10/0/0	0/29/17/13/17/24/0	0/0/31/17/12/17/23	<0.001

Abbreviations: HCC, hepatocellular carcinoma; CTP, Child-Turcotte-Pugh; SD, standard deviation; HBV, hepatitis B virus; HCV, hepatitis C virus; BUN, blood urea nitrogen; INR, international normalized ratio; PT, prothrombin time; ALT, alanine aminotransferase; AFP, α-fetoprotein; IQR, interquartile range; MELD, model for end-stage liver disease; No., number; TTV, total tumor volume; TACE, transcatheter arterial chemoembolization; BCLC, Barcelona Clinic Liver Cancer; CLIP, Cancer of the Liver Italian Program; TIS, Taipei Integrated Scoring.

Patient Characteristics

The baseline characteristics of all HCC patients and patients with modified CTP class 0, A, B and C are shown in Table 3. The study patients were predominantly male (77%) with a mean age of 64 years. The most common etiology for chronic liver disease is HBV only (42%). The mean and median CTP scores of all patients were 6.1 and 5, respectively, and the mean and median MELD scores were 9.8 and 8.3, respectively. Patients with CTP class 0 had a higher percentage of HBV infection in etiology, higher serum albumin and sodium levels, lower serum bilirubin, creatinine, INR of PT, alanine aminotransferase (ALT), lower serum α-fetoprotein (AFP) level, better general well-being, lower mean CTP and MELD scores, smaller tumor burden with more solitary nodules, lower rates of vascular invasion, ascites formation, hepatic encephalopathy, more frequently treated with curative interventions and better BCLC, CLIP and TIS stages (all $p<0.001$).

Survival Analysis

During a median follow up period of 18 [range 0.5–129, interquartile range (IQR) 40] months, the cumulative 3- and 5-year survival of patients with original CTP class A, B and C were 70% and 50%, 36% and 26% and 17% and 15%, respectively ($p<0.001$; Fig. 1A).

The 3- and 5- year survival of patients with modified CTP class 0, A, B and C were 80% and 71%, 67% and 52%, 36% and 26% and 17% and 15%, respectively ($p<0.001$; Fig. 1B). Survival comparisons of other baseline characteristics are shown in Table 4. Patients with a high serum creatinine and AFP levels, low serum sodium level, large TTV, poor performance status, presence of vascular invasion and receiving non-curative treatments were associated with a worse long-term outcome in the univariate analysis (all $p<0.001$). In the Cox proportional hazards model, the adjusted hazard ratio for CTP class A, B and C were 1.739 [95% confidence interval (CI):1.395–2.168; $p<0.001$], 3.120 (CI:2.442–3.986; $p<0.001$) and 5.107 (CI:3.758–6.940; $p<0.001$), respectively, when compared to CTP class 0. Moreover, other independent prognostic predictors identified in the Cox model were serum creatinine and AFP levels, TTV, performance status, vascular invasion and receiving non-curative treatments (all $p\leq 0.001$).

The long-term survival of different treatment strategies stratified by CTP class 0 and A were analyzed. In patients with CTP class 0, the 3-year survival rates for patients with SR, local ablation, TACE, sorafenib and other treatments were 84%, 88%, 73%, 50% and 36%, respectively ($p<0.001$). In patients with modified CTP class A, the 3-year survival rates for the corresponding groups were 80%, 76%, 57%, 22% and 26%, respectively ($p<0.001$).

Proposals of Modified BCLC, CLIP and TIS Staging Systems Based on the New CTP Classification

The staging and scoring criteria were re-defined based on the new CTP classification in the 9 modified BCLC, CLIP and TIS models (Table 5&6). In modified BCLC model A, CTP class 0, A, A, B and C were assigned to stage 0-D, respectively. In modified BCLC model B, CTP class 0, A, B, B and C were assigned to stage 0-D, respectively. In modified BCLC model C, CTP class 0, A–B, B, B and C were assigned to stage 0-D, respectively. Criteria of other factors remained the same.

In the modified CLIP and TIS model A patients, scores of 0, 1, 2 and 3 were assigned to CTP class 0, A, B and C, respectively. Scores of 0, 1 and 2 were assigned to patients with CTP class 0, A and B–C and class 0, A–B and C, respectively, in patients with modified CLIP and TIS model B and C patients. Scores for other factors remained the same.

Comparison of Prognostic Ability of the Original and Modified BCLC, CLIP and TIS Systems

The distributions of patients with different stages of the original and modified BCLC, CLIP and TIS staging systems are shown in Table 7. Among the 4 BCLC-based staging systems, the modified model B showed the lowest AIC value, followed by the modified model C and the modified model A, and lastly, the original system. Among the 4 CLIP-based staging systems and the 4 TIS-based staging systems, the modified model A had the best prognostic ability, followed by the modified model B, the original systems, and lastly, the modified model C. Among all 12 original and modified staging systems, the modified CLIP model A had the lowest AIC value.

Long-term Survival among Patients with Different Stages of BCLC, CLIP and TIS

The survival distributions among patients with different stages of original and modified BCLC, CLIP and TIS models with the lowest AIC scores are shown in Fig. 2A–2F. Patients with a more advanced stage were associated with a worse long-term survival in the original and modified model B BCLC systems, the original and modified model A CLIP systems, the original and modified model A TIS systems (Fig. 2A–2F; all $p<0.001$).

Table 4. Univariate and multivariate Cox regression survival analysis in HCC patients.

		Univariate analysis			Multivariate analysis		
	N	3-year survival (%)	5-year survival (%)	p	HR	95% CI	p
Sex (male/female)	2054/600	61/63	48/50	0.283			
Age (≤65/>65 years)	1362/1292	61/61	52/46	0.254			
HBsAg (negative/positive)	1187/1467	61/61	46/51	0.54			
Creatinine (≤1.0/>1.0 mg/dL)	1563/1091	64/56	53/43	<0.001	1.226	1.079–1.392	0.002
Sodium (≤139/>139 mmol/L)	1513/1141	53/71	44/55	<0.001			
AFP (≤50/>50 ng/mL)	1333/1321	73/47	58/38	<0.001	1.679	1.469–1.919	<0.001
TTV (≤50/>50 cm^3)	1325/1329	75/44	61/33	<0.001	1.544	1.326–1.798	<0.001
Performance status (ECOG 0/1–4)	1536/1118	74/38	61/19	<0.001	1.959	1.679–2.287	<0.001
Vascular invasion (No/Yes)	1726/928	70/39	56/34	<0.001	1.703	1.467–1.977	<0.001
Treatment (curative/non-curative)	1242/1412	78/42	65/30	<0.001	2.319	2.005–2.681	<0.001
Modified CTP class				<0.001			
0	441	80	71		1		
A	1483	67	52		1.739	1.395–2.168	<0.001
B	583	36	26		3.120	2.442–3.986	<0.001
C	147	17	15		5.107	3.758–6.940	<0.001

Abbreviations: HCC, hepatocellular carcinoma; HR, hazard ratio; CI, confidence interval; HBsAg, hepatitis B surface antigen; AFP, α-fetoprotein; TTV, total tumor volume; ECOG, Eastern Cooperative Oncology Group; CTP, Child-Turcotte-Pugh.

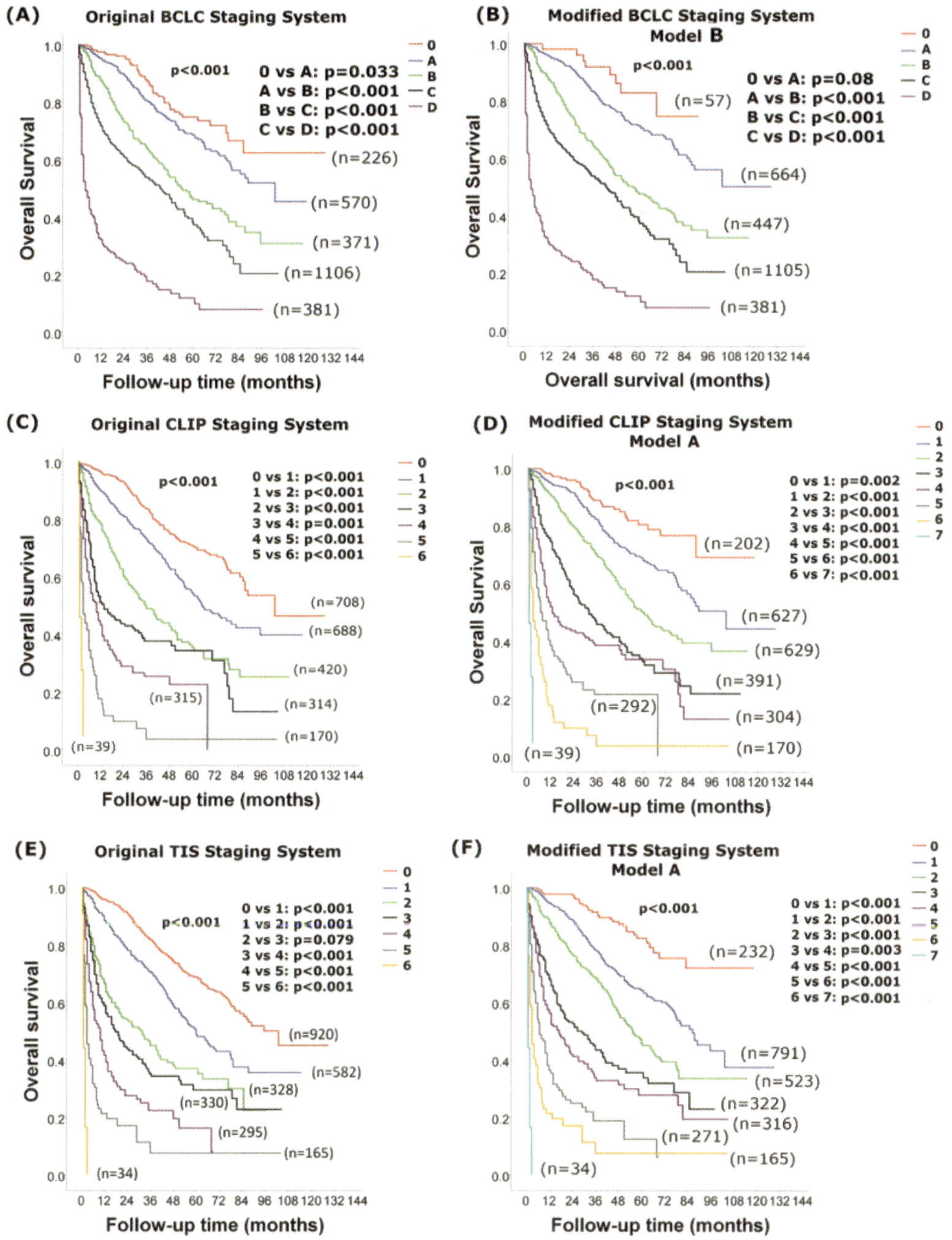

Figure 2. Comparison of survival between stages in the original and modified models BCLC, CLIP and TIS with the lowest AIC score. Patients with a more advanced stage were associated with a worse long-term survival in the original (panel A) and modified model B (panel B) BCLC systems, the original (panel C) and modified model A (panel D) CLIP systems, the original (panel E) and modified model A (panel F) TIS systems (all $p < 0.001$). Pairwise comparison of survival differences between all stages in the modified BCLC, CLIP and TIS staging systems showed significant differences between each stage (all $p < 0.05$), except for patients with modified BCLC stage 0 and A ($p = 0.08$).

Discussion

The CTP classification has been used to estimate liver functional reserve and predict survival among chronic liver disease patients. In our study, a total of 1924 (72%) patients belonged to the original CTP class A. The lack of the ability to discriminate liver function and outcome among patients with well-preserved liver function is a major drawback of the original CTP classification. The proposal of the new CTP class 0 in the modified CTP classification, which is aimed to more specifically define early stage patients, showed more accurate outcome prediction for HCC patients. In the modified CTP classification, 441 (23%) of patients with very-well preserved liver function in the original CTP class A were re-classified as CTP class 0. Notably, CTP class 0 was associated with a better long-term survival, with a 74% to 4-fold decrease in mortality when compared with patients with CTP class A to C (Fig. 1A & Table 4).

Patients with CTP class 0 were characterized by distinct clinical presentations. These patients had higher prevalence of HBV infection, very well-preserved liver function, lower serum AFP

Table 5. The proposed criteria for original and modified models of the BCLC staging system.

Stage	BCLC	Modified BCLC Model A	Modified BCLC Model B	Modified BCLC Model C
0 (Very early)	Performance status (PS) 0; one small tumor ≤2 cm;			
	Original Child-Turcotte-Pugh (CTP) class A	Modified CTP class 0		
A (Early)	PS 0; single tumor ≤5 cm or 3 or few nodules ≤3 cm;			
	Original CTP class A–B	Modified CTP class A	Modified CTP class A	Modified CTP class A–B
B (Intermediate)	PS 0; large/multiple HCC;			
	Original CTP class A–B	Modified CTP class A	Modified CTP class B	Modified CTP class B
C (Advanced)	PS 1–2; vascular invasion or extrahepatic spread;			
	Original CTP class A–B	Modified CTP class B		
D (End stage)	PS 3–4; any tumor burden;			
	Original CTP class C	Modified CTP class C		

Original BCLC stage 0, A and B: all criteria should be fulfilled; stage C and D: at least one criterion should be fulfilled.
Modified BCLC stage 0: all criteria should be fulfilled; stage A, B, C and D: at least one criterion should be fulfilled.
Abbreviations: CTP, Child-Turcotte-Pugh; BCLC, Barcelona Clinic Liver Cancer; PS, performance status.

level, better general well-being, smaller tumor burden with more solitary nodule, lower rate of vascular invasion and more frequently treated with curative interventions. It should be noted that advanced CTP classes usually represent a worse residual liver function resulting from chronic inflammation and fibrosis and thus affect the growth and behavior of HCC [25]. Reversely, in patients with large tumors, the large tumor burden may compromise liver functional reserve and have a more advanced cirrhosis stage at presentation. Furthermore, the complications of cirrhosis may influence the general well-being of the patient [26] and the applicability of receiving aggressive treatment for HCC [27]. Importantly, modified CTP classification was not only independently associated with long-term survival; its impact on mortality outweighed most other prognostic factors in the multivariate Cox model after adjusting the confounding effect of treatment strategy. This result strongly implies that modified CTP classification is a powerful and comprehensive indicator in predicting the survival of patients with HCC.

The current tumor staging systems used the original CTP classification in stratification of the tumor stages. After identifying patients with very well-preserved liver function as CTP class 0, the modified CTP classification may be more applicable for tumor staging stratification and treatment allocation. In this regard, we have modified the currently used cancer staging systems for HCC, based on the modified CTP classification, in order to enhance the prognostic ability of these systems. Of all the BCLC-based models, the 3 modified models had better prognostic ability than the original BCLC staging system, indicating that the original system is not informative enough to discriminate the outcome of these HCC patients. In the original BCLC staging systems, the criteria for evaluating liver function are all CTP A–B in patients of stage A, B and C. The same definition for CTP classification would sacrifice a very important parameter in assessing the cancer stages and predicting outcome among patients with original BCLC stage A to C. Reassigning CTP class 0, A, B, B and C to stage 0 to D may enhance the prognostic ability of the original BCLC model and was the most informative one among all modified models. In this modified model, only 2% of patients were selected as stage 0. This group indicates patients with very small tumor size, better liver functional reserve and general well-being, and had 5-year survival rate of 75%. Taken together, the modification of the BCLC system further enhances their prognostic ability in patients with early to advanced cancer stage (Fig. 2 & Table 7).

One of the advantages of the BCLC system is that it can also be used for treatment allocation. Whether the new modified system has a better ability in assigning treatment still needs to be validated in future studies. However, our results imply that the modified BCLC model is more informative in treatment allocation. In the very early stage (stage 0) of the original BCLC system, patients with CTP class A and single tumor nodule with size ≤2 cm are suggested to undergo RFA therapy due to its high complete response rate and good long-term outcome [8,28–31]. However, whether RFA is superior to SR in this group of patients is under intense debate [32–34]. In our study, we have further selected patients with very-well preserved liver function for patients receiving RFA. Well preservation of liver function for the applicability of repeated therapy due to tumor recurrence after primary RFA is considered to predict a good long-term survival [35,36]. Therefore, reassigning CTP class 0 patients to stage 0 may better select candidates with adequate liver functional reserve to receive RFA. Furthermore, in the modified early stage (stage A) of the BCLC model, modified CTP class A replaced the original CTP class A–B for assessing liver function. Surgical resection was considered with a higher risk of mortality among patients with CTP class B [37–40] and re-defining the BCLC staging may better select patients for surgical resection.

The CLIP staging system was well validated for its prognostic ability in HCC [4,41], but early studies disclosed its limitations in discriminating patients with early stage HCC [42]. In our modified CLIP model A, scores of 0–7 were proposed for better discrimination of the patients in terms of outcome prediction. A total of 8% of patients were selected with very-well preserved liver function, small tumor burden and good tumor behavior and predicted a 5-year survival of 81%. The new modified CLIP model showed significant improvements in discriminative ability and prognostic power from very early to advanced cancer stages. Interestingly, consistent with our previous study [41], the modified CLIP model A had the lowest AIC score among all original and modified BCLC, CLIP and TIS staging systems and was considered to be the best prognostic model for outcome prediction in HCC patients. The TIS model was initially proposed to use TTV as the main indicator for tumor burden [6] and its modified

Table 6. The proposed criteria for original and modified models of the CLIP and TIS staging systems.

	Prognostic predictors for hepatocellular carcinoma patients								Scores
	Tumoral factor		Liver function				Tumor behavior		
	Total tumor volume	Tumor number and size	Original Child-Turcotte-Pugh (CTP) classification	Modified CTP classification			α-fetoprotein	Vascular invasion	
	<50/50–250/250–500/>500	Single and <50% liver span/ multiple and <50% liver span/≥50% liver span	A/B/C	0/A/B/C	0/A/B-C	0/A–B/C	<400/>400	Absence/ presence	
Scores	0/1/2/3	0/1/2	0/1/2	0/1/2/3	0/1/2	0/1/2	0/1	0/1	
CLIP		V	V				V	V	0–6
Modified CLIP Model A		V		V			V	V	0–7
Modified CLIP Model B		V			V		V	V	0–6
Modified CLIP Model C		V				V	V	V	0–6
TIS	V		V				V		0–6
Modified TIS Model A	V			V			V		0–7
Modified TIS Model B	V				V		V		0–6
Modified TIS Model C	V					V			0–6

Abbreviations: CTP, Child-Turcotte-Pugh; CLIP, Cancer of the Liver Italian Program; TIS, Taipei Integrated Scoring.

Table 7. Comparison of the prognostic ability among 4 BCLC-, 4 CLIP- and 4 TIS-based staging systems.

N = 2654	Distribution of patients (%)	Homogeneity (Likelihood ratio χ^2)	Akaike information criterion
BCLC models (0/A/B/C/D)			
Original	9/22/14/42/14	492.449	13695.982
Modified A	2/25/13/46/14	500.669	13687.762
Modified B	2/25/17/42/14	518.292	13670.139
Modified C	2/28/14/42/14	502.622	13685.809
CLIP models [0/1/2/3/4/5/6(/7)]			
Original	27/26/16/12/12/6/2	710.818	13477.613
Modified A	8/24/24/15/12/11/6/2	762.847	13425.584
Modified B	8/24/25/15/11/11/7	714.275	13474.156
Modified C	8/28/25/14/13/12/2	622.205	13566.226
TIS models [0/1/2/3/4/5/6(/7)]			
Original	35/22/12/12/11/6/1	685.371	13503.060
Modified A	9/30/20/12/12/10/6/1	745.476	13442.955
Modified B	9/30/21/11/12/11/7	691.347	13497.084
Modified C	9/36/19/10/13/12/1	595.013	13593.418

Abbreviations: BCLC, Barcelona Clinic Liver Cancer; CLIP, Cancer of the Liver Italian Program; TIS, Taipei Integrated Scoring.

model A also showed great discriminatory ability in comparison with the modified BCLC models.

This study has a few limitations. Firstly, HBV is the most common etiology of HCC in Taiwan. This feature is different from most Western countries, where HCV infection and alcoholism are the predominant causes of chronic liver disease. It is our concern whether our results can be applied to patients in the Western countries. Secondly, another important limitation of our study was that the cutoff values for the definition of CTP class 0 were set arbitrary aiming to identify patients with very well-preserved liver function. Thus, validation in future studies is needed. Thirdly, the calculation of TTV for the TIS staging systems was based on the assumption that all tumor nodules were spherical. Therefore, TTV could be slightly overestimated in patients with non-spherical tumor nodules.

In conclusion, the newly proposed CTP classification, aimed to identify patients without overt liver dysfunction as CTP class 0, could accurately predict survival among HCC patients. This proposal is consistently supported by the findings that the modified cancer staging systems of BCLC, CLIP and TIS according to the modified CTP classification have better discriminatory ability and prognostic power when compared with the original models. Treatment strategy according to the modified BCLC model needs to be validated in future studies.

Author Contributions

Conceived and designed the experiments: YHL C. Hsu CWC TIH. Performed the experiments: C. Hsia YHH CWS YYC. Analyzed the data: YHL HCL. Contributed reagents/materials/analysis tools: PHL C. Hsu. Wrote the paper: YHL TIH.

References

1. Bosch FX, Ribes J, Diaz M, Cleries R (2004) Primary liver cancer: worldwide incidence and trends. Gastroenterology 127: S5–S16.
2. Child CG, Turcotte JG (1964) Surgery and portal hypertension. In: The liver and portal hypertension. Edited by CG Child. Philadelphia: Saunders 50–64.
3. Pugh RN, Murray-Lyon IM, Dawson JL, Pietroni MC, Williams R (1973) Transection of the oesophagus for bleeding oesophageal varices. Br J Surg 60: 646–649.
4. (1998) A new prognostic system for hepatocellular carcinoma: a retrospective study of 435 patients: the Cancer of the Liver Italian Program (CLIP) investigators. Hepatology 28: 751–755.
5. Llovet JM, Fuster J, Bruix J (2004) The Barcelona approach: diagnosis, staging, and treatment of hepatocellular carcinoma. Liver Transpl 10: S115–120.
6. Hsu CY, Huang YH, Hsia CY, Su CW, Lin HC, et al. (2010) A new prognostic model for hepatocellular carcinoma based on total tumor volume: the Taipei Integrated Scoring System. J Hepatol 53: 108–117.
7. Cabrera R, Nelson DR (2010) Review article: the management of hepatocellular carcinoma. Aliment Pharmacol Ther 31: 461–476.
8. (2012) EASL-EORTC clinical practice guidelines: management of hepatocellular carcinoma. J Hepatol 56: 908–943.
9. Lee YH, Hsu CY, Hsia CY, Huang YH, Su CW, et al. (2012) Defining the severity of liver dysfunction in patients with hepatocellular carcinoma by the model for end-stage liver disease-derived systems. Dig Liver Dis 44: 868–874.
10. Silva MF, Sapisochin G, Strasser SI, Hewa-Geeganage S, Chen J, et al. (2013) Liver resection and transplantation offer similar 5-year survival for Child-Pugh-Turcotte A HCC-patients with a single nodule up to 5 cm: a multicenter, exploratory analysis. Eur J Surg Oncol 39: 386–395.
11. Chen X, Zhai J, Cai X, Zhang Y, Wei L, et al. (2012) Severity of portal hypertension and prediction of postoperative liver failure after liver resection in patients with Child-Pugh grade A cirrhosis. Br J Surg 99: 1701–1710.
12. Yamakado K, Miyayama S, Hirota S, Mizunuma K, Nakamura K, et al. (2014) Subgrouping of intermediate-stage (BCLC stage B) hepatocellular carcinoma based on tumor number and size and Child-Pugh grade correlated with prognosis after transarterial chemoembolization. Jpn J Radiol (in press).
13. Hsu KF, Chu CH, Chan DC, Yu JC, Shih ML, et al. (2012) Superselective transarterial chemoembolization vs hepatic resection for resectable early-stage hepatocellular carcinoma in patients with Child-Pugh class a liver function. Eur J Radiol 81: 466–471.
14. Takahashi S, Kudo M, Chung H, Inoue T, Nagashima M, et al. (2007) Outcomes of nontransplant potentially curative therapy for early-stage hepatocellular carcinoma in Child-Pugh stage A cirrhosis is comparable with liver transplantation. Dig Dis 25: 303–309.
15. Hsu CY, Lee YH, Liu PH, Hsia CY, Huang YH, et al. (2014) Decrypting cryptogenic hepatocellular carcinoma: clinical manifestations, prognostic factors and long-term survival by propensity score model. PLoS One 9: e89373.
16. Bruix J, Sherman M (2011) Management of hepatocellular carcinoma: an update. Hepatology 53: 1020–1022.
17. Song P, Tobe RG, Inagaki Y, Kokudo N, Hasegawa K, et al. (2012) The management of hepatocellular carcinoma around the world: a comparison of guidelines from 2001 to 2011. Liver Int 32: 1053–1063.

18. Grant BF, Dufour MC, Harford TC (1988) Epidemiology of alcoholic liver disease. Semin Liver Dis 8: 12–25.
19. Kamath PS, Wiesner RH, Malinchoc M, Kremers W, Therneau TM, et al. (2001) A model to predict survival in patients with end-stage liver disease. Hepatology 33: 464–470.
20. Torzilli G, Makuuchi M, Inoue K, Takayama T, Sakamoto Y, et al. (1999) No-mortality liver resection for hepatocellular carcinoma in cirrhotic and noncirrhotic patients: Is there a way? A prospective analysis of our approach. Arch Surg 134: 984–992.
21. de Lope CR, Tremosini S, Forner A, Reig M, Bruix J (2012) Management of HCC. J Hepatol 56 Suppl 1: S75–87.
22. Feinstein AR (1972) Clinical biostatistics. XVI. The process of prognostic stratification. 2. Clin Pharmacol Ther 13: 609–624.
23. Hosmer DW, Hosmer T, Le Cessie S, Lemeshow S (1997) A comparison of goodness-of-fit tests for the logistic regression model. Stat Med 16: 965–980.
24. Forster MR (2000) Key Concepts in Model Selection: Performance and Generalizability. J Math Psychol 44: 205–231.
25. Lee YH, Hsu CY, Huang YH, Hsia CY, Chiou YY, et al. (2014) Vascular Invasion in Hepatocellular Carcinoma: Prevalence, Determinants and Prognostic Impact. J Clin Gastroenterol (in press).
26. Hsu CY, Lee YH, Hsia CY, Huang YH, Su CW, et al. (2012) Performance status in patients with hepatocellular carcinoma: Determinants, prognostic impact and ability to improve the BCLC system. Hepatology 57: 112–119.
27. Bruix J, Sherman M (2005) Management of hepatocellular carcinoma. Hepatology 42: 1208–1236.
28. Livraghi T, Meloni F, Di Stasi M, Rolle E, Solbiati L, et al. (2008) Sustained complete response and complications rates after radiofrequency ablation of very early hepatocellular carcinoma in cirrhosis: Is resection still the treatment of choice? Hepatology 47: 82–89.
29. Shiina S, Tateishi R, Arano T, Uchino K, Enooku K, et al. (2012) Radiofrequency ablation for hepatocellular carcinoma: 10-year outcome and prognostic factors. Am J Gastroenterol 107: 569–577.
30. Komorizono Y, Oketani M, Sako K, Yamasaki N, Shibatou T, et al. (2003) Risk factors for local recurrence of small hepatocellular carcinoma tumors after a single session, single application of percutaneous radiofrequency ablation. Cancer 97: 1253–1262.
31. Ikeda K, Kobayashi M, Kawamura Y, Imai N, Seko Y, et al. (2011) Stage progression of small hepatocellular carcinoma after radical therapy: comparisons of radiofrequency ablation and surgery using the Markov model. Liver Int 31: 692–699.
32. Chen MS, Li JQ, Zheng Y, Guo RP, Liang HH, et al. (2006) A prospective randomized trial comparing percutaneous local ablative therapy and partial hepatectomy for small hepatocellular carcinoma. Ann Surg 243: 321–328.
33. Huang J, Yan L, Cheng Z, Wu H, Du L, et al. (2010) A randomized trial comparing radiofrequency ablation and surgical resection for HCC conforming to the Milan criteria. Ann Surg 252: 903–912.
34. Pompili M, Saviano A, de Matthaeis N, Cucchetti A, Ardito F, et al. (2013) Long Term Effectiveness of Resection and Radiofrequency Ablation for Single Hepatocellular Carcinoma ≤3 cm. Results of a Multicenter Italian Survey. J Hepatol 59: 89–97.
35. Okuwaki Y, Nakazawa T, Kokubu S, Hidaka H, Tanaka Y, et al. (2009) Repeat radiofrequency ablation provides survival benefit in patients with intrahepatic distant recurrence of hepatocellular carcinoma. Am J Gastroenterol 104: 2747–2753.
36. Cabibbo G, Maida M, Genco C, Alessi N, Peralta M, et al. (2013) Survival of patients with hepatocellular carcinoma (HCC) treated by percutaneous radio-frequency ablation (RFA) is affected by complete radiological response. PLoS One 8: e70016.
37. Nagasue N, Kohno H, Tachibana M, Yamanoi A, Ohmori H, et al. (1999) Prognostic factors after hepatic resection for hepatocellular carcinoma associated with Child-Turcotte class B and C cirrhosis. Ann Surg 229: 84–90.
38. Harada N, Shirabe K, Ikeda Y, Korenaga D, Takenaka K, et al. (2012) Surgical management of hepatocellular carcinoma in Child-Pugh class B cirrhotic patients: hepatic resection and/or microwave coagulation therapy versus living donor liver transplantation. Ann Transplant 17: 11–20.
39. Grazi GL, Cescon M, Ravaioli M, Ercolani G, Gardini A, et al. (2003) Liver resection for hepatocellular carcinoma in cirrhotics and noncirrhotics. Evaluation of clinicopathologic features and comparison of risk factors for long-term survival and tumour recurrence in a single centre. Aliment Pharmacol Ther 17 Suppl 2: 119–129.
40. Zhong JH, Xiang BD, Gong WF, Ke Y, Mo QG, et al. (2013) Comparison of long-term survival of patients with BCLC stage B hepatocellular carcinoma after liver resection or transarterial chemoembolization. PLoS One 8: e68193.
41. Hsu CY, Hsia CY, Huang YH, Su CW, Lin HC, et al. (2010) Selecting an optimal staging system for hepatocellular carcinoma: comparison of 5 currently used prognostic models. Cancer 116: 3006–3014.
42. Kudo M, Chung H, Osaki Y (2003) Prognostic staging system for hepatocellular carcinoma (CLIP score): its value and limitations, and a proposal for a new staging system, the Japan Integrated Staging Score (JIS score). J Gastroenterol 38: 207–215.

2

Gene Expression Profiling Unravels Cancer-Related Hepatic Molecular Signatures in Steatohepatitis but Not in Steatosis

Julia Starmann[1], Maria Fälth[1,2], Walter Spindelböck[3], Katja-Lauren Lanz[3], Carolin Lackner[4], Kurt Zatloukal[4], Michael Trauner[3,5], Holger Sültmann[1]*

1 Unit Cancer Genome Research, German Cancer Research Center and National Center for Tumor Diseases, Heidelberg, Germany, **2** Cellzome/GlaxoSmithKline, Heidelberg, Germany, **3** Laboratory of Experimental and Molecular Hepatology, Division of Gastroenterology and Hepatology, Department of Internal Medicine, Medical University of Graz, Austria, **4** Institute of Pathology, Medical University of Graz, Austria, **5** Division of Gastroenterology and Hepatology, Department of Internal Medicine III, Medical University of Vienna, Vienna, Austria

Abstract

Background: Pathogenesis and factors for determining progression of alcoholic and non-alcoholic steatosis to steatohepatitis with risk of further progression to liver cirrhosis and cancer are poorly understood. In the present study, we aimed to identify potential molecular signatures for discrimination of steatohepatitis from steatosis.

Methodology and Results: Global microarray gene expression analysis was applied to unravel differentially expressed genes between steatohepatitis compared to steatosis and control samples. For functional annotation as well as the identification of disease-relevant biological processes of the differentially expressed genes the gene ontology (GO) database was used. Selected candidate genes (n = 46) were validated in 87 human liver samples from two sample cohorts by quantitative real-time PCR (qRT-PCR). The GO analysis revealed that genes down-regulated in steatohepatitis were mainly involved in metabolic processes. Genes up-regulated in steatohepatitis samples were associated with cancer progression and proliferation. In surgical liver resection samples, 39 genes and in percutaneous liver biopsies, 30 genes were significantly up-regulated in steatohepatitis. Furthermore, immunohistochemical investigation of human liver tissue revealed a significant increase of AKR1B10 protein expression in steatohepatitis.

Conclusions: The development of steatohepatitis is characterized by distinct molecular changes. The most striking examples in this respect were *KRT23* and *AKR1B10*, which we found to be highly differentially expressed in steatohepatitis compared to steatosis and normal liver. We propose that *KRT23* and *AKR1B10* may serve as future potential biomarkers for steatohepatitis as well as markers for progression to HCC.

Editor: Wing-Kin Syn, Institute of Hepatology London, United Kingdom

Funding: This work was supported by the funding of the Austria Wirtschaftsservice GmbH (AWS) and the Austrian Nationalstiftung through the framework of the IMGuS research program (Institute for Medical and Genome Research and Systems Biology, Vienna). The funders had no role in study design, data collection and analysis, decision to publish, or preparation of the manuscript.

Competing Interests: The authors have declared that no competing interests exist. Austria Wirtschaftsservice GmbH is a non commercial public funding agency organised as a non profit GmbH. It was neither involved in any decisions on the direction of the funded research nor in the study design; collection, analysis, and interpretation of data; writing of the paper; and decision to submit for publication.

* E-mail: h.sueltmann@dkfz.de

Introduction

Fatty liver diseases comprise a spectrum of severity ranging from simple steatosis over steatohepatitis to cirrhosis and hepatocellular cancer (HCC) [1,2]. There are two major etiologies for fatty liver disease, namely alcohol and metabolic syndrome-associated disorders such as obesity and type 2 diabetes mellitus (T2DM). Due to its high prevalence and potential for severe hepatic outcomes such as liver cirrhosis and HCC in a substantial fraction of affected individuals, fatty liver disease has become a major issue of public health. Up to 30% of the general population is affected by non-alcoholic fatty liver disease (NAFLD), reaching up to 70% among diabetic patients [3,4]. The prevalence of steatosis and steatohepatitis in obese patients undergoing bariatric surgery is as high as 76% and 37%, respectively [3,5]. Steatohepatitis develops in about 20% of alcoholics and up to 50% of T2DM who are also obese (BMI>30). This places fatty liver disease as the most common liver disease of the 21st century accounting for the majority of liver cirrhosis and HCC in Western countries. Its prevalence is expected to further rise in light of the ongoing epidemic of diabetes and obesity [1,2].

While simple steatosis has a relatively benign course and is principally reversible, steatohepatitis carries a poor prognosis and can lead to severe liver damage with progresson to cirrhosis and HCC. Conventional non-invasive markers such as serum transaminases correlate poorly with the risk of development as well as progression of liver disease, and currently available routine liver tests may even be unremarkable in a significant proportion of patients with steatohepatitis [6]. Therefore in current standard clinical practice, non-invasive serum and imaging markers do not allow the distinction of relatively benign fatty liver from progressive steatohepatitis. This situation results in underdiagnosis and undertreatment of these disorders. The development of efficient diagnostic, prognostic and therapeutic strategies has been substantially hampered by the fact that our understanding of the molecular pathogenesis of steatohepatitis is still incomplete. Several studies showed that the different forms of steatohepatitis (alcoholic – ASH, non-alcoholic – NASH) cannot be morphologically distinguished, which suggests a common pathogenetic mechanism despite different etiologies of the disease [7]. A major unsolved problem is the marked difference in the individual risk to develop steatohepatitis and to progress to cirrhosis (e.g., only 20% of heavy drinkers or 50% of obese type II diabetic patients develop steatohepatitis; Hispanics and Caucasians are more susceptible than Afro-Americans [8,9]). However, the factors responsible for disease progression across the spectrum of fatty liver disease are poorly understood. Why some patients are protected against developing steatohepatitis or simple steatosis, while others are not, is still unclear [10]. It is currently even debated whether steatosis and steatohepatitis represent two consecutive disease stages; alternatively, individuals may *a priori* be predetermined to develop either a rather benign steatosis or prognostically unfavorable steatohepatitis [4].

In the present study, we performed microarray-based gene expression profiling analysis of steatosis and steatohepatitis and compared them with normal human liver samples. We focused on analyzing transcriptional changes of genes relevant in steatohepatitis but not in steatosis and normal liver to identify potential signatures as basis for further development of biomarkers in the discrimination of steatohepatitis as a prognostically more relevant disease entity. Notably, we aimed at investigating molecular changes between steatohepatitis and steatosis, rather than to differentiate between disease etiologies of NALFD. Overall, we validated the expression of 46 target genes in human liver samples from two cohorts. We demonstrate a hitherto unknown molecular signature for cancer-related changes in steatohepatitis but not in steatosis. Several genes were highly significantly expressed in steatohepatitis compared to steatosis and normal liver. The associated protein of one gene (*AKR1B10*) was expressed in steatohepatitis tissue. The gene signature reported in this study may serve as a valuable tool to distinguish between steatosis and steatohepatitis as well as for future development of diagnostic and prognostic biomarkers. Moreover, the results offer important insights into the pathogenesis of the disease, which may also be relevant for design of future therapeutic strategies.

Methods

Patient tissue samples

The detailed clinical, biochemical and histological data of the studied patients are given in table 1, 2 and 3. The study was approved by the ethical review committee at the University of Graz (EK number: 20-119 ex 08/09). The diagnoses of all samples used were histologically validated by a board certified pathologist (C.L.) prior to molecular analysis. For histological analysis, hematoxylin and eosin (H&E) and chromotrope aniline blue

Table 1. Clinical, biochemical and histopathological patient characteristics.

Microarray samples

	Steatohepatitis (n = 8)	Steatosis (n = 14)	Controls (n = 10)	p-value
Sex (m:f)	6:2	8:6	5:5	
Age (y)	55 (46–72)	61.5 (37–78)	51 (25–73)	0.37
BMI (kg/m2)	25.5 (19.8–39.2)	31 (21.4–30.8)	22.8 (18.3–30.1)	0.17
ALT (IU/l)	34 (16–56)	25 (12–359)	20 (5–156)	0.57
AST (IU/l)	59 (38–92)	27 (9–398)	22 (10–240)	0.02 a,b
GGT (IU/l)	60 (24–804)	46 (14–136)	36 (15–146)	0.26
AP (IU/l)	88 (60–261)	88 (42–146)	77 (45–157)	0.55
Bilirubin (mg/dl)	3.2 (0.8–7.8)	0.8 (0.3–2.5)	1 (0.2–2)	0.01 a,b
Cholesterol (mg/dl)	112 (57–177)	226 (117–270)	174 (44–240)	0.00 a
Triglycerides (mg/dl)	97 (57–203)	159 (117–270)	97 (32–172)	0.04 a,c
Diabetes II (Y/N)	2/6	3/11	0/10	
Hyperlipidaemia (Y/N)	2/6	5/9	0/10	
Hypertension (Y/N)	6/2	8/6	0/10	
Histological steatosis grade (0:1:2:3)	3*:1:4:0	0:10:3:1	10:0:0:0	
Lobular inflammation (0:A1:A2:A3)	1:3:3:1	1:7:5:1	6:3.1:0	
Ballooning (0:1:2)	0:4:4	14:0:0	10:0:0	
Matteoni (points)	3 (0–4)	2 (1–2)	n/a	
Fibrosis (0:F1:F2:F3:F4)	0:0:0:2:6	9:4:1:0:0	9:1:0:0:0	
Apoptosis (0:1:2)	4:4:0	7:5:2	6:4:0	
Alcoholic/non-alcoholic	5:3	0:14	n/a	

***...steatosis present, albeit <5% of parenchymal area.**

Samples from the Biobank cohort investigated by microarray analysis. (p-value: a. steatohepatitis vs. steatosis, b. steatohepatitis vs. control, c. steatosis vs. control).

(CAB) stained sections were used. A histological diagnosis of steatosis was made if more than 5% of the parenchymal area was occupied by steatosis using routine H&E stain, whereas the diagnosis of steatohepatitis (SH) was based on the presence of hepatocellular ballooning in combination with variable degrees of steatosis and/or inflammation [11,12]. Stage of liver fibrosis was assessed according to the NASH Clinical Research Network Scoring System for NAFLD [13].

Eighty-seven samples from two independent cohorts of human liver samples with alcoholic and non-alcoholic fatty liver disease were used for this study (table 4). The first cohort ('Biobank cohort', n = 58) consisted of non-neoplastic liver tissue samples (controls, i.e. normal liver, n = 18; steatosis, n = 30; steatohepatitis, n = 10, of these 8/2 cirrhotic/non-cirrhotic) obtained from patients who underwent liver resections because of HCC (n = 7), other malignant liver lesions (n = 33, 20/33 colon cancer) or benign liver tumors (n = 7) (table 1 and 2). Eight patients from whom steatosis samples were obtained had received a platin-containing chemotherapy (7/8 FOLFOX) three months prior to resection. Although steatosis can be a side effect of FOLFOX treatment, there was no indication that these cases were related to the chemotherapy. In addition, tissue samples from explanted donor livers not utilized for transplantation (n = 11) were included.

The second cohort ('Biopsy cohort', n = 29) encompassed percutaneous liver biopsy samples including steatosis (n = 13), steatohepatitis (n = 11, of these, 5/6 cirrhotic/non-cirrhotic), and chronic hepatitis C (CHC, n = 5, all genotype 1) as disease controls with absence of steatosis. In the Biopsy cohort, CHC samples were used as controls since patients with normal liver tissue do not undergo percutaneous liver biopsy (table 3). Informed consent was obtained from all patients prior to use of an aliquot of the liver biopsy tissue for molecular analysis.

RNA extraction and quality control

Total RNA was isolated from the samples using TRI Reagent® (Molecular Research Center, Cincinnati, OH, USA) according to the manufacturer's protocols. The RNA quality was analyzed using microcapillary electrophoresis (Agilent 2100 Bioanalyzer, Agilent Technologies, Böblingen, Germany). Only samples with RIN (RNA integrity number) of 5.0 or higher were subjected to gene expression array analysis.

Illumina microarray experiments and data analysis

Global gene expression screenings were performed using Biobank samples only (steatohepatitis n = 8 (6/2 cirrhotic/non-cirrhotic), steatosis n = 14 and controls n = 10). For gene expression analysis, we used whole genome expression microarray Sentrix® Human-6 v3 expression bead chips (Illumina®, San Diego, CA, USA) encompassing 49577 features. The experiments were performed at the Genomics and Proteomics Core Facility of DKFZ Heidelberg using 300 ng/µl RNA and protocols recommended by the supplier.

The raw data was log2-transformed and quantile-normalized. Principal Components Analysis (PCA) was performed to investigate the internal data structure in a way which best explained the variance in the data and to identify potential outliers. The R-package "limma" was used to identify differentially expressed genes [14]. With "limma", a linear model is fitted for each gene and a t-test is used to identify differential expressed genes. P-values were adjusted for multiple testing using the Benjamini-Hochberg

Table 2. Clinical, biochemical and histopathological patient characteristics.

qRTPCR biobank samples	Steatohepatitis (n = 10)	Steatosis (n = 30)	Controls (n = 18)	p-value
Sex (m:f)	7:03	14:16	9:09	
Age (y)	54 (44–72)	64 (37–78)	52.5 (22–73)	0.02 c
BMI (kg/m2)	26.1 (19.8–39.2)	25.7 (21–33.5)	23.2 (18.3–30.1)	0.03 c
ALT (IU/l)	39 (16–204)	25 (11–359)	21.5 (5–311)	0.33
AST (IU/l)	65 (38–441)	28 (9–398)	23.5 (7–240)	0.00 a,b
GGT (IU/l)	98 (24–804)	40 (14–286)	35 (9–223)	0.03 a,b
AP (IU/l)	132 (60–342)	87 (42–161)	77 (45–157)	0.14
Bilirubin (mg/dl)	3.43 (0.8–8.5)	0.72 (0.3–3.3)	0.87 (0.2–2.4)	0.00 a,b
Cholesterol (mg/dl)	114 (57–180)	219 (87–301)	160 (44–240)	0.00 a,c
Triglycerides (mg/dl)	103 (57–231)	149 (54–712)	95.5 (10–184)	0.02 c
Diabetes II (Y/N)	2/8	8/22	1/17	
Hyperlipidaemia (Y/N)	3/7	7/23	1/17	
Hypertension (Y/N)	3/7	18/12	1/17	
Histological Steatosis grade (0:1:2:3)	3*:1:5:1	0:19:8:3	17:0:0:0	
Lobular inflammation (0:A1:A2:A3)	2:3:3:2	2:18:9:1	11:5:1:0	
Ballooning (0:1:2)	0:5:5	30:0:0	17:0:0	
Matteoni (points)	4 (0–4)	2 (1–3)	n/a	
Fibrosis (0:F1:F2:F3:F4)	0:0:0:2:8	23:6:1:0:0	11:5:1:0:0	
Apoptosis (0:1:2)	4:6:0	9:15:6	12:5:0	
Alcoholic/non-alcoholic	7:3	0:30	n/a	

***...steatosis present, albeit <5% of parenchymal area.**
Samples from the Biobank cohort analyzed by qRT-PCR (p-value: a. steatohepatitis vs. steatosis, b. steatohepatitis vs. control, c. steatosis vs. control).

Table 3. Clinical, biochemical and histopathological patient characteristics.

qRTPCR biopsy samples				
	Steatohepatitis (n = 11)	**Steatosis (n = 13)**	**Controls (n = 5)**	**p-value**
sex (m:f)	6:05	9:04	4:01	
age (y)	54 (34–69)	45 (25–62)	43 (28–50)	0.07
BMI (kg/m2)	28.8 (25.2–31.6)	28.3 (22.8–35.5)	26.7 (24.3–27.7)	0.19
ALT (IU/l)	83 (43–154)	75 (21–253)	66 (39–130)	0.59
AST (IU/l)	68 (35–520)	42 (19–137)	41 (33–65)	0.07
GGT (IU/l)	426 (98–2195)	171 (17–536)	40 (27–69)	0.00 a, c
AP (IU/l)	118 (76–267)	87 (37–224)	55 (38–69)	0.01 b
Bilirubin (mg/dl)	1 (0.4–1.7)	0.68 (0.3–3.6)	0.46 (0.4–1.5)	0.27
Cholesterol (mg/dl)	258 (131–326)	206 (146–259)	142 (125–177)	0.04 b,c
Triglycerides (mg/dl)	185 (127–488)	161 (51–324)	43 (20–56)	0.01 b,c
Diabetes II (Y/N)	4/7	3/8	0/5	
Hyperlipidaemia (Y/N)	3/8	3/8	0/5	
Hypertension (Y/N)	5/6	4/7	0/5	
Steatosis grade (0:1:2:3)	0:3:3:4	0:5:3:3	4:1:0:0	
Lobular inflammation (0:A1:A2:A3)	0:2:5:3	1:5:5:0	n/a	
Ballooning (0:1:2)	0:9:1	11:0:0	5:0:0	
Matteoni (points)	4 (2–4)	2 (1–2)	n/a	
Fibrosis (0:F1:F2:F3:F4)	0:5:1:0:4	7:2:1:0:1	n/a	
Apoptosis (0:1:2)	4:6:0	8:3:0	n/a	
Alcoholic/non-alcoholic	3:8	0:13	n/a	

Samples from the Biopsy cohort used for the validation by qRT-PCR (p-value: a. steatohepatitis vs. steatosis, b. steatohepatitis vs. control, c. steatosis vs. control).

(BH) procedure. In addition, a fold change of at least 30% was required to designate a gene as differentially expressed. Resulting data was imported into Ingenuity Pathway analysis (IPA) software (Ingenuity Systems, Redwood City, CA, USA) to identify over- or underrepresented pathways as well as potential biomarkers.

The data discussed in this publication have been deposited in NCBI's Gene Expression Omnibus [15] and are accessible through GEO Series accession number GSE33814 (http://www.ncbi.nlm.nih.gov/geo/query/acc.cgi?token = nrmdhyayykcgavo&acc = GSE33814).

Quantitative real-time PCR

Quantitative gene expression analysis was performed with 87 human liver tissue samples (Biobank samples: 10 steatohepatitis, 8/2 cirrhotic/non-cirrhotic; 30 steatosis and 18 controls; Biopsy samples: 11 steatohepatitis, 5/6 cirrhotic/non-cirrhotic; 13 steatosis; 5 disease controls from patients with chronic hepatitis C) using real-time PCR (LightCycler®480 Real-Time PCR System, Roche Applied Science, Mannheim, Germany). We applied gene specific primer and probe TaqMan® gene expression assays (Applied Biosystems, Weiterstadt, Germany) and performed relative quantification of all genes. *HPRT1* was used as a housekeeping gene to normalize the data. The Cp value was extracted from the Lightcycler®480 software 1.5.0 and the expression level was calculated with the $2^{-\Delta Cp}$ method [16,17].

Table 4. Overview of samples applied to screening and validation of deregulated genes in steatohepatitis and steatosis.

	Microarray screen	**Validation of selected target genes**
Biobank cohort	N = 32	N = 58
Biopsy cohort		N = 29
total	**N = 32**	**N = 87**

Sample from the screen were also included in the validation.

Immunohistochemistry

For immunohistochemical analysis 3 µm thick paraffin sections of liver tissue of chronic hepatitis C, NAFLD associated steatosis (NAFL) and steatohepatitis were dewaxed and rehydrated following standard procedures. For antigen retrieval the sections were microwaved in Target Retrieval Solution, pH 9.0 (Dako REAL ™ S2367; Dako, Glostrup, Denmark), for 40 min at 160 W followed by cooling down for 20 min at RT. The sections were then washed in water and PBS. Blocking was carried out with Dako REAL ™ Blocking Solution for 10 min prior to incubation with antibodies against the aldose reductase AKR1B10 (Novus Biologicals, Littleton, CO, USA) diluted 1:500 in Dako REAL ™ Antibody Diluent for 60 min at RT. Binding of the antibodies was detected with the Dako REAL ™ EnVision ™ Detection System Peroxidase/DAB⁺, Rabbit/Mouse leading to a reddish-brown reaction product.

AKR1B10 protein expression detected in the cytoplasm of hepatocytes was assessed semiquantitatively as outlined below. The intensity of immunostaining was classified as mild to moderate (score A) or marked (score B), and the amount of

Table 5. Immunohistochemical expression of AKR1B10 in liver parenchyma of patients with steatohepatitis, steatosis and chronic hepatitis C.

Histological diagnosis		Score A*	Score B**	AKR1B10 score (A+B)	M-W-U test
Steatohepatitis (SH) (n = 9)	Median	2	2	4	
	Range	1–3	1–5	2–5	
Steatosis (S) (n = 11)	Median	1	1	2	SH vs.S: *P* = *0.003*
	Range	0–2	0–2	0–4	
Chronic hepatitis C (CHC) (n = 7)	Median	1	0	1	S vs. CHC: *P* = *0.351* SH vs. CHC: *P* = *0.006*
	Range	0–3	0–1	0–4	

*Weak and moderate AKR1B10 expression (% of parenchymal area): 0: no expression; 1: 1–10%; 2:>10–30%; 3:>30%.
**Marked AKR1B10 expression (% of parenchymal area): 0: no expression; 1: 1–10%; 2:>10–30%; 3:>30%.

positive hepatocytes was estimated by application of numerical scores which were defined as:

Score A or B 0: – AKR1B10 immunostaining in hepatocytes not detected

Score A or B 1: – AKR1B10 positive hepatocytes comprise less than 10% of liver parenchyma

ScoreA or B 2: – AKR1B10 positive hepatocytes comprise between 10–30% of liver parenchyma

Score A or B 3: – AKR1B10 positive hepatocytes comprise more than 30% of liver parenchyma

The AKR1B10 score was then derived from the sum of scores A and B and represents an estimate of the amount and the intensity of immunohistochemically detectable AKR1B10 protein expression in liver parenchyma (table 5).

Results

Gene expression pattern clearly separates steatohepatitis from steatosis and controls

To screen for changes in hepatic gene expression distinguishing steatohepatitis from steatosis, liver samples from patients with both alcoholic and nonalcoholic fatty liver disease obtained by surgery (Biobank) were subjected to Illumina gene expression bead chip-based analysis. A total of 32 Biobank samples were investigated (table 1). For the analysis of the microarray data, ASH and NASH cases were grouped together in one "steatohepatitis" group. Importantly, we aimed at investigating the molecular changes between steatohepatitis and steatosis only, not between their etiologies. This appears appropriate since both of the diseases, ASH as well as NASH, are characterized by a greatly overlapping spectrum of morphological changes [18]. Gene expression data

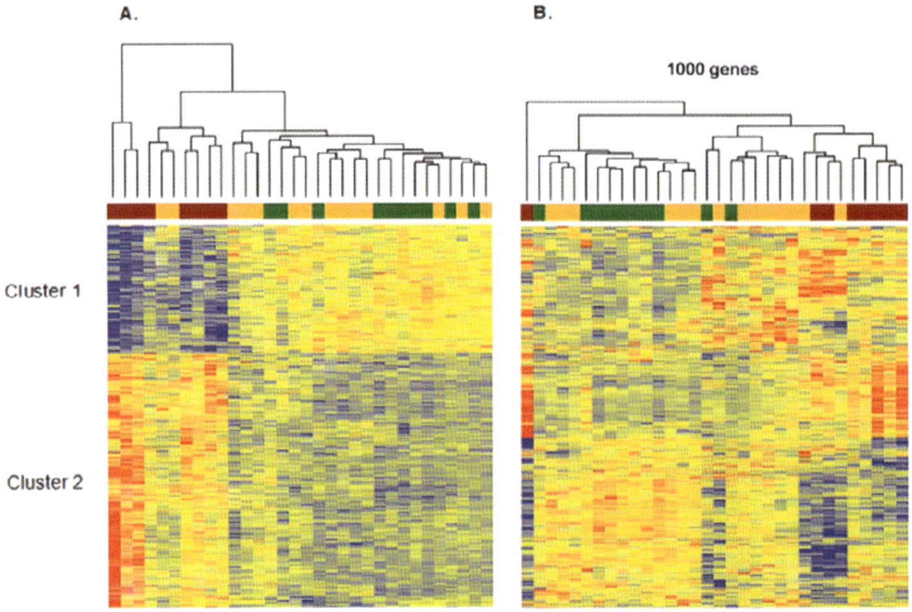

Figure 1. Supervised (A) and unsupervised (B) clustering of differentially expressed genes in the three groups of liver samples. A. Common differentially expressed genes were used for supervised clustering. B. Unsupervised clustering was performed with the 1000 most variable genes in the three groups of liver samples (steatohepatitis, red; steatosis, orange; controls, green).

were subsequently explored by two data analysis procedures, consisting of (i) identification of differentially expressed genes using limma and (ii) selection of the 1000 genes with the highest variance in the entire data set. In the pair-wise comparisons, we identified 4963 and 2543 genes as significantly (FDR<0.05) differentially expressed between steatohepatitis and controls, and steatohepatitis and steatosis, respectively. The two comparisons, shared 1931 differentially expressed genes. The differences between the gene expression profiles of the normal and steatosis samples are small. The variance within the groups is high and due to that, the power of the statistical test is not sufficient to identify significantly differentially expressed genes between the two groups. The number of differentially expressed genes indicates that steatohepatitis, when compared to normal liver tissue, is characterized by more profound molecular changes than steatosis.

Hierarchical clustering was used to visualize the 1931 common genes in a heat map (figure 1A). With two exceptions, steatosis and control samples clustered together whereas steatohepatitis samples clustered in a separate branch. Notably, the combination of NASH and ASH did not affect the hierarchical clustering. The common genes were divided into two branches, down-regulated genes in steatohepatitis compared to steatosis and controls (figure 1A, cluster 1) or up-regulated in steatohepatitis compared to steatosis and controls (figure 1A, cluster 2).

The 1000 genes with the highest variance were used for an unsupervised clustering and a visualization of the results in a heat map (figure 1B). Again, with one exception, steatohepatitis samples clustered in a branch separated from steatosis samples and controls. The highly variant genes fell into two classes, characterized by up- and down-regulation in steatohepatitis compared to the remaining samples. Taken together, both types of analyses yielded differential gene expression signatures, which clearly separated steatohepatitis from steatosis and control samples.

Gene ontology [19] analysis was performed for cluster 1 and cluster 2 (table 6 and 7, respectively) to identify disease-relevant biological processes from differentially expressed genes. Notably, cluster 1 (upregulated in controls and steatosis) was characterized by metabolism only (oxidation reduction, metabolic processes, and biosynthesis). In contrast, several GO classes in cluster 2 (upregulated in steatohepatitis) belonged to molecular processes, which are characteristic for malignant diseases and tumor progression (cell adhesion, extracellular matrix, cell motion, integrin signaling). This finding suggests that steatohepatitis is accompanied by entirely different gene expression programs when compared to steatosis and controls. Notably, the programs upregulated in steatohepatitis are characteristic for malignant diseases.

Table 6. Gene Ontology (GO) analysis.

	GO.ID	Term	pvalue
1	GO:0006805	xenobiotic metabolic process	3.0e-07
2	GO:0055114	oxidation-reduction process	3.7e-07
3	GO:0032787	monocarboxylic acid metabolic process	7.1e-07
4	GO:0006569	tryptophan catabolic process	1.9e-05
5	GO:0042559	pteridine-containing compound biosynthetic process	7.5e-05
6	GO:0009437	carnitine metabolic process	8.9e-05
7	GO:0046874	quinolinate metabolic process	0.0002
8	GO:0070646	protein modification by small protein removal	0.0005
9	GO:0016098	monoterpenoid metabolic process	0.0008
10	GO:0006542	glutamine biosynthetic process	0.0012

Over-represented GO terms for down regulated genes in the common gene list in steatohepatitis samples (Fig. 1A, cluster 1).

qRT-PCR validation of microarray data

A total of 87 human liver samples were used for PCR-based validation of the array data (table 8 and 9). To optimally select candidate genes for validation, three strategies were employed. First, 265 common genes between the 1931 differentially expressed genes and the 1000 genes with the highest variation were identified. This group of common genes was analyzed by the web-based software IPA® (Ingenuity® systems). IPA-Biomarker® was applied to identify relevant biomarker candidates that could be useful to distinguish between steatohepatitis and steatosis. A total of 126 genes were detected after filtering. From this group, 13 genes were selected for further validation, due to their significant fold change in the microarray analysis. Second, GO terms from the two defined clusters were systematically analyzed for potential targets and three genes were chosen. Third, 17 differentially expressed genes were identified by a significant p-value and fold change from the microarray data. Furthermore, five genes were used as positive controls and additionally, eight genes were chosen due to known function on protein level in steatohepatitis (table 8). Within the selection process of applicable candidates, we mainly focused on genes linked to metabolism, oxidative stress, inflammation, and their relevance in fatty liver disease. In summary, 46 genes were selected for further validation by qRT-PCR. *HPRT1* was used as a housekeeping gene. Figure 2 summarizes the fold changes of the expression of the selected genes. The rates of verification of differential gene expression were high: The changes – as determined by qRT-PCR - of differential expression for 39 genes in Biobank steatohepatitis samples were significant. Only

Table 7. Gene Ontology (GO) analysis.

	GO.ID	Term	pvalue
1	GO:0007155	cell adhesion	1.7e-15
2	GO:0006415	translational termination	1.7e-10
3	GO:0006414	translational elongation	1.8e-10
4	GO:0006935	chemotaxis	2.7e-10
5	GO:0007409	axonogenesis	4.4e-10
6	GO:0030198	extracellular matrix organization	8.4e-09
7	GO:0019083	viral transcription	2.5e-08
8	GO:0016477	cell migration	1.0e-07
9	GO:0031018	endocrine pancreas development	1.0e-07
10	GO:0042060	wound healing	1.1e-06

Over-represented GO terms for up regulated genes in common gene list in steatohepatitis samples (Fig. 1A, cluster 2).

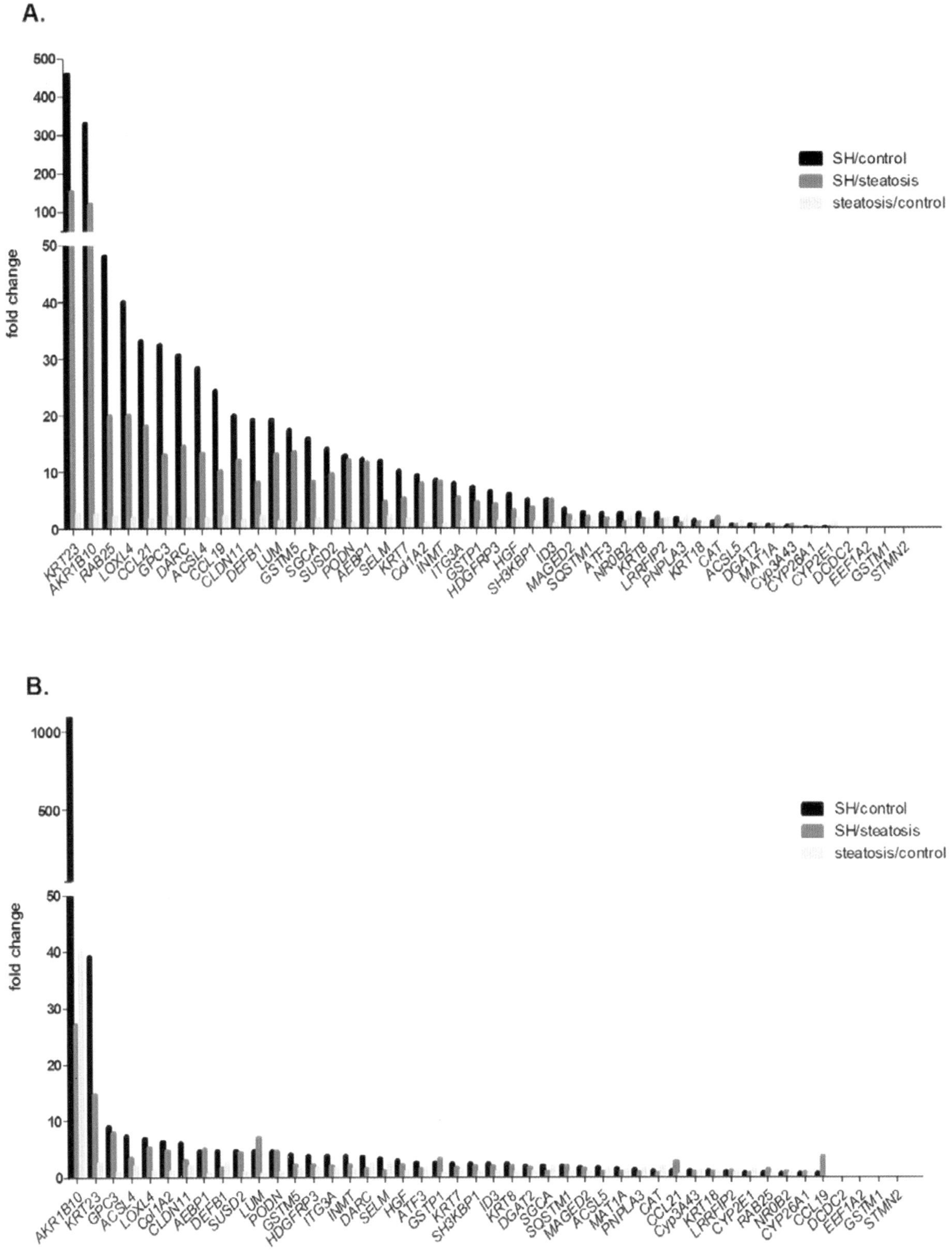

Figure 2. Fold changes of selected genes validated by qRT-PCR. The expression of selected target genes was determined in surgically collected samples (A) and in liver samples obtained by biopsy (B). The fold change was calculated by comparing the three groups of liver samples against each other.

Table 8. Candidate genes for qRT-PCR validation.

				Biobank samples					
Gene	**Reference**	**Chip/FC (SH/ctrl)**	**Chip/FC (SH/steatosis)**	**FC q-RT-PCR (SH/ctrl)**	**p-value (SH/ctrl)**	**FC q-RT-PCR (SH/steatosis)**	**p-value (SH/steatosis)**	**FC q-RT-PCR (steatosis/ctrl)**	**p-value (steatosis/ctrl)**
KRT23	This study	1.261	1.253	460.482	2.29E-10	155.130	9.57E-09	2.968	0.011
AKR1B10	IPA biomarker	4.473	4.123	331.812	2.12E-11	121.404	4.29E-11	2.733	0.079
RAB25	This study	1.427	1.331	48.235	9.56E-11	20.135	9.44E-10	2.396	0.025
LOXL4	This study	3.503	2.564	40.122	7.16E-08	20.196	1.50E-06	1.987	0.018
CCL21	IPA biomarker	2.683	2.347	33.277	8.17E-10	18.341	2.13E-08	1.814	0.061
GPC3	This study	1.590	1.439	32.522	1.17E-10	13.147	2.02E-08	2.474	3.54E-04
DARC	This study	0.804	0.926	30.678	4.88E-07	14.726	1.86E-05	2.083	0.044
ACSL4	[20,21]	1.993	1.825	28.509	1.16E-08	13.526	3.57E-07	2.108	0.029
CCL19	IPA biomarker	2.587	2.177	24.562	1.62E-10	10.147	1.75E-08	2.421	0.004
CLDN11	IPA biomarker	1.699	1.690	20.043	5.11E-08	12.173	1.88E-06	1.646	0.064
DEFB1	This study	2.257	1.661	19.309	4.88E-11	8.200	8.81E-09	2.355	0.001
LUM	IPA biomarker	2.509	2.262	19.256	7.43E-08	13.272	2.20E-07	1.451	0.061
GSTM5	This study [21]	0.676	0.758	17.483	8.43E-06	13.658	2.18E-05	1.280	0.494
SGCA	This study	0.677	0.586	15.864	3.57E-09	8.378	2.06E-07	1.893	0.013
SUSD2	IPA biomarker	2.076	1.673	14.207	4.24E-07	9.669	1.16E-06	1.469	0.069
PODN	This study	2.046	1.949	12.954	1.72E-08	12.109	1.32E-08	1.070	0.803
AEBP1	IPA biomarker	2.277	2.068	12.309	1.25E-07	11.841	6.90E-08	1.040	0.887
SELM	This study	1.208	1.224	12.061	5.23E-08	4.938	1.90E-05	2.442	0.002
KRT7	This study	1.456	1.083	10.156	3.43E-06	5.372	1.32E-04	1.891	0.026
COL1A2	IPA biomarker	1.406	1.588	9.552	2.23E-07	8.076	6.84E-07	1.183	0.482
INMT	IPA biomarker	2.038	2.095	8.593	4.03E-06	8.380	5.31E-06	1.025	0.919
ITGA3	This study	-	-	8.164	1.99E-07	5.632	2.21E-06	1.450	0.133
GSTP1	IPA biomarker	1.457	1.246	7.418	9.03E-07	4.747	1.87E-05	1.563	0.053
HDGFRP3	This study	0.157	0.231	6.710	5.51E-06	4.423	9.26E-05	1.517	0.032
HGF	This study	0.244	0.260	6.068	3.56E-06	3.324	2.68E-04	1.825	0.002
SH3KBP1	This study	0.587	0.539	5.236	9.67E-06	3.789	9.27E-05	1.382	0.143
ID3	This study	1.171	1.659	5.206	6.46E-05	5.174	7.44E-05	1.006	0.968
MAGED2	This study	0.400	0.389	3.610	1.10E-05	2.476	3.66E-04	1.458	0.010
SQSTM1	This study	-	-	2.993	1.50E-04	2.260	0.002	1.324	0.130
ATF3	[20]	-	-	2.782	0.001	1.768	0.104	1.573	0.174
NR0B2	This study [21]	-	-	2.776	0.008	1.223	0.531	2.270	0.001
KRT8	This study	-	-	2.689	0.001	1.628	0.049	1.652	0.041
LRRFIP2	This study	−0.398	−0.535	2.665	9.07E-05	1.482	0.037	1.799	0.005

Table 8. Cont.

				Biobank samples					
Gene	**Reference**	**Chip/FC (SH/ctrl)**	**Chip/FC (SH/steatosis)**	**FC q-RT-PCR (SH/ctrl)**	**p-value (SH/ctrl)**	**FC q-RT-PCR (SH/steatosis)**	**p-value (SH/steatosis)**	**FC q-RT-PCR (steatosis/ctrl)**	**p-value (steatosis/ctrl)**
PNPLA3	This study	-	-	1.917	0.029	0.894	0.641	2.145	0.002
KRT18	This study	-	-	1.434	0.030	1.218	0.209	1.178	0.306
CAT	IPA biomarker [20]	−1.389	-	1.406	0.079	1.948	0.197	0.722	0.521
ACSL5	This study	−0.896	−0.983	0.780	0.282	0.565	0.026	1.380	0.049
DGAT2	This study	-	-	0.715	0.324	0.544	0.074	1.313	0.231
MAT1A	IPA biomarker	−1.245	−1.007	0.556	0.012	0.650	0.051	0.855	0.321
CYP3A43	This study	−2.113	−1.499	0.435	0.000	0.560	0.060	0.777	0.405
CYP26A1	This study	-	-	0.301	0.018	0.288	0.009	1.043	0.916
CYP2E1	This study	-	-	0.296	0.021	0.213	0.006	1.388	0.051
DCDC2	This study	0.740	0.710	-	-	-	-	-	-
EEF1A2	IPA biomarker	3.408	3.158	-	-	-	-	-	-
GSTM1	This study	-	-	-	-	-	-	-	-
STMN2	IPA biomarker	2.581	2.249	-	-	-	-	-	-

FCs (fold changes) of selected target genes were calculated from gene expression array data for the Biobank cohort. Gene expression from selected target genes was validated by qRT-PCR in the Biobank cohort.. FC was calculated between steatohepatitis (SH) and controls (ctrl) as well as between SH and steatosis.

Table 9. Candidate genes for qRT-PCR validation.

	biopsy samples					
Gene	FC q-RT-PCR (SH/ctrl)	p-value (SH/ctrl)	FC q-RT-PCR (SH/ steatosis)	p-value (SH/steatosis)	FC q-RT-PCR (steatosis/ctrl)	p-value (steatosis/ctrl)
AKR1B10	1095.838	4.98E-10	27.173	6.79E-05	40.328	1.23E-05
KRT23	39.302	0.001	14.809	0.006	2.654	0.049
GPC3	9.060	0.010	8.043	0.004	1.126	0.862
ACSL4	7.444	0.001	3.491	0.004	2.132	0.103
LOXL4	6.939	1.58E-05	5.274	0.001	1.316	0.449
Col1A2	6.362	1.94E-05	4.852	1.67E-04	1.311	0.408
CLDN11	6.251	0.001	2.968	0.003	2.106	0.078
AEBP1	4.862	3.18E-04	5.130	0.001	0.948	0.894
DEFB1	4.794	8.99E-06	1.767	0.066	2.713	0.001
SUSD2	4.786	2.50E-04	4.478	2.93E-04	1.069	0.846
LUM	4.735	1.54E-04	7.045	4.00E-05	0.672	0.213
PODN	4.650	0.001	4.661	4.00E-04	0.998	0.995
GSTM5	4.037	0.014	2.291	0.119	1.762	0.283
HDGFRP3	3.986	7.93E-05	2.337	0.006	1.706	0.075
ITG3A	3.909	0.009	2.170	0.046	1.801	0.221
INMT	3.860	0.005	2.389	0.003	1.616	0.208
DARC	3.841	1.11E-04	1.591	0.139	2.415	0.010
SELM	3.386	2.98E-04	1.240	0.454	2.729	0.005
HGF	3.039	2.74E-06	2.291	0.003	1.326	0.215
ATF3	2.732	0.005	1.603	0.138	1.704	0.051
GSTP1	2.694	0.044	3.364	0.001	0.801	0.599
KRT7	2.519	0.014	1.694	0.201	1.487	0.310
SH3KBP1	2.472	0.012	2.148	0.003	1.151	0.632
ID3	2.456	5.48E-05	1.913	0.013	1.284	0.266
KRT8	2.442	0.007	2.146	0.013	1.138	0.637
DGAT2	2.207	0.019	1.823	0.041	1.211	0.504
SGCA	2.161	0.063	1.138	0.750	1.900	0.125
SQSTM1	2.085	0.001	2.089	0.001	0.998	0.991
MAGED2	1.821	0.001	1.664	0.025	1.094	0.655
ACSL5	1.725	0.016	1.055	0.810	1.635	0.034
MAT1A	1.599	0.035	1.098	0.684	1.456	0.046
PNPLA3	1.443	0.304	0.932	0.805	1.548	0.177
CAT	1.329	0.389	0.682	0.233	1.950	0.003
CCL21	1.295	0.539	2.826	0.035	0.458	0.094
Cyp3A43	1.216	0.502	1.037	0.906	1.173	0.296
KRT18	1.178	0.397	1.101	0.646	1.070	0.719
LRRFIP2	1.114	0.723	1.188	0.392	0.938	0.835
CYP2E1	0.956	0.875	0.708	0.264	1.351	0.045
RAB25	0.916	0.903	1.451	0.616	0.632	0.318
NROB2	0.765	0.557	1.097	0.757	0.698	0.432
CYP26A1	0.643	0.348	0.859	0.709	0.749	0.466
CCL19	0.634	0.385	3.689	0.032	0.172	0.002
DCDC2	-	-	-	-	-	-
EEF1A2	-	-	-	-	-	-
GSTM1	-	-	-	-	-	-
STMN2	-	-	-	-	-	-

Gene expression from selected target genes was validated in the Biopsy cohort. FC was calculated between steatohepatitis (SH) and controls (ctrl) as well as between SH and steatosis.

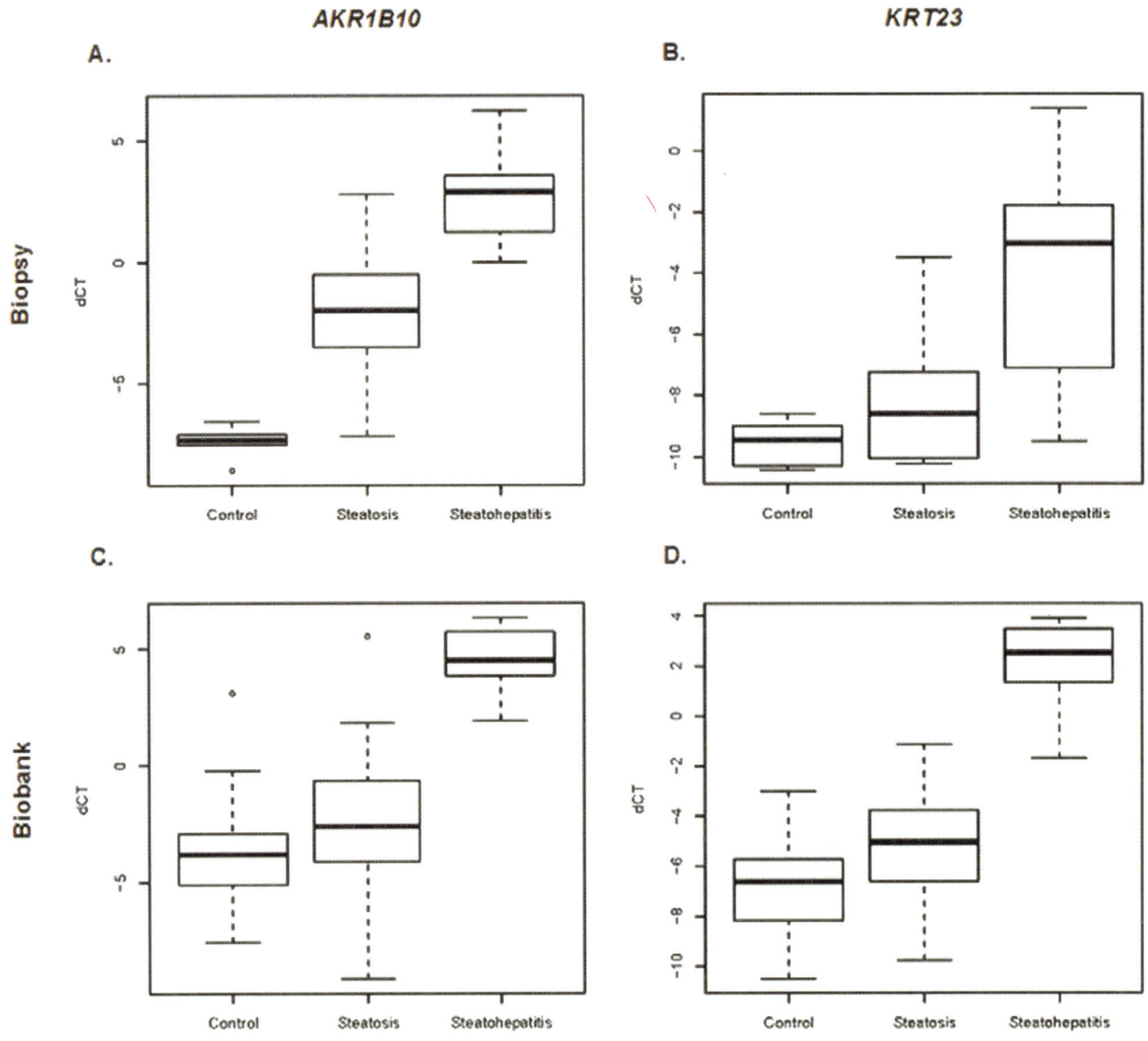

Figure 3. Validation of *AKR1B10* (A and C) and *KRT23* (B and D) mRNA expression by qRT-PCR in biopsy (top) and biobank (bottom) samples. *HPRT1* was chosen to normalize the gene expression in the analyzed samples. Mean normalized expression levels are given in log2.

three genes were not significantly deregulated. In biopsies, 30 genes were significant, and twelve genes were not significantly deregulated. The reasons for the lower verification rate in biopsies may be that most of the analyzed Biobank samples had already been used for the whole genome microarray experiment (no independent sample cohort). Four genes (*DCDC2*, *EEF1A2*, *GSTM1* and *STMN2*) could not be reliably measured in any of the samples.

The genes *ACSL4*, *ATF3*, *CAT*, *GSTM5* and *NR0B2* were previously described in fatty liver disease [20,21] and served as positive controls for the quantitative validation of candidate genes in the present study. The significant up-regulation of these positive control genes was validated in either one or both of the analyzed cohorts (table 8 and 9).

The major finding supports the notion of a striking alteration of molecular programs in steatohepatitis when compared to steatosis and control samples. The most strikingly deregulated genes in this respect were *AKR1B10* and *KRT23* (figure 3) since our data showed a highly significant overexpression of both genes in steatohepatitis.

Immunohistochemical analysis of AKR1B10 expression in steatosis, steatohepatitis and chronic hepatitis C

Weak to moderate or marked cytoplasmic and sometimes nuclear reactivity with antibodies against AKR1B10 was detected in hepatocytes of almost all of the liver tissue samples of patients with steatosis and steatohepatitis of both, alcoholic and non alcoholic etiology, as well as chronic hepatitis C controls (figure 4 A–F, table 5). AKR1B10 expression in cases with steatohepatitis as assessed by the immunohistochemical AKR1B10 score was significantly higher as compared to the AKR1B10 expression in the steatosis and chronic hepatitis C cases ($p = 0.003$ and 0.006, respectively). However, AKR1B10 expression in liver tissues with steatosis or chronic hepatitis C was not different ($p = 0.351$) (Table 5). AKR1B10 expression was also detected in the

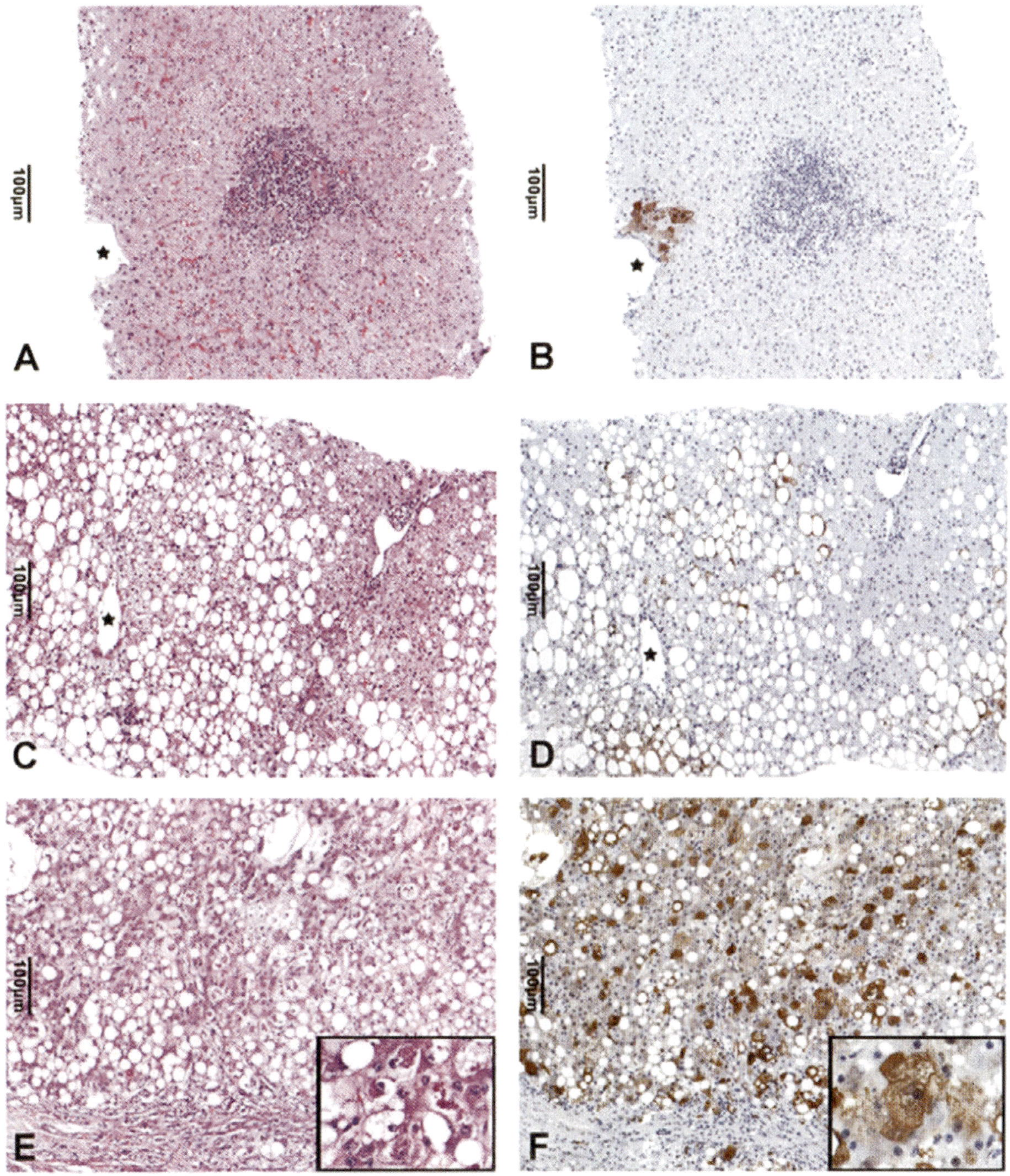

Figure 4. Immunohistochemical detection of the expression of AKR1B10 in chronic hepatitis C (A,B), fatty liver (C,D) and (cirrhotic) steatohepatitis (E,F). Only representative areas are shown. (A) Case of chronic hepatitis C with an inflamed portal tract with lymphocytic infiltrates and mild interphase hepatitis (central vein marked by asterisk, H&E stained section). (B) Consecutive section of the area shown in (A). Only a group of few centrilobular hepatocytes exhibit cytoplasmic and nuclear AKR1B10 immunostaining (central vein marked by asterisk). (C) Case of fatty liver with marked macro- and mediovacuolar steatosis predominantly of centrilobular and mid-zonal hepatocytes (central vein marked by asterisk; H&E stained section). (D) Consecutive section of the area shown in (C) of the hepatocytes with fatty change show staining of the rim of cytoplasm not occupied by fat with AKR1B10 antibodies (central vein marked by asterisk). (E) Case of steatohepatitis in a cirrhotic liver with parenchymal nodule abuting a fibrous septum with mild ductular reaction. Many hepatocytes show fatty change and some of them are characterized by an enlarged, lightly stained cytoplasm (ballooned hepatocytes) and irregular eosinophilic cytoplasmic inclusions (Mallory-Denk bodies, MDBs; inset with higher magnification showing ballooned hepatocytes containing MDBs; H&E stained section). (F) Consecutive section of the area shown in (E). Many of the normal-sized as well as the ballooned hepatocytes show moderate cytoplasmic immunostaining with AKR1B10 antibodies whereas the MDBs remain unstained (inset with higher magnification shows ballooned hepatocytes with MDB).

epithelium of some of the large or medium sized bile ducts (data not shown).

Discussion

The present study unravels gene expression signatures profoundly distinguishing steatohepatitis from steatosis and normal liver. Notably, normal tissue and steatosis clustered more closely together when compared to the steatohepatitis samples. Since the hierarchical clustering clearly demonstrated common expression profiles for NASH and ASH samples, no further distinction was made between the different etiologies. Furthermore, both etiologies manifest with a broadly overlapping spectrum of histological key features (e.g. centrilobular based features of steatosis, inflammation and hepatocellular ballooning as well as pericellular fibrosis) [7,18].

The gene expression data suggests that steatohepatitis exhibits molecular profiles which are characteristic for processes relevant in malignant tumors and may therefore reflect a premalignant state of liver disease already at the precirrhotic stage (table 7.). Indeed, increasing evidence supports the fact that steatohepatitis can progress to HCC already in precirrhotic stage [22]. Obesity and diabetes are not only established risk factors for developing steatohepatitis and cirrhosis, but have also been implicated in the formation of HCC. Other major risk factors for HCC in steatohepatitis are advanced age and tissue fibrosis. The mechanisms underlying the progression from steatohepatitis to HCC are still unclear, and targets for the treatment of steatohepatitis and HCC are missing. However, signaling pathways involved in inflammation and insulin resistance promoting steatohepatitis, may contribute to its carcinogenic potential.

The gene expression of the 46 selected genes was validated by qRT-PCR for both of the tested sample cohorts. Although the analyzed samples were collected by different approaches, and for the biopsy samples chronic hepatitis C samples were used as controls (since percutaneous liver biopsy is not performed in individuals with normal liver), many significantly deregulated genes were found in all three tested groups of liver samples in both independent sample cohorts (table 1 to 3). Despite a difference in the percentage of cirrhotic cases between the two cohorts (80% in surgical samples, and 45% in biopsies), *AKR1B10* as well as *KRT23* were significantly high expressed in both sample cohorts. This indicates common pathogenetic mechanisms in both alcoholic and non-alcoholic steatohepatitis. Among the differentially expressed genes, *AKR1B10* and *KRT23* were the most prominent ones. AKR1B10 belongs to the aldose reductases and was first described in human HCC [23,24]. It is a monomeric enzyme reducing aldehydes and ketones to the corresponding alcohols. The protein is expressed in cervical cancer and non-small cell lung cancer, where it is considered as a potential diagnostic biomarker [25,26,27]. Several findings also support the hypothesis that *AKR1B10* may be a useful marker for differentiation and proliferation of liver, colon, lung and breast cancer [28,29,30]. In addition, AKR1B10 protein plays a role in the detoxification of toxic aldehydes. Free radicals generated by reactive oxygen species oxidize fatty acids of the lipid membrane resulting in the production of reactive aldehydes, which are rapidly reduced by AKR1B10 thereby protecting cells from toxification [31,32]. Lipotoxicity of fatty acid and lipid intermediary metabolites may be a key event in the progression of fatty liver disease by inducing hepatocellular death. In the present study, we report the significant overexpression of *AKR1B10* in steatohepatitis which could be caused by the increased need to inactivate toxic components in hepatocytes. This suggests that *AKR1B10* may be a molecular marker accompanying the progression of steatohepatitis to HCC.

Genes involved in lipid partitioning by keeping potentially lipotoxic fatty acids stored in neutral triglycerides (TG) may counteract/protect from lipotoxicity as a potentially important factor in progression of NAFLD to steatohepatitis [33]. Notably, some of the genes which were found to be deregulated included enzymes involved in FA homeostasis such as DGAT2 (responsible for FA esterification to TGs) and PNPLA3 (adiponutrin), recently identified as a key determinant for pathogenesis and progression of alcoholic and non-alcoholic fatty liver disease [34,35].

Furthermore, we describe the highly significant overexpression of *KRT23* in steatohepatitis compared to steatosis and normal liver. *KRT23* has been detected in different cancer types. In microsatellite stable colon cancer, *KRT23* expression is highly increased, and this may have a protective function counteracting the proliferation and survival of cells [36]. Another study identified KRT23 as a HCC-associated antigen in patient sera [37]. *KRT23* has not yet been described to be expressed in liver or liver disease. The role of KRT23 under physiological conditions and in steatohepatitis is unknown. However, mutations of other members of the keratin multigene family, namely keratins 8 and 18, were found to be associated with chronic human liver disease. Furthermore, disturbances of the expression levels of keratins 8 and 18 led to formation of Mallory-Denk bodies, an important morphological characteristic of steatohepatitis [38,39]. Nevertheless, the functional role of *KRT23* in liver or liver diseases needs to be resolved.

In summary, we propose that *AKR1B10* and *KRT23* may represent pre-malignant markers in the progression of steatohepatitis to HCC. These marker genes can be useful to test patients for a potential development of HCC and for therapeutic decisions in clinical practice. However, further studies will be needed to address the use of these signatures in predicting prognosis and disease course in patients with fatty liver disease.

Acknowledgments

We thank Dr. G. Bernhardt and Prof. H.J. Mischinger for their support with providing clinical patient data and help with obtaining surgical samples. For excellent technical assistance, we thank Sabrina Balaguer Puig and Simon John Ogrodnik.

Author Contributions

Conceived and designed the experiments: JS HS CL. Performed the experiments: JS CL. Analyzed the data: JS MF. Contributed reagents/materials/analysis tools: JS MF WS KLL CL KZ MT HS. Wrote the paper: JS CL MT HS.

References

1. Angulo P (2002) Nonalcoholic fatty liver disease. N Engl J Med 346: 1221–1231.
2. Cohen JC, Horton JD, Hobbs HH (2011) Human fatty liver disease: old questions and new insights. Science 332: 1519–1523.
3. Lazo M, Clark JM (2008) The epidemiology of nonalcoholic fatty liver disease: a global perspective. Semin Liver Dis 28: 339–350.
4. Trauner M, Arrese M, Wagner M (2010) Fatty liver and lipotoxicity. Biochim Biophys Acta 1801: 299–310.
5. Machado M, Marques-Vidal P, Cortez-Pinto H (2006) Hepatic histology in obese patients undergoing bariatric surgery. J Hepatol 45: 600–606.
6. Williams CD, Stengel J, Asike MI, Torres DM, Shaw J, et al. (2011) Prevalence of nonalcoholic fatty liver disease and nonalcoholic steatohepatitis among a largely middle-aged population utilizing ultrasound and liver biopsy: a prospective study. Gastroenterology 140: 124–131.

7. Syn WK, Teaberry V, Choi SS, Diehl AM (2009) Similarities and differences in the pathogenesis of alcoholic and nonalcoholic steatohepatitis. Semin Liver Dis 29: 200–210.
8. Browning JD, Szczepaniak LS, Dobbins R, Nuremberg P, Horton JD, et al. (2004) Prevalence of hepatic steatosis in an urban population in the United States: impact of ethnicity. Hepatology 40: 1387–1395.
9. Cossrow N, Falkner B (2004) Race/ethnic issues in obesity and obesity-related comorbidities. J Clin Endocrinol Metab 89: 2590–2594.
10. Day CP, James OF (1998) Steatohepatitis: a tale of two "hits"? Gastroenterology 114: 842–845.
11. Neuschwander-Tetri BA, Caldwell SH (2003) Nonalcoholic steatohepatitis: summary of an AASLD Single Topic Conference. Hepatology 37: 1202–1219.
12. Yip WW, Burt AD (2006) Alcoholic liver disease. Semin Diagn Pathol 23: 149–160.
13. Kleiner DE, Brunt EM, Van Natta M, Behling C, Contos MJ, et al. (2005) Design and validation of a histological scoring system for nonalcoholic fatty liver disease. Hepatology 41: 1313–1321.
14. Smyth GK (2004) Linear models and empirical bayes methods for assessing differential expression in microarray experiments. Stat Appl Genet Mol Biol 3: Article3.
15. Edgar R, Domrachev M, Lash AE (2002) Gene Expression Omnibus: NCBI gene expression and hybridization array data repository. Nucleic Acids Res 30: 207–210.
16. Pfaffl MW (2001) A new mathematical model for relative quantification in real-time RT-PCR. Nucleic Acids Res 29: e45.
17. Livak KJ, Schmittgen TD (2001) Analysis of relative gene expression data using real-time quantitative PCR and the 2(-Delta Delta C(T)) Method. Methods 25: 402–408.
18. Brunt EM (2006) Non-alcoholic fatty liver disease. In: Burt AD, Portmann BC, Ferrell LD, editors. MacSween's Pathology of the Liver. Philadelphia: Churchill Livingstone. pp. 367–397.
19. Alexa A, Rahnenfuhrer J, Lengauer T (2006) Improved scoring of functional groups from gene expression data by decorrelating GO graph structure. Bioinformatics 22: 1600–1607.
20. Younossi ZM, Gorreta F, Ong JP, Schlauch K, Del Giacco L, et al. (2005) Hepatic gene expression in patients with obesity-related non-alcoholic steatohepatitis. Liver Int 25: 760–771.
21. Stepanova M, Hossain N, Afendy A, Perry K, Goodman ZD, et al. (2010) Hepatic Gene Expression of Caucasian and African-American Patients with Obesity-Related Non-Alcoholic Fatty Liver Disease. Obes Surg 20(5): 640–650.
22. Hashimoto E, Yatsuji S, Tobari M, Taniai M, Torii N, et al. (2009) Hepatocellular carcinoma in patients with nonalcoholic steatohepatitis. J Gastroenterol 44 Suppl 19: 89–95.
23. Cao D, Fan ST, Chung SS (1998) Identification and characterization of a novel human aldose reductase-like gene. J Biol Chem 273: 11429–11435.
24. Scuric Z, Stain SC, Anderson WF, Hwang JJ (1998) New member of aldose reductase family proteins overexpressed in human hepatocellular carcinoma. Hepatology 27: 943–950.
25. Fukumoto S, Yamauchi N, Moriguchi H, Hippo Y, Watanabe A, et al. (2005) Overexpression of the aldo-keto reductase family protein AKR1B10 is highly correlated with smokers' non-small cell lung carcinomas. Clin Cancer Res 11: 1776–1785.
26. Yoshitake H, Takahashi M, Ishikawa H, Nojima M, Iwanari H, et al. (2007) Aldo-keto reductase family 1, member B10 in uterine carcinomas: a potential risk factor of recurrence after surgical therapy in cervical cancer. Int J Gynecol Cancer 17: 1300–1306.
27. Penning TM (2005) AKR1B10: a new diagnostic marker of non-small cell lung carcinoma in smokers. Clin Cancer Res 11: 1687–1690.
28. Heringlake S, Hofdmann M, Fiebeler A, Manns MP, Schmiegel W, et al. (2010) Identification and expression analysis of the aldo-ketoreductase1-B10 gene in primary malignant liver tumours. J Hepatol 52: 220–227.
29. Wang C, Yan R, Luo D, Watabe K, Liao DF, et al. (2009) Aldo-keto reductase family 1 member B10 promotes cell survival by regulating lipid synthesis and eliminating carbonyls. J Biol Chem 284: 26742–26748.
30. Ma J, Yan R, Zu X, Cheng JM, Rao K, et al. (2008) Aldo-keto reductase family 1 B10 affects fatty acid synthesis by regulating the stability of acetyl-CoA carboxylase-alpha in breast cancer cells. J Biol Chem 283: 3418–3423.
31. Martin HJ, Maser E (2009) Role of human aldo-keto-reductase AKR1B10 in the protection against toxic aldehydes. Chem Biol Interact 178: 145–150.
32. Mattson MP (2009) Roles of the lipid peroxidation product 4-hydroxynonenal in obesity, the metabolic syndrome, and associated vascular and neurodegenerative disorders. Exp Gerontol 44: 625–633.
33. Neuschwander-Tetri BA (2010) Hepatic lipotoxicity and the pathogenesis of nonalcoholic steatohepatitis: the central role of nontriglyceride fatty acid metabolites. Hepatology 52: 774–788.
34. Romeo S, Kozlitina J, Xing C, Pertsemlidis A, Cox D, et al. (2008) Genetic variation in PNPLA3 confers susceptibility to nonalcoholic fatty liver disease. Nat Genet 40: 1461–1465.
35. Tian C, Stokowski RP, Kershenobich D, Ballinger DG, Hinds DA (2010) Variant in PNPLA3 is associated with alcoholic liver disease. Nat Genet 42: 21–23.
36. Birkenkamp-Demtroder K, Mansilla F, Sorensen FB, Kruhoffer M, Cabezon T, et al. (2007) Phosphoprotein Keratin 23 accumulates in MSS but not MSI colon cancers in vivo and impacts viability and proliferation in vitro. Mol Oncol 1: 181–195.
37. Wang K, Xu X, Nie Y, Dai L, Wang P, et al. (2009) Identification of tumor-associated antigens by using SEREX in hepatocellular carcinoma. Cancer Lett 281: 144–150.
38. Stumptner C, Heid H, Fuchsbichler A, Hauser H, Mischinger HJ, et al. (1999) Analysis of intracytoplasmic hyaline bodies in a hepatocellular carcinoma. Demonstration of p62 as major constituent. Am J Pathol 154: 1701–1710.
39. Stumptner C, Fuchsbichler A, Zatloukal K, Denk H (2007) In vitro production of Mallory bodies and intracellular hyaline bodies: the central role of sequestosome 1/p62. Hepatology 46: 851–860.

3

Prediction of Liver-Related Events Using Fibroscan in Chronic Hepatitis B Patients Showing Advanced Liver Fibrosis

Seung Up Kim[1,2,5]§, Ji Hoon Lee[1]§, Do Young Kim[1,2,5], Sang Hoon Ahn[1,2,5,6], Kyu Sik Jung[1], Eun Hee Choi[3], Young Nyun Park[4,6], Kwang-Hyub Han[1,2,5,6], Chae Yoon Chon[1,2,5], Jun Yong Park[1,2,5]*

1 Department of Internal Medicine, Yonsei University College of Medicine, Seoul, Korea, **2** Institute of Gastroenterology, Yonsei University College of Medicine, Seoul, Korea, **3** Department of Biostatistics, Yonsei University College of Medicine, Seoul, Korea, **4** Department of Pathology, Yonsei University College of Medicine, Seoul, Korea, **5** Liver Cirrhosis Clinical Research Center, Seoul, Korea, **6** Brain Korea 21 Project of Medical Science, Seoul, Korea

Abstract

Background: Liver stiffness measurement (LSM) using transient elastography (FibroScan®) can assess liver fibrosis noninvasively. This study investigated whether LSM can predict the development of liver-related events (LREs) in chronic hepatitis B (CHB) patients showing histologically advanced liver fibrosis.

Methods: Between March 2006 and April 2010, 128 CHB patients with who underwent LSM and liver biopsy (LB) before starting nucleot(s)ide analogues and showed histologically advanced fibrosis (≥F3) with a high viral loads [HBV DNA ≥2,000 IU/mL] were enrolled. All patients were followed regularly to detect LRE development, including hepatic decompensation (variceal bleeding, ascites, hepatic encephalopathy, spontaneous bacterial peritonitis, hepatorenal syndrome) and hepatocellular carcinoma (HCC).

Results: The mean age of the patient (72 men, 56 women) was 52.2 years. During the median follow-up period [median 27.8 (12.6–61.6) months], LREs developed in 19 (14.8%) patients (five with hepatic decompensation, 13 with HCC, one with both). Together with age, multivariate analysis identified LSM as an independent predictor of LRE development [$P<0.044$; hazard ratio (HR), 1.038; 95% confidence interval (CI), 1.002–1.081]. When the study population was stratified into two groups using the optimal cutoff value (19 kPa), which maximized the sum of sensitivity (61.1%) and specificity (86.2%) from a time-dependent receiver operating characteristic curve, patients with LSM>19 kPa were at significantly greater risk than those with LSM≤19 kPa for LRE development (HR, 7.176; 95% CI, 2.257–22.812; $P=0.001$).

Conclusion: LSM can be a useful predictor of LRE development in CHB patients showing histologically advanced liver fibrosis.

Editor: James Fung, The University of Hong Kong, Hong Kong

Funding: This study was supported by a grant of the Korea Healthcare Technology R & D project, Ministry of Health and Welfare, Republic of Korea (A102065). The funders had no role in study design, data collection and analysis, decision to publish, or preparation of the manuscript.

Competing Interests: The authors have declared that no competing interests exist.

* E-mail: DRPJY@yuhs.ac

§ These authors contributed equally to this work.

Introduction

Chronic infection with hepatotropic viruses is the main cause of chronic liver disease (CLD) worldwide, and hepatitis B virus (HBV) is predominant in the Far East [1,2]. Approximately 10–20% of patients with chronic hepatitis B (CHB) infection have liver cirrhosis at first presentation, and an additional 20–30% of patients will eventually develop this condition and its complications within one or more decades [3,4]. Previous studies indicated an annual risk of developing hepatocellular carcinoma (HCC) of 1–6%, and a similar or higher risk of hepatic decompensation after the development of cirrhosis [5,6]. Although antiviral treatment using nucleot(s)ide analogues (NUCs) suppresses HBV effectively [7], liver-related events (LREs) including hepatic decompensation, HCC, and liver-related death still occur and remain an important watershed in the management algorithm of patients with CHB.

Because LREs usually develop in patients with advanced liver fibrosis and cirrhosis, the early detection of advanced liver fibrosis and cirrhosis and the assessment of their severity for the design of optimal surveillance and intervention strategies are important. Although liver biopsy (LB) has been the gold standard for assessing liver fibrosis to date [8], it is prone to sampling error and interpretational variability [9]. Recently, liver stiffness measurement (LSM) using transient elastography (FibroScan®) has been introduced for assessing liver fibrosis with accurate, reproducible, and reliable results [10,11]. Furthermore, because LSM can be expressed numerically as a continuous variable, clinicians can grade the degree of liver fibrosis, even in patients with cirrhosis,

Table 1. Baseline Characteristics (n = 128).

Variables	Values
Demographic data	
Age (years)	52.2±9.3
Male	72 (56.3)
Diabetes mellitus	11 (8.6)
Body mass index (kg/m^2)	24.0±2.9
Laboratory data	
Serum albumin (g/dL)	4.2±0.5
Total bilirubin (mg/dL)	0.8±0.3
Alanine aminotransferase (IU/L)	44.4±21.6
Prothrombin time (%)	90.9±9.8
Platelet count (10^9/L)	148.5±48.4
Alpha-fetoprotein (ng/mL)	4.7 (0.8–50.6)
Histological data	
Fibrosis stage, 3/4	18 (14.1)/110 (85.9)
Activity grade, 1–2/3–4	97 (75.8)/31 (24.2)
Liver stiffness measurement	
LSM values (kPa)	12.9 (4.4–57.1)
Success rate (%)	100 (63–100)
Interquartile range/median value (kPa)	0.15 (0.01–0.30)
Antiviral agent	
Lamivudine	49 (38.3)
Entecavir	79 (61.7)

Variables are expressed as mean ± SD, median (range), or n (%).
HBeAg, hepatitis B e antigen; LSM, liver stiffness measurement; kPa, kilopascal.

and assess the risk of developing liver-related complications and HCC [12–14]. Thus, we hypothesized that LSM could predict the development of LREs in CHB patients who were receiving antiviral treatment using NUCs due to histologically advanced liver fibrosis or cirrhosis with a high viral load.

Previous cross-sectional studies have reported an association between LSM and the presence of liver-related complications or HCC in patients with CLD [12,13,15,16]. However, few prospective longitudinal studies have investigated the role of LSM as a predictor of LRE development in patients with advanced liver fibrosis. Thus, we evaluated the usefulness of LSM in assessing the risk of LRE development in CHB patients showing histologically advanced liver fibrosis with a high viral load.

Methods

Patients

Between March 2006 and April 2010, a total of 178 NUC-naïve CHB patients underwent LB to assess the degree of liver fibrosis and necroinflammation before starting antiviral treatment at Severance Hospital, Yonsei University College of Medicine, Seoul, Korea. CHB was defined as the persistent presence of serum hepatitis B surface antigen (HBsAg) for more than 6 months and HBV DNA positivity on a polymerase chain reaction (PCR) assay. Patients who provided written informed consent and received LB and LSM were consecutively enrolled in this prospective study. The study protocol conformed to the ethical guidelines of the 1975 Declaration of Helsinki and was approved by the institutional review board of Severance Hospital.

Exclusion criteria were as follows: 1) LSM failure (no valid shots; $n = 0$), 2) invalid LSM [defined as an interquartile range (IQR) to median value ratio (IQR/M) >0.3, success rate <60%, or <10 valid measurements; $n = 6$] [17], 3) a history of hepatic decompensation or antiviral treatment ($n = 0$), 4) co-infection with hepatitis C, hepatitis D, or HIV ($n = 1$), 5) heavy alcohol consumption (>30 g/day for >5 years; $n = 4$), 6) right-sided heart failure, ascites, or pregnancy ($n = 0$), 7) F0–2 fibrosis stage on LB ($n = 20$), 8) low viral load (<2,000 IU/mL; $n = 7$), 9) LB specimen shorter than 15 mm ($n = 9$), and 10) follow-up loss ($n = 3$) (**Figure S1**).

A total of 50 patients were excluded; the remaining 128 CHB patients showing advanced (≥F3) liver fibrosis on LB with a high viral load (HBV DNA ≥2,000 IU/L) were selected for the final statistical analysis (**Figure S1**).

Laboratory tests

On the same day as LB and LSM, blood parameters including serum albumin, total bilirubin, alanine aminotransferase (ALT), prothrombin time, platelet count, and alpha-fetoprotein (AFP) were recorded. HBsAg and hepatitis B e antigen (HBeAg) were measured using standard enzyme-linked immunosorbent assays (Abbott Diagnostics, Abbott Park, IL, USA). HBV DNA levels were measured by quantitative PCR assay (Amplicor HBV Monitor Test; Roche Diagnostics, Basel, Switzerland) with a detection limit of 12 IU/mL. The upper normal range of ALT was 40 IU/L.

Liver stiffness measurement

On the same day as LB, LSM was performed on the right lobe of the liver through the intercostal spaces on patients lying in the dorsal decubitus position with the right arm in maximal abduction [17]. One experienced technician (>10,000 examinations) who was blinded to the patients' clinical data performed all LSMs. The

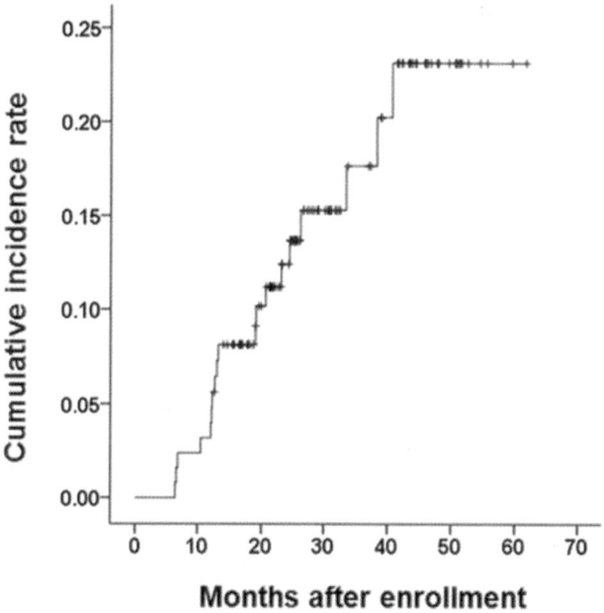

Figure 1. The cumulative incidence rates of LREs (Kaplan-Meier plot). The cumulative incidence rates of LREs at 1, 2, and 3 years were 3.1%, 11.7%, and 16.2%, respectively. LRE, liver-related event.

success rate was calculated by dividing the number of valid measurements by the total number of measurements. IQR was defined as an index of intrinsic variability of LSM corresponding to the interval of LSM results containing 50% of the valid measurements between the 25th and 75th percentiles [14]. LSM scores are expressed as kilopascals (kPa). When LSM showed an IQR/M >0.3, success rate <60%, or <10 valid measurements, it was regarded as invalid and was excluded from the final analysis.

Liver biopsy and liver histology evaluation

LB specimens were fixed in formalin and embedded in paraffin. Four-micrometer-thick sections were stained with hematoxylin & eosin and Masson's trichrome. All liver tissue samples were evaluated by an experienced hepatopathologist who was blinded to the clinical data of the study population, including LSM results. Liver fibrosis and necroinflammation were evaluated semiquantitatively according to the Batts scoring system [18]. Fibrosis was staged on a 0–4 scale: F0, no fibrosis; F1, portal fibrosis; F2, periportal fibrosis; F3, septal fibrosis; and F4, cirrhosis. The activity grade referred to the degree of hepatocellular necroinflammatory activity: A0, no activity; A1, minimal; A2, mild; A3, moderate; and A4, severe activity. Steatosis in the liver specimen was graded on a four-point scale: S0 (non-significant, <5%), S1 (mild, 5–33%), S2 (moderate, 34–66%) and S3 (severe, ≥66% of hepatocytes with fat deposits) [19]. LB specimens shorter than 15 mm were considered ineligible and excluded from the final analysis. The median length of LB specimens was 17 mm (range, 15–23 mm).

Follow up

All patients underwent LB and LSM and were screened ultrasonographically for HCC at their initial visit. NUCs, such as lamivudine and entecavir, were chosen non-randomly after enrollment according to the patient's economic status and physicians' judgment, and an HCC surveillance program was initiated in all patients. Patients were followed up with AFP and ultrasonography every 3 or 6 months. Furthermore, patients were assessed at baseline and every 3 months thereafter for clinical evidence of hepatic decompensation, including variceal bleeding, ascites, hepatic encephalopathy (HE), spontaneous bacterial

Table 2. Comparison Between Patients with and without LRE Development.

Variables	Patients with LRE development (n = 19, 14.8%)	Patients without LRE development (n = 109, 85.2%)	*P* value
Demographic data			
Age (years)	56.2±6.5	51.5±9.6	0.043
Male	12 (63.2)	60 (55.0)	0.511
Diabetes mellitus	3 (15.8)	8 (7.3)	0.210
Body mass index (kg/m^2)	24.1±2.9	23.9±2.9	0.794
HBeAg positivity	12 (63.2)	58 (53.2)	0.422
HBV DNA (log_{10} IU/mL)	5.7±1.1	5.6±1.2	0.610
Laboratory data			
Serum albumin (g/dL)	3.9±0.6	4.3±0.4	0.003
Total bilirubin (mg/dL)	0.9±0.3	0.8±0.3	0.181
Alanine aminotransferase (IU/L)	39.4±16.0	45.3±22.4	0.279
Prothrombin time (%)	85.1±12.7	91.9±9.0	0.037
Platelet count (10^9/L)	124.7±37.4	152.7±49.0	0.019
Alpha-fetoprotein (ng/mL)	6.7 (2.4–38.2)	4.4 (0.8–50.6)	0.020
Histological data			
Fibrosis stage, 3/4	4 (21.1)/15 (78.9)	14 (12.8)/95 (87.2)	0.342
Activity grade, 1–2/3–4	12 (63.2)/7 (36.8)	85 (78.0)/24 (22.0)	0.164
Liver stiffness measurement			
LSM values (kPa)	21.1 (7.8–57.1)	11.8 (4.4–48.0)	0.011
Antiviral treatment			
Antiviral agent			0.515
Lamivudine	6 (31.6)	43 (39.4)	
Entecavir	13 (68.4)	66 (60.6)	
HBV DNA negativity			
At 3 months	10 (52.6)	67 (61.5)	0.468
At 6 months	13 (68.4)	80 (73.4)	0.654
At 12 months	15 (78.9)	92 (84.4)	0.515
YMDD mutation	2(10.5)	15(13.8)	1.000

Variables are expressed as mean ± SD, median (range), or n (%).
LRE, liver-related event; HBeAg, hepatitis B e antigen; LSM, liver stiffness measurement; kPa, kilopascal.

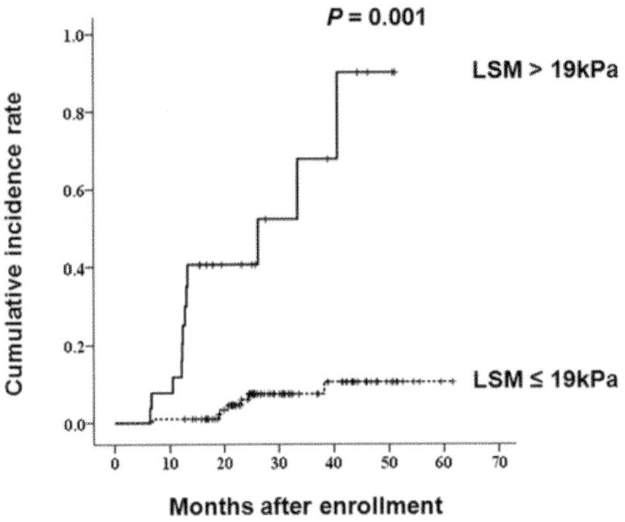

Figure 2. Cumulative incidence rates of LREs based on stratified LSM values (Kaplan-Meier plot). Patients with LSM value >19 kPa were at a significantly greater risk of LREs development with a hazard ratio of 7.176 [95% confidence interval, 2.257–22.812; P=0.001], as compared to those with LSM value ≤19 kPa. LSM, liver stiffness measurement; kPa, kilopascal. LRE, liver-related event.

peritonitis (SBP), and hepatorenal syndrome (HRS). At the end of the follow-up period (March 2011), one patient had died due to HCC and another had undergone liver transplantation after ascitic decompensation.

Primary endpoint

The primary endpoint was the development of LREs, including hepatic decompensation (variceal bleeding, ascites, HE, SBP, and HRS) and HCC.

Definition of hepatic decompensation

Variceal bleeding was diagnosed endoscopically if hemorrhage from the dilated veins in the distal esophagus or proximal stomach caused by elevated pressure in the portal venous system was noted [20]. Ascites was diagnosed by imaging, such as computed tomography (CT) or ultrasonography, if fluid collection within the abdominal cavity associated with cirrhosis was noted [21]. HE was diagnosed if confusion, altered level of consciousness, and coma developed as a result of liver failure, after the exclusion of known brain disease [22]. SBP was defined as an ascitic fluid infection without an intra-abdominal, surgically treatable source [23]. Diagnosis was established by a positive ascitic fluid bacterial culture and an elevated ascitic fluid absolute polymorphonuclear leukocyte count (≥250 cells/mm3). HRS was diagnosed when acute renal failure developed in association with advanced chronic liver disease, after the exclusion of other causes of renal failure [24].

Diagnosis of HCC

HCC was diagnosed based on the guidelines of the American Association for the Study of Liver Diseases (AASLD) [25]. Briefly, patients were diagnosed with HCC if they had a tumor with a maximum diameter >2 cm, features typical of HCC on dynamic CT (hyperattenuation in the arterial phase and early washout in the portal phase), and AFP >200 ng/mL. If the maximum diameter of the tumor was 1–2 cm, dynamic CT and magnetic resonance imaging were performed and HCC was diagnosed if coincidental typical features of HCC were noted. If the tumor did not satisfy the above criteria, a biopsy was performed. When the tumor was <1 cm, ultrasonographic examination was repeated after 3 months.

Statistical analyses

Data are expressed as the mean ± standard deviation (SD), median (range), or *n* (%), as appropriate. Baseline characteristics of patients with and without LRE development were compared using the chi-squared and Fisher's exact tests. To identify independent predictors of LRE development, univariate and subsequent multivariate Cox proportional hazard regression analyses were used. Hazard ratios (HRs) and corresponding 95% confidence intervals (CIs) are indicated. Time-dependent receiver operating characteristic (ROC) curves and areas under the ROC (AUROC) were used to calculate the optimal LSM cutoff value for the prediction of LRE development, which maximized the sum of sensitivity and specificity. The annual incidence rates of HCC were expressed in person-years. The cumulative incidence rates of HCC were calculated using the Kaplan–Meier method. A P value<0.05 on a two-tailed test was considered statistically significant. Statistical analyses were performed using SPSS software (ver. 18.0; SPSS Inc., Chicago, IL, USA).

Results

Baseline characteristics

The baseline characteristics of 128 patients at enrollment are summarized in **Table 1**. The mean age of the patients (72 men and 56 women) was 52.2 years. All patients with cirrhosis showed preserved liver function of Child–Pugh class A. The mean body mass index (BMI) and ALT were 24.0 kg/m^2 and 44.4 IU/L, respectively, and the median LSM value was 12.9 kPa.

F3 and F4 fibrosis stages were noted in 18 (14.1%) and 110 (85.9%) patients, respectively, and most patients (n = 97, 75.8%) had a necroinflammatory activity grade of 1–2 (**Table 1**). S0–1 steatosis was identified in 127 (99.2%) patients and S2 in one (0.8%), whereas none showed S3 steatosis.

LRE development and comparisons between patients with and without LREs

During the follow-up period [median, 27.8 (range, 12.6–61.6) months] constituting a total of 297 person-years, LREs developed in 19 (14.8%) patients (6.4/100 person-years; five cases with decompensation, 13 with HCC, and one with both decompensation and HCC; **Table 2**). The six cases of hepatic decompensation included variceal bleeding in two patients, ascites development in two, and HE in two. SBP and HRS did not develop during the follow-up period. The cumulative incidence rates of LREs at 1, 2, and 3 years were 3.1%, 11.7%, and 16.2%, respectively (**Figure 1**). The incidence rate of HCC and hepatic decompensation was 4.7/100 and 2.0/100 person-years, respectively.

When we compared the baseline characteristics of patients with and without LRE development, serum albumin, prothrombin time, and platelet count were significantly higher in patients without LREs, whereas age, AFP, and LSM values were significantly higher among those with LRE development (all P<0.05; **Table 2**). No significant difference was observed in the proportion of fibrosis stage, activity grade, or steatosis between patients with and without LRE development (all P>0.05; **Table 2**).

Table 3. Independent Risk Factors for LRE Development.

Variables	Univariate	Multivariate	
	P value	Hazard ratio (95% CI)	*P* value
Demographic data			
Age	0.045	1.083 (1.008–1.164)	0.030
Male	0.421		
Diabetes mellitus	0.192		
Body mass index	0.667		
Laboratory data			
Serum albumin	0.002	0.549 (0.168–1.794)	0.321
Total bilirubin	0.188		
Alanine aminotransferase	0.321		
Prothrombin time	0.005	0.979 (0.935–1.025)	0.363
Platelet count	0.015	0.996 (0.983–1.009)	0.581
Alpha-fetoprotein	0.041	0.984 (0.907–1.067)	0.694
HBeAg positivity	0.517		
HBV DNA	0.623		
HBV DNA negativity at 3 months	0.750		
Liver biopsy data			
Fibrosis stage, 3/4	0.352		
Activity grade, 1–2/3–4	0.208		
Liver stiffness measurement	<0.001	1.038 (1.002–1.081)	0.044
Antiviral treatment			
Lamivudine vs. entecavir	0.442		
HBV DNA negativity at 3 months	0.750		
HBV DNA negativity at 6 months	0.834		
HBV DNA negativity at 12 months	0.681		
YMDD mutation	0.522		

LRE, liver-related event; CI, confidence interval; ALT, alanine aminotransferase; HBeAg, hepatitis B e antigen; kPa, kilopascal.

Antiviral treatment

All patients received antiviral treatment with either lamivudine ($n=49$, 38.3%) or entecavir ($n=79$, 61.7%; **Table 1**). Baseline characteristics, including demographic, laboratory, and histologic data, did not differ between patients who received lamivudine and those who received entecavir (all $P>0.05$). Furthermore, the treatment period until the end of follow-up was similar (median 29.1 months for lamivudine *vs.* 27.2 months for entecavir; $P=0.785$). HBV DNA negativity at 3, 6, and 12 months of antiviral treatment, type of antiviral agent, and the development of the YMDD mutation did not influence LRE development (all $P>0.05$; **Table 2**).

Six (12.2%) of the 49 patients treated with lamivudine and 13 (16.5%) patients treated with entecavir developed LREs ($P=0.614$). During antiviral treatment, the YMDD mutation developed in 17 (13.3%) patients who received lamivudine after a median of 18.5 months; however, no genotypic antiviral resistance was identified in patients treated with entecavir. Of the 17 patients with the YMDD mutation, two experienced LRE development (HCC). Add-on treatment with adefovir was administered to all patients with the YMDD mutation.

Independent risk factors for LRE development

Together with age, multivariate analysis identified LSM as an independent predictor of LRE development ($P=0.044$; HR, 1.038; 95% CI, 1.002–1.081; **Table 3**). When we used a time-dependent ROC curve analysis to identify the optimal LSM cutoff values for stratifying our study population into two groups, 19 kPa showed the greatest accuracy (AUROC, 0.722; 95% CI, 0.582–0.864; $P=0.003$; sensitivity, 61.1%; specificity, 86.2%). Twenty-seven patients with LSM values >19 kPa were found to be at a significantly greater risk of LRE development (HR, 7.176; 95% CI, 2.257–22.812; $P=0.001$) in comparison with 101 patients with LSM values ≤19 kPa (**Figure 2**).

Incidence of LREs according to fibrosis stage and LSM values

The median LSM values of patients with F3 and F4 fibrosis stages were 9.0 (5.7–19.8) kPa and 14.1 (4.4–57.1) kPa, respectively. LSM values were significantly higher in patients with F4 fibrosis stage than in those with F3 (10.1±3.7 *vs.* 15.8±8.8 kPa; $P<0.001$; **Figure 3**).

The mean follow-up periods of patients with F3 and F4 fibrosis stages were similar (24.0 *vs.* 24.7 months; $P=0.827$). The incidence of LREs was similar in patients with F3 and F4 fibrosis stages (4/18, 22.2% *vs.* 15/110, 13.6%; $P=0.472$), whereas it

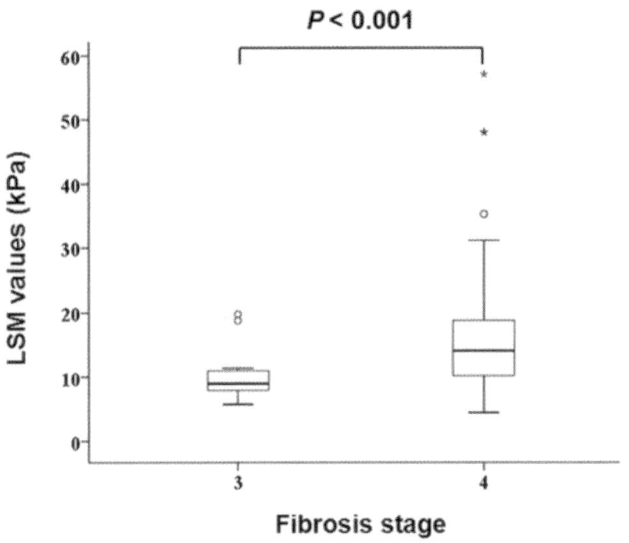

Figure 3. Box plots of LSM values in patients with F3 and F4 fibrosis stage. Median LSM value of patients with F3 and F4 were 9.0 (range, 5.7–19.8) kPa and 14.1 (range, 4.4–57.1) kPa, respectively and LSM values in patients with F4 fibrosis stage were significantly higher than those with F3 (10.1±3.7 *vs.* 15.8±8.8 kPa, $P<0.001$). LSM, liver stiffness measurement; kPa, kilopascal.

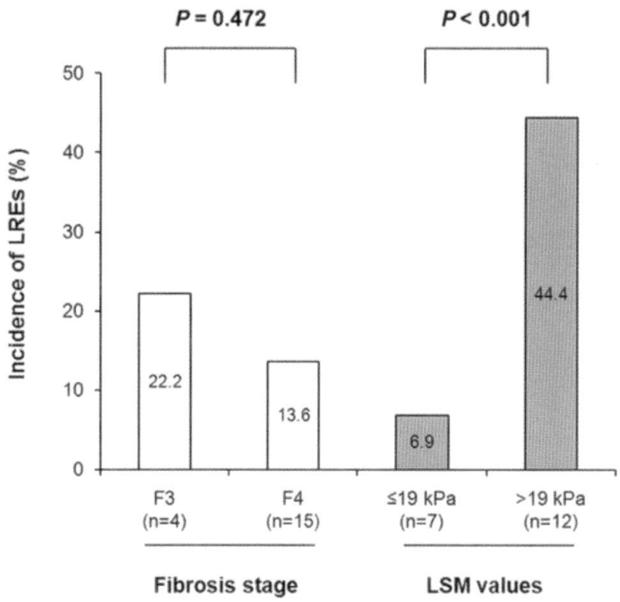

Figure 4. Incidence of LREs according to fibrosis stage and LSM values. The incidence of LREs was similar between patients with F3 fibrosis stage and those with F4 (22.2% *vs.* 13.6%, $P=0.472$) whereas it was signficanly different between patients with LSM value ≤19 kPa and those with LSM value >19 kPa (6.9% *vs.* 44.4%, $P<0.001$). LRE, liver-related event; LSM, liver stiffness measurement; kPa, kilopascal.

differed significantly between patients with LSM values ≤19 kPa and those with LSM values >19 kPa (7/101, 6.9% *vs.* 12/27, 44.4%; $P<0.001$; **Figure 4**).

Discordance between baseline LSM value and LRE development

As shown in **Figure 4**, discordant results between LSM values and LRE development were identified in 15/27 (55.6%) patients who did not experience LRE development despite baseline LSM values >19 kPa and 7/101 (6.9%) patients who developed LREs despite LSM values ≤19 kPa. However, no independent variable that could predict this discordance between LSM value and LRE development was identified.

Influence of dynamic LSM changes on LRE development

With the exception of 14 patients without follow-up LSMs before LRE development, 114 patients underwent a second LSM before LRE development at a median interval of 13.1 (range, 3.8–51.6) months. Of these, LREs developed in 10 (8.8%) patients.

To estimate the LRE incidence according to LSM change, we stratified the patients into three groups as follows: baseline and follow-up LSM values ≤19 kPa ($n=91$), baseline LSM >19 kPa and follow-up LSM ≤19 kPa ($n=11$), and any baseline and follow-up LSM values >19 kPa ($n=12$). The overall incidence of LRE development did not differ among groups ($P>0.05$). Although we further stratified the study population [LSM value increased by >30% of baseline LSM ($n=10$), change in LSM values ≤30% of baseline LSM ($n=70$), and LSM decreased by >30% of baseline LSM ($n=34$)] [26]. no difference in LRE development was identified ($P>0.05$).

Discussion

Advanced liver fibrosis or cirrhosis is significantly related to an increased risk of hepatic decompensation and HCC development, which, in turn, can worsen the prognosis of patients with CLD [27]. At a time when the natural course of chronic viral hepatitis could be observed due to the absence of antiviral agents, the incidence of HCC in highly endemic areas was approximately 1/100 person-years for CHB patients without cirrhosis [28,29]. Other Asian studies reported that the incidence of HCC in untreated patients with compensated cirrhosis increased to 3–8/100 person-years [30,31]. Moreover, the 5-year cumulative incidence of hepatic decompensation was reported as 16–20% (3.3–4/100 person-years) [32,33]. In our study, the incidence of HCC and hepatic decompensation seemed relatively low (4.7/100 and 2.0/100 person-years, respectively), which can be explained in part by the relative short follow-up period and the inclusion of patients with F3 fibrosis stages.

However, effective antiviral agents such as NUCs and interferon (IFN) have emerged and are actively used to prevent or delay disease progression in patients with chronic viral hepatitis [34–36]. Hence, the natural course of chronic viral hepatitis has changed and some recent studies have demonstrated improved prognosis in such patients. George *et al.* [37] concluded that CHB patients receiving NUCs had a significantly lower incidence of HCC compared with untreated controls (2.4% *vs.* 6.4%). The regression of liver fibrosis due to the long-term use of antiviral agents may explain the improved long-term prognosis [38,39]. However, because not all patients receiving antiviral treatment experience liver fibrosis regression [40], hepatic decompensation and HCC can eventually occur in some patients despite antiviral treatment.

Baseline HBV DNA level is the most important risk factor for HCC development without antiviral treatment [41]. However, we identified a significant predictive role for LSM with 19 kPa as an optimal cutoff value when appropriate suppression of HBV DNA using antiviral treatment was available. Similarly, Zakareya *et al.* identified a significant association between LSM and the development of cirrhosis-related complications in patients with CLD, and concluded that LSM values >32 kPa was associated with HCC development [42]. Because 19–32 kPa for predicting LRE development is much higher than the generally accepted cutoff LSM value for cirrhosis (10.3–11.0 kPa) [43,44], it can be postulated that cirrhosis can be further sub-classified, which indicates that all patients with cirrhosis do not have identical prognoses according to severity.

Because our study enrolled only patients with available histology before starting antiviral treatment, our results cannot be directly applied to patients who will receive antiviral treatment without baseline LBs. However, the purpose of this study was to evaluate the additional clinical implications of LSM value, when compared with histologic data as a reference standard, for CHB patients before starting antiviral treatment using NUCs. We demonstrated that LSM with an optimal cutoff value might be useful in assessing the risk of LRE development in these patients, which is impossible using histologic data alone. Thus, LSM is not only a noninvasive tool for the one-time evaluation of the degree of liver fibrosis, but also a significant predictor of LRE development, which should be checked before antiviral treatment regardless of LB data, in CHB patients. Our results also suggest that LSM is more useful than LB, and that the incidence of LREs could only be identified using LSM, not histologic data. Since LSM values perform better than histology, further studies investigating the predictive ability of LSM in patients undergoing antiviral treatment using NUCs without baseline LB data are needed.

In our study, there was a significant overlap in LSM values between patients with F3 (5.7–19.8 kPa) and F4 (4.4–57.1 kPa), although the overall LSM values were significantly higher in F4 fibrosis stage. This can be explained in part by the overestimating influence of necroinflammatory activity on LSM [45]. Indeed, the proportion of high activity (A3–4) in F3 showed a trend to be higher than those of F4 (35.0% vs. 26.9%). Furthermore, LSM values of patients with F3 and high activity (A3–4) was statistically similar with those of patients with F4 and low activity (A1–2) (mean 12.7 vs. 14.6 kPa, $P>0.05$). All these results might have caused some overlapping values between patients with F3 and F4.

The prediction of LRE development using LSM was imperfect. Although patients with baseline LSM values >19 kPa were at a significantly greater risk of LRE development (HR, 7.176) than were those with baseline LSM values ≤19 kPa, 55.6% of patients with LSM values >19 kPa developed no LRE and 6.9% of those with LSM values ≤19 kPa did. In the sub-group analysis, we found no significant predictor of discordant results regarding LRE development. Because this finding might be related to statistical error due to the short-term follow-up period and the low number of LREs, large-scale studies with long-term follow-up are needed to elucidate a novel serological predictor of LRE development. When we increased the sensitivity of cutoff LSM value up to 89.5%, 9.1 kPa was selected. Using this cutoff value, we can clinically identify the sub-group of patients at low risk of LRE development (1.6%), such that these patients can be reassured.

LSM has been known to predict fibrosis regression in response to long-term antiviral treatment [46]. Thus, we further analyzed the role of LSM as a dynamic indicator of LRE development using cutoff LSM values of 19 kPa or relative change in LSM values from baseline, but the results were negative. However, small sample size of some groups (n = 11 and 12, respectively) might be related to type II error. Furthermore, because the study by Jung *et al.* [14] revealed that LSM change, similar to baseline LSM value, can influence HCC development, large cohorts with sufficient events will likely be required to investigate the usefulness of serial LSM value follow-up in patients with chronic viral hepatitis.

We included only patients with histologically advanced liver fibrosis (≥F3). However, because histologic evaluation grades liver fibrosis categorically, it cannot exactly represent the continuous spectrum of liver fibrosis, especially between adjacent fibrosis grades. Furthermore, because histologic evaluation of liver fibrosis can be influenced by intra- and interobserver variability, the over- or underestimation of liver fibrosis inevitably occurs. Considering these limitations of histologic evaluation, some patients who were excluded due to F0–F2 liver fibrosis may represent underestimations of F3 or F4 fibrosis, which might have resulted in selection bias, a major limitation of this study. Thus, further validation of LSM cutoff values for predicting advanced liver fibrosis regardless of histologic data should be performed. Furthermore, the significantly higher proportion of patients with F4 fibrosis may be another bias of this study.

In conclusion, our data suggest that LSM can be a useful predictor of LRE development in CHB patients showing histologically advanced liver fibrosis. However, this finding should be confirmed in CHB patients without baseline histologic data before the widespread application of LSM to all patients undergoing antiviral treatment.

Acknowledgments

The authors are grateful to Dong-Su Jang, (Medical Illustrator, Medical Research Support Section, Yonsei University College of Medicine, Seoul, Korea) for his help with the figures.

Author Contributions

Conceived and designed the experiments: SUK JHL JYP. Analyzed the data: SUK JHL EHC JYP. Contributed reagents/materials/analysis tools: YNP. Wrote the paper: SUK JHL DYK SHA KHH CYC KSJ JYP.

References

1. Margolis HS, Alter MJ, Hadler SC (1991) Hepatitis B: evolving epidemiology and implications for control. Semin Liver Dis 11: 84–92.
2. WHO (1999) Global surveillance and control of hepatitis C. Report of a WHO Consultation organized in collaboration with the Viral Hepatitis Prevention Board, Antwerp, Belgium. J Viral Hepat 6: 35–47.
3. Di Marco V, Lo Iacono O, Camma C, Vaccaro A, Giunta M, et al. (1999) The long-term course of chronic hepatitis B. Hepatology 30: 257–264.
4. Ikeda K, Saitoh S, Suzuki Y, Kobayashi M, Tsubota A, et al. (1998) Disease progression and hepatocellular carcinogenesis in patients with chronic viral hepatitis: a prospective observation of 2215 patients. J Hepatology 28: 930–938.
5. Colombo M, de Franchis R, Del Ninno E, Sangiovanni A, Tommasini M, et al. (1991) Hepatocellular carcinoma in Italian patients with cirrhosis. N Engl J Med 325: 675–680.
6. Tanaka R, Itoshima T, Nagashima H (1987) Follow-up study of 582 liver cirrhosis patients for 26 years in Japan. Liver 7: 316–324.
7. Fattovich G, Giustina G, Schalm SW, Hadziyannis S, Sanchez-Tapias J, et al. (1995) Occurrence of hepatocellular carcinoma and decompensation in western European patients with cirrhosis type B. The EUROHEP Study Group on Hepatitis B Virus and Cirrhosis. Hepatology 21: 77–82.
8. Bravo AA, Sheth SG, Chopra S (2001) Liver biopsy. N Engl J Med 344: 495–500.

9. Regev A, Berho M, Jeffers LJ, Milikowski C, Molina EG, et al. (2002) Sampling error and intraobserver variation in liver biopsy in patients with chronic HCV infection. Am J Gastroenterol 97: 2614–2618.
10. Foucher J, Chanteloup E, Vergniol J, Castera L, Le Bali B, et al. (2006) Diagnosis of cirrhosis by transient elastography (FibroScan): a prospective study. Gut 55: 403–408.
11. Ganne-Carrie N, Ziol M, de Ledinghen V, Douvin C, Marcellin P, et al. (2006) Accuracy of liver stiffness measurement for the diagnosis of cirrhosis in patients with chronic liver diseases. Hepatology 44: 1511–1517.
12. Kazemi F, Kettaneh A, N'Kontchou G, Pinto E, Ganne-Carrie N, et al. (2006) Liver stiffness measurement selects patients with cirrhosis at risk of bearing large oesophageal varices. J Hepatology 45: 230–235.
13. Kim BK, Han KH, Park JY, Ahn SH, Kim JK, et al. (2010) A liver stiffness measurement-based, noninvasive prediction model for high-risk esophageal varices in B-viral liver cirrhosis. Am J Gastroenterology 105: 1382–1390.
14. Jung KS, Kim SU, Ahn SH, Park YN, Kim do Y, et al. (2011) Risk assessment of hepatitis B virus-related hepatocellular carcinoma development using liver stiffness measurement (FibroScan). Hepatology 53: 885–894.
15. Kim HS, Kim JK, Park YN, Nyung SM, Pang MS, et al. (2007) Non-invasive assessment of liver fibrosis by measuring the liver stiffness and biochemical markers in chronic hepatitis B patients. Korean J Med 72: 459–469.
16. Masuzaki R, Tateishi R, Yoshida H, Yoshida H, Sato S, et al. (2008) Risk assessment of hepatocellular carcinoma in chronic hepatitis C patients by transient elastography. J Clin Gastroenterol 42: 839–843.
17. Sandrin L, Fourquet B, Hasquenoph JM, Yon S, Fournier C, et al. (2003) Transient elastography: a new noninvasive method for assessment of hepatic fibrosis. Ultrasound Med Biol 29: 1705–1713.
18. Batts KP, Ludwig J (1995) Chronic hepatitis. An update on terminology and reporting. Am J Surg Pathol 19: 1409–1417.
19. Brunt EM, Janney CG, Di Bisceglie AM, Neuschwander-Tetri BA, Bacon BR (1999) Nonalcoholic steatohepatitis: a proposal for grading and staging the histological lesions. Am J Gastroenterology 94: 2467–2474.
20. Patch D, Dagher L (2001) Acute variceal bleeding: general management. World J Gastroenterol 7: 466–475.
21. Moore KP, Aithal GP (2006) Guidelines on the management of ascites in cirrhosis. Gut 55 Suppl 6: vi1–12.
22. Prakash R, Mullen KD (2010) Mechanisms, diagnosis and management of hepatic encephalopathy. Nat Rev Gastroenterol Hepatol 7: 515–525.
23. Such J, Runyon BA (1998) Spontaneous bacterial peritonitis. Clin Infect Dis 27:669–674; quiz 675–6.
24. Gines P, Arroyo V (1999) Hepatorenal syndrome. J Am Soc Nephrol 10: 1833–1839.
25. Bruix J, Sherman M (2005) Management of hepatocellular carcinoma. Hepatology 42: 1208–1236.
26. Wong GL, Wong VW, Choi PC, Chan AW, Chim AM, et al. (2011) On-treatment monitoring of liver fibrosis with transient elastography in chronic hepatitis B patients. Antiviral ther 16: 165–172.
27. Min AD, Dienstag JL (2007) Oral antivirals for chronic hepatitis B. Clin Liver Dis 11:851–868, ix.
28. Lin SM, Sheen IS, Chien RN, Chu CM, Liaw YF (1999) Long-term beneficial effect of interferon therapy in patients with chronic hepatitis B virus infection. Hepatology 29: 971–975.
29. Liaw YF, Tai DI, Chu CM, Lin DY, Sheen IS, et al. (1986) Early detection of hepatocellular carcinoma in patients with chronic type B hepatitis. A prospective study. Gastroenterology 90: 263–267.
30. Kato Y, Nakata K, Omagari K, Furukawa R, Kusumoto Y, et al. (1994) Risk of hepatocellular carcinoma in patients with cirrhosis in Japan. Analysis of infectious hepatitis viruses. Cancer 74: 2234–2238.
31. Oon CJ (1992) Long-term survival following treatment of hepatocellular carcinoma in Singapore: evaluation of Wellferon in the prophylaxis of high-risk pre-cancerous conditions. Cancer Chemother Pharmacol 31 Suppl. pp S137–142.
32. Fattovich G, Pantalena M, Zagni I, Realdi G, Schalm SW, et al. (2002) Effect of hepatitis B and C virus infections on the natural history of compensated cirrhosis: a cohort study of 297 patients. Am J Gastroenterology 97: 2886–2895.
33. Liaw YF, Lin DY, Chen TJ, Chu CM (1989) Natural course after the development of cirrhosis in patients with chronic type B hepatitis: a prospective study. Liver 9: 235–241.
34. Sobesky R, Mathurin P, Charlotte F, Moussalli J, Olivi M, et al. (1999) Modeling the impact of interferon alfa treatment on liver fibrosis progression in chronic hepatitis C: a dynamic view. The Multivirc Group. Gastroenterology 116: 378–386.
35. Mazzella G, Accogli E, Sottili S, Festi D, Orsini M, et al. (1996) Alpha interferon treatment may prevent hepatocellular carcinoma in HCV-related liver cirrhosis. J Hepatol 24: 141–147.
36. Suzuki Y, Kumada H, Ikeda K, Chayama K, Arase Y, et al. (1999) Histological changes in liver biopsies after one year of lamivudine treatment in patients with chronic hepatitis B infection. J Hepatol 30: 743–748.
37. Papatheodoridis GV, Lampertico P, Manolakopoulos S, Lok A (2010) Incidence of hepatocellular carcinoma in chronic hepatitis B patients receiving nucleos(-t)ide therapy: a systematic review. J Hepatol 53: 348–356.
38. Liaw YF, Sung JJ, Chow WC, Farrell G, Lee CZ, et al. (2004) Lamivudine for patients with chronic hepatitis B and advanced liver disease. N Eng J Med 351: 1521–1531.
39. Fung SK, Lok AS (2005) Management of patients with hepatitis B virus-induced cirrhosis. J Hepatol 42 Suppl. pp S54–64.
40. Dienstag JL, Goldin RD, Heathcote EJ, Hann HW, Woessner M, et al. (2003) Histological outcome during long-term lamivudine therapy. Gastroenterology 124: 105–117.
41. Chen CJ, Yang HI, Su J, Jen CL, You SL, et al. (2006) Risk of hepatocellular carcinoma across a biological gradient of serum hepatitis B virus DNA level. JAMA 295: 65–73.
42. Zakareya T, Razek WA, Allam N, Gabal AA, Rewisha E, et al. (2010) The utility of transient elastography in predicting complications of chronic liver disease. Nile Liver J 1: 49–57.
43. Kim do Y, Kim SU, Ahn SH, Park JY, Lee JM, et al. (2009) Usefulness of FibroScan for detection of early compensated liver cirrhosis in chronic hepatitis B. Dig Dis Sci 54: 1758–1763.
44. Marcellin P, Ziol M, Bedossa P, Douvin C, Poupon R, et al. (2009) Non-invasive assessment of liver fibrosis by stiffness measurement in patients with chronic hepatitis B. Liver Int 29: 242–247.
45. Kim SU, Kim JK, Park YN, Han KH (2012) Discordance between liver biopsy and FibroScan® in assessing liver fibrosis in chronic hepatitis B: Risk factors and influence of necroinflammation. PLoS One 7: e322233.
46. Kim SU, Park JY, Kim do Y, Ahn SH, Kim HM, et al. (2010) Non-invasive assessment of changes in liver fibrosis via liver stiffness measurement in patients with chronic hepatitis B: impact of antiviral treatment on fibrosis regression. Hepatol Int 4: 673–680.

4

Cytokinome Profile of Patients with Type 2 Diabetes and/or Chronic Hepatitis C Infection

Susan Costantini[1]*, Francesca Capone[1], Eliana Guerriero[1], Raffaele Marfella[2], Angela Sorice[1], Patrizia Maio[3], Michele Di Stasio[4], Giuseppe Paolisso[2], Giuseppe Castello[1], Giovanni Colonna[5]

1 INT "G. Pascale" - Oncology Research Centre of Mercogliano, Mercogliano, Italy, **2** Department of Geriatrics and Metabolic Diseases, Second University of Naples, Naples, Italy, **3** Unità Operativa Malattie Infettive, Azienda Ospedaliera di Rilievo Nazionale "San Giuseppe Moscati", Avellino, Italy, **4** Institute of Food Science - CNR, Avellino, Italy, **5** Department of Biochemistry and Biophysics and Interdepartmental Research Center for Computational and Biotechnological Sciences, Second University of Naples, Naples, Italy

Abstract

Both type 2 diabetes (T2D) and chronic hepatitis C (CHC) infection are associated with increased risk of developing hepatocellular carcinoma (HCC). Cytokines are known to play an important role not only in the mechanisms of insulin resistance and glucose disposal defects but also in the pathological processes occurring in the liver during viral infection. We evaluated the serum levels of many cytokines, chemokines, adipokines and growth factors in patients with type 2 diabetes, CHC, CHC-related cirrhosis, CHC and type 2 diabetes and CHC-related cirrhosis and type 2 diabetes by BioPlex assay. The obtained data evidenced that the serum levels of some proteins are significantly up-regulated in all the patients or in those with only one disease and are often higher, even if in different amounts, when both diseases are associated. In particular, our results can be useful for the clinical monitoring of patients because they give specific information in regard to the progression from CHC to LC and CHD to LCD. Moreover, some molecules have shown significant correlations with clinical/biochemical data, suggesting the possibility to define mini-panels that can be used as specific markers for the different disease staging. However, our observations demonstrate that an integrated approach is much more powerful than isolated measurements to evaluate specific stages of these two complex pathologies (type 2 diabetes and chronic CHC hepatitis) alone or when they are concomitant in a patient. In fact it has emerged as an accurate, simple, specific, noninvasive, reproducible and less expensive method that, in future, could be included in routine clinical practice to monitor the association of type 2 diabetes and/or CHC to liver cirrhosis and, possibly, to cancer, and to improve the prognosis of these diseases.

Editor: Patricia Fitzgerald-Bocarsly, University of Medicine and Dentistry of New Jersey - New Jersey Medical School, United States of America

Funding: The authors have no funding or support to report.

Competing Interests: The authors have declared that no competing interests exist.

* E-mail: susan.costantini@unina2.it

Introduction

Recent epidemiological studies suggest that profound alterations in glucose homeostasis, as occurs in type 2 diabetes mellitus or metabolic syndrome, increase the risk of fatty liver disease as well as of hepatocellular carcinoma (HCC) [1]. In fact, many clinical and experimental data have demonstrated that type 2 diabetes is more common among patients with chronic hepatitis C virus than in those with hepatitis B virus or in the general population [2–4] and that CHC infection is associated with increased risk of developing insulin resistance and its major late feature, type 2 diabetes [5–6].

In general, CHC infection itself also increases the risk of HCC, leading to complications such as chronic hepatitis, hepatocellular necrosis and inflammation, fibrosis, cirrhosis and HCC. For patients with CHC-related cirrhosis the risk for development of HCC is 0.54 to 2.0% per year [7].

Recently type 2 diabetes has been recognized as a cofactor that can modify the course of CHC infection and can be used as an independent predictor of HCC. Recent studies have shown that type 2 diabetes was associated with hepatocarcinogenesis in patients with CHC infection without liver cirrhosis [8–9]. Therefore, there has been a great interest in the search of possible specific immunological markers able to follow the progression of CHC to cirrhosis and HCC also in association with type 2 diabetes.

It is well known that cytokines and chemokines are signaling molecules involved in the inflammatory as well as in cancer-related processes [10]. Hence, understanding in patients affected from cancers the dynamics of the complex interaction network of cytokines [11], defined "cytokinome" [12], should be very useful to follow the disease progression and evolution from its early stages as well as to define therapeutic strategies by using systems biology approaches [11]. However, many data on cytokines have been reported in the literature and sometimes their correlation appears to be difficult. In fact, in the most part of these papers, the researchers have evaluated only few cytokines by single measurements and, therefore, both the global inflammation mechanism and the cytokine relationships are understandable with difficulty [12–13].

In our approach, the serum levels of a panel of numerous cytokines, chemokines, adipokines and growth factors were evaluated at the same time by BioPlex assay in patients with chronic hepatitis C (CHC), CHC-related cirrhosis (LC), type 2 diabetes (T2D), CHC hepatitis and type 2 diabetes (CHD), CHC-related cirrhosis and type 2 diabetes (LCD) and in healthy controls, to identify those molecules that might be useful for discriminating the various stages of these diseases. In other hands, the simultaneous quantitative determination of a large panel of cytokines, able to report the correct ratios and dynamics between highly and poorly represented molecules, has emerged as an accurate, simple, specific, noninvasive, reproducible and less expensive method that, in future, could be included in routine clinical practice to monitor the association of type 2 diabetes and/or CHC to liver cirrhosis and, possibly, to cancer, and to improve the prognosis of these diseases.

Materials and Methods

Patients

In this study we enrolled seventeen patients (6 women, 11 men) with type 2 diabetes (T2D), twenty patients (11 women, 9 men) with CHC, twenty patients (12 women, 8 men) with LC, ten patients (4 women, 6 men) with CHD, ten patients (4 women, 6 men) with LCD, and 20 healthy control subjects (11 women, 9 men). In Table 1 we report the clinical characteristics of all patients. This choice depended from our interest to study the association of chronic liver damage leading to cirrhosis in presence or absence of type 2 diabetes. The ADA criteria were used to classify patients with the type 2 diabetes [14]: i) fasting plasma glucose 126 mg/dl (7.0 mmol/l) where fasting is defined as no caloric intake for at least 8 h or ii) symptoms of hyperglycemia and a casual plasma glucose 200 mg/dl (11.1 mmol/l) where casual is defined as any time of day without regard to time since last meal whereas the classic symptoms of hyperglycemia include polyuria, polydipsia, and unexplained weight loss, or iii) 2-h plasma glucose 200 mg/dl (11.1 mmol/l) during an OGTT where the test has been performed as described by the World Health Organization, using a glucose load containing the equivalent of 75 g anhydrous glucose dissolved in water.

Moreover, the cirrhosis was defined by clinical diagnosis in presence of liver functional insufficiency (Child Pügh = B and C) or by liver biopsies in the case of initial chronic hepatopathy without clear liver laboratoristic function tests of cirrhotic evolution (Child Pügh = A). All patients with CHC, LC, CHD and LCD had transaminase values (AST and ALT) higher than control range, evaluated in healthy donors. Moreover, liver cirrhosis patients presented higher birilubin values and lower albumin and platelets count (PLT) respect to control range. Both CHD and LCD had hyperglycemia. All patients had normal alpha-fetoprotein (AFP) values and did not present cancer. The patients with T2D, CHD and LCD were overweight with BMI values in the range between 25–29 kg/m^2 whereas those with only CHC and LC have BMI of about 25 kg/m^2. The smoking status was known only for T2D patients.

For this study we obtained ethics approval from the ethics committee at our institution (INT "G. Pascale" – CROM) and obtained written informed consent from all involved participants.

BioPlex Assay

Blood samples were collected from a peripheral vein and kept on ice. Serum was collected by centrifugation (3,000 rpm for 10 min at 4°C), aliquoted, and stored at −80°C until analyzed. A multiplex biometric ELISA-based immunoassay, containing dyed microspheres conjugated with a monoclonal antibody specific for a target protein was used according to the manufacturer's instructions (Bioplex, Bio-Rad Lab., Inc., Hercules, CA, USA). Soluble molecules were measured using three commercially available kits: i) 21-Plex panel: IL-1α, IL-2R, IL-3, IL-12p40, IL-16, IL-18, CCL27, CXCL1, CXCL9, CXCL12, HGF, IFN-α2, LIF, MCP-3, M-CSF, MIF, β-NGF, SCF, SCGF-β, TNF-β, TRAIL; ii) 10-Plex panel: C-peptide, ghrelin, GIP, glp-1, glucagon, insulin, leptin, PAI-1, resistin, visfatin and iii) 2-Plex panel: adiponectin and adipsin.

Each experiment was performed in duplicate using the same procedure described in our recent papers [10,13]. Serum levels of all proteins were determined using a Bio-Plex array reader (Luminex, Austin, TX) that quantifies multiplex immunoassays in a 96-well plate with very small fluid volumes. The analytes concentration was calculated using a standard curve, with software provided by the manufacturer (Bio-Plex Manager Software).

Data Analysis and Statistics

The nonparametric Mann-Whitney U test was used to evaluate differences between cytokine, chemokine and growth factor ratios in the patients and healthy controls. In particular $p<0.05$ is indicated with *, $p<0.01$ with **, and $p<0.001$ with ***. T-test was used to compare the serum levels of these proteins evaluated in different patients groups. The correlations between the cytokine levels and clinical/biochemical data were determined using the Pearson correlation coefficient. Values of $p<0.05$ were considered to be statistically significant. Multivariate logistic regression analysis was performed to evaluate associations between levels of significant cytokines/adipokines and smoking status, hypertension, BMI, and hypercholesterolemia. Odds ratios (OR) and 95% confidence intervals (95% CI) for association between each cytokine and four parameters were estimated using unconditional logistic regression models. In details, OR represent a measure of the strength of association between variables and, when OR is greater then 1, it indicates that the association is significant. The statistical programs Prism 4 (GraphPad Software, San Diego, CA, USA) and MedCalc (MedCalc software, Mariakerke, Belgium) were employed.

Results

Comparison between Patients with Type 2 Diabetes and Healthy Donors

In Figures 1–2 and in Table 2 we report the proteins that show different serum levels in the type 2 diabetes (T2D) patients respect to controls; data that were not statistically significant are not reported. Greater amounts of IL-1α, IL-2R, IL-12, IL-18, HGF, MIF, glucagon, insulin, leptin, PAI-1, resistin and adipsin and lower of ghrelin were secreted by T2D patients. The significantly increased serum levels of four pro-inflammatory interleukins (IL-1α, IL-2R, IL-12 and IL-18) are in agreement with already published data [15–16] that showed and confirmed how the inflammation course is more severe in diabetic patients than in non-diabetic subjects. Elevated HGF and MIF levels were indicated as markers of atherosclerotic and cardiomyopathic complications in T2D patients, respectively [17–18]. On the other hand, the increased levels of leptin, insulin, resistin and adipsin and the decreased levels of ghrelin are certainly correlated between them because adipsin is activated by insulin, whereas ghrelin and leptin exert antagonistic effects via their specific receptors. In fact, in hepatocytes ghrelin reduces and leptin augments insulin signal transduction [19]. Also, it has recently shown that the levels of resistin are correlated to those of leptin and that both these adipokines induce increased procoagulability in diabetes mellitus [20,21]. Certainly, the elevated concentrations of glucagon in T2D patients depend from its role in dysregulated

Table 1. Biochemical characteristics of all patients.

	T2D	CHC	CHD	LC	LCD	Control range
Age	61,8	62,54	65,2	70	71,8	60,92
Gender	11M/6F	10M-10F	7M-3F	8M-12F	5M-5F	9M-11F
Hypertension	17	10	3	11	3	
Hypercholesterolemia	17	5	6	5	7	
Cigarette smoking	12	n.d.	n.d.	n.d.	n.d.	
BMI (kg/m^2)	27,4±1	24,2±0,9	28,1±1,2	24,4±0,8	27,9±1,4	<25
Total cholesterol (mg/dL)	192±21	170±5,8	181±4,6	182±7,2	200±2,1	130–200
Triglycerides (mg/dL)	179±21	98±23	111±35	105±27	117±36	40–165
AST (IU/L)	31±4	71,43±2,3	66,4±4,5	81,25	112,1	5–40
ALT (IU/L)	33±6	121,1	104	71,96	106,7	7–56
TotBilirubin (mg/dL)	1,01±0,06	0,94	1,03	1,72	1,58	0,20–1,30
Albumin (g/dL)	4,2±0,9	4,01	4,44	2,61	3,4	3,5–5
PLT (mL)	198464±10221	187413	162000	113875	114833	150000–400000
CHC – PCR RNA	negative	positive	positive	positive	positive	
CHC genot	negative	1:11; 2:9	1:6; 2:4	1:12; 2:8	1:7; 2:3	
Glycemia (mg/dL)	145,9±12,3	86	139,2	88,3	132,5	70–105
Creatinine (mg/dL)	0,9±0,01	0,9	0,8	1	1,1	0,6–1,36
AFP (ng/mL)	<10	<10	<10	<20	<20	
Child Pügh				A:8; B:7;C:5	A:3; B3;C:4	

§n.d. = not detected.
We report the number of patients to which some parameters refer. For clinical data the mean value and the related control range, evaluated in healthy donors, are shown.

hepatic glucose production and abnormal glucose homeostasis [22]. Finally, since the platelet function is enhanced in T2D patients, the increased levels of PAI-1 (plasminogen activator inhibitor type 1) are considered to be a risk factor of cardiovascular diseases in these patients [23]. Since smoking status was known for T2D patients, we have subdivided them in two different subgroups, i.e. smokers and not smokers, and compared their cytokine levels to understand what proteins were related to cigarette smoking. The analysis showed that there were no statistically significant differences for the cytokines between the two subgroups of patients.

Then, we have correlated the serum levels of all the significant proteins in T2D patients with clinical/biochemical data by Pearson correlation coefficient (Table 3). In these patients, IL-18, resistin and MIF showed a significant correlation with BMI and glycemia levels (see Table 2). This result confirms these three proteins can be considered as predictors of inflammatory activation during the progression of T2D, as recently reported [21].

Comparison between Patients with Chronic CHC Hepatitis and Healthy Donors

In CHC patients greater amounts of IL-1α, IL-2R, IL-12, IL-18, CXCL1, CXCL9, MIF, β-NGF, C-peptide, GIP, insulin, leptin, PAI-1, resistin, adiponectin and adipsin and lower of ghrelin were secreted with respect to healthy controls (Figures 1–2 and Table 2).

The increased serum levels of IL-1α, IL-2R, CXCL1, CXCL9, MIF and β-NGF agree with our recently published data [13] since they are all pro-inflammatory cytokines involved in the immune response to CHC and drive liver damage. Moreover, during inflammation both IL-12 and IL-18 are produced by macrophages, work together in inducing cell-mediated immunity and stimulate the production of CXCL9 [24].

Also in literature, increased levels of leptin, resistin and adiponectin as well as of PAI-1 have been found in CHC patients and they have been correlated to the severity of fibrosis and, hence, indicated as marker in detecting HCC when the carcinogenesis is affected by CHC infection [25–26].

In general, C-peptide serves as an important link between the insulin chains and facilitates the efficient assembly, the folding and the processing of insulin in the endoplasmic reticulum. Higher C-peptide and insulin levels in CHC patients were already reported supporting the hypothesis that insulin resistance may contribute to fibrotic progression in CHC infection [5]. The secretion of adipsin, as reported above, is activated by insulin [19] whereas GIP (called gastrointestinal inhibitory peptide) induces insulin secretion [27]. Hence the increased levels of GIP, adipsin and insulin as well as of leptin, that augments insulin signal transduction, are mainly correlated not only between them but also with the decreased levels of ghrelin that has been indicated as marker of the liver fibrosis progression [19].

However, no data have been found in literature related to GIP and adipsin evaluations in CHC patients and our integrated analysis suggests, for the first time, a role for GIP and adipsin in CHC-related chronic inflammation.

From the correlation of the serum levels of all the significant proteins in CHC group with clinical/biochemical data, it is resulted that IL-2R, MIF and β-NGF showed a positive correlation coefficient with the transaminase values (Table 3), which were higher in these patients than in healthy controls. This confirms the role of these proteins as index of immune activation according to our recently published data [13].

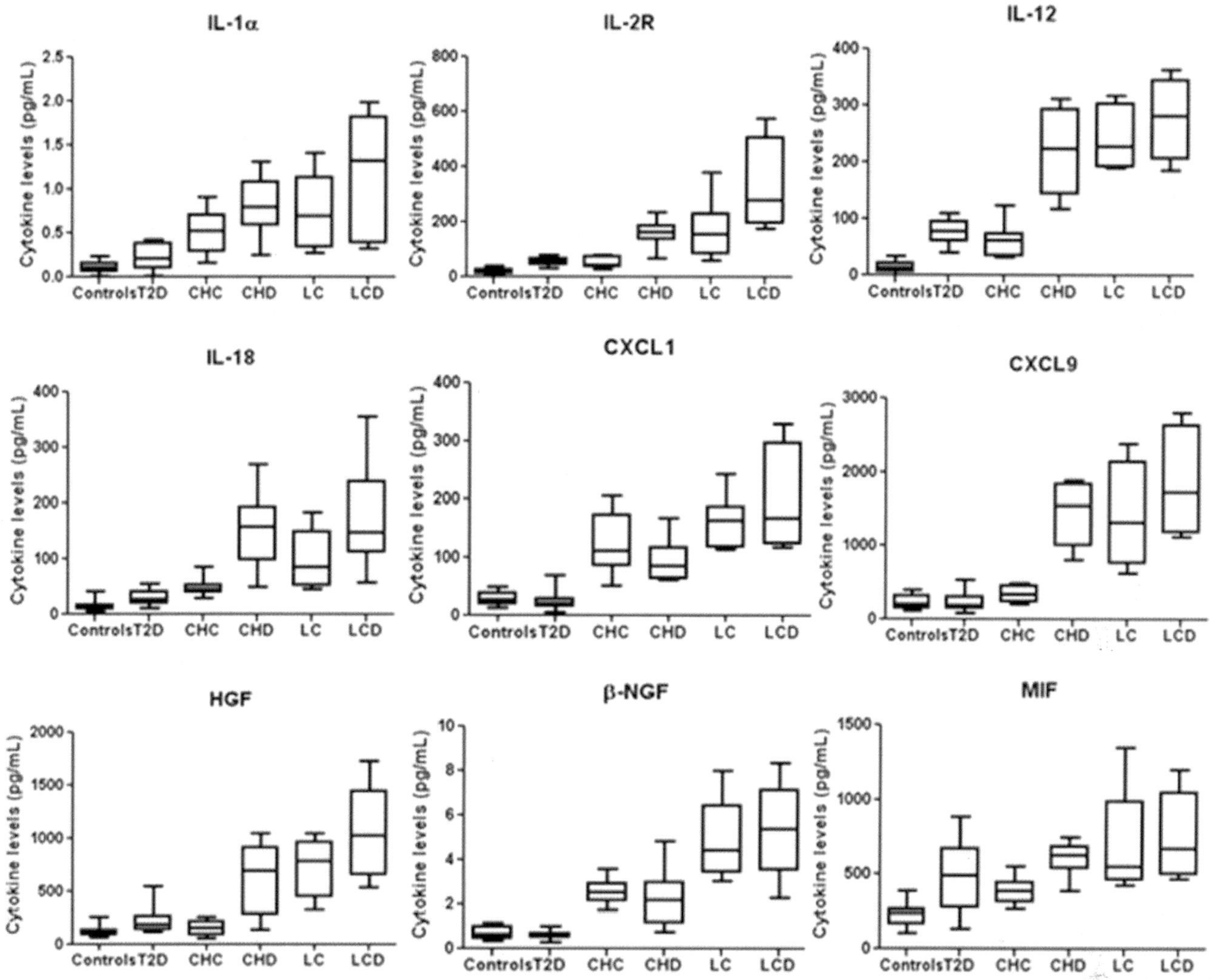

Figure 1. Significant cytokines in some patient groups. We report the significant molecule levels from controls and patients with type 2 diabetes (T2D), chronic hepatitis C (CHC), CHC-related cirrhosis (LC), CHC hepatitis and type 2 diabetes (CHD) and CHC-related cirrhosis and type 2 diabetes (LCD), evaluated by 21-Plex panel, are plotted with box-and-whisker graphs. The boxes extend from the 25th to the 75th percentile, and the line in the middle is the median. The error bars extend down to the lowest value and up to the highest.

Comparison between Patients with Type 2 Diabetes and those with Chronic CHC Hepatitis

In both T2D and CHC patients, IL-1α, IL-2R, IL-12, IL-18, MIF, insulin, leptin, PAI-1, resistin and adipsin are increased whereas ghrelin is decreased with respect to healthy controls (Table 2 and Figures 1–2). We used T-test to compare the serum levels of these proteins evaluated in different patients groups. In particular, IL-2R, IL-12, IL-18, MIF, resistin and adipsin have similar concentrations in both diseases. In CHC patients ghrelin and leptin levels are lower than those with T2D (with p-value <0.05) whereas IL-1α, insulin and PAI-1 levels are higher (with p-value <0.05).

Moreover, CXCL1, CXCL9, β-NGF, C-peptide, GIP and adiponectin are higher only in CHC patients in agreement with previous studies in which these molecules were found elevated only in diabetic patients with complications (nephropathy, retinopathy and atherosclerotic lesions) [28–32].

On the other hand, HGF and glucagon are higher only in T2D patients and this confirms that glucagon and HGF play a specific role in glucose production and homeostasis [23] and in the progression of chronic inflammation to liver cirrhosis and cancer [13], respectively.

Patients with Chronic CHC Hepatitis and Type 2 Diabetes (CHD)

In CHD patients greater amounts of IL-1α, IL-2R, IL-12, IL-18, CXCL1, CXCL9, HGF, MIF, β-NGF, C-peptide, GIP, glucagon, insulin, leptin, PAI-1, resistin, adiponectin and adipsin and lower of ghrelin were secreted than in healthy controls (Figures 1–2 and Table 2). Since in CHD patients there are increased levels of the same molecules resulted significant in type 2 diabetes and/or CHC patients, we compared by T-test the serum concentrations in CHD patients and those evaluated in patients having only type 2 diabetes or CHC to understand what cytokines change or unchange in presence of both diseases.

The levels of MIF, insulin, ghrelin, leptin, glucagon, resistin and adipsin are similar in type 2 diabetes and CHD patients whereas IL-1α, IL-2R, IL-12, IL-18, HGF, and PAI-1 are higher in CHD patients than in type 2 diabetes patients (with p-value <0.01).

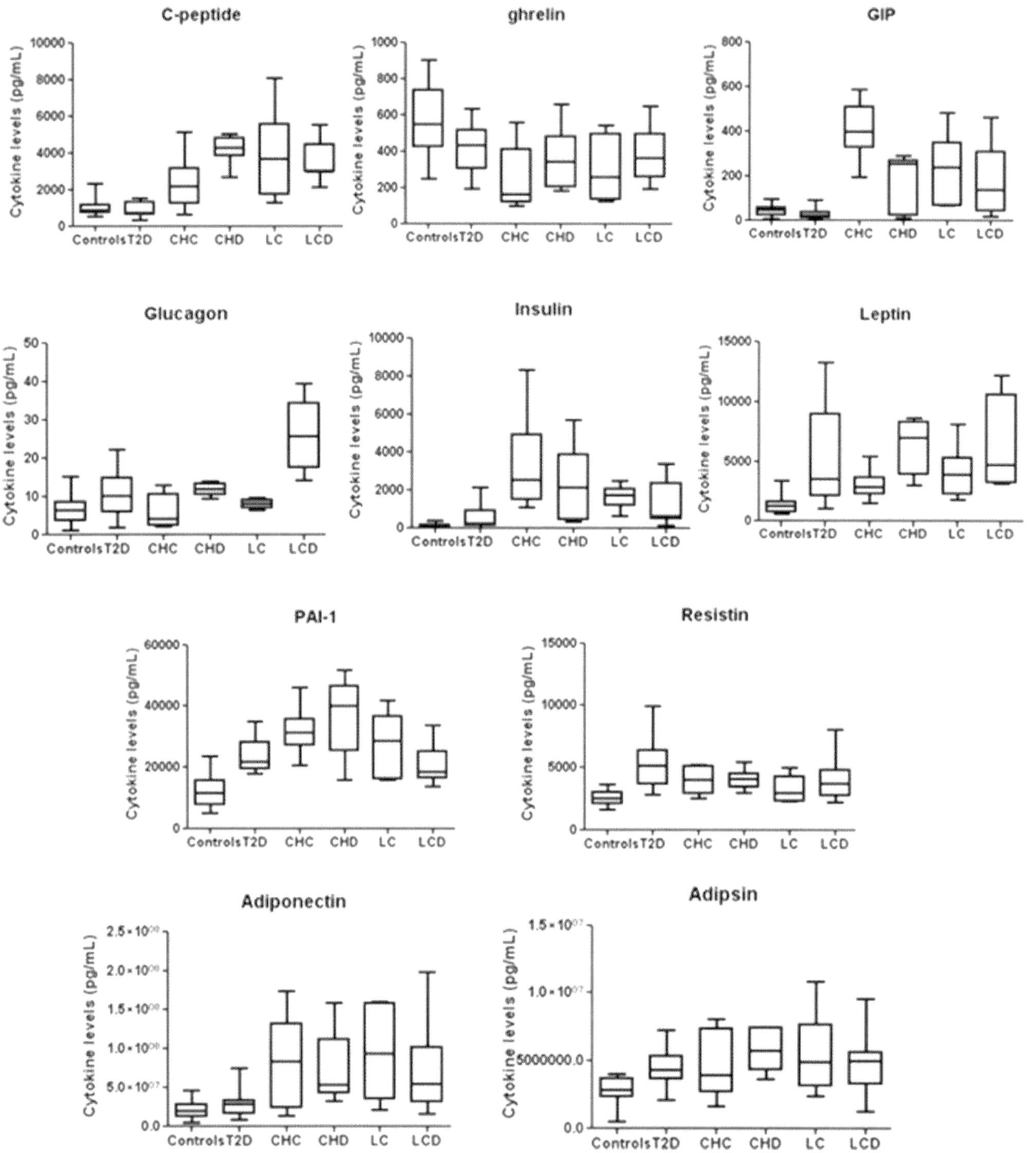

Figure 2. Significant cytokines in some patient groups. We report the significant molecule levels from controls and patients with type 2 diabetes (T2D), chronic hepatitis C (CHC), CHC-related cirrhosis (LC), CHC hepatitis and type 2 diabetes (CHD) and CHC-related cirrhosis and type 2 diabetes (LCD), evaluated by 10+2-Plex panel, are plotted with box-and-whisker graphs. The boxes extend from the 25th to the 75th percentile, and the line in the middle is the median. The error bars extend down to the lowest value and up to the highest.

On the other hand, the levels of CXCL1, β-NGF, resistin, adiponectin, adipsin and PAI-1 are similar in CHC and CHD patients whereas IL-1α, IL-2R, IL-12, IL-18, leptin, C-peptide, ghrelin and CXCL9 are higher in CHD patients than in CHC patients and GIP is lower in CHD patients than in CHC patients (with p-value <0.01).

Overall these data highlight that the simultaneous presence of CHC and type 2 diabetes induces an evident increase of the following proinflammatory cytokines: IL-1α, IL-2R, IL-12, IL-18, CXCL9, MIF and HGF. In fact, in CHD patients their levels are higher than in type 2 diabetes or CHC patients suggesting an associative effect of two diseases. In particular, in comparison to C-

Table 2. Comparison of cytokine serum levels in all patients and healthy controls.

Cytokines	Controls vs T2D	Controls vs CHC	Controls vs CHD	Controls vs LC	Controls vs LCD
21-Plex					
IL-1α	*	**	***	***	***
IL-2R	*	*	**	**	***
IL-12	*	*	***	***	***
IL-18	*	*	***	**	***
CXCL1		**	**	**	**
CXCL9		*	***	***	***
HGF	*		**	**	**
β-NGF		**	**	***	***
MIF	*	*	***	***	***
10-Plex					
C-peptide		*	**	**	**
Ghrelin	*	**	*	*	*
GIP		**	*	*	*
Glucagon	*		*		**
Insulin	*	**	**	**	**
Leptin	**	*	**	**	**
PAI-1	*	**	**	**	**
Resistin	*	*	*	*	*
2-Plex					
Adiponectin		*	*	*	*
Adipsin	*	*	*	*	*

We report P-values (p) obtained for all significant molecules in patients with type 2 diabetes (T2D), chronic hepatitis C (CHC), CHC-related cirrhosis (LC), CHC hepatitis and type 2 diabetes (CHD) and CHC-related cirrhosis and type 2 diabetes (LCD), with respect to healthy control subjects using the nonparametric Mann-Whitney U test. In particular $p<0.05$ is indicated with *, $p<0.01$ with **, and $p<0.001$ with ***.

peptide, ghrelin, GIP, insulin and adiponectin, it is worth noting that CXCL9, HGF and glucagon levels are increased in CHD patients even if they were resulted significant in patients affected by one only disease.

As in the case of T2D and CHC patients, we have correlated the serum levels of all the significant proteins in CHD group with clinical/biochemical data. In these patients both IL-18 and C-peptide showed a significant positive correlation with transaminases and BMI values (Table 3). Moreover, IL-18 correlated also with glycemia as in type 2 diabetes patients. Certainly, these data are interesting since IL-18 is increased in both CHC and type 2 diabetes patients whereas C-peptide is increased only in CHC patients. Therefore, an increased concentration of C-peptide associated with elevated serum levels of transaminases can be used as index of viral infection in diabetic hyperglycemic patients.

Table 3. Significant correlations between cytokines and clinical/biochemical data in all patients.

Disease	Cytokines	Clinical Data
T2D	IL-18, resistin, MIF	glycemia, BMI
CHC	IL-2R, MIF, β-NGF	transaminase
CHD	IL-18, C-peptide	glycemia, transaminasi, BMI
LC	CXCL1, CXCL9, HGF	albumin
LCD	Glucagon, HGF	glycemia, BMI, albumin

We report in patients with type 2 diabetes (T2D), chronic hepatitis C (CHC), CHC-related cirrhosis (LC), CHC hepatitis and type 2 diabetes (CHD) and CHC-related cirrhosis and type 2 diabetes (LCD) the cytokines and the clinical/biochemical data that correlate between them.

Patients with CHC-related Cirrhosis (LC)

Greater amounts of IL-1α, IL-2R, IL-12, IL-18, CXCL1, CXCL9, MIF, β-NGF, HGF, C-peptide, GIP, insulin, PAI-1, adiponectin, leptin, resistin and adipsin and lower of ghrelin were secreted by LC patients respect to controls (Figures 1–2). These results have evidenced that high circulating levels of these molecules are correlated to the presence of fasting glucose in cirrhotic patients due to reduced liver function and altered hepatic glucose metabolism in agreement to previous papers [33–39]. However, it is important to underline that the same molecules increased in CHC and LC patients with the sole exception of HGF that can be used for predicting the progression to HCC in patients with CHC-related liver disease and low albumin.

We have used the T-test to compare the levels of all the significant proteins in CHC as well as LC patients. Insulin, PAI-1, adiponectin, resistin and adipsin levels are similar in both groups whereas GIP is lower in LCs than in CHC patients (with p-value <0.05) and C-peptide, IL-1α, IL-2R, IL-12, IL-18, CXCL9, MIF, β-NGF, HGF and leptin are higher in LCs than in CHC patients (with p-value <0.05). These data suggest that these pro-inflammatory cytokines increase during the chronic inflammation leading to LC and, then, to cancer. Since it has been reported in the literature that T2D can be associated with HCC in CHC patients without cirrhosis [1,4,9], we have also compared by T-test the levels of significant molecules in CHD and LC patients to separate cytokines in two groups (similar or different) in order to use them as specific markers of the two different processes. In particular, only three molecules behave differently in CHD and LC patients: β-NGF is higher in LC whereas glucagon and IL-18 are higher in CHD (with p-value <0.05) (Figure 3). This suggests that β-NGF is a pro-inflammatory protein and index of inflammatory process related to chronic infection leading to cirrhosis and then to cancer, whereas glucagon and IL-18 are mainly due to diabetes that occurs as part of the metabolic syndrome with an increased risk of HCC. Moreover, in agreement with our recent results [13], the levels of CXCL1, CXCL9 and HFG in patients with LC showed a significant positive correlation among them, and a negative correlation with the albumin values (Table 3), which are lower in these patients in respect to controls.

Patients with CHC-related Cirrhosis and Type 2 Diabetes (LCD)

Greater amounts of IL-1α, IL-2R, IL-12, IL-18, CXCL1, CXCL9, MIF, β-NGF, HGF, C-peptide, GIP, insulin, PAI-1, adiponectin, leptin, resistin, ghrelin, and adipsin and lower amounts of ghrelin were found in LCD patients compared with healthy donors (Figures 1–2 and Table 2). It is also evident that the same molecules are significant in LC and LCD patients. The only difference is represented from glucagon (with p-value <0.05) that is significant in LCD patients and not in LC patients. Concerning the levels of all the significant molecules we can underline that they are similar in two groups with the exception of IL-2R, IL-18 and glucagon that are higher in LCD patients. This indicates that the levels of the three molecules are due to the presence of type 2 diabetes in LC patients. Finally, from the correlation of the serum levels of all the significant proteins in LCD group with clinical/biochemical data (Table 3), we observe that glucagon and HGF show a significant positive correlation among them and with glycemia and BMI values while correlate negatively with albumin values, which are lower in these patients compared to controls.

Discussion

In this paper we report a simultaneous and comparative analysis of serum levels of a large panel of cytokines, chemokines, adipokines and growth factors in patients with type 2 diabetes, CHC, CHC-related cirrhosis, CHC and type 2 diabetes and CHC-related cirrhosis and type 2 diabetes by BioPlex assay. Our interest for these diseases depends from the fact that Southern Italy shows the highest rates of type2 diabetes/obesity [40] and, also, of liver cancer for Europe, mainly related to infection with hepatitis viruses (i.e. CHC) [41].

A general view of the results in Table 2, shows that β-NGF, CXCL1, CXCL9, C-peptide, GIP and adiponectin resulted up-expressed in all the patient groups except in those with T2D suggesting that they can be associated to the chronic CHC infection leading to fibrotic, cirrhotic and cancer progression, also in presence of type 2 diabetes (CHD and LCD). In fact, β-NGF is involved in cancer growth and metastasis and it has also been detected in diseased liver tissues [11], CXCL1 and CXCL9 have chemotactic activities and roles in angiogenesis, inflammation and tumor genesis [10], adiponectin is expressed on monocytes and macrophages that mediate the stimulation of protein kinase activated by AMP, the oxidation of fatty acids and the uptake of glucose [42], whereas C-peptide is implicated in insulin resistance [5] and GIP induces insulin secretion [27].

Since type 2 diabetes has been recognized as a cofactor that can modify the course of chronic CHC infection and can be used as an independent predictor of HCC [8], we have compared the significant molecules in patients with T2D and CHC. In details, we have evidenced that: i) ghrelin and leptin levels are lower in CHC patients than in those with T2D, ii) IL-1α, insulin and PAI-1 levels are higher in CHC patients than in those with T2D, iii) CXCL1, CXCL9, β-NGF, C-peptide, GIP and adiponectin are higher only in CHC patients and iv) HGF and glucagon are higher only in T2D patients.

All these molecules were analysed by Ingenuity Pathway Analysis 7.1 (Ingenuity Systems, Inc., Redwood City, CA, USA) that created a network on the basis of associated functions and data mining from experimental studies reported in literature (Figure 4 and Table S1). This graph presents five hub genes such as STAT3 (signal transducer and activator of transcription), NR3C1 (nuclear receptor subfamily 3, group C, member 1), NF-kB (called also RELA), TP53 (tumor p53) and USF1 (upstream stimulatory factor 1). In particular, STAT3 is induced from the leptin [43] and has a role in suppressing IFN induction of STAT1-dependent inflammatory genes, such as CXCL9 [44]. Therefore, we can hypothesize that in T2D patients the higher level of leptin induces the STAT3 increased expression and the related CXCL9 suppression. On the other hand, NR3C1 is the receptor to which cortisol and other glucocorticoids bind and interacts with STAT3 and RELA [45]. The network reported in Figure 4 shows that RELA modulates the expression of TP53, MIF, CXCL9 and IL-1α whereas TP53 that of CXCL1, IL2R, IL-1α, MIF, PAI-1 (called also SERPINE1) and IL18. In literature it is reported that two RELA and TP53 genes are up-expressed in CHC and liver fibrosis [46] and this can explain because CXCL1, IL-1α IL18 and PAI-1 as well as CXCL9 are higher in CHC patients. As regards USF1, it is involved in the regulation of numerous genes of glucose and lipid metabolism as well as hepatic metabolism. USF1 resulted down-expressed during the progression of liver fibrosis in CHC patients [47] and this explains the lower ghrelin expression in CHC patients in respect to those with T2D.

Moreover, it is worth of note that HGF has been found normal only in CHC patients. This growth factor stimulates mitogenic, motogenic (including metastogenesis) and morphogenic effects on epithelial and endothelial cells via its receptor, proto-oncogene Met. The activation of Met by HGF binding is linked to cell growth and survival, through activation of both the PI3-kinase/PDK/Akt and the Ras/Raf/MEK/ERK pathways, and to cell mobility and cytoskeletal organization via activation of the Rho-GTPases, Rho, Rac and CDC42. HGF and Met have been associated with progression, invasiveness and metastasis in a number of cancer types and for these reasons their signaling is a major target for cancer therapeutics development [48]. Hence, HGF increased levels in all patient groups except in CHC confirm and suggest that this protein can be used as index for predicting, in patients with T2D, the progression of chronic inflammation to cancer [13].

The analysis of how molecule levels change during the progression to more advanced stages, showed that IL-1α, IL-2R, IL-12, IL-18, CXCL9, MIF and HGF are higher in CHD, LC and LCD than in patients with only type 2 diabetes or CHC suggesting that these proteins are associative markers of these two diseases and implicated in their complicance and progression.

Furthermore, we have compared cytokinomes of LC and CHD patients to realize what molecules were significantly different in these two stages because in literature it has been reported that patients with chronic CHC infection and type 2 diabetes without liver cirrhosis can evolve into hepatocarcinogenesis [8–9]. In

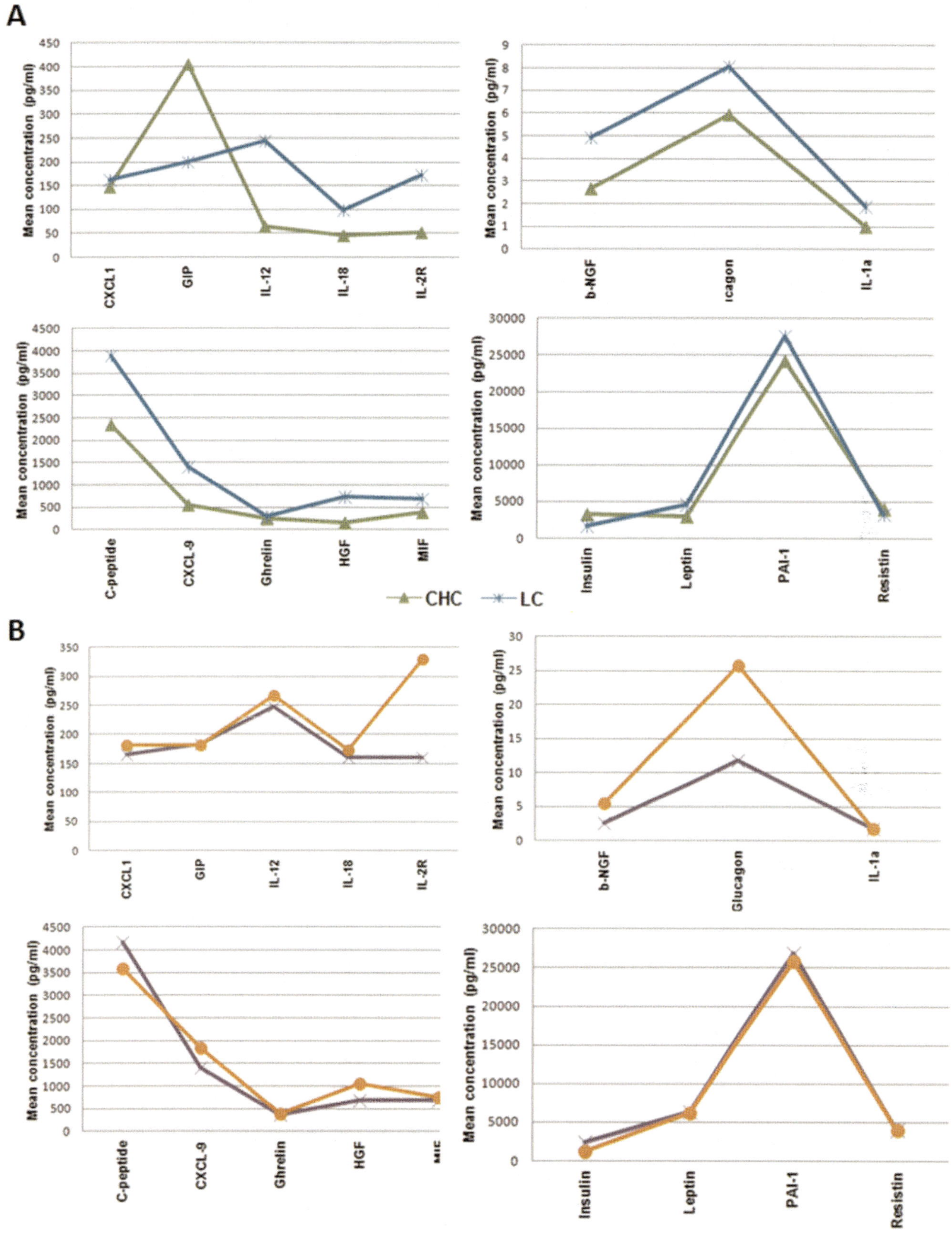

Figure 3. Mean concentrations of significant cytokines. We report the mean levels of the molecules evaluated in patients with chronic hepatitis C (CHC) and CHC-related cirrhosis (LC) (A), and with CHC hepatitis and type 2 diabetes (CHD) and CHC-related cirrhosis and type 2 diabetes (LCD) (B). The legends evidence the different colors used for the analyzed groups.

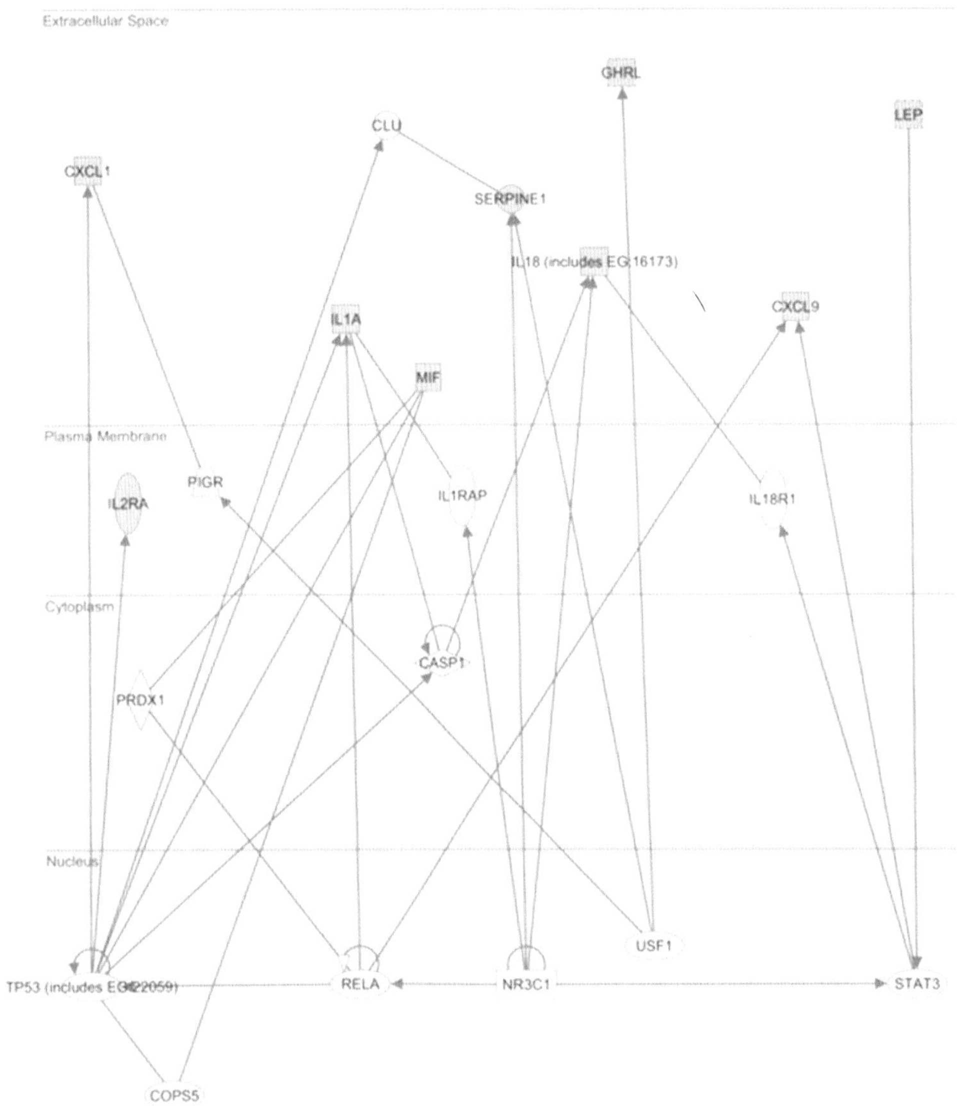

Figure 4. Ingenuity Pathway Analysis (IPA) of significant molecules. The graph shows the closely associated network for significant cytokines, reported also in Table 2, (evidenced with grey symbols) and other molecules (evidenced with white symbols) obtained by IPA software.

details, β-NGF is higher in LC patients whereas glucagon and IL-18 are higher in CHD patients (Figure 3). Hence, data evidence that these three molecules can be associated to two different stages of the pathological processes (CHD and LC) that may lead to cancer. Therefore, we suggest that β-NGF can be helpful as index of that chronic infection stage able to evolve into cirrhosis and, then, HCC while glucagon and IL-18 can be index of the diabetes association that occurs as part of the metabolic syndrome leading to HCC.

In overall the obtained results evidence that the serum levels of some cytokines, chemokines, adipokines and growth factors can be useful for the clinical monitoring of patients because they give specific information in regard to the progression from CHC and LC and to that from CHD to LCD. In fact, we have evaluated the ratio between the mean concentrations of significant molecules in LC versus CHC patients and in LCD vs CHD patients (see Table S2) and in Figures 3A and B the mean concentrations of all the significant molecules are reported in order to compare quickly the different cytokinome profiles in the disease progression of these patients. In details, the levels of GIP are lower in LC patients than in CHC patients whereas those of C-peptide, IL-1α, IL-2R, IL-12, IL-18, CXCL9, MIF, β-NGF, HGF and leptin are higher in LC patients than in CHC patients. This suggests that these proteins can be used to monitor and follow the CHC patients and to understand whether they are leading to LC. Comparing CHD and LCD patients we can observe that four proteins, i.e. β-NGF, glucagon, IL-2R and HGF, present in LCD patients concentrations significantly higher than those with CHD. Therefore we suggest that the monitoring of these four molecules can be useful to improve the prognosis of CHD patients.

At present our data are only indicative of HCC risk only showing that cytokines are up-expressed in CHD, LCD and LC as stage before cancer. However, we have already planned to collect sera of HCC patients with or without T2D to identify the cytokinome profile of these patients and explain what cytokines can be marker of HCC risk.

Moreover, we have correlated the serum levels of all the significant proteins in each group with clinical/biochemical data by Pearson correlation coefficient (Table 3). This analysis has evidenced that: i) in T2D patients IL-18, resistin and MIF correlated positively with glycemia and BMI levels, ii) in CHC patients IL-2R, MIF and β-NGF correlated positively with transaminase values, iii) in CHD patients IL-18 and C-peptide correlated positively with transaminase, BMI and glycemia values, iv) in LC patients CXCL1, CXCL9 and HFG correlated negatively with albumin values and v) in LCD patients glucagon and HGF correlated positively with BMI and glycemia values and negatively with albumin values. All the results have suggested the possibility to use mini-panels composed from cytokines and biochemical data for discriminating the various stages of these diseases.

To evaluate the possible association between the serum levels of all the significant proteins in each group and smoking status, hypertension, BMI, and hypercholesterolemia, we performed a multivariate regression analysis using the cytokines as dependent variables and these parameters as independent variables (Table 4). In particular, the smoking status was known only for T2D patients. As evidenced from odds ratios (OR) higher than 1, BMI values resulted positively related to high levels of IL-8, resistin and MIF in T2D patients, of IL-18 and C-peptide in CHD patients and of glucagon and HGF in LCD patients. On the other hand, cytokine levels were not associated with hypertension and hypercholesterolemia in all the groups as well as with the smoking status in T2D patients (*data not shown*).

In overall, our observations demonstrate that an integrated approach (multiplex bead-based assays) is much more powerful than isolated measurements to evaluate specific stages of these two complex pathologies (type 2 diabetes and chronic CHC hepatitis) alone or when they are concomitant in a patient. Reproducibility (coefficient of variance), degree of multiplexing (plex level), reliability (publication history) and higher sensitivity are the best feature of this assay. The interconnected, vital extracellular signaling networks of cytokines, are at least as complex as intracellular signaling pathways. Cellular signals when released into the extracellular milieu are strongly diluted and, hence, the detection of multiple cytokines is necessary to get a more global view of these signals. The less that is known about a particular physiologic or pathologic mechanism directed by cytokine signaling, the greater the need to use multiplexed cytokine detection. However, when we are monitoring changes in levels in certain disease conditions, what is important is to have a correct ratio between the cytokines expressed at high concentration compared to those expressed at very low concentrations to the limits of detectability in experiments which follow these changes dynamically over time. The correct ratio is much more important than single measured quantities because it represents the balance of population among the signaling molecules, also it makes the results more significant because internally consistent. Therefore, the multiplex assay has emerged as an accurate, simple, specific, noninvasive, reproducible and less expensive method that, in

Table 4. Multivariate regression analysis using the cytokines as dependent variables and smoking status, hypertension, BMI, and hypercholesterolemia as independent variables.

Cytokines	OR (95% CI)				
	T2D	CHC	CHD	LC	LCD
21-Plex					
IL-1α	0.66 (0.32–1.12)	0.72 (0.44–1.06)	0.69 (0.39–1.02)	0.88 (0.69–1.11)	0.79 (0.49–1.08)
IL-2R	0.65 (0.21–1.01)	0.79 (0.48–1.04)	0.72 (0.42–1.01)	0.85 (0.48–1.10)	0.81 (0.55–1.10)
IL-12	0.74 (0.50–1.05)	0.78 (0.52–1.01)	0.65 (0.49–1.11)	0.77 (0.48–1.05)	0.80 (0.58–1.09)
IL-18	**5.36 (3.51–7.65)**	0.81 (0.56–1.15)	**4.51 (3.95–5.23)**	0.79 (0.45–1.21)	1.01 (0.89–1.20)
CXCL1		0.77 (0.42–1.05)	1.01 (0.72–1.41)	0.94 (0.55–1.29)	0.95 (0.78–1.20)
CXCL9		0.81 (0.49–1.07)	0.99 (0.58–1.09)	0.95 (0.51–1.28)	0.91 (0.79–1.13)
HGF	1.06 (0.52–1.55)		1.01 (0.71–1.44)	0.88 (0.71–1.15)	**3.45 (2.74–4.76)**
β-NGF		0.74 (0.47–1.08)	0.79 (0.50–1.13)	0.79 (0.50–1.09)	0.89 (0.71–1.10)
MIF	**2.36 (1.91–4.01)**	0.80 (0.59–1.04)	0.81 (0.57–1.11)	0.90 (0.68–1.12)	0.94 (0.75–1.12)
10-Plex					
C-peptide		0.69 (0.41–1.00)	**1.86 (1.55–3.92)**	0.87 (0.75–1.13)	1.00 (0.78–1.22)
Ghrelin	0.71 (0.44–1.10)	0.78(0.49–1.09)	0.80 (0.64–1.00)	0.93 (0.73–1.22)	0.92 (0.79–1.10)
GIP		0.75 (0.44–1.10)	0.78 (0.52–1.09)	0.76 (0.59–1.12)	0.89 (0.70–1.08)
Glucagon	0.73 (0.41–1.07)		0.99 (0.59–1.14)		**2.77 (1.98–3.89)**
Insulin	0.92 (0.56–1.45)	0.74 (0.45–1.05)	1.01 (0.79–1.23)	0.89 (0.66–1.11)	0.88 (0.75–1.06)
Leptin	0.65 (0.43–0.99)	0.84 (0.50–1.10)	1.00 (0.77–1.19)	0.91 (0.76–1.21)	0.89 (0.66–1.09)
PAI-1	0.44 (0.21–1.01)	0.90 (0.74–1.11)	1.03 (0.75–1.30)	0.79 (0.54–1.13)	0.95 (0.79–1.19)
Resistin	**1.99 (1.52–3.21)**	0.71 (0.52–1.02)	1.05 (0.75–1.28)	0.85 (0.57–1.09)	0.99 (0.78–1.21)
2-Plex					
Adiponectin		0.69 (0.40–0.99)	0.98 (0.79–1.19)	0.79 (0.60–1.07)	0.70 (0.51–1.00)
Adipsin	0.55 (0.38–1.04)	0.73 (0.50–1.03)	1.01 (0.68–1.19)	0.84 (0.51–1.05)	0.72 (0.49–1.08)

We report odds ratios (OR) and 95% confidence intervals (95% CI) evaluated for association between each significant cytokine (shown in Table 2) and BMI in patients with type 2 diabetes (T2D), chronic hepatitis C (CHC), CHC hepatitis and type 2 diabetes (CHD), CHC-related cirrhosis (LC), and CHC-related cirrhosis and type 2 diabetes (LCD). OR being positively associated (higher than 1) to cytokines are evidenced in bold.

future, could be included in routine clinical practice to monitor the association of type 2 diabetes and/or CHC to liver cirrhosis, and to improve the prognosis of these diseases. Work is already in progress to collect in specialized databanks as much data is possible on cytokinomes determined by multiplexing as well as clinical/biochemical data to distinguish and evaluate quantitatively the pathological patterns of these patients by a neural network approach [49]. Of course the presence of protein chips able to evaluate comparatively the amounts of a high number of cytokines is an important prerequisite to improve the discriminating ability of this approach as well as the decision-making ability of the neural networks.

In conclusion our working hypothesis was i) to understand if the cytokinome profiles can be used to distinguish the patients with only CHC or T2D or with both diseases, ii) to identify what cytokines present concentrations similar or different in CHD and LC patients because in the literature it has reported that T2D can be associated with HCC in HCV patients without cirrhosis iii) to identify what cytokines can be useful for the clinical monitoring of patients in the progression from CHC and LC and to that from CHD to LCD and iv) to define the prognostic mini-panels for these diseases based on biochemical data and cytokines. The results obtained in our paper have evidenced that some cytokines are significantly up-regulated in patients with only CHC or T2D whereas other cytokines increase when both the diseases are present. Moreover, from the comparison between the levels of significant molecules in CHD and LC patients, it is resulted that three molecules present different behavior in these patients: β-NGF is higher in LC whereas glucagon and IL-18 are higher in CHD. Therefore we suggest that β-NGF is a pro-inflammatory protein and index of inflammatory process related to chronic infection leading to cirrhosis and, then, to cancer whereas glucagon and IL-18 are due mainly to the diabetes and occurs as part of the metabolic syndrome that can increase the risk of HCC. Also our results have evidenced what cytokines change in the progression from CHC and LC and to that from CHD to LCD. Finally our studies have demonstrated that some molecules have significant correlations and associations with clinical/biochemical data (see Tables 3 and 4), and defined mini-panels that can be used as specific markers for the different disease staging.

Supporting Information

Table S1 List of molecules involved in the network reported in figure 4. For each gene the table shows the symbol, Entrez Gene Name, Cellular Location and the type.

Table S2 Ratio between the mean concentrations of significant molecules in LC versus CHC patients and in LCD vs CHD patients. We have evidenced in bold the ratio >1.5

Author Contributions

Conceived and designed the experiments: SC G. Colonna G. Castello RM PM GP. Performed the experiments: EG FC AS. Analyzed the data: EG FC SC MDS. Contributed reagents/materials/analysis tools: FC EG AS MDS SC. Wrote the paper: SC GC RM PM.

References

1. Lai MS, Hsieh MS, Chiu YH, Chen TH (2006) Type 2 diabetes and hepatocellular carcinoma: A cohort study in high prevalence area of hepatitis virus infection. Hepatology 43: 1295–1302.
2. Veldt BJ, Chen W, Heathcote EJ, Wedemeyer H, Reichen J, et al. (2008) Increased risk of hepatocellular carcinoma among patients with hepatitis C cirrhosis and diabetes mellitus. Hepatology 47: 1856–62.
3. Chen CL, Yang HI, Yang WS, Liu CJ, Chen PJ, et al. (2008) Metabolic factors and risk of hepatocellular carcinoma by chronic hepatitis B/C infection: a follow-up study in Taiwan. Gastroenterology 135: 111–21.
4. Hung CH, Lee CM, Chen CH, Hu TH, Jiang SR, et al. (2009) Association of inflammatory and anti-inflammatory cytokines with insulin resistance in chronic hepatitis C. Liver Int 29(7): 1086–93.
5. Hui JM, Sud A, Farrell GC, Bandara P, Byth K, et al. (2003) Insulin resistance is associated with chronic hepatitis C virus infection and fibrosis progression. Gastroenterology 125: 1695–704.
6. Huang JF, Dai CY, Hwang SJ, Ho CK, Hsiao PJ, et al. (2007) Hepatitis C viremia increases the association with type 2 diabetes mellitus in a hepatitis B and C endemic area: an epidemiological link with virological implication. Am J Gastroenterol 102: 1237–43.
7. Castello G, Costantini S, Scala S (2010) Targeting the inflammation in CHC-associated hepatocellular carcinoma: a role in the prevention and treatment. J Transl Med 8: 109.
8. Hung CH, Lee CM, Wang JH, Hu TH, Chen CH, et al. (2011) Impact of diabetes mellitus on incidence of hepatocellular carcinoma in chronic hepatitis C patients treated with interferon-based antiviral therapy. Int J Cancer 128(10): 2344–52.
9. Paradis V, Zalinski S, Chelbi E, Guedj N, Degos F, et al. (2009) Hepatocellular carcinomas in patients with metabolic syndrome often develop without significant liver fibrosis: a pathological analysis. Hepatology 49: 851–9.
10. Capone F, Costantini S, Guerriero E, Calemma R, Napolitano M, et al. (2010) Serum cytokine levels in patients with hepatocellular carcinoma. Eur Cyt Net 21(2): 99–104.
11. Costantini S, Autiero I, Colonna G (2008) On new challenge for the Bioinformatics. Bioinformation 3: 238–239.
12. Costantini S, Castello G, Colonna G (2010) Human Cytokinome: a new challenge for systems biology. Bioinformation 5: 166–167.
13. Costantini S, Capone F, Guerriero E, Maio P, Colonna G, et al. (2010) Serum cytokine levels as putative prognostic markers in the progression of chronic CHC hepatitis leading to cirrhosis. Eur Cyt Netw 21: 251–6.
14. Standard of Medical Care in Diabetes (2009) Diabetes Care 32: S62–S67.
15. Chao PC, Huang CN, Hsu CC, Yin MC, Guo YR (2010) Association of dietary AGEs with circulating AGEs, glycated LDL, IL-1α and MCP-1 levels in type 2 diabetic patients. Eur J Nutr 49: 429–34.
16. Yao K, Lu H, Huang R, Zhang S, Hong X, et al. (2011) Changes of dendritic cells and fractalkine in type 2 diabetic patients with unstable angina pectoris: a preliminary report. Cardiovasc Diabetol 10: 50.
17. Yu XY, Chen HM, Liang JL, Lin QX, Tan HH, et al. (2011) Hyperglycemic myocardial damage is mediated by proinflammatory cytokine: macrophage migration inhibitory factor. PLoS One 6: e16239.
18. Anan F, Masaki T, Jikumaru K, Iwao T, Eshima N, et al. (2010) Hepatocyte growth factor is a significant risk factor for white matter lesions in Japanese type 2 diabetic patients. Eur J Clin Invest 40: 585–90.
19. Fantuzzi G (2005) Adipose tissue, adipokines, and inflammation. Journal of Allergy and Clinical Immunology 115: 911–919.
20. Bobbert P, Eisenreich A, Weithäuser A, Schultheiss HP, Rauch U 2(011) Leptin and resistin induce increased procoagulability in diabetes mellitus. Cytokine.
21. Netea MG, Joosten LAB, Lewis E, Jensen DR, Voshol PJ, et al. (2006) Deficiency of interleukin-18 in mice leads to hyperphagia, obesity and insulin resistance. Nature Medicine 12: 650–656.
22. D'Alessio D (2011) The role of dysregulated glucagon secretion in type 2 diabetes. Diabetes Obes Metab 13: 126–32.
23. Konya H, Hasegawa Y, Hamaguchi T, Satani K, Umehara A, et al. (2010) Effects of gliclazide on platelet aggregation and the plasminogen activator inhibitor type 1 level in patients with type 2 diabetes mellitus. Metabolism 59: 1294–9.
24. Coma G, Peña R, Blanco J, Rosell A, Borras FE, et al. (2006) Treatment of monocytes with interleukin (IL)-12 plus IL-18 stimulates survival, differentiation and the production of CXC chemokine ligands CXCL8, CXCL9 and CXCL10. Clin Exp Immunol 145: 535–44.
25. Divella R, Lacalamita R, Tommasi S, Coviello M, Daniele A, et al. (2008) PAI-1, t-PA and circulating hTERT DNA as related to virus infection in liver carcinogenesis. Anticancer Res 28: 223–8.
26. Marra F, Bertalani C (2009) Adipokines in liver diseases. Hepatology 50: 957–969.
27. Thorens B (1995) Glucagon-like peptide-1 and control of insulin secretion. Diabète & métabolisme 21: 311–8.
28. Alfadda AA, Alzoghaibi MA (2008) Circulatory neutrophil chemokines in statin-treated diabetic patients. Saudi Med J 29: 584–8.
29. Osei K, Falko JM, O'Dorisio TM, Fields PG, Bossetti B (1986) Gastric inhibitory polypeptide responses and glucose turnover rates after natural meals in type II diabetic patients. J Clin Endocrinol Metab 62: 325–30.

30. Wong CK, Ho AW, Tong PC, Yeung CY, Kong AP, et al. (2007) Aberrant activation profile of cytokines and mitogen-activated protein kinases in type 2 diabetic patients with nephropathy. Clin Exp Immunol 149: 123–31.
31. Park KS, Kim SS, Kim JC, Kim HC, Im YS, et al. (2008) Serum and tear levels of nerve growth factor in diabetic retinopathy patients Am J Ophthalmol 145(3): 432–7.
32. Kim ST, Kim BJ, Lim DM, Song IG, Jung JH, et al. (2011) Basal C-peptide Level as a Surrogate Marker of Subclinical Atherosclerosis in Type 2 Diabetic Patients. Diabetes Metab J 35(1): 41–9.
33. Montoliu C, Piedrafita B, Serra MA, del Olmo JA, Urios A, et al. (2009) IL-6 and IL-18 in Blood May Discriminate Cirrhotic Patients With and Without Minimal Hepatic Encephalopathy. Journal of Clinical Gastroenterology 43: 272–279.
34. Sharma A, Chakraborti A, Das A, Dhiman RK, Chawla Y (2009) Elevation of interleukin-18 in chronic hepatitis C: implications for hepatitis C virus pathogenesis. Immunology 128: e514–e522.
35. Kalaitzaki E, Bosaeus I, Öhman L, Björnsson E (2007) Altered postprandial glucose, insulin, leptin, and ghrelin in liver cirrhosis: correlations with energy intake and resting energy expenditure. American Journal of Clinical Nutrition 85: 808–815.
36. Kruszynska YT, Ghatei MA, Bloom SR, McIntyre N (1995) Insulin secretion and plasma levels of glucose-dependent insulinotropic peptide and glucagon-like peptide 1 [7–36 amide] after oral glucose in cirrhosis. Hepatology 21: 933–941.
37. Raya-Sánchez JM, González-Reimers E, Rodríguez-Martín JM, Santolaria-Fernández F, Molina-Pérez M, et al. (1998) Coagulation inhibitors in alcoholic liver cirrhosis. Alcohol 15: 19–23.
38. Tietge, U J F, Böker KHW, Manns MP, Bahr MJ (2004) Elevated circulating adiponectin levels in liver cirrhosis are associated with reduced liver function and altered hepatic hemodynamics. American Journal of Physiology 287: E82–E89.
39. Bahr MJ, Ockenga J, Böker KHW, Manns MP, Tietge UJF (2006) Elevated resistin levels in cirrhosis are associated with the proinflammatory state and altered hepatic glucose metabolism but not with insulin resistance. American Journal of Physiology 291: E199–E206.
40. Classen JB (2011) Italian pediatric data support hypothesis that simultaneous epidemics of type 1 diabetes and type 2 diabetes/metabolic syndrome/obesity are polar opposite responses (i.e., symptoms) to a primary inflammatory condition. J Pediatr Endocrinol Metab 24: 455–6.
41. Fusco M, Girardi E, Piselli P, Palombino R, Polesel J, et al. (2008) Epidemiology of viral hepatitis infections in an area of southern Italy with high incidence rates of liver cancer. Eur J Cancer 44: 847–53.
42. Kadowaki T, Yamauchi T. (2005) Adiponectin and adiponectin receptors. Endocr Rev 26: 439–51.
43. Carvalheira JBC, Siloto RMP, Ignacchitti I, Brenelli SL, Carvalho CRO, et al. (2001) Insulin modulates leptin-induced STAT3 activation in rat hypothalamus. Febs Letters 500: 119–124.
44. Ho HH, Ivashkiv LB. (2006) Role of STAT3 in Type I Interferon Responses. JBC 281: 14111–14118.
45. Hollenberg SM, Weinberger C, Ong ES, Cerelli G, Oro A, et al. (1985) Primary structure and expression of a functional human glucocorticoid receptor cDNA. Nature 318: 635–41.
46. Schuppan D, Krebs A, Bauer M, Hahn EG (2003) Hepatitis C and liver fibrosis. Cell Death and Differentiation 10: S59–S67.
47. Takahara Y, Takahashi M, Zhang Q-W, Wagatsuma H, Mori M, et al. (2008) Serial changes in expression of functionally clustered genes in progression of liver fibrosis in hepatitis C patients. World J Gastroenterol 14: 2010–2022.
48. Gentile A, Trusolino L, Comoglio PM. (2008) The Met tyrosine kinase receptor in development and cancer. Cancer Metastasis Rev 27: 85–94.
49. Evangelista D, Colonna G, Miele M, Cutugno F, Castello G, et al. (2010) CDMS (Clinical Data Mining Software): a cytokinome data mining system for a predictive medicine of chronic inflammatory diseases. PEDS 123: 899–902.

COMMD1-Deficient Dogs Accumulate Copper in Hepatocytes and Provide a Good Model for Chronic Hepatitis and Fibrosis

Robert P. Favier[1]*, Bart Spee[1], Baukje A. Schotanus[1], Ted S. G. A. M. van den Ingh[2], Hille Fieten[1], Bas Brinkhof[1], Cornelia S. Viebahn[1], Louis C. Penning[1], Jan Rothuizen[1]

1 Department of Clinical Sciences of Companion Animals, Faculty of Veterinary Medicine, Utrecht University, Utrecht, The Netherlands, **2** TCCI Consultancy BV, Utrecht, The Netherlands

Abstract

New therapeutic concepts developed in rodent models should ideally be evaluated in large animal models prior to human clinical application. COMMD1-deficiency in dogs leads to hepatic copper accumulation and chronic hepatitis representing a Wilson's disease like phenotype. Detailed understanding of the pathogenesis and time course of this animal model is required to test its feasibility as a large animal model for chronic hepatitis. In addition to mouse models, true longitudinal studies are possible due to the size of these dogs permitting detailed analysis of the sequence of events from initial insult to final cirrhosis. Therefore, liver biopsies were taken each half year from five new born COMMD1-deficient dogs over a period of 42 months. Biopsies were used for H&E, reticulin, and rubeanic acid (copper) staining. Immunohistochemistry was performed on hepatic stellate cell (HSC) activation marker (alpha-smooth muscle actin, α-SMA), proliferation (Ki67), apoptosis (caspase-3), and bile duct and liver progenitor cell (LPC) markers keratin (K) 19 and 7. Quantitative RT-PCR and Western Blots were performed on gene products involved in the regenerative and fibrotic pathways. Maximum copper accumulation was reached at 12 months of age, which coincided with the first signs of hepatitis. HSCs were activated (α-SMA) from 18 months onwards, with increasing reticulin deposition and hepatocytic proliferation in later stages. Hepatitis and caspase-3 activity (first noticed at 18 months) increased over time. Both HGF and TGF-β1 gene expression peaked at 24 months, and thereafter decreased gradually. Both STAT3 and c-MET showed an increased time-dependent activation. Smad2/3 phosphorylation, indicative for fibrogenesis, was present at all time-points. COMMD1-deficient dogs develop chronic liver disease and cirrhosis comparable to human chronic hepatitis, although at much higher pace. Therefore they represent a genetically-defined large animal model to test clinical applicability of new therapeutics developed in rodent models.

Editor: Erica Villa, University of Modena & Reggio Emilia, Italy

Funding: These authors have no support or funding to report.

Competing Interests: The authors have read the journal's policy and have the following interests: Ted S.G.A.M. van den Ingh is employed by TCCI Consultancy BV. The dogs in this study received normal non-copper restricted commercial dog food (Nobless, Purina). There are no patents, products in development or further marketed products to declare.

* E-mail: r.p.favier@uu.nl

Introduction

Chronic hepatic injury activates a general aetiology-independent process characterized by liver regeneration and fibrogenesis. The sequence of events starts with the primary insult, followed by hepatocyte proliferation and activation of non-parenchymal cells, including hepatic stellate cells (HSCs), liver progenitor cells (LPCs) and macrophages, leading to fibrosis, concomitant failure of regeneration, and finally cirrhosis [1,2].

HSCs are situated in the space of Disse along the sinusoids. Quiescent HSCs contain vitamin-A loaded lipid droplets. Upon cytokine-induced activation HSCs rapidly loose the lipid droplets, increase the expression of alpha-smooth muscle actin (α-SMA), and secrete extracellular matrix (ECM) components [3–5]. HSCs, together with other mesenchymal liver cells and hepatocytes, produce transforming growth factor β (TGF-β) [6]. A transient increase of TGF-β1 in the liver promotes fibrosis with the formation of ECM components, and suppresses hepatocyte proliferation [7]. The hallmark of TGF-β signaling is Smad2/3 phosphorylation [8]. Oppositely, HSCs play an important role in hepatic regeneration as they secrete growth factors including hepatocyte growth factor (HGF). HGF is a potent mitogen for hepatocytes and induces a plethora of other physiological activities comprising anti-apoptosis, morphogenesis and angiogenesis [9,10]. When mature hepatocytes are extensively damaged or hampered in their replication, the LPCs become activated [11]. LPCs are bipotential and can differentiate both into cholangiocytes and hepatocytes [1,12,13].

Chronic liver disease is a worldwide health problem, which in later stages leads to ineffective regeneration, fibrosis, cirrhosis and tumour formation, and can only be solved by organ transplantation. New therapeutic options like anti-fibrotic strategies, or growth factor-mediated interventions are being developed in rodent model studies [2,14]. The step from *principle-to-practice*, however, remains considerable. The availability of a suitable large animal model with a pathogenesis and pathophysiology of chronic liver disease comparable to that in man is lacking. The availability of such a model would greatly enhance the understanding of possibilities and drawbacks of new clinical interventions. Furthermore it could be tailored to develop effective and safe protocols prior to clinical application [14]. Recently, canine fibrotic liver diseases have been demonstrated to be highly comparable to their human counterparts in both pathophysiological and molecular mechanisms [13,15]. Comparable pathophysiology itself is not sufficient to become a model animal. A defined etiology allows for more standardized experimental conditions. A dog model with a well-defined genetic aetiology is the Bedlington terrier (BT) which lacks the COMMD1 protein. The absence of the COMMD1 protein in BT, due to a deletion of exon-2 of the *COMMD1* gene, results in a progressive accumulation of copper in hepatocytes leading to chronic hepatitis and cirrhosis [16,17]. This canine disease was discussed as a potential model for human Wilson's disease (WD), an autosomal recessive inherited copper storage disorder due to a reduced or absent *ATP7B* gene expression [18,19,20,21]. COMMD1 and ATP7B proteins interact and ATP7B function and stability are impaired upon COMMD1 depletion [22,23]. These dogs therefore could serve as model for Wilson's disease and in general for chronic liver disease leading to end-stage liver cirrhosis. Because of their size and life-span, the availability of molecular tools, the possibility and easiness to approach the liver with comparable procedures as performed in man, *e.g.* to take multiple and sequential liver biopsies, combined with a known genetic aetiology these dogs are potentially well-suited for evaluation of new protocols aimed at enhancing liver regeneration and reduction of fibrosis/cirrhosis. A requirement for an accepted model is that the pathogenesis of the disease is known in detail and highly comparable to the human pathology. Therefore we provide a detailed longitudinal analysis of clinical, clinicopathological, and molecular aspects focusing on regenerative and fibrotic pathways of COMMD1-deficient dogs.

Results

Physical Examination and Blood Examination

During the entire follow-up period dogs showed no abnormalities at physical examination. Serum ALT was significantly increased at 24, 36, and 42 months of age (2–3-fold), whereas serum AP significantly increased at 18 and 42 months of age. During the 42 months follow-up period, bile acids and albumin remained within reference limits (Table 1).

Table 1. Blood examinations.

Parameter & Reference Range	ALT 0–54 U/l	AP 0–73 U/l	Bile acids 0–10 μmol/l	Albumin 26–37 g/L
Age (months)				
12	44 (34–75)	73 (66–109)	7 (3–11)	33 (30–34)
18	45 (35–60)	111 * (91–209)	1 (1–2)	30 (28–32)
24	66 * (43–257)	115 (61–120)	7 (6–12)	29 (27–31)
30	83 * (62–153)	87 (68–140)	4 (1–8)	30 (30–32)
36	180 (69–225)	94 (59–153)	2 (0–3)	29 (29–30)
42	112 * (55–201)	101 * (72–219)	2 (1–3)	28 (27–30)

ALT: alanine aminotransferase; AP: alkaline phosphatase.
Blood examinations during aging in five COMMD1-deficient dogs. Values are expressed as median (range).
*significantly increased serum concentration compared with 12 months of age.

Histopathological Findings

At six months of age all dogs showed a moderate centrilobular hepatic copper accumulation; however no evidence of copper laden Kupffer cells (phagocytosis of copper from destruction of copper laden hepatocytes) or other evidence of hepatitis was observed at this stage (Figure 1). At 12 months of age all animals had extensive copper accumulation diffuse throughout the lobules and in two animals a mild hepatitis was present. At 18 months all dogs showed a slight to mild hepatitis. Although there was some individual variation, the activity of hepatitis progressed to mild and moderate at older age (>24 months) in all dogs.

Fibrogenesis

α-SMA showed an increasing presence similarly in the COMMD1-deficient dogs and normal age matched controls between 6 (grade 0–1) and 18 months (grade 2). Pathologically increased α-SMA-immunopositivity positivity was seen in all COMMD1-deficient dogs in the centrilobular areas starting from 18 months of age (Figure 1 & Table 2).

The reticulin stain showed progressive centrilobular fibrosis starting in one of the five dogs at 24 months of age (Figure 1 & Table 2) and present in all COMMD1-deficient dogs at 42 months of age, finally resulting in centro-central bridging fibrosis and cirrhosis in three of the five animals (at 42 months). Sirius red staining was similar to reticulin staining (data not shown).

Apoptosis and Regeneration

Active caspase-3 remained undetectable up to 24 months and became visible in the hepatocytes from 30 months of age until 42 months (Table 3). A 2-fold increased median number of Ki67 positive hepatocytes was seen at 36 and 42 months (Table 3), particularly in the three dogs with centro-central bridging fibrosis and cirrhosis, and in the areas with the least copper storage. Both K7 and K19 stainings showed a doubling (median number) of LPCs at 30 months of age and further increase later on, but they showed no differentiation into intermediate cells (Table 3).

Gene-expression Profiling

The mRNA levels of TGF-β1 and both its receptors increased significantly starting at 24 months and decreased gradually afterwards (Figure 2A). The increase in relative mRNA levels of HGF and its receptor c-MET was sharp and strong (15 and 11-fold, respectively) occurring at 24 months of age in all dogs (Figure 3A). These levels decreased gradually over time and returned to basal levels at 36 months of age.

Western Blot Analysis

Western blots were performed at the time points 12 (prior to elevation of mRNA levels of TGF-β1, HGF and their respective receptor), 30 (elevated mRNA levels), and 42 (mRNA levels returned to basal levels) months of age. Smad2/3 was detectable at all time-points. Phosphorylated Smad2 was present in the COMMD1-deficient dogs at all time-points (Figure 2B). HGF was variably present at all measured time-points in COMMD1-

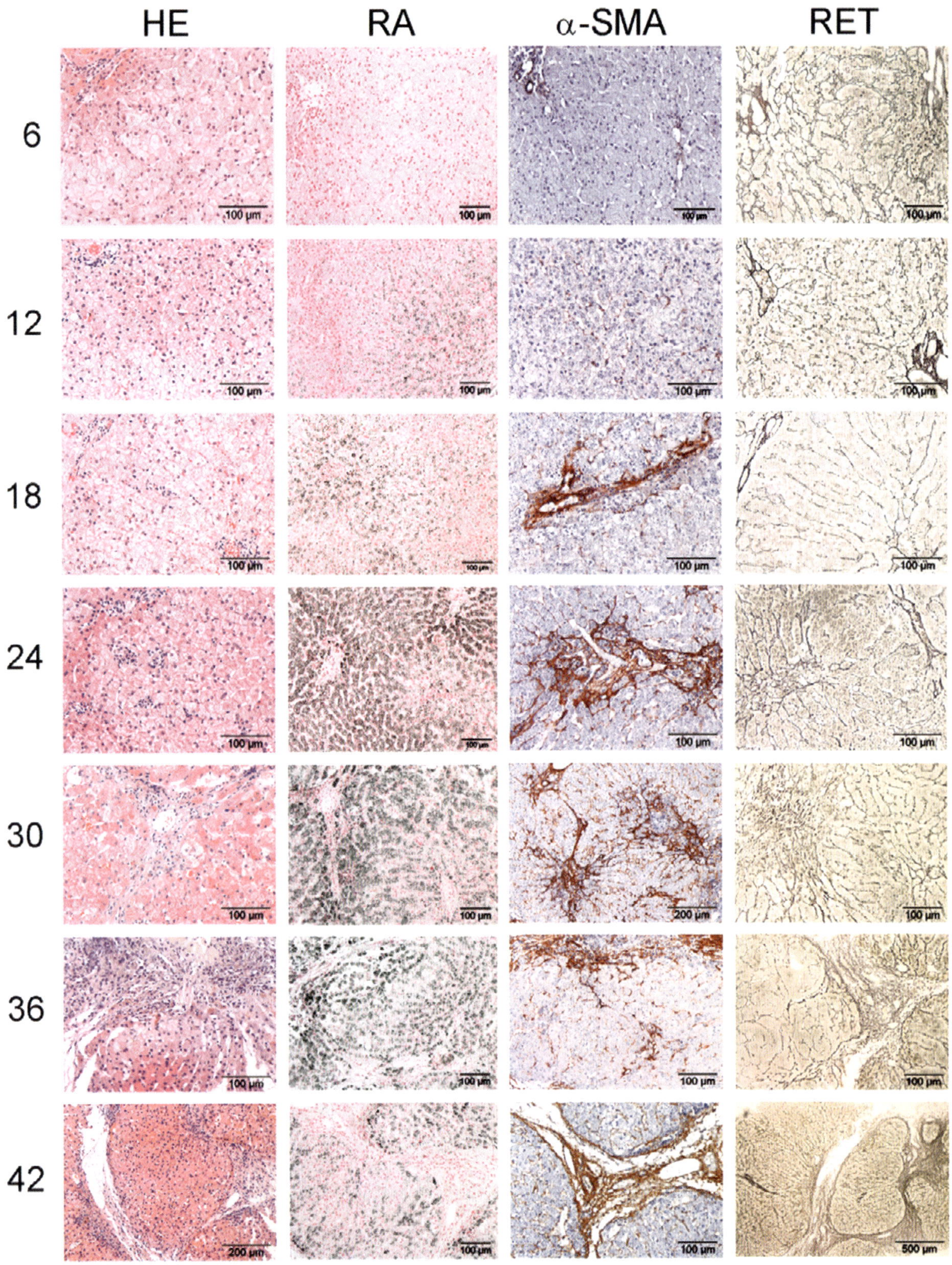

Figure 1. Histological description. COMMD1-deficient dog livers were stained with H&E and RA to assess inflammation and copper accumulation, respectively, and stained for α-SMA and reticulin (collagen type III) to assess fibrosis. Representative pictures of a COMMD1-deficient dog over a period of 42 months are shown. Numbers indicate age in months.

Table 2. Fibrosis.

Age (months)	6	12	18	24	30	36	42
α-SMA grading (0–4)	1 (–)	2 (1–2)	2 (2–2.5)	3 (2–4)	3 (3–4)	4 (2–4)	3 (2–4)
p-value	–	0.15	0.048	0.057	0.053	0.054	0.057
Reticulin grading (0–3)	0 (–)	1 (0–1)	0 (0–1)	1 (0–2.5)	0 (0–2.5)	2.5 (0–3)	2 (1–3)
p-value	–	0.15	1	0.17	0.37	0.17	0.058

Fibrosis scoring: α-SMA (hepatic stellate cell activation) and reticulin grading (collagen type III) in five COMMD1-deficient dogs in a time-dependent copper-induced hepatitis. Data are presented as median (range).
α-SMA grading; 0: no staining of HSCs; 1: a few positive HSCs; 2: diffuse staining of HSCs; 3: mild increased staining of HSCs; 4: marked increased staining of HSC and compared with age matches normal controls.
Reticulin grading; grade 0: normal, grade 1: local mild centrilobular increase, grade 2: multifocal mild to moderate centrilobular increase, grade 3: moderate increase with centro-central bridging or nodular transformation. The uncorrected p-values for comparison of each time point with 6 months of age are reported in the table. No significant differences are present when correcting these p-values for the number of tests.

Table 3. Apoptosis and regeneration.

Age (months)	6	12	18	24	30	36	42
Casp3	0 (–)	0 (–)	0 (–)	0 (–)	0.1 (0–3)	0.1 (0–1.1)	0.1 (0–0.1)
p-value	–	NA	NA	NA	0.15	0.17	0.35
Ki67	0.9 (0.6–2.9)	0.8 (0.4–1.1)	1.1 (0.7–2.0)	0.5 (0.3–1.3)	0.7 (0.1–1.0)	2.3 (0.1–4.4)	2.1 (1–4.6)
p-value	–	0.79	0.88	0.25	0.13	0.88	0.5
K19	1.9 (1.2–3.2)	2.5 (1–3.3)	3.2 (2.7–3.4)	1.8 (1.5–3.3)	3.7 (2.5–5.3)	3.6 (2.8–7.4)	5.2 (4–9.6)
p-value	–	0.10	0.063	0.58	0.058	0.063	0.125

NA: not available.
Number of (active) caspase-3 (Casp3) positive hepatocytes per 10-times objective (manual count), number of Ki67 positive hepatocytes per 10-times objective (manual count), and number of K19 positive cells in the limiting plate per portal area in five COMMD1-deficient dogs in a time-dependent copper-induced hepatitis. Data are presented as median (range).
The uncorrected p-values for comparison of each time point with 6 months of age are reported in the table. No significant differences are present when correcting these p-values for the number of tests.

deficient dogs. Phosphorylated c-MET was increased age-dependently as was phosphorylated STAT3 (Figure 3B).

Discussion

We evaluated COMMD1-deficient dogs as a possible large animal model for chronic hepatitis, in a 42 month lasting longitudinal study. A clear sequence of events occurred and explains in molecular terms the histological finding: copper accumulation, followed by hepatocellular damage, increased plasma ALT activity, hepatitis, HSC activation and fibrosis and further progression towards centro-central bridging fibrosis and cirrhosis. At the latest stages increased HGF proteins and activated STAT3 proteins were present.

Free copper is highly toxic due to its ability to generate hydroxyl radicals and it has been demonstrated that hepatocellular apoptosis is triggered by copper-induced cell damage [24,25,26]. Signs of regeneration appeared when the inflammatory process had progressed. This was mainly associated with hepatocytic regeneration shown by Ki67 immunostaining. LPC activation, reflected by non-cholangiocytic K19 immunostaining, was also present. In acute hepatitis LPCs differentiate through intermediate hepatocytes into hepatocytes within one week after the insult [27]. The fact that no intermediate hepatocytes were seen near the activated LPCs in the COMMD1-deficient dogs indicates a minor contribution of these cells to liver regeneration in this stage of hepatitis. The slow onset of disease and regenerative capacity of hepatocytes may explain that the endogenous LPCs do not contribute to the regeneration process in this model. One important multifunctional cytokine during liver regeneration is HGF [9,10]. In this study, mRNA-expressions of HGF and its receptor c-MET peaked at 24 months of age. This coincided with hepatic stellate cell activation (α-SMA), and the expression of TGF-β1 and its receptors. Although HGF and c-MET expression were temporarily present, HGF, c-MET activation, and the downstream time-dependent increase in phospho-STAT3 indicated a continuous activation of the regenerative pathway. High HGF protein levels at 42 months, most likely from an extra-hepatic source, stimulated STAT3 activation but cannot rule out increased inflammatory signaling via *e.g.* the IL-6 receptor towards STAT3 phosphorylation.

TGF-β1 signalling components (at mRNA and activated protein level) increased transiently from 24 months and coincided expectedly with an increased fibrosis (reticulin staining). The presence of pSMAD2/3 already at 12 months remains unexplained.

Until now COMMD1-deficient Bedlington terriers have been the best described dog model for hepatic copper toxicosis. Copper storage in COMMD1-deficient dogs causes chronic hepatitis, fibrosis and cirrhosis causing hepatic failure, portal hypertension, ascites, portosystemic collateral circulation, and hepatic encephalopathy. Therewith all features of chronic hepatitis and cirrhosis, not only copper-associated, are displayed. This experimentally reproducible autosomal recessive genetic disease may thus serve as an appropriate large animal model for chronic hepatitis and cirrhosis in man. Our study adds to the understanding of the sequence of pathophysiological events occurring in copper-associated hepatitis in COMMD1-deficient dogs and agrees with a semi-longitudinal study performed in $ATP7B^{-/-}$ mice [28]. COMMD1 mutations have so far not been associated with unexplained copper storage diseases in man [29,30]. Although COMMD1 function remains puzzling [31], the major effects of its absence in the dog model seem to be impaired ATP7B-mediated copper export from the hepatocytes [22]. The COMMD1-deficient dog model is thus not the exact copy of Wilson's disease, but shows all relevant features of human chronic hepatitis. This is the first well-defined large animal model of chronic hepatitis. We anticipate that it may provide an important instrument for the evaluation of future regenerative and anti-fibrotic therapies in a preclinical model and helps to close the gap between commonly used rodent models and human pathology.

In December 2011 a PlosOne paper described copper accumulation in liver-specific COMMD1 KO mouse [32] and confirmed the siRNA-based conclusion that COMMD1 plays an essential role in hepatic copper homeostasis [20,33]. Surprisingly, these mice did not develop an obvious liver pathology under excessive copper diet. This clearly underscores the importance of

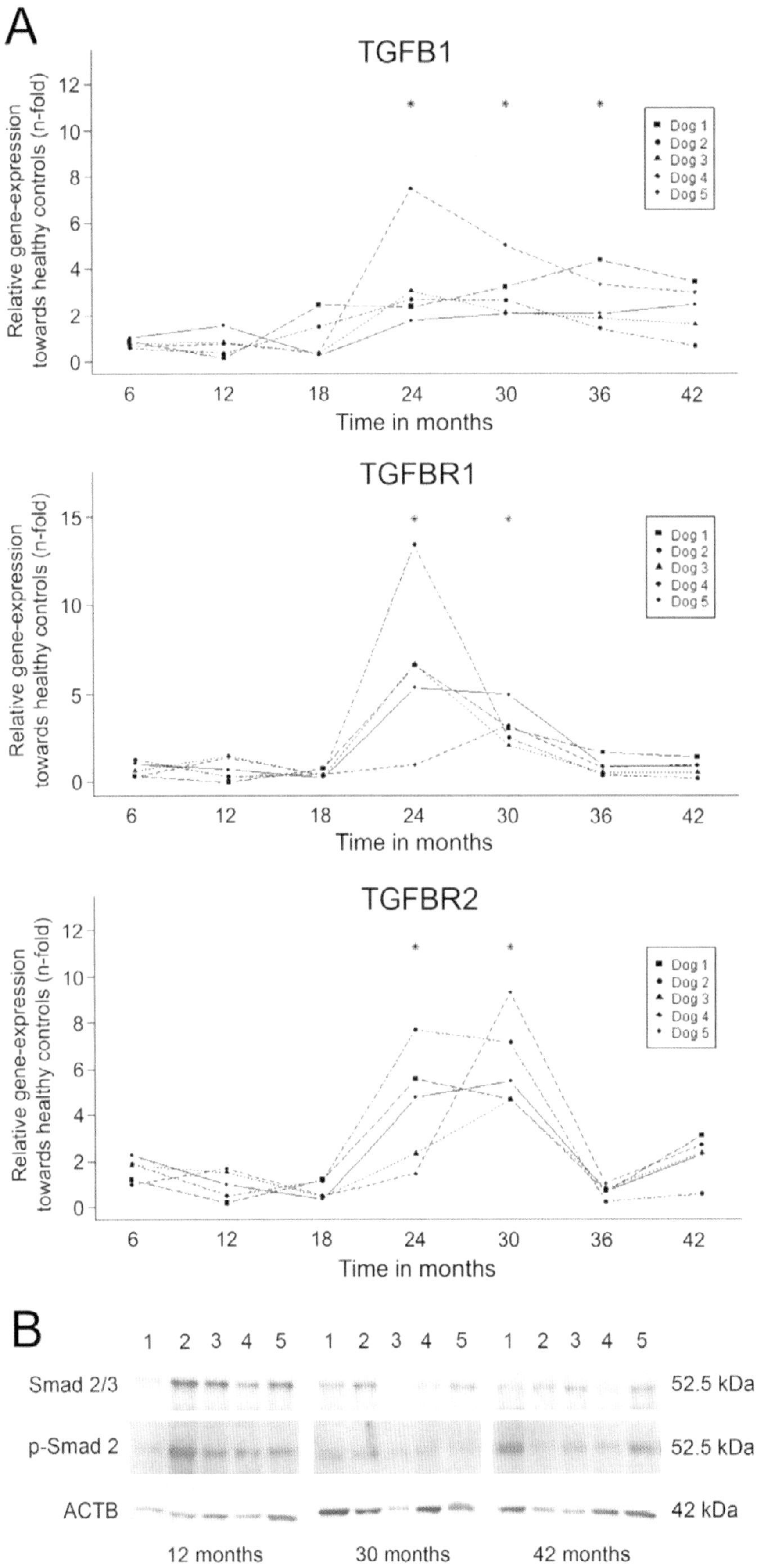
A
TGFB1
Relative gene-expression towards healthy controls (n-fold)
Dog 1
Dog 2
Dog 3
Dog 4
Dog 5
Time in months
TGFBR1
Relative gene-expression towards healthy controls (n-fold)
Dog 1
Dog 2
Dog 3
Dog 4
Dog 5
Time in months
TGFBR2
Relative gene-expression towards healthy controls (n-fold)
Dog 1
Dog 2
Dog 3
Dog 4
Dog 5
Time in months
B
Smad 2/3
p-Smad 2
ACTB
52.5 kDa
52.5 kDa
42 kDa
12 months
30 months
42 months

Figure 2. TGF-β1 pathway. (**A**) Gene-expression profiling. Interaction plots of Q-PCR data of important mediators of fibrogenesis in a time-dependent copper-induced hepatitis in five COMMD1-deficient dogs. Q-PCR results were normalized against the expression of six control dogs (one to three years of age). Linear mixed-effect modeling was used; * significant difference corrected for multiple testing. (**B**) Western blot analysis on the activation of TGF-beta signalling (total Smad2 and phosphorylated Smad2 (Ser727)) of five COMMD1-deficient dogs at 12, 30, and 42 months. β-actin (ACTB) served as loading control.

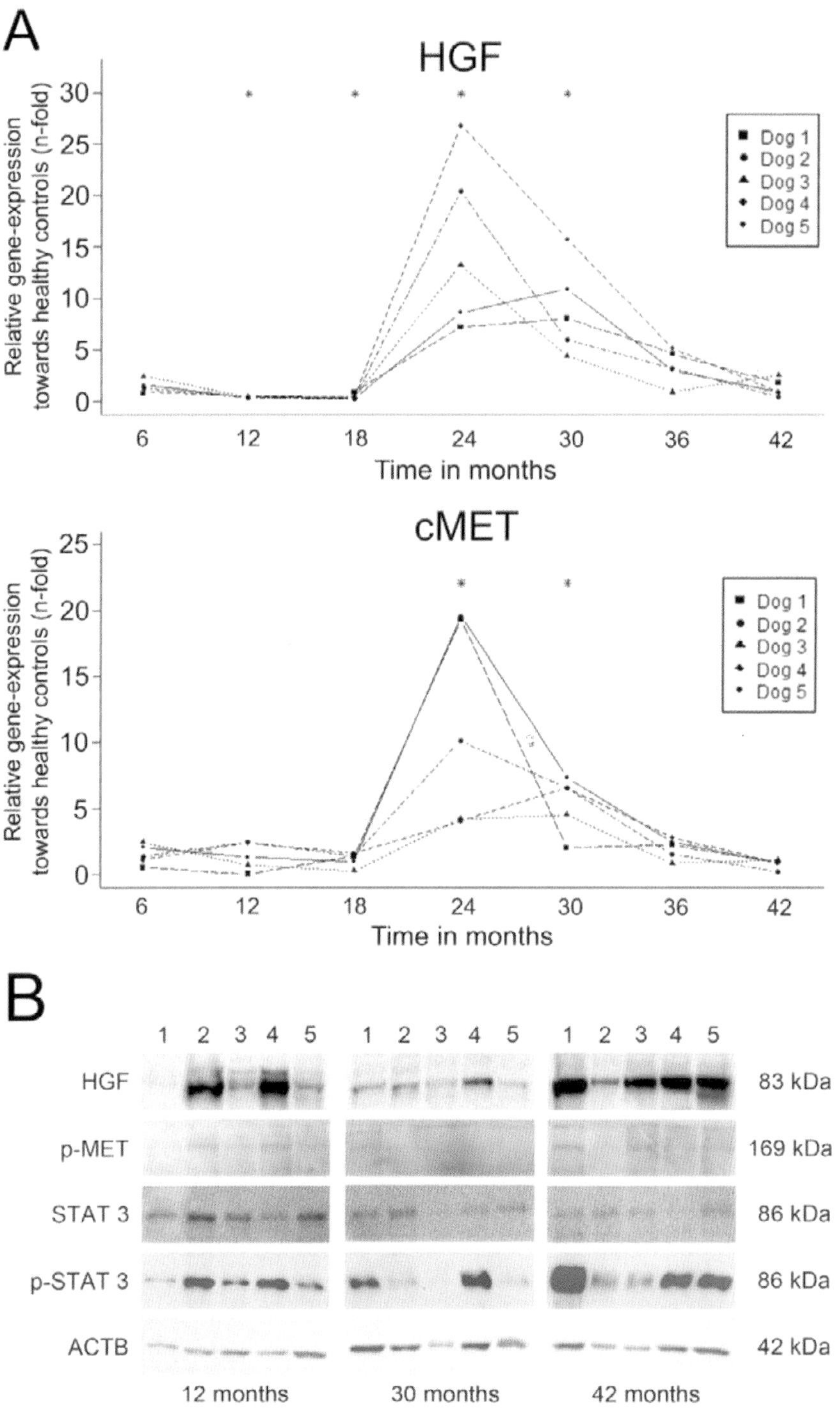

Figure 3. HGF pathway. (**A**) Gene-expression profiling. Interaction plots of Q-PCR data of important mediators of regeneration in a time-dependent copper-induced hepatitis in five COMMD1-deficient dogs. Q-PCR results were normalized against the expression of six control dogs (one to three years of age). Linear mixed-effect modeling was used; * significant difference corrected for multiple testing. (B) Western blot analysis on the activation HGF-signalling (HGF, phosphorylated c-Met, (phosphorylated) STAT3) of five COMMD1-deficient dogs at 12, 30, and 42 months. β-actin (ACTB) served as loading control.

this canine model as a long-term model for (therapeutic interventions into) chronic hepatitis.

Materials and Methods

Animals

Five new born COMMD1-deficient dogs with confirmed COMMD1 status (two males, three females) were used for longitudinal follow-up [34]. Dogs were examined every six months until the age of 42 months. At each occasion the clinical symptoms were scored, physical and blood examinations were performed, and liver biopsies were taken. Dogs were housed individually and received normal non-copper restricted commercial dog food (Noblesse, Purina), once a day and water *ad libitum*. The procedures were approved by Utrecht University's Ethical Committee, as required under Dutch legislation (ID 2007.III.06.080).

Blood Examinations

Serum alanine aminotransferase (ALT), alkaline phosphatase (AP), bile acids, and albumin were determined using a DXC-600 Beckman (Beckman Coulter, Woerden, the Netherlands). Reference ranges for ALT, AP, bile acids, and albumin are 0–54 U/l, 0–73 U/l, 0–10 μmol/l, and 26–37 g/L, respectively.

Liver Tissue Sampling and Histopathology

Liver biopsies (five per dog per time-point) were obtained using a 14G Menghini needle [35]. Two biopsies were formalin-fixed and paraffin-embedded, and 4 μm thick paraffin sections were stained with haematoxylin and eosin (H&E), rubeanic acid (RA) for copper quantification, reticulin (Gordon and Sweet), and Sirius red. Hepatitis and fibrosis scoring were performed by one board-certified veterinary pathologist (TvdI) according to the WSAVA classification [36]. Copper accumulation (RA) was evaluated semi-quantitatively using a scale from 0 to 5 as previously described [37], and localization within the liver lobule was assessed. Three biopsies were fixed in RNAlater (Ambion, Austin, TX, USA) for a maximum of 24 hours and stored at −70°C.

Immunohistochemistry

Alpha-smooth muscle actin (α-SMA), activated caspase-3 (Casp3), proliferation marker Ki67, Keratin 7 (K7), and Keratin 19 (K19) were stained as described elsewhere with slight modifications [5,38]. The antibodies used for IHC are described in Table S1. Three μm sections were mounted on poly-L lysine coated slides and stored for a maximum of 48 hours at room temperature (RT). Sections were deparaffinised followed by antigen retrieval (AR). Enzymatic AR was performed with proteinase K (DAKO, Glostrup, Danmark) for 40 minutes (K7) or 15 minutes (K19). AR for Ki67 was achieved in 10 mM citric acid buffer (pH 6) for 15 minutes in a microwave. Activated casp3 and α-SMA staining needed no AR. Endogenous peroxidase and unspecific binding were blocked in 0.3% H_2O_2 and 10% non-immune goat serum for 30 min, respectively. After application of the primary antibody over-night (Casp3 and K7) or 1 h at RT (α-SMA, Ki67, and K19), slides were washed in PBS and incubated with the appropriate secondary antibody (Envision (DAKO) HRP-labeled polymer, anti-mouse or -rabbit) for 45 minutes at RT. After washing staining was detected using 3-3′-diaminobenzidine and counterstained with 10% Mayer's haematoxylin.

α-SMA grading was performed as follows; 0: no staining of HSCs; 1: a few positive HSCs; 2: diffuse staining of HSCs; 3: mild increased staining of HSCs; 4: marked increased staining of HSCs. Results were compared with normal aged matched controls. The quantity of liver tissues from two needle biopsies was equal at all time points and in all animals; therefore both Ki67 and Casp3 were expressed as the number of positive hepatocytes per slide. K19 and K7 were graded as the number of positive cells in the limiting plate per portal area, either solitary or as small groups.

RNA Isolation and Quantitative RT-PCR (q-PCR)

RNA was isolated from RNAlater (Ambion, Austin, TX, USA) fixed biopsies, using Qiagen RNeasy Mini Kit (Qiagen, Leusden, the Netherlands). RNA quality was analysed with the Agilent BioAnalyzer 2100 (Agilent, Palo Alto, CA, USA). A SYBR green I-based Q-PCR was performed on TFG-β1, TGF-β receptor type I (TGF-βR1), TGF-β receptor type II (TGF-βR2), hepatocyte growth factor (HGF), and c-MET protooncogene (c-MET) (Table S2) [15]. Normalisation was performed using four reference-genes (glyceraldehyde-3-phosphate dehydrogenase (GAPDH), hypoxanthine phosphoribosyl transferase (HPRT), ribosomal protein S5 (RPS5) and S19 (RPS19)) [39]. Q-PCR results were related to the expression of six clinically and histologically determined healthy control dogs (one to three years of age). Minus RT and water controls remained negative.

Western Blot Analysis

Liver biopsies were lysed in RIPA buffer containing 50 mM Tris–HCl, 150 mM NaCl, 1% NP-40, 0.25% sodium deoxycholate, 1 mM EDTA, 1 mM sodium orthovanadate, 1 μg/ml aprotinin, and 1 mM PMSF. Extracted protein was quantified using a Lowry based assay (DC Protein Assay, Bio-Rad, Veenendaal, the Netherlands). To detect HGF, phospho-c-MET, (phospho-)STAT3 and (phospho-)Smad2/3 protein levels, 7.5 μg protein was denatured for 3 minutes at 95°C, subsequently run on a Criterion Tris-HCl polyacrylamide gel (Bio-Rad), transferred to Hybond-C nitrocellulose membranes (Amersham Biosciences, Roosendaal, the Netherlands) and blocked with the ECL Advance Western Blotting Detection Kit (Amersham, Little Chalfont, UK) or with non-fat dry milk (HGF). The blots were incubated overnight at 4°C with the appropriate primary antibodies (Table S3) and subsequently incubated with HRP-conjugated anti-mouse antibodies (R&D Systems Europe, Abingdon, UK; dilution 1:20,000) or HRP-conjugated anti-rabbit antibodies (Santa Cruz Biotechnology, Santa Cruz, CA, USA; dilution 1:20,000). All secondary antibodies were incubated for 1 hour at RT. Luminescence induced by the ECL Advanced Western Blotting Detection Kit (Amersham) was measured with a ChemiDoc XRS Imager (BioRad) and analyzed with provided software (Quantity-One 4.6.5).

Statistical Analysis

Statistical analysis was performed in R (version 2.11.1) [40]. Q-PCR data and results of blood examination were analyzed using linear mixed-effect modeling with the R package "nlme". When necessary, the outcome variables were transformed by their natural logarithm in order to fulfill the criteria of normality and constant variance. Restricted maximum likelihood method was used to estimate the best fitting model with a random intercept, a random slope, or both based on Akaike's information criteria. Maximum likelihood was used to estimate the fixed effect of the time in months (included in the model as a factor). Residuals were checked for normality and constancy of variance. The Wilcoxon signed rank test with continuity correction was performed for comparisons of all time points with the reference time point (6 months) for differences in immunohistochemical data. Uncorrected p-values were reported in Table 2 and 3. P-values were considered significant, when the p-value times the number of comparisons was <0.05.

Supporting Information

Table S1 Used antibodies in immunohistochemical experiments.

Table S2 Nucleotide Sequences of dog specific primers for Quantitative Real-Time PCR.

Table S3 Used antibodies in Western blot experiments.

Acknowledgments

We thank of J.A. Drie–van Putten, R. Kisjes and H.G.H. van Engelen for technical assistance. H. Vernooij (Centre for Biostatistics, Utrecht University) assisted with statistical analysis.

Author Contributions

Conceived and designed the experiments: RPF BS LCP JR. Performed the experiments: RPF BS BAS BB. Analyzed the data: RPF BS TSGAMvdI HF LCP. Wrote the paper: RPF BS TSGAMvdI CSV LCP JR.

References

1. Bird TG, Lorenzini S, Forbes SJ (2008) Activation of stem cells in hepatic diseases. Cell Tissue Res 331: 283–300.
2. Henderson NC, Forbes SJ (2008) Hepatic fibrogenesis: From within and outwith. Toxicology 254: 130–135.
3. Cassiman D, Libbrecht L, Desmet V, Denef C, Roskams T (2002) Hepatic stellate cell/myofibroblast subpopulations in fibrotic human and rat livers. J Hepatol 36: 200–209.
4. Bedossa P, Paradis V (2003) Liver extracellular matrix in health and disease. J Pathol 200: 504–515.
5. Mekonnen GA, IJzer J, Nederbragt H (2007) Tenascin-C in chronic canine hepatitis : immunohistochemical localization and correlation with necro-inflammatory activity, fibrotic stage, and expression of alpha-smooth muscle actin, cytokeratin 7, and CD3+ cells. Vet Pathol 44: 803–813.
6. Iredale JP (2007) Models of liver fibrosis: exploring the dynamic nature of inflammation and repair in a solid organ. J Clin Invest 117: 539–548.
7. Koniaris LG, McKillop IH, Schwartz SI, Zimmers TA (2003) Liver regeneration. J Am Coll Surg 197: 634–659.
8. Liu C, Gaca MD, Swenson ES, Vellucci VF, Reiss M, et al. (2003) Smad 2 and 3 are differentially activated by transforming growth factor-beta (TGF-beta) in quiescent and activated hepatic stellate cells. J Biol Chem 278: 11721–11728.
9. Michalopoulos GK, DeFrances MC (1997) Liver regeneration. Science 276: 60–66.
10. Huh CG, Factor VM, Sánchez A, Uchida K, Conner EA, et al. (2004) Hepatocyte growth factor/c-met signalling pathway is required for efficient liver regeneration and repair. Proc Natl Acad Sci USA 101: 4477–4482.
11. Shibata C, Mizuguchi T, Kikkawa Y, Nobuoka T, Oshima H, et al. (2006) Liver repopulation and long-term function of rat small hepatocyte transplantation as an alternative cell source for hepatocyte transplantation. Liver Transpl 12: 78–87.
12. Roskams T (2006) Different types of liver progenitor cells and their niches. J Hepatol 45: 1–4.
13. Schotanus BA, van den Ingh TSGAM, Penning LC, Rothuizen J, Roskams TA, et al. (2009) Cross-species immunohistochemical investigation of the activation of the liver progenitor cell niche in different types of liver disease. Liver Int 29: 1241–1252.
14. Sancho-Bru P, Najimi M, Caruso M, Pauwelyn K, Cantz T, et al. (2009) Stem and progenitor cells for liver repopulation: can we standardise the process form bench to bedside? Gut 58: 594–603.
15. Spee B, Arends B, van den Ingh TSGAM, Brinkhof B, Nederbragt H, et al. (2006) Transforming growth factor B-1 signalling in canine hepatic diseases: new models for human fibrotic liver pathologies. Liver Int 26: 716–725.
16. van de Sluis B, Rothuizen J, Pearson PL, van Oost BA, Wijmenga C (2002) Identification of a new copper metabolism gene by positional cloning in a purebred dog population. Hum Mol Genet 15: 165–173.
17. Klomp AE, van de Sluis B, Klomp LW, Wijmenga C (2003) The ubiquitously expressed MURR1 protein is absent in canine copper toxicosis. J Hepatol 39: 703–709.
18. Su LC, Ravanshad S, Owen CA Jr, McCall JT, Zollman PE, et al. (1982) A comparison of copper-loading disease in Bedlington terriers and Wilson's disease in humans. Am J Physiol 243: G226–G230.
19. Hoogenraad TU, Rothuizen J (1986) Compliance in Wilson's disease and in copper toxicosis of Bedlington terriers. Lancet 19: 170.
20. Spee B, Arends B, van Wees AM, Bode P, Penning LC, et al. (2007) Functional consequenses of RNA interference targeting COMMD1 in a canine hepatic cell line in relation to copper toxicosis. Anim Genet 38: 168–170.
21. Tanzi RE, Petrukhin K, Chernov I, Pellequer JL, Wasco W, et al. (1993) The Wilson's disease gene is a copper-transporting ATPase with homology to the Menkes's disease gene. Nat Genet 5: 344–350.
22. Tao TY, Liu F, Klomp L, Wijmenga C, Gitlin JD (2003) The copper toxicosis gene product Murr1 directly interacts with the Wilson disease protein. J Biol Chem 278: 41593–41596.
23. de Bie P, van de Sluis B, Burstein E, van de Berghe PV, Muller P, et al. (2007) Distinct Wilson's disease mutations in ATP7B are associated with enhanced binding to COMMD1 and reduced stability of ATP7B. Gastroenterology 133: 1316–1326.
24. Valko M, Leibfritz D, Moncol J, Cronin MT, Mazur M, et al. (2007) Free radicals and antioxidants in normal physiological functions and human disease. Int J Biochem Cell Biol 39: 44–84.
25. Ferenci P, Gilliam TC, Gitlin JD, Packman S, Schilsky ML, et al. (1996) An international symposium on Wilson's and Menkes'diseases. Hepatology 24: 952–958.
26. Strand S, Hofmann WJ, Grambihler A, Hug H, Volkmann M, et al. (1998) Hepatic failure and liver cell damage in acute Wilson's disease involve CD95 (APO-1/Fas) – mediated apoptosis. Nat Med 4: 588–593.
27. Katoonizadeh A, Nevens F, Verslype C, Pirenne J, Roskams T (2006) Liver regeneration in acute severe liver impairment: a clinicopathological correlation study. Liver Int 26: 1225–1233.
28. Huster D, Finegold MJ, Morgan CT, Burkhead JL, Nixon R, et al. (2006) Consequences of copper accumulation in the livers of the Atp7b−/− (Wilson disease gene) knockout mice. Am J Pathol 168: 423–434.
29. Müller T, van de Sluis B, Zhernakova A, van Binsbergen E, Janecke AR, et al. (2003) The canine copper toxicosis gene MURR1 does not cause non-Wilsonian hepatic copper toxicosis. J Hepatol 38: 164–168.
30. Lovicu M, Dessi V, Lepori MB, Zappu A, Zancan L, et al. (2006) The canine copper toxicosis gene MURR1 is not implicated in the pathogenesis of Wilson disease. J Gastroenterol 41: 582–587.
31. Sarkar B, Roberts AE (2011) The puzzle posed by COMMD1, a newly discovered protein binding Cu(II). Metallomics 3: 20–27.
32. Vonk WI, Bartuzi P, de Bie P, Kloosterhuis N, Wichers CG, et al. (2011) Liver-specific commd1 knockout mice are susceptible to hepatic copper accumulation. PLoS One 6: 29183.
33. Burstein E, Ganesh L, Dick RD, van de Sluis B, Wilkinson JC, et al. (2004) A novel role for XIAP in copper homeostasis through regulation of MURR1. EMBO J 23: 244–254.
34. Favier RP, Spee B, Penning LC, Brinkhof B, Rothuizen J (2005) Quantitative PCR method to detect a 13-kb deletion in the MURR1 gene associated with copper toxicosis and HIV-1 replication. Mamm Genome 16: 460–463.
35. Hoffmann G, van den Ingh TS, Bode P, Rothuizen J (2006) Copper-associated chronic hepatitis in Labrador Retrievers. J Vet Intern Med 20: 856–861.
36. Van den Ingh TSGAM, Van Winkle TJ, Cullen JM, Charles JA, Desmet VJ (2006) Morphological classification of parenchymal disorders of the canine and feline liver. In Rothuizen J, Bunch SE, Charles JA, Cullen ME, Desmet VJ, Szatmári V, Twedt DC, van den Ingh TSGAM, Van Winkle T, Washabau RJ, editors. WSAVA Standards for Clinical and Histological Diagnosis of Canine and Feline Liver Diseases, 1st edition, Saunders Elsevier, Philadelphia PA, USA. 85–101.
37. van den Ingh TSGAM, Rothuizen J, Cupery R (1988) Chronic active hepatitis with cirrhosis in the Doberman pinscher. Vet Q 10: 84–89.
38. van Sprundel RG, van den Ingh TS, Desmet VJ, Katoonizadeh A, Penning LC, et al. (2010) Keratin 19 marks poor differentiation and a more aggressive behaviour in canine and human hepatocellular tumours. Comp Hepatol 18: 4.
39. Brinkhof B, Spee B, Rothuizen J, Penning LC (2006) Development and evaluation of canine reference genes for accurate quantification of gene expression. Anal Biochem 356: 36–43.
40. R Development Core Team (2010) R: A language and environment for statistical computing. R Foundation for Statistical Computing, Vienna, Austria. ISBN 3-900051-07-0. Available: http://www.R-project.org. Accessed 2012 Jun 26.

Soluble Serum CD81 Is Elevated in Patients with Chronic Hepatitis C and Correlates with Alanine Aminotransferase Serum Activity

Martin-Walter Welker[1], David Reichert[1], Simone Susser[1], Christoph Sarrazin[1], Yolanda Martinez[1], Eva Herrmann[2], Stefan Zeuzem[1], Albrecht Piiper[1], Bernd Kronenberger[1]*

1 Medizinische Klinik 1, Klinikum der Johann Wolfgang Goethe-Universität, Theodor-Stern-Kai 7, Frankfurt am Main, Germany, **2** Fachbereich Medizin, Institut für Biostatistik und mathematische Modellierung, Johann Wolfang Goethe-Universität, Frankfurt am Main, Germany

Abstract

Aim: Cellular CD81 is a well characterized hepatitis C virus (HCV) entry factor, while the relevance of soluble exosomal CD81 in HCV pathogenesis is poorly defined. We performed a case-control study to investigate whether soluble CD81 in the exosomal serum fraction is associated with HCV replication and inflammatory activity.

Patients and Methods: Four cohorts were investigated, patients with chronic hepatitis C ($n = 37$), patients with chronic HCV infection and persistently normal ALT levels ($n = 24$), patients with long term sustained virologic response (SVR, $n = 7$), and healthy volunteers ($n = 23$). Concentration of soluble CD81 was assessed semi-quantitatively after differential centrifugation ranging from 200 g to 100,000 g in the fifth centrifugation fraction by immunoblotting and densitometry.

Results: Soluble CD81 was increased in patients with chronic hepatitis C compared to healthy subjects ($p = 0.03$) and cured patients ($p = 0.017$). Patients with chronic HCV infection and persistently normal ALT levels and patients with long term SVR had similar soluble CD81 levels as healthy controls ($p > 0.2$). Overall, soluble CD81 levels were associated with ALT levels ($r = 0.334$, $p = 0.016$) and severe liver fibrosis ($p = 0.027$).

Conclusion: CD81 is increased in the exosomal serum fraction in patients with chronic hepatitis C and appears to be associated with inflammatory activity and severity of fibrosis.

Editor: Johan K. Sandberg, Karolinska Institutet, Sweden

Funding: This study was supported by the clinical research unit KFO 129, funded by the German Research Foundation (DFG), and by the Scolari Stiftung. The funders had no role in study design, data collection and analysis, decision to publish, or preparation of the manuscript.

Competing Interests: The authors have declared that no competing interests exist.

* E-mail: Bernd.Kronenberger@kgu.de

Introduction

Chronic hepatitis C virus (HCV) infection is a major cause of liver cirrhosis, and hepatocellular carcinoma worldwide [1,2]. Recently the protease inhibitors boceprevir and telaprevir, which are associated with considerably enhanced sustained virologic response (SVR) rates in HCV genotype 1 infected patients in combination with pegylated interferon-alfa and ribavirin, have been approved by the European Medicines Agency and the Food and Drug Administration [3–5]. Nevertheless, approximately one quarter of patients with HCV genotype 1 infection are assumed not to achieve SVR even with triple therapy including either boceprevir or telaprevir [6].

HCV is a plus-strand RNA virus without known ability to integrate its genome into the host genome. Chronic hepatitis C is characterized by high turnover of infected cells and persistence of HCV requires continuous *de novo* infection [7–10]. Therefore, inhibition of cell entry is a promising approach in antiviral therapy against HCV. Moreover, cell entry inhibitors may be useful in prevention of otherwise inevitable graft infection after orthotopic liver transplantation in HCV associated liver cirrhosis and hepatocellular carcinoma. Proof-of-concept studies suggest that the new class of HCV entry inhibitors has a substantial capability to widen preventive and therapeutic options in HCV infection [11].

Four essential HCV hepatocyte entry receptors, CD81, the scavenger receptor B1, claudin-1, and occludin have been identified, yet [12–15]. CD81 is of particular interest because CD81 is not only expressed on hepatocytes but also on peripheral blood mononuclear cells (PBMC). Interaction of HCV with CD81 expressed on PBMC was suggested to be involved in an attenuated innate and adaptive immune response against HCV as well as in development of extrahepatic HCV manifestations [16–20]. However, these results were challenged by a recent study showing that HCV envelope 2 proteins have no modulatory effect on natural killer cell functions when expressed as part of cell culture infectious viral particles [21]. The different observations could be explained by differences in the configuration of viral envelope proteins in protein expression systems compared to systems using compete HCV particles [20,21].

Yet well known as a cell surface protein, CD81 is also a typical component of exosomes. Exosomes are membrane vesicles secreted by different eukaryotic cells, e.g. hepatocytes and lymphocytes [22–24]. In two studies, exosomes were enriched by differential centrifugation from human plasma from patients with chronic hepatitis C [23,25]. Exosomal CD81 was reliably detectable in the pellet of the fifth fraction of the centrifugation process. Moreover, CD81 exosomes were found to be associated with HCV RNA in plasma obtained from patients chronically infected with HCV [25]. However, neither CD81 levels nor HCV RNA were quantified in enriched plasma or serum, which makes it difficult to assess clinical importance of these findings. Nevertheless, exosomal CD81 may be of relevance in chronic HCV infection as HCV particles bound to exosomal CD81 could represent an additional HCV compartment with putative impact on the HCV infection rate or viral persistence, respectively [8].

Aim of the present study was to perform a comprehensive analysis if soluble CD81 is increased in patients with chronic hepatitis C compared to healthy controls, patients with chronic HCV infection but persistently normal alanine transaminase (ALT) levels, and patients with cured hepatitis C. Therefore, a method to quantify soluble CD81 in the exosomal serum fraction was established, and the association of soluble CD81 in the exosomal serum fraction with clinical and virological parameters within the different cohorts was investigated.

Methods

Patients

The present study is a case control study with 23 healthy controls and 37 patients with chronic hepatitis C and elevated alanine aminotransferase (ALT) level measured at least at 2 time points 14 days or more apart within 6 months before study entry. Furthermore, 24 patients with chronic HCV infection and persistently normal ALT serum levels as documented by three occasional measurements within the last 6 months before study entry and a minimum interval of 4 weeks between measurements, and 7 patients with long-term sustained virologic response 5 years after antiviral therapy with pegylated interferon-alfa 2a and ribavirin were included. All cohorts were independently recruited. Patients with decompensated liver cirrhosis or co-infection with hepatitis B virus or human immunodeficiency virus were excluded. Diagnosis of chronic HCV infection (>6 months) was confirmed by positive anti-HCV antibodies by third-generation enzyme immunoassay and detectable HCV RNA in serum. Grading and staging of chronic hepatitis C was done by a local, experienced pathologist according to the histological activity index described by Knodell et al. [26]. Patient cohorts with persistently normal ALT levels and patients with elevated ALT levels were derived from clinical trials performed at the university hospitals Frankfurt/Main, Germany and Homburg/Saar, Germany. Study protocols were conform to the ethical guidelines of the 1975 Declaration of Helsinki and were approved by the ethic committees of the university hospitals Frankfurt/M, Germany and Homburg/Saar, Germany. Written, informed consent was obtained from every human subject when the samples were collected under the terms of study protocol.

Isolation of CD81 from serum and plasma

Serum and plasma for ALT and AST levels, CD81 assessment, and HCV-RNA quantification were collected at the same time point and stored at −80°C until use. Enrichment of exosomes was performed according to Masciopinto et al. [25]. In this former study, the CD81 enriched exosomal fraction was identified by immunoblotting in the pellets from the fourth (p4) and - mainly - the fifth (p5) centrifugation fraction from plasma [25]. In the current study, differential centrifugation was performed at 200 g for 10 min (p1), at 500 g (p2), at 2000 g for 15 min (p3), at 10,000 g for 30 min (p4), and finally 100,000 g for 30 min (p5). The corresponding pellets (p1, p2, etc.) were each resuspended in 50 µl lysis buffer (100 mL 0.5 M TrisHCl pH 7.4, 1.5 mM NaCl, 2.5% desoxycholic acid, 10% NP-40, 10 mM ethylenediamine-tetraacetic acid, diluted 1:10 in aqua bidest., Merck, Darmstadt, Germany, and Sigma-Aldrich, Taufkirchen, Germany) and stored at −20°C until further analysis. As usage of serum may have some advantages over plasma, e.g. better reflection of biological conditions and easier sample processing, we further optimized detection of CD81 in enriched serum. Therefore, we first compared isolation of not cell-bound CD81 from plasma and serum samples, and then tested different volumes of serum (30 mL, 15 mL, 7 mL, and 1 mL) to evaluate a possible minimum amount for reliable detection of CD81. In contrast to plasma, serum samples were allowed to clot for 10 min before centrifugation. After that, serum specimen of the healthy controls and distinct patient groups were processed using the developed optimized serum sample processing protocol.

Immunoblotting of CD81

Serum derived proteins from different centrifugation steps were separated by dodecylsulfate polyacrylamide gel electrophoresis (SDS-PAGE). As thiol compounds may have a negative impact on anti-CD81 antibody binding [27], a thiol free SDS sample buffer was used. In detail, after dilution of specimens in loading buffer (5 mL glycerin, 2 mL 0.625 M TrisHCl, pH 6,8, 0.2 g SDS, 0.1 mL bromphenoleblue as 1% ethanol dilution, 2.4 mL aqua bidest.), the samples were separated by SDS-page (50 mA, 90 min) and electrophoretic transferred (110 mA, 90 min) to nitrocellulose membranes Whatman Schleicher & Schell, Dassel, Germany). Nonspecific binding sites were blocked by incubation in 5% skim milk in buffer TBST (150 mM NaCl; 30 mM Tris, pH 7.4; 0.05% Tween20) for 12 hours at +4°C. Primary anti-CD81 antibody (mouse-anti-human antibody, clone JS-81, Pharmingen, Heidelberg, Germany) were allowed to bind for a minimum of 2 hours. Detection of CD81/antibody immune complexes was performed using horse radish peroxidase-conjugated antibodies (Bio-Rad Laboratories, Hercules CA, U.S.A.) and enhanced chemiluminescence (Millipore GmbH, Schwalbach, Germany). By staining with monoclonal anti-CD81 antibodies and consecutive polyclonal horse raddish peroxidase-conjugated antibodies or staining with polyclonal horse raddish peroxidase-conjugated antibodies only, specific detection of CD81 was confirmed (data not shown). Further semi-quantitative analysis was performed by automated densitometry.

Quantification of CD81

Huh7 cells are characterized by high CD81 expression [28]. Serial dilutions of a cell lysate of 10^4 Huh7 were used as standard for semi-quantitative assessment of serum CD81. Aliquots of the lysate were stored at −80°C until use, and applied as the same standard for all experiments. CD81 in Huh7 cell lysates was detected by immunoblotting and densitometric analysis by use of an analysis program (Gelscan 5, BioSciTec GmbH, Frankfurt, Germany). Concentration of serum derived CD81 was assessed semi-quantitatively in relation to the standard curve obtained from the Huh7 cell lysate dilutions by densitometry and expressed as relative units (RU).

Measurement of HCV RNA from native serum and HCV genotyping

Quantitative assessment of HCV RNA in serum was performed by a quantitative reverse transcription polymerase chain reaction assay (Cobas Amplicor HCV MonitorTM 2.0, Roche Diagnostic Systems, Branchburg, NJ; lower detection limit, 600 IU/mL). Samples with HCV RNA concentration above the upper detection limit above 800.000 IU/mL were diluted appropriately. HCV genotyping was performed by reverse hybridization assay (Inno LiPA HCV II, Innogenetics, Gent, Belgium). All contamination prevention measures suggested by Kwok and Higuchi were strictly applied [29].

Measurement of HCV RNA in enriched serum

For comparison with serum HCV RNA and correlation to CD81 concentration within enriched serum fraction p5, HCV RNA was assessed in enriched serum, also. Therefore, differential centrifugation was performed in accordance to the CD81 enrichment protocol. Each pellet from a given centrifugation step was resuspended in 0.25 mL PBS, and HCV RNA was extracted fully automatic (COBAS-Ampliprep, Roche, Mannheim, Germany). Quantification of HCV RNA was performed standardized by real-time polymerase chain reaction (COBAS-Taqman 48 Analyzer Roche, Mannheim, Germany).

Statistical analyses

Unless indicated otherwise, all tests were two tailed and p values<0.05 were considered significant. Clinical and biochemical characteristics of patients were expressed as mean ± standard deviation (SD) or median and range as appropriate. Correlations between two variables were calculated by the spearman test. Furthermore, Kruskal-Wallis test, Friedman test, Wilcoxon-paired sample test and Wilcoxon Mann-Whitney U test were applied as appropriate. A Bonferroni correction was applied, if multiple comparisons were performed. A receiver operating characteristic analysis was performed to compare CD81-p5 and severity of liver fibrosis.

Results

Detection of CD81 in the exosomal serum fraction

Detection of exosomal CD81 in plasma from patients with chronic hepatitis C has been previously described by Masciopinto et al. [25]. In the present study, we investigated whether exosomal CD81 is also detectable in human serum. For this purpose, differential centrifugation for enrichment of exosomal CD81 was performed with human plasma and serum as previously described for plasma, followed by immunoblotting with CD81 specific monoclonal antibodies [25]. Lysates from Huh7 cells characterized by high CD81 expression were used as positive control. Consistently, CD81 was absent in fractions p2 and p3, weakly detectable in fraction p4 and reliably detectable in the exosomal fraction p5 of both plasma and serum samples (Figure 1 A, B). The only difference in detection of CD81 in serum vs. plasma samples was found in the p1 fraction corresponding to the cellular fraction. Here, CD81 was detectable in plasma samples only. Fraction p5 containing exosomal CD81 was used for subsequent analyses. Enrichment of CD81 from different volumes of serum ranging from 1 mL to 30 mL showed that robust detection of CD81 was feasible with the smallest tested volume of 1 mL serum. This volume was used in all further analyses.

Quantification of serum CD81

We next investigated whether CD81 concentration in the p5 fraction can be quantified. For this purpose, different dilutions of Huh7cell lysates were detected by Western blot analysis and quantified by densitometry. As shown in Figure 1 C and D, this approach allowed semiquantitative assessment of CD81 in the p5 fraction (CD81-p5). In the subsequent experiments, different dilutions of Huh7 lysates covering the range of serum CD81-p5 were used as reference standard. Stock solutions from the same lysate were used for all analyses (Figure 2A).

Association of serum CD81-p5 with chronic hepatitis C virus infection

Aim of this study was to investigate whether soluble CD81 levels are increased in patients with chronic hepatitis C. Therefore, the concentration of soluble CD81 in the exosomal fraction p5 was compared between a cohort of 23 healthy controls and 37 patients with chronic hepatitis C. As shown in Figure 2, the serum CD81 concentration in fraction p5 was significantly higher in patients with chronic hepatitis C compared with healthy controls (Figure 2 A, B). In patients with chronic hepatitis C, CD81-p5 was neither associated with patients characteristics such as age and gender (Table 1). Apparently, there was no association between CD81-p5 and HCV genotype, however, reliable conclusions on the association between HCV genotype and soluble CD81 cannot be drawn due to imbalanced genotype distribution in the different cohorts. To investigate whether HCV infection is associated with an increase of serum obtained CD81, CD81-p5 was analyzed in a cohort of patients with long term cure of HCV after pegylated interferon-alfa based antiviral therapy and compared with CD81-p5 in healthy controls and in patients with chronic hepatitis C. In patients with cured hepatitis C the CD81-p5 level was similar to healthy controls and significantly lower than in patients with chronic hepatitis C (Figure 2 B).

CD81-p5 concentration and inflammatory activity

Exosomal CD81 may also be associated with inflammatory activity. To investigate a potential association between the CD81 concentration in the p5 fraction and liver inflammation, CD81-p5 was analyzed in a cohort of patients with chronic hepatitis C and persistently normal ALT levels. In the present study, patients with chronic hepatitis C and persistently normal ALT levels showed lower CD81-p5 levels than patients with chronic hepatitis C and elevated ALT levels and comparable levels of CD81-p5 with healthy controls and patients with cured HCV.

Overall, the CD81-p5 level was associated with serum ALT activity in patients with chronic hepatitis C with or without ALT elevation ($r = 0.372$, $p = 0.003$, Figure 2C). Furthermore, we observed a significant association between CD81-p5 and aspartate aminotransferase serum levels ($r = 0.306$, $p = 0.017$; Figure 2D). Both associations were significant for the complete cohort of patient with chronic HCV infection only, but not for subgroups with normal or elevated ALT levels, respectively ($p>0.2$ for both). Gamma-glutamyl transferase levels were significantly associated with ALT and AST serum levels but not with CD81-p5 ($r = 0.589$; $p<0.001$; $r = 0.576$, $p<0.001$; $r = 0.228$, $p = 0.08$, respectively).

We also analyzed the association between CD81-p5 and histological liver damage. CD81-p5 was significantly associated with severe vs. non severe fibrosis (area under curve 0.699, $p = 0.027$, Figure 3). However, no correlation was noticed between CD81-p5 and histological necroinflammatory activity ($p>0.2$).

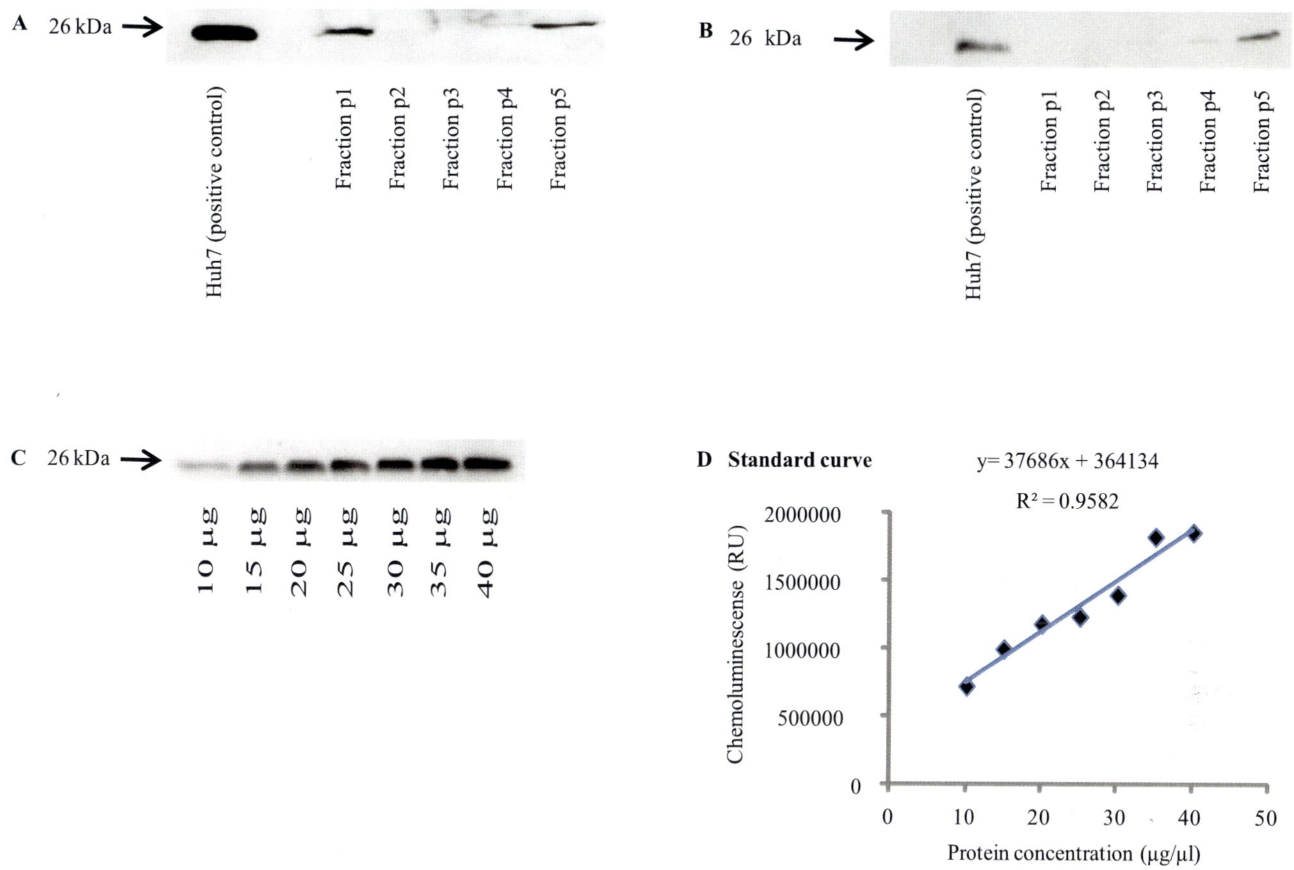

Figure 1. Enrichment and quantification of soluble CD81. (A, B) Immunoblotting of soluble CD81 is shown after enrichment by differential centrifugation of frozen (A) plasma and (B) serum samples. Huh7 cells served as positive control, and HepG2 cells as negative control. While only a marginal fraction was detectable in fraction p4, the main portion was detectable in fraction p5, comparable between plasma and serum samples. (C, D). Soluble CD81 concentration was assessed semi-quantitatively by use of dilutions from a Huh7 cell lysate by densitometric analysis. The lysate dilution immunoblot analysis and the corresponding obtained standard curve are shown in (C) and (D), respectively.

Serum ALT and AST levels also did not show significant correlations with necroinflammatory activity ($p>0.2$ for both).

CD81-p5 and HCV RNA

As HCV binds to CD81, the CD81 concentration in fraction p5 may be associated with the HCV RNA level. The HCV RNA concentration was quantified in unfractionated serum and in the enriched serum fraction p5 in all patients with chronic HCV infection (Figure 4 A, B). The HCV RNA concentration in unfractionated serum was significantly correlated with the HCV RNA concentration in fraction p5 ($p<0.001$; $r=0.696$, Figure 4C). However, the CD81 concentration in fraction p5 neither correlated with the HCV RNA concentration in unfractionated serum ($p=0.373$; $r=0.135$, Figure 4A) nor with the HCV RNA concentration in fraction p5 ($p=0.39$; $r=0.15$, Figure 4D). Accordant analyses of the subgroups of patients with persistently normal or elevated ALT serum levels showed no correlation between HCV RNA concentration in serum or HCV RNA concentration in fraction p5 with CD81-p5, respectively ($p>0.2$ for both subgroups).

Discussion

The tetraspanin CD81 is an essential HCV hepatocyte cell entry receptor [13,14]. Interplay between HCV and CD81 expressed on PBMC has been related to HCV persistence as well as modulation of extrahepatic manifestations of chronic HCV infection [16–20,27].

CD81 containing exosomes have not been studied in larger cohorts of patients with chronic hepatitis C, so far. Exosomes are small vesicles secreted by vital cells only, amongst others considered to modify immune response in viral and malignant diseases [23,30–33]. For instance, exosome mediated infection of cells has been described in human immunodeficiency virus infection [32]. Moreover, exosome mediated intercellular transfer of CD81 and enhancement of CD81 concentration on cell surfaces by mergence has been observed [23]. Therefore, exosomal CD81 taken up by target cells, e.g. hepatocytes, could increase HCV receptor density and facilitate HCV entry, and HCV particles bound to exosomal CD81 could moreover represent an additional HCV compartment with putative relevance for the HCV infection rate. Aim of the present study was to quantify and compare CD81 in the exosomal serum fraction in patients with chronic hepatitis C compared to healthy controls and patients with cured hepatitis, and furthermore to investigate whether soluble CD81 in the exosomal serum fraction is associated with inflammatory activity in chronic hepatitis C.

Enrichment of exosomes from plasma or serum, as performed within the current study, can be performed by differential centrifugation [23,25]. Here, CD81 is an exosomal marker

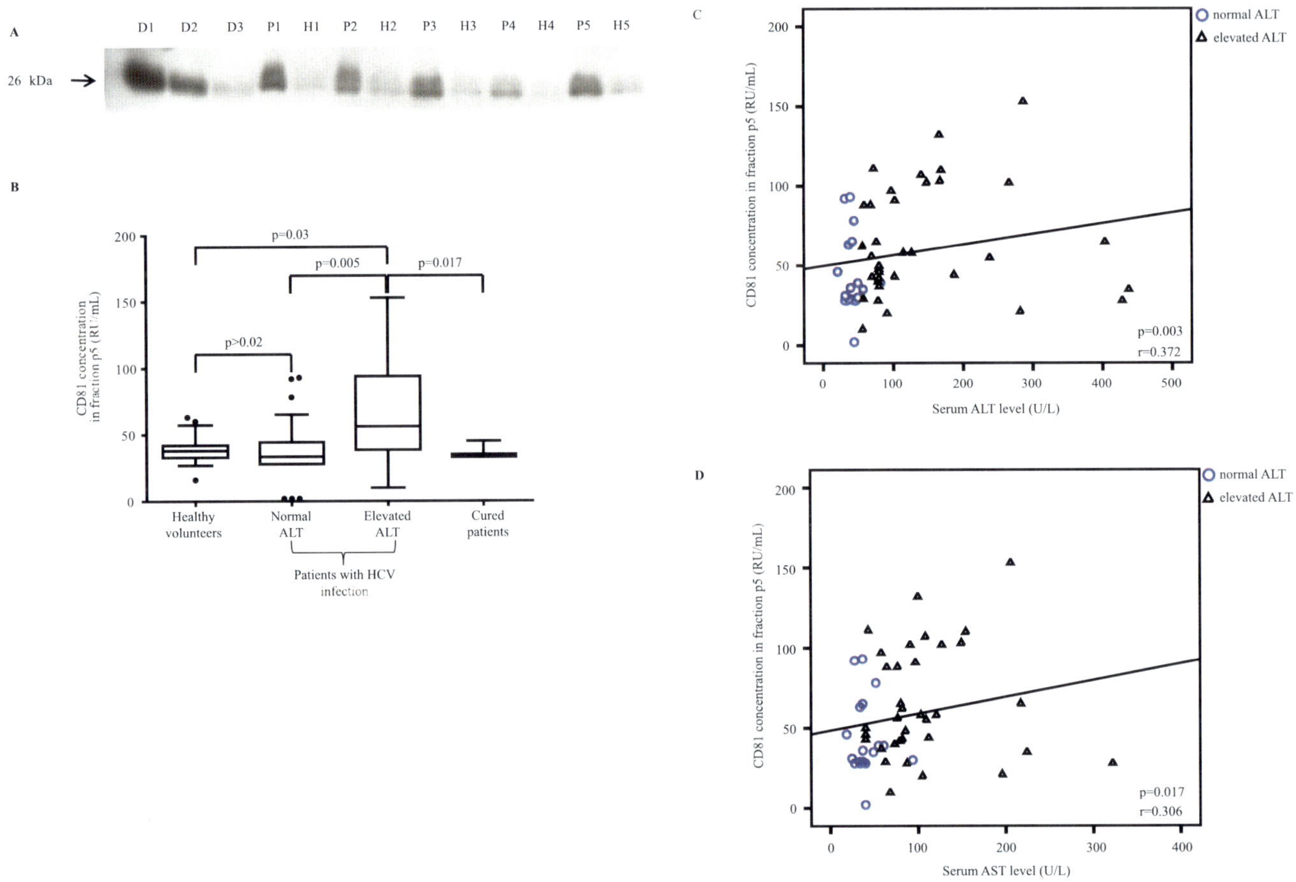

Figure 2. Quantification of soluble CD81 serum levels in different populations and correlation to serum ALT and AST levels. (A) Immunoblot analysis from representative patient samples (P1–P5) and healthy controls (H1–H5) as well as Huh7 dilution series (D1–D3). Enrichment of soluble CD81 had been standardized before sample processing, and a standardized volume of 1 mL serum was used for CD81 enrichment and quantification in all study samples analyzed. (B) Enriched CD81 serum concentrations given in healthy volunteers (n = 23), patients with chronic HCV infection and persistently normal ALT levels (n = 24), patients with chronic hepatitis C and elevated ALT levels (n = 37), and patients with long-term SVR (n = 7). The CD81 concentration is given in relative units (RU)/mL as box-and-whisker plot showing median, 25 and 75 quartiles as well as the total range. Differences between two groups were calculated by the Mann-Whitney U test. (C) Correlation of CD81 concentration in fraction p5 given in RU/mL and serum ALT level given in U/mL in all patients with chronic HCV infection, including patients with elevated (△) and persistently normal (○) ALT levels (n = 61). Correlations between two variables were assessed by the Spearman's rank correlation test. (D) Correlation of CD81 concentration in fraction p5 given in RU/mL and serum AST level given in U/mL in all patients with chronic HCV infection, including patients with elevated (△) and persistently normal (○) ALT levels (n = 61). Correlations between two variables were assessed by the Spearman's rank correlation test.

protein, and the CD81 content in the exosomal fraction can be considered to be mainly of exosomal origin [23,25]. Therefore, we measured the concentration of soluble CD81 after differential centrifugation of a standardized volume of 1 mL serum.

In the present study, soluble CD81 levels were increased in the exosomal serum fraction p5 in patients with chronic hepatitis C compared to healthy volunteers. Moreover, in patients cured from hepatitis C, CD81 levels normalized to levels found in healthy subjects. Overall these results suggest that infection with the hepatitis C virus is associated with increase of soluble CD81.

Soluble CD81 could be associated with HCV replication. Therefore, we assessed whether soluble CD81 correlates with the HCV RNA level. In the present study, however, HCV RNA serum levels were not correlated with the CD81 concentration in the exosomal serum fraction p5. HCV RNA may also bind to exosomal CD81 which is suggested by data from Masciopinto et al., who have shown an association of HCV envelope proteins and HCV RNA with exosomal CD81 *in vitro* [25]. In the present study, HCV RNA was enriched in the exosomal serum fraction; however, the concentration of HCV RNA in the exosomal serum fraction was not correlated with the soluble CD81 concentration. Therefore, it may be concluded that exosomal CD81 is not directly involved in HCV replication.

Recently, proinflammatory exosomes have been described to contribute to inflammation e.g. in sarcoidosis [34]. To investigate whether increased soluble CD81 levels are associated with disease activity in chronic HCV infection, we compared soluble CD81 serum levels in patients with chronic hepatitis C to a cohort of patients with HCV infection but persistently normal ALT levels as ALT is a surrogate marker for apoptosis and necroinflammation in chronic hepatitis C. It is estimated that approximately 30% of patients with HCV show normal ALT levels [35]. The reason therefore is unknown, but it was suggested that an arbitrary high upper limit of normal range may contribute to this phenomenon [36]. The long term clinical outcome is not completely known.

Patients with HCV infection and persistently normal ALT levels may show a more benign course than patients with elevated ALT levels. Nevertheless, several studies described significant histological liver lesions and increased ALT levels over time in these patients [36–40], indicating that this specific cohort may develop

Table 1. Baseline characteristics of patients and healthy controls.

		Patients with chronic HCV infection		Patients with SVR	Healthy volunteers
		normal ALT	elevated ALT		
		(n = 24)	(n = 37)	(n = 7)	(n = 23)
Demography					
Age (mean ± SD)		50.8±11.8	53.3±10.2	63.6±11.8	29.4±5.7
Gender (male/female)		10/14	15/22	4/3	12/11
Biochemistry					
ALT (U/L; mean ± SD)		41.4±12.8	145.3±108.3	28.7±10.8	26.5±4.9
AST (U/L; mean ± SD)		39.9±16.9	106.7±61.8	38.4±4.1	29.1±5.5
GGT (U/L; mean ± SD)		49.3±48.1	99.8±71.3	24.5±10.6	30.0±6.8
Histological activity index					
I	(median [min., max.])	1 (1, 1)	1 (1, 3)	n.d.	n.a.
II	(median [min., max.])	1 (1, 1)	1 (1, 1)	n.d.	n.a.
III	(median [min., max.])	3 (1, 3)	3 (1,3)	n.d.	n.a.
IV	(median [min., max.])	1 (1, 3)	3 (1,3)	n.d.	n.a.
Virology					
Genotype distribution (1/2/3)		17/4/3	32/1/4	n.d.	n.a.
HCV RNA (log IU/mL, mean ± SD)		5.8±0.6	6.1±0.6	n.d.	n.a.

ALT, alanine transaminase; AST, aspartate transaminase; GGT, gamma-glutamyl transferase (the upper limit of normal was 50 U/L, 50 U/L, 39 U/L for ALT, AST and GGT); max., maximum; min; minimum; n.a., not applicable; n.d., not done NR, nonresponse SD, standard deviation; SVR, sustained virologic response.

liver damage in the absence of surrogate cell death markers. In the current study, soluble CD81 levels were significantly higher in patients with hepatitis C compared to patients with HCV infection and normal ALT levels. This may indicate that increase of soluble CD81 in patients with chronic hepatitis C is mostly related with HCV associated necroinflammation.

To further investigate the observed correlation between soluble CD81 levels and necroinflammatory activity, we compared CD81 levels to ALT and AST levels. Here, a significant correlation between serum ALT as well as AST levels and soluble CD81 was observed. This may indicate an association between hepatocyte cell death and higher CD81 serum levels. The association between soluble CD81 and surrogate markers of cell death could be due to release of CD81 containing exosomes or cell detritus from hepatocytes during the necroinflammatory process. However, the correlation coefficients between soluble CD81 levels and biochemical markers of liver damage, even though statistically significant, were weak. A final conclusion that soluble CD81 levels are mostly derived from inflammatory processes in patients with hepatitis C cannot be drawn from the results of the current study.

Another explanation for the increase of soluble CD81 levels in patients with chronic hepatitis C is secretion of CD81 containing exosomes by lymphocytes. Interaction of HCV particles with CD81 expressed on PBMC as well as alteration of CD81 expression on PBMC during HCV infection is well known and of clinical importance [18,19,41]. Potential interaction of PBMC released CD81 exosomes with HCV particles may occur and influence hepatic inflammation in chronic hepatitis C. Here, further studies defining the source of soluble CD81 in HCV infection are necessary.

In summary, the results of the present study show that chronic HCV infection is associated with increase of soluble CD81 in the exosomal serum fraction. CD81 in the exosomal fraction in patients with chronic hepatitis C appears to be associated with inflammatory activity. This is a new finding with potential implications in the understanding of HCV persistence and HCV-associated necroinflammation. In concordance, soluble CD81 levels were associated with higher stage liver fibrosis.

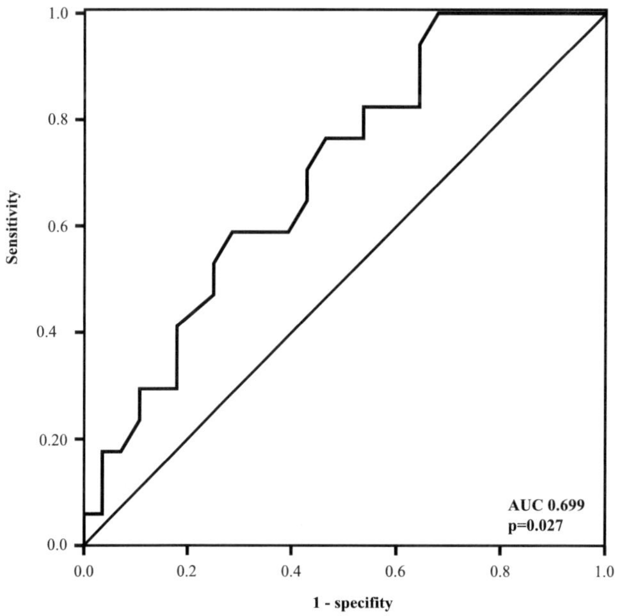

Figure 3. Receiver operating characteristic showing the association between soluble CD81 serum concentration and fibrosis. Higher CD81-p5 levels were associated with sever fibroses (area under curve, AUC, 0.699; p = 0.027).

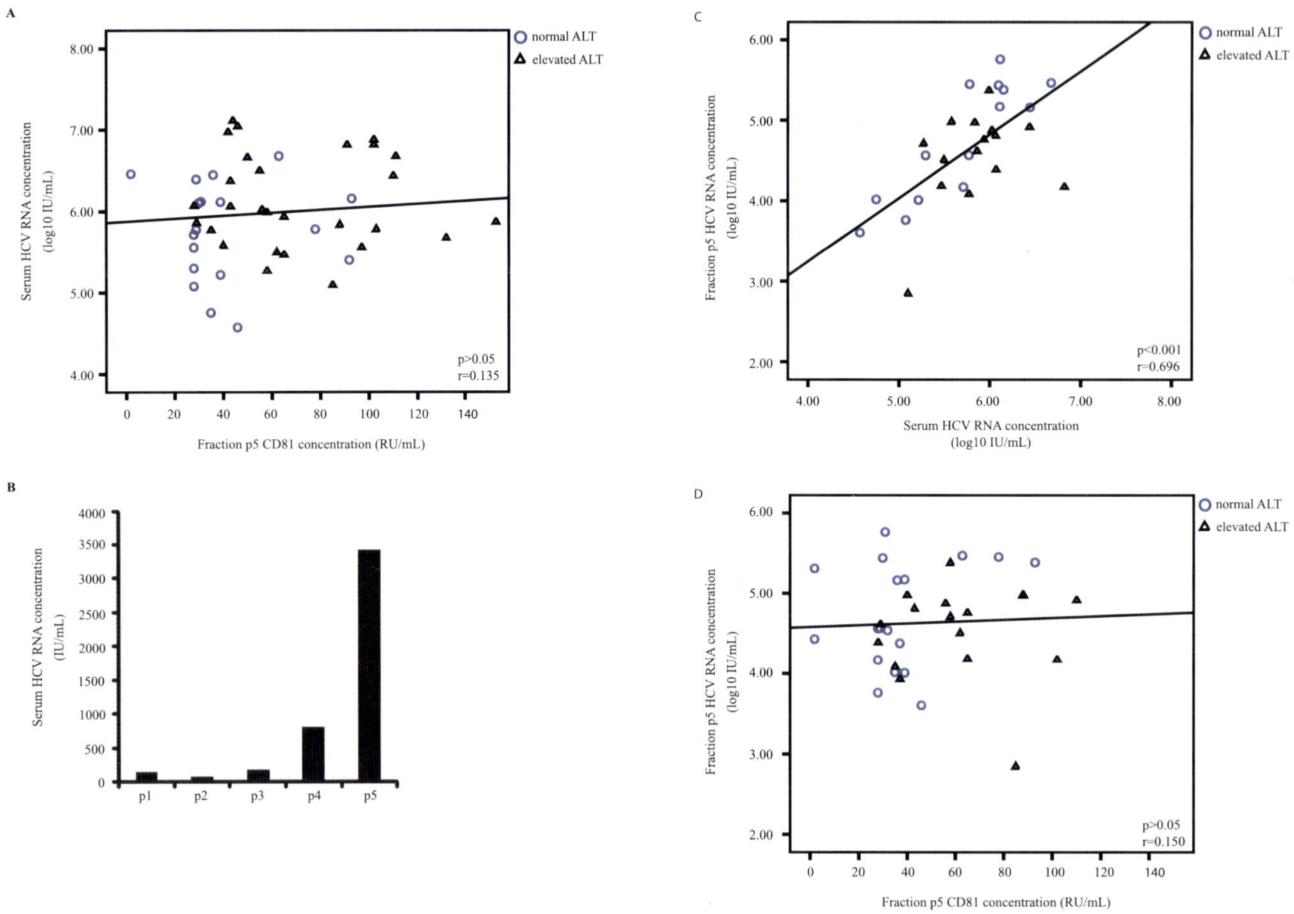

Figure 4. Association of HCV RNA levels and the concentration of CD81 in serum fraction p5 in patients with chronic hepatitis C and persistently normal (○) and elevated (△) ALT levels. Correlations between two variables were assessed by the Spearman's rank correlation test. (A) Serum HCV RNA and CD81 concentration in fraction p5 were not correlated. (B) Quantification of HCV RNA in the different serum fractions showing the highest HCV RNA concentration in fraction p5. (C) Correlation between HCV RNA concentration in fraction p5 and serum showing high correlation between HCV RNA concentration in unfractionated and enriched serum. (D) Concentrations of HCV RNA in fraction p5 and CD81 fraction p5 showed no correlation. P values and correlation coefficient r are given for each correlation.

Author Contributions

Conceived and designed the experiments: MWW CS EH SZ AP BK. Performed the experiments: DR SS YM. Analyzed the data: MWW DR CS EH SZ AP BK. Contributed reagents/materials/analysis tools: CS EH SZ AP BK. Wrote the paper: MWW CS SZ AP BK.

References

1. Alter MJ, Margolis HS, Krawczynski K, Judson FN, Mares A, et al. (1992) The natural history of community-acquired hepatitis C in the United States. The Sentinel Counties Chronic non-A, non-B Hepatitis Study Team. N Engl J Med 327: 1899–1905.
2. Saito I, Miyamura T, Ohbayashi A, Harada H, Katayama T, et al. (1990) Hepatitis C virus infection is associated with the development of hepatocellular carcinoma. Proc Natl Acad Sci U S A 87: 6547–6549.
3. Lange CM, Sarrazin C, Zeuzem S (2010) Review article: specifically targeted anti-viral therapy for hepatitis C - a new era in therapy. Aliment Pharmacol Ther 32: 14–28.
4. Jacobson IM, McHutchison JG, Dusheiko G, Di Bisceglie AM, Reddy KR, et al. (2011) Telaprevir for Previously Untreated Chronic Hepatitis C Virus Infection. New England Journal of Medicine 364: 2405–2416.
5. Poordad F, McCone J, Bacon BR, Bruno S, Manns MP, et al. (2011) Boceprevir for Untreated Chronic HCV Genotype 1 Infection. New England Journal of Medicine 364: 1195–1206.
6. Kronenberger B, Zeuzem S (2009) Current and future treatment options for HCV. Annals of Hepatology 8: 103–112.
7. Wakita T, Pietschmann T, Kato T, Date T, Miyamoto M, et al. (2005) Production of infectious hepatitis C virus in tissue culture from a cloned viral genome. Nat Med 11: 791–796.
8. Welker MW, Zeuzem S (2009) Occult Hepatitis C: How Convincing Are the Current Data? Hepatology 49: 665–675.
9. Moradpour D, Penin F, Rice CM (2007) Replication of hepatitis C virus. Nat Rev Microbiol 5: 453–463.
10. Perelson AS, Herrmann E, Micol F, Zeuzem S (2005) New kinetic models for the hepatitis C virus. Hepatology 42: 749–754.
11. Zeisel MB, Fofana I, Fafi-Kremer S, Baumert TF (2011) Hepatitis C virus entry into hepatocytes: Molecular mechanisms and targets for antiviral therapies. Journal of Hepatology 54: 566–576.
12. Ploss A, Evans MJ, Gaysinskaya VA, Panis M, You H, et al. (2009) Human occludin is a hepatitis C virus entry factor required for infection of mouse cells. Nature 457: 882–886.
13. Pileri P, Uematsu Y, Campagnoli S, Galli G, Falugi F, et al. (1998) Binding of hepatitis C virus to CD81. Science 282: 938–941.
14. Bartosch B, Vitelli A, Granier C, Goujon C, Dubuisson J, et al. (2003) Cell entry of hepatitis C virus requires a set of co-receptors that include the CD81 tetraspanin and the SR-B1 scavenger receptor. J Biol Chem 278: 41624–41630.
15. Evans MJ, von Hahn T, Tscherne DM, Syder AJ, Panis M, et al. (2007) Claudin-1 is a hepatitis C virus co-receptor required for a late step in entry. Nature 446: 801–805.

16. Crotta S, Stilla A, Wack A, D'Andrea A, Nuti S, et al. (2002) Inhibition of natural killer cells through engagement of CD81 by the major hepatitis C virus envelope protein. J Exp Med 195: 35–41.
17. Wack A, Soldaini E, Tseng C, Nuti S, Klimpel G, et al. (2001) Binding of the hepatitis C virus envelope protein E2 to CD81 provides a co-stimulatory signal for human T cells. Eur J Immunol 31: 166–175.
18. Kronenberger B, Herrmann E, Hofmann WP, Wedemeyer H, Sester M, et al. (2006) Dynamics of CD81 expression on lymphocyte subsets during interferon-alpha-based antiviral treatment of patients with chronic hepatitis C. J Leukoc Biol 80: 298–308.
19. Zuckerman E (2003) Expansion of CD5+ B-cell overexpressing CD81 in HCV infection: towards better understanding the link between HCV infection, B-cell activation and lymphoproliferation. J Hepatol 38: 674–676.
20. Tseng CT, Klimpel GR (2002) Binding of the hepatitis C virus envelope protein E2 to CD81 inhibits natural killer cell functions. J Exp Med 195: 43–49.
21. Yoon JC, Shiina M, Ahlenstiel G, Rehermann B (2009) Natural killer cell function is intact after direct exposure to infectious hepatitis C virions. Hepatology 49: 12–21.
22. Conde-Vancells J, Rodriguez-Suarez E, Embade N, Gil D, Matthiesen R, et al. (2008) Characterization and comprehensive proteome profiling of exosomes secreted by hepatocytes. J Proteome Res 7: 5157–5166.
23. Fritzsching B, Schwer B, Kartenbeck J, Pedal A, Horejsi V, et al. (2002) Release and intercellular transfer of cell surface CD81 via microparticles. J Immunol 169: 5531–5537.
24. Lykke-Andersen S, Brodersen DE, Jensen TH (2009) Origins and activities of the eukaryotic exosome. J Cell Sci 122: 1487–1494.
25. Masciopinto F, Giovani C, Campagnoli S, Galli-Stampino L, Colombatto P, et al. (2004) Association of hepatitis C virus envelope proteins with exosomes. Eur J Immunol 34: 2834–2842.
26. Knodell RG, Ishak KG, Black WC, Chen TS, Craig R, et al. (1981) Formulation and application of a numerical scoring system for assessing histological activity in asymptomatic chronic active hepatitis. Hepatology 1: 431–435.
27. Levy S, Todd SC, Maecker HT (1998) CD81 (TAPA-1): a molecule involved in signal transduction and cell adhesion in the immune system. Annu Rev Immunol 16: 89–109.
28. Koutsoudakis G, Herrmann E, Kallis S, Bartenschlager R, Pietschmann T (2007) The level of CD81 cell surface expression is a key determinant for productive entry of hepatitis C virus into host cells. Journal of Virology 81: 588–598.
29. Kwok S, Higuchi R (1989) Avoiding false positives with PCR. Nature 339: 237–238.
30. Thery C, Zitvogel L, Amigorena S (2002) Exosomes: composition, biogenesis and function. Nat Rev Immunol 2: 569–579.
31. Rana S, Zoller M (2011) Exosome target cell selection and the importance of exosomal tetraspanins: a hypothesis. Biochemical Society Transactions 39: 559–562.
32. Wiley RD, Gummuluru S (2006) Immature dendritic cell-derived exosomes can mediate HIV-1 trans infection. Proc Natl Acad Sci U S A 103: 738–743.
33. Whiteside TW, Mandapathil M, Szczepanski M, Szajnik M (2011) Mechanisms of tumor escape from the immune system: Adenosine-producing Treg, exosomes and tumor-associated TLRs. Bulletin du Cancer 98: E25–E31.
34. Qazi KR, Paredes PT, Dahlberg B, Grunewald J, Eklund A, et al. (2010) Proinflammatory exosomes in bronchoalveolar lavage fluid of patients with sarcoidosis. Thorax 65: 1016–1023.
35. Bacon BR (2002) Treatment of patients with hepatitis C and normal serum aminotransferase levels. Hepatology 36: S179–S184.
36. Prati D, Taioli E, Zanella A, Della Torre E, Butelli S, et al. (2002) Updated definitions of healthy ranges for serum alanine aminotransferase levels. Annals of Internal Medicine 137: 1–9.
37. Puoti C, Bellis L, Guarisco R, Dell' Unto O, Spilabotti L, et al. (2010) HCV carriers with normal alanine aminotransferase levels: Healthy persons or severely ill patients? Dealing with an everyday clinical problem. European Journal of Internal Medicine 21: 57–61.
38. Alberti A, Noventa F, Benvegnu L, Boccato S, Gatta A (2002) Prevalence of liver disease in a population of asymptomatic persons with hepatitis C virus infection. Annals of Internal Medicine 137: 961–964.
39. Martinot-Peignoux M, Boyer N, Cazals-Hatem D, Pham BN, Gervais A, et al. (2001) Prospective study on anti-hepatitis C virus-positive patients with persistently normal serum alanine transaminase with or without detectable serum hepatitis C virus RNA. Hepatology 34: 1000–1005.
40. Zeuzem S, Diago M, Gane E, Reddy KR, Pockros P, et al. (2004) Peginterferon alfa-2a (40 kilodaltons) and ribavirin in patients with chronic hepatitis C and normal aminotransferase levels. Gastroenterology 127: 1724–1732.
41. Zuckerman E, Kessel A, Slobodin G, Sabo E, Yeshurun D, et al. (2003) Antiviral treatment down-regulates peripheral B-cell CD81 expression and CD5 expansion in chronic hepatitis C virus infection. J Virol 77: 10432–10436.

Unhealthy Alcohol Use, HIV Infection and Risk of Liver Fibrosis in Drug Users with Hepatitis C

Roberto Muga[1]*, Arantza Sanvisens[1], Daniel Fuster[1,2], Jordi Tor[1], Elisenda Martínez[1], Santiago Pérez-Hoyos[3], Alvaro Muñoz[4]

1 Department of Internal Medicine, Hospital Universitari Germans Trias i Pujol, Universitat Autònoma Barcelona, Barcelona, Spain, **2** Section of General Internal Medicine, Boston Medical Center, Boston University School of Medicine, Boston, Massachusetts, United States of America, **3** Department of Public Health, Institut de Recerca Hospital Vall d'Hebrón, Universitat Autònoma Barcelona, Barcelona, Spain, **4** Department of Epidemiology, Johns Hopkins University, Bloomberg School of Public Health, Baltimore, Maryland, United States of America

Abstract

Aim: To analyze alcohol use, clinical data and laboratory parameters that may affect FIB-4, an index for measuring liver fibrosis, in HCV-monoinfected and HCV/HIV-coinfected drug users.

Patients and Methods: Patients admitted for substance abuse treatment between 1994 and 2006 were studied. Socio-demographic data, alcohol and drug use characteristics and clinical variables were obtained through hospital records. Blood samples for biochemistry, liver function tests, CD4 cell count, and serology of HIV and HCV infection were collected at admission. Multivariate linear regression was used to analyze the predictors of FIB-4 increase.

Results: A total of 472 (83% M, 17% F) patients were eligible. The median age at admission was 31 years (Interquartile range (IQR) 27–35 years), and the median duration of drug use was 10 years (IQR 5.5–15 years). Unhealthy drinking ($>$50 grams/day) was reported in 32% of the patients. The FIB-4 scores were significantly greater in the HCV/HIV-coinfected patients (1.14, IQR 0.76–1.87) than in the HCV-monoinfected patients (0.75, IQR 0.56–1.11) ($p<0.001$). In the multivariate analysis, unhealthy drinking ($p=0.034$), lower total cholesterol ($p=0.042$), serum albumin ($p<0.001$), higher GGT ($p<0.001$) and a longer duration of addiction ($p=0.005$) were independently associated with higher FIB-4 scores in the HCV-monoinfected drug users. The effect of unhealthy drinking on FIB-4 scores disappeared in the HCV/HIV-coinfected patients, whereas lower serum albumin ($p<0.001$), a lower CD4 cell count ($p=0.006$), higher total bilirubin ($p<0.001$) and a longer drug addiction duration ($p<0.001$) were significantly associated with higher FIB-4 values.

Conclusions: Unhealthy alcohol use in the HCV-monoinfected patients and HIV-related immunodeficiency in the HCV/HIV-coinfected patients are important risk factors associated with liver fibrosis in the respective populations

Editor: Michael Alan Polis, National Institute of Allergy and Infectious Diseases, United States of America

Funding: This work was funded by grants from Ministry of Science and Innovation, Spain (grants RD06/001, RD06/006 and PI05/1550), the Agència de Gestió d'Ajuts Universitaris i de Recerca (AGAUR) (grant 2008 BE-2 00269), Ministry of Health (grant EC11-042) and Ministry of Education (grant 2010-0945). The funders had no role in study design, data collection and analysis, decision to publish, or preparation of the manuscript.

Competing Interests: The authors have declared that no competing interests exist.

* E-mail: rmuga.germanstrias@gencat.cat

Introduction

Liver fibrosis is the main predictor of whether chronic hepatitis C will progress to cirrhosis and end-stage liver disease [1]. Because the complications of liver disease mainly occur in patients with advanced-stage fibrosis, assessing chronic hepatitis C early is essential when evaluating at-risk patients [2]. In Western countries, more than 50% of new HCV infections are associated with drug abuse. However, this particular population also has lower rates of clinical assessment and chronic hepatitis C treatment. Given the likelihood of new and more effective treatments, drug abusers with chronic hepatitis C would benefit from simple, non-invasive measurements of liver fibrosis.

The cofactors associated with chronic hepatitis C progression differ among studies; alcohol abuse, male gender, age at infection, body mass index, and coinfection with human immunodeficiency virus infection (HIV) and Hepatitis B virus infection (HBV) have been related to more rapid disease progression [1–5]. In HCV/HIV-coinfected individuals, CD4 cell counts below 200 cells/μL have been associated with liver fibrosis progression [6]. In parallel, highly active antiretroviral therapy (HAART) has been shown to reduce liver-related deaths [7,8].

In HIV-negative patients, it is well established that alcohol abuse and HCV infection have a synergistic effect on liver fibrosis. However, there are conflicting results regarding the independent effect of alcohol on liver damage in HCV/HIV-coinfected patients [6,9,10].

Liver biopsy is the gold standard for assessing fibrosis [11]. However, assessing liver disease through an invasive procedure is unlikely in patients with substance abuse [12]. Furthermore, eligibility for chronic hepatitis C treatment in this population is low compared with eligibility in other populations [13,14]. To a certain extent, the evolution of liver disease in drug abusers parallels the natural history of chronic hepatitis C.

Several non-invasive markers of liver fibrosis have been proposed as alternatives to liver biopsy. Some of these markers reflect the modified extracellular matrix turnover that occurs during fibrogenesis [15,16], whereas others reflect alterations in hepatic function [17,18]. FIB-4 was initially described in 2006 [18], and since then, it has been proposed as reliable marker of fibrosis in both HCV-monoinfected and HCV/HIV-coinfected individuals [18,19]. FIB-4 correlates well with liver biopsy in patients with and without advanced fibrosis [20,21]. Moreover, non-invasive markers of liver fibrosis have been proposed as predictors of all-cause and liver-related mortality [22,23].

Although abuse of alcohol and illegal drugs is frequent in patients with HIV infection and HCV infection, it is unclear how non-invasive liver fibrosis tests may reflect disease progression. In this study, we hypothesize that certain clinical and laboratory characteristics may influence a simple index of fibrosis and that the cofactors associated with elevated FIB-4 scores may differ between HCV-monoinfected patients and HCV/HIV-coinfected patients. Hence, the primary objective of the study was to characterize the putative differences in risk factors for elevated liver function biomarkers between HCV-monoinfected and HCV/HIV-coinfected patients.

Patients and Methods

Study Population

This was a cross-sectional study of patients admitted for substance abuse treatment between 1994 and 2006. The demographic and drug use characteristics were recorded through a structured questionnaire administered by a physician the day of admission. Questions related to drug and alcohol abuse included: (i) the main drug of abuse (type of drug, age at first use, duration of drug use and route of administration), (ii) poly-drug use (yes/no) (iii) alcohol consumption: do you regularly drink alcohol? (yes/no); if yes, do you drink 5 or more standard drinks per day?. A standard drink unit contains 12–14 grams of alcohol and unhealthy alcohol consumption was defined as a daily alcohol intake ≥50 grams (g) [24,25] in the 6-month period prior to admission. All participants gave written informed consent. The methods used in this study complied with the ethical standards for medical research and principles of good clinical practice defined by the World Medical Association's Declaration of Helsinki. The study was approved by the Ethics Committee of the Hospital Universitari Germans Trias i Pujol.

Routine laboratory parameters, including liver function tests and serology for HIV infection and HCV infection, were analyzed at admission. Other characteristics of admission for substance abuse treatment have been described elsewhere [26].

The liver function tests and biochemical parameters were assessed using an Olympus 5200 Multichannel chemistry analyzer. The procedure, which remained the same throughout the study, was based on the reference method recommended by the International Federation of Clinical Chemistry.

HIV infection was identified by an enzyme-linked immunosorbent assay. Repeatedly reactive samples were confirmed by the Western immunoblot technique.

HCV infection was assessed prior to or during admission by a second- or later-generation enzyme immunoassay (Ortho Diagnostics, Raritan, NJ). The positive samples were confirmed by either a recombinant immunoblot assay (RIBA HCV 2 SIA, Chiron Corporation, Emeryville, CA) or a qualitative/quantitative assay (COBAS AMPLICOR, Roche Diagnostic Systems, Branchburg, NJ).

Outcome

The primary outcome was the FIB-4 score, which was calculated as

$$FIB4 = \frac{Age[years] \times AST[U/L]}{Platelet[10^9/L] \times \sqrt{ALT[U/L]}}$$

FIB-4 scores lower than 1.45 indicate lack of liver fibrosis with a negative predictive value of 90% and a sensitivity of 70% [18]. FIB-4 scores greater than 3.25 indicate significant liver fibrosis with a positive predictive value of 65% and a specificity of 97% [18].

Statistical Analysis

All of the analyses were conducted separately for the HCV-monoinfected (N = 228) and the HCV/HIV-coinfected (N = 244) individuals. We used medians and interquartile ranges (IQRs) to describe the quantitative variables and absolute frequencies and percentages to describe the qualitative variables.

The distribution of FIB-4 score was strongly skewed to the right (i.e., there were several very high values); we therefore normalized it for analysis purposes using a logarithmic transformation.

We used multiple linear regression models to determine the FIB-4 predictive values of the variables. There were three types of predictors: (1) binary, which included sex, alcohol use, and HBsAg; (2) continuous on a natural (additive) scale, which included body mass index (BMI), CD4 cell count, total cholesterol, alkaline phosphatase, and duration of drug use; and (3) continuous on a logarithmic (multiplicative) scale, which included total bilirubin, serum albumin, and GGT. The decision to analyze a variable using a logarithmic scale was based on the need to reduce the undue influence of high values in predictors with strong right skewness.

The interpretation of the regression coefficients differed among the three types of predictors. Specifically, the regression coefficients of the binary variables represented the percentage FIB-4 difference between those with and without the condition; the regression coefficients of the additive continuous variables represented the percentage FIB-4 difference associated with an unitary increase or decrease in the variables, and the regression coefficients of the multiplicative continuous variables represented the percentage FIB-4 difference associated with an increment or decrement in the variables.

The intercept represented the expected FIB-4 score in an individual with zero values for all of the predictors.

The test results were considered to be statistically significant if the resulting *P-value* was <.05. The statistical analysis was performed using the SPSS software, version 15.0.1 (SPSS, Chicago, IL, USA).

Results

Patients were eligible for this study if they had chronic HCV infection (N = 544). Patients with aminotransferase levels 10 times greater than the upper limit of the normal range (N = 5,1.0%), patients who had received HCV antiviral therapy (N = 6,1.1%) and patients with antecedent of decompensated liver cirrhosis (N = 10,1.8%) were excluded. In addition, patients with an HCV-RNA level below the limit of detection (<50 IU/mL) were excluded (N = 9, 1.7%). Finally, patients with outlier laboratory values and those with incomplete data for calculating FIB-4 score were also excluded (N = 42, 7.7%). After these exclusions, the study population consisted of 472 patients and 244 patients (52%) were coinfected with HIV. Table 1 shows the descriptive statistics at admission for the entire group and for the HCV-monoinfected (N = 228) and HCV/HIV-coinfected (N = 244) subgroups. Overall, 17% of the patients were women, the median age at admission was 31 years (IQR 27–35 years), the median BMI was 22 kg/m^2, the median duration of drug use was 10 years, and unhealthy drinking was reported in 32% of the patients. In addition to decreased CD4 cell counts, the HCV/HIV-coinfected patients had a longer median drug use duration, an increased frequency of unhealthy alcohol intake, lower levels of total cholesterol, higher levels of GGT and a higher prevalence of HBsAg than those infected with HCV only. The median AST and ALT levels and platelet counts were 35 U/L, 47 U/L, and 180 × 10^9/L, respectively.

Thirty-one percent of the HIV-positive patients were receiving antiretroviral therapy at admission, and 48% had never received antiretroviral therapy.

The median FIB-4 score at admission was 0.93 (IQR 0.65–1.46); it was significantly higher in the HCV/HIV-coinfected patients (1.14, IQR 0.76–1.87) than in the HCV-monoinfected patients (0.75, IQR 0.56–1.11). Figure 1 shows the distribution of the FIB-4 scores in the two groups on both natural and logarithmic scales. As can be seen in the bottom panels of Figure 1, the log-transformed FIB-4 scores approximately followed a normal distribution, rendering normally based methods appropriate for the analysis.

Regression Analysis of FIB-4 (Log Scale)

We conducted univariate regressions of the variables shown in Table 1 against the log-transformed FIB-4 scores; only the variables that define FIB-4 were not used in the univariate regressions. The two columns with univariate headings in Table 2 show the results of the univariate analyses separately for the monoinfected and coinfected patients.

In the univariate models for the HCV-monoinfected patients, unhealthy alcohol use, higher BMI, longer duration of drug use, lower cholesterol, higher bilirubin, lower albumin, and higher GGT were significantly associated ($p<0.05$) with higher FIB-4 scores. In the coinfected patients, higher FIB-4 scores were found to be significantly associated ($p<0.05$) with a longer drug use duration, lower cholesterol, higher alkaline phosphatase, lower CD4 cell count, higher bilirubin, lower albumin, and higher GGT.

For each group, the variables that showed significant relationships in the univariate analyses were used in a multivariate model. In the multivariate model for the HCV-monoinfected patients, unhealthy alcohol use ($p = 0.034$), longer drug use duration ($p = 0.005$), lower cholesterol ($p = 0.042$), lower albumin ($p<0.001$), and higher GGT ($p = 0.001$) continued to be significantly associated with higher FIB-4 scores.

In the coinfected patients, longer drug use duration ($p<0.001$), lower CD4 cell count ($p = 0.007$), higher bilirubin ($p<0.001$), and lower albumin ($p<0.001$) were significantly associated with higher FIB-4 scores.

Longer drug use duration and lower albumin levels were significantly associated with increased FIB-4 scores in both groups. By contrast, unhealthy alcohol use was strongly predictive of high FIB-4 scores only in the HCV-monoinfected group; similarly, high

Table 1. Descriptive statistics (median [IQR] or n (%)) of HCV-monoinfected and HCV/HIV-coinfected patients at admission to substance abuse treatment.

	HCV	HCV/HIV		Total
	N = 228	N = 244	p_value*	N = 472
Socio-demographic and anthropometric				
Females	35 (15.4%)	45 (18.4%)	0.371	80 (16.9%)
Age, years	30 [26,34]	31.5 [28, 35]	0.008	31 [27, 35]
Body mass index, kg/m^2 (N = 421)	22.3 [20.7, 24.6]	21.6 [19.6, 23.6]	0.000	21.9 [20.2, 23.9]
Drug use				
Unhealthy alcohol use (N = 440)	62 (28.2%)	79 (35.9%)	0.082	141 (32.0%)
Duration of drug use, years (N = 463)	7.6 [3.5, 12.0]	12.0 [7.6, 16.0]	0.000	10.0 [5.5, 15.0]
Laboratory parameters				
Hepatitis B surface Antigen (N = 440)	9 (4.2%)	15 (6.7%)	0.243	24 (5.5%)
Total cholesterol, mg/dL	162 [143, 178]	149 [128, 170]	0.001	155 [135, 174]
Alkaline Phosphatase, U/L	70 [55, 82]	70 [59, 86]	2.664	70 [56, 84]
Total bilirubin, mg/dL	0.4 [0.3, 0.6]	0.4 [0.3, 0.6]	0.297	0.4 [0.3, 0.6]
Albumin, g/L (N = 438)	39 [36, 42]	38 [35, 41]	0.013	39 [36, 41]
GGT, U/L	33 [19, 62]	44.5 [24, 93]	0.052	38 [22, 76]
CD4 lymphocytes, cells/μL (N = 456)	1225 [933, 1428]	383 [204, 661]	0.000	742 [350, 1225]
Laboratory components of FIB-4				
Platelets, 10^9/L	197 [166, 243]	163 [127, 196]	0.000	180 [146, 224]
AST, U/L	33.5 [21.0, 61.0]	37.5 [24.2, 61.0]	0.907	35.0 [23.0, 61.0]
ALT, U/L	54.0 [23.0, 98.0]	43.0 [25.0, 71.0]	0.001	47.0 [24.0, 84.0]

*p value for the comparison between HCV-monoinfected and HCV/HIV-coinfected patients; p values correspond to χ square test in categorical variables and t test for differences of mean values in continuous variables.

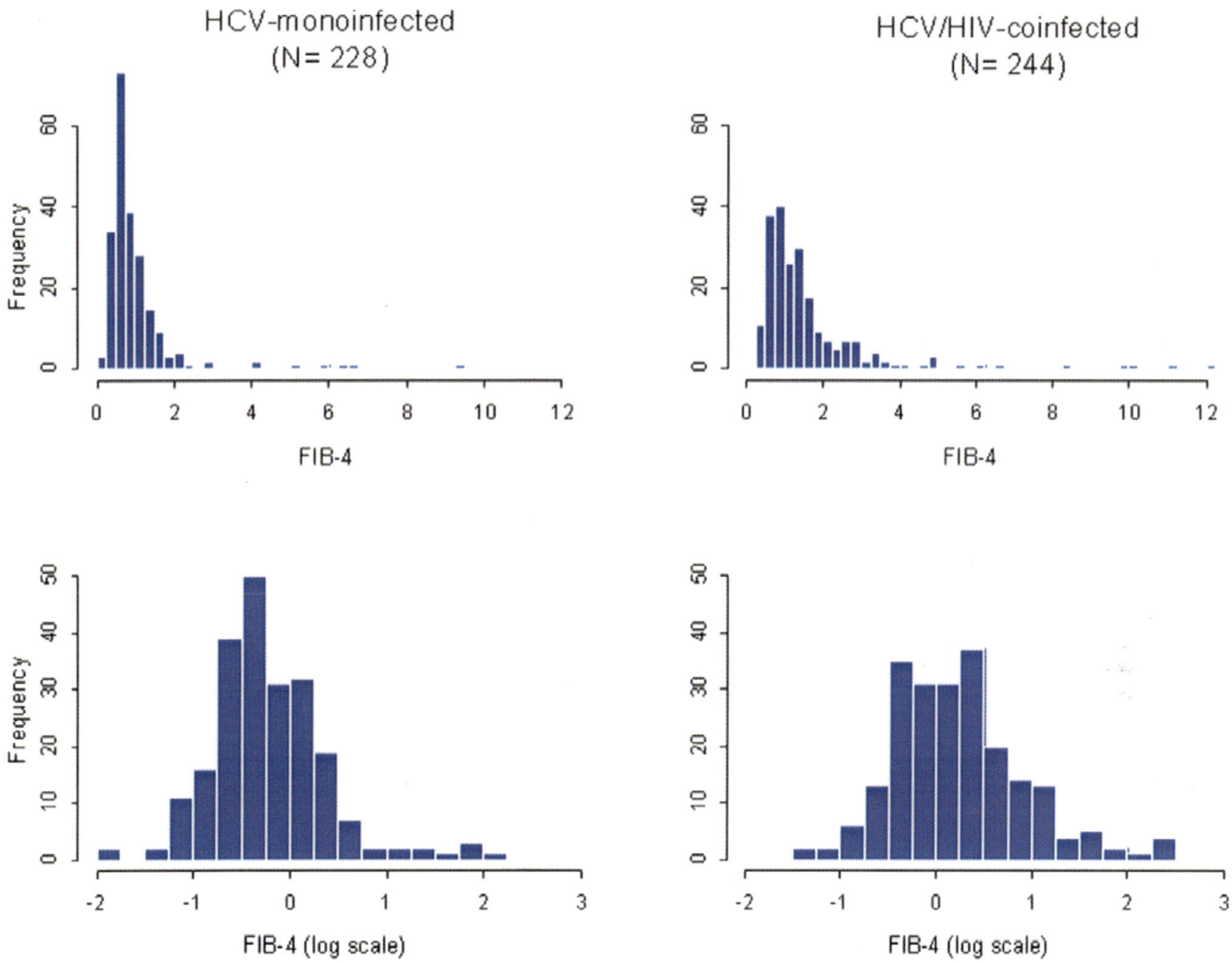

Figure 1. Distribution of FIB-4 score and log FIB-4 score according to HCV-monoinfection and HCV/HIV-coinfection.

total bilirubin levels were associated with higher FIB-4 scores only in the coinfected patients.

Although the primary aim of the study was the characterization of the variables that were associated with FIB-4 increase in HCV-monoinfected and HCV/HIV-coinfected, the intercepts of the multivariate models provide a means of comparing a hypothetical HCV-monoinfected individual with a hypothetical HCV/HIV-coinfected individual, assuming that both have 900 CD4 cells/μL and that all of the other variables are equal. The slightly increased FIB-4 intercept value (0.778 in the monoinfected and 0.875 in the coinfected patients) was not statistically significant ($p = 0.218$). However, for each decline of 100 CD4 cells/μL among the coinfected patients, there was a significant FIB-4 increase of 3.6% ($p = 0.007$) (Table 2).

To further characterize the differential effect of unhealthy alcohol use on FIB-4 scores, Figure 2 shows the distributions of the FIB-4 scores in the four groups by alcohol consumption and HIV coinfection. Figure 2 shows box plots that are graphically enhanced to show the 2.5th, 5th, 10th, 25th, 50th, 75th, 90th, 95th and 97.5th percentiles of the FIB-4 distribution. It is clear from Figure 2 that the primary difference was between the non-drinking HCV-monoinfected patients and the other three groups. In particular, the increased FIB-4 score due to unhealthy alcohol use among the HCV-monoinfected patients was similar to the effect of HIV-related immunodeficiency among the non-drinkers. The additional increase in FIB-4 among the coinfected individuals with unhealthy alcohol use was small and not significant ($p = 0.695$).

Discussion

Individuals with histories of drug use account for the majority of new hepatitis C infections in Western countries. This population is at risk for liver fibrosis, and a number of disease progression cofactors highlight the relevance of medical assessment. Evaluating liver fibrosis via non-invasive tests early in the course of drug addiction may increase the proportion of patients who are eligible for treatment. This study of young adults with chronic hepatitis C shows that the factors associated with higher FIB-4 scores clearly differed between the HCV-monoinfected and HCV/HIV-coinfected individuals.

The main contribution of the study is related to the fact that unhealthy alcohol use had a differential effect on FIB-4 values if patients have hepatitis C alone or HCV/HIV coinfection. Unhealthy alcohol drinking has been regarded as a major contributor to the progression of liver disease in the setting of chronic hepatitis C [27] and, a synergistic effect between HCV and alcohol has been proposed [28]. However, even though

Table 2. Percentage change in FIB-4 score associated with differences in predictors of higher FIB-4 scores.

	HCV-monoinfected		HCV/HIV-coinfected	
	N = 228		N = 244	
	Univariate	Multivariate	Univariate	Multivariate
Variable	**% (p_value)**	**% (p_value)**	**% (p_value)**	**% (p_value)**
Intercept	NA	0.778* (95% CI : 0.705, 0.861)	NA	0.875** (95% CI: 0.762, 1.005)
Female to Male	−11.6% (0.266)		+11.5% (0.343)	
Unhealthy alcohol use	**+46.7% (<.001)**	**+20.6% (0.034)**	+3.9% (0.695)	
HBsAg positive	+25.1% (0.268)		+31.3% (0.155)	
BMI: increase of 1 kg/m^2	**+4.3% (0.001)**	+2.2% (0.069)	+0.8% (0.609)	
Duration of drug use: increase of 5 years	**+9.4% (0.007)**	**+10.0% (0.005)**	**+21.5% (<.001)**	**+13.9% (<.001)**
Cholesterol: decrease of 20 mg/100 mL	**+5.4% (0.018)**	**+4.5% (0.042)**	**+6.6% (0.006)**	+2.4% (0.318)
Alkaline Phosphatase: increase of 10 U/L	+2.7% (0.108)		**+4.9% (0.001)**	+0.9% (0.618)
CD4: decrease of 100 cells/μL	NA	NA	**+5.2% (<.001)**	**+3.6% (0.007)**
Bilirubin: 1.5-fold increment	**+12.7% (<.001)**	+5.7% (0.097)	**+22.8% (<.001)**	**+22.2% (<.001)**
Albumin: 1.1-fold decrement	**+19.8% (<.001)**	**+19.1% (<.001)**	**+15.4% (<.001)**	**+12.9% (<.001)**
GGT: 2-fold increment	**+20.3% (<.001)**	**+12.3% (0.001)**	**+16.4% (<.001)**	+7.3% (0.061)

*Expected value of FIB-4 for individuals with predictors at BMI = 22 kg/m^2, no alcohol consumption, total cholesterol = 155 mg/100 mL, Total bilirubin = 0.4 mg/dL, albumin = 39 g/L, GGT = 38 U/L, and duration of IDU = 10 years.
**Expected value of FIB-4 for individuals with predictors at CD4 = 900 cells/μL, total cholesterol = 155 mg/100 mL, total bilirubin = 0.4 mg/dL, albumin = 39 g/L, Alkaline Phosphatase = 70 U/L, GGT = 38 U/L, and duration of IDU = 10 years.

alcohol use is among the cofactors related with liver fibrosis in coinfection in studies with liver biopsy [6,29], the present and other studies that have used non- invasive methods to estimate fibrosis [9,10], does not detect an additional effect of alcohol drinking on the FIB-4 of HCV/HIV-coinfected patients.

In coinfected patients with unhealthy alcohol consumption, the FIB-4 does not reflect the negative impact of alcohol intake on liver fibrosis. Therefore, clinicians may not be able to assess the impact of ethanol nor can advise the patient on the risk of disease progression. On the contrary, unhealthy alcohol use is reflected in

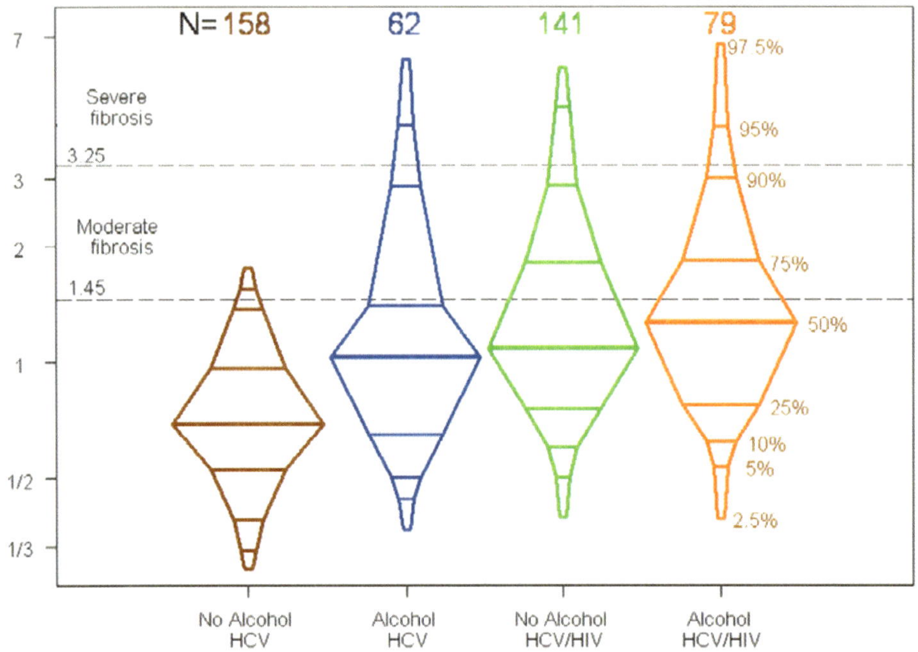

Figure 2. Distribution of FIB-4 scores according to unhealthy alcohol use in HCV-monoinfected and HCV/HIV-coinfected patients.

the FIB-4 of the monoinfected patients thus making possible preventive interventions to reduce harm.

Unhealthy alcohol use in the HCV-monoinfected patients and HIV-related immunodeficiency in the HCV/HIV-coinfected patients are the most important cofactors associated with fibrosis progression in the respective populations. In addition, we found that drug use duration and serum albumin were correlated with the FIB-4 scores of both the monoinfected and coinfected patients, whereas unhealthy alcohol use, GGT and total cholesterol were associated with higher FIB-4 scores only in the monoinfected patients. The effect of HIV-related immunodeficiency in the coinfected patients was strong (an increase of 3.5% in the FIB-4 score for every 100 CD4 cells/μL decrease). Furthermore, we did not observe differing FIB-4 values between the HCV-mono-infected and coinfected individuals with CD4 cell counts above 900 cells/μL. This observation suggests that FIB-4 elevation is associated with immunoactivation and the resulting decrease of CD4 cell counts in HCV/HIV-coinfected drug users.

The relationship between HIV-related immunodeficiency and liver fibrosis progression has been described in coinfected patients [6,29,30]; in fact, treating HIV/AIDS with HAART has been shown to reverse the effect of HIV-related immunodeficiency in patients with chronic hepatitis C [7,26,29,31].

In this study, decreased serum albumin and increased total bilirubin were associated with elevated FIB-4 scores. This finding may facilitate identifying a subpopulation of patients at increased risk for cirrhosis. It is well known that albumin and bilirubin are key components of the Child-Turcotte-Pugh score that clinicians use to assess decompensated liver cirrhosis.

In individuals with history of injection drug use, the duration of injection use is a surrogate for the duration of HCV infection [32]. As expected, the duration of drug addiction in this study was related to increased FIB-4 scores.

It has been reported that HCV infection itself lowers both low-density lipoprotein (LDL) and total cholesterol and that patients treated for chronic hepatitis C had larger increases in LDL and total cholesterol from baseline [33]. Interestingly, the current study did not find a significant association between cholesterol levels and FIB-4 scores among the HCV/HIV-coinfected patients.

This study has a number of limitations that should be mentioned. First, the alcohol intake assessment was limited to one categorical variable (>50 g/day, ≤50 g/day in the 6-month period before admission), and there was no information on the history and complications of alcohol consumption. In previous studies, however, recent alcohol consumption has been treated as a dichotomous variable using a threshold of 40–50 grams of ethanol per day or using the definition of heavy alcohol intake provided by the US National Institute on Alcohol Abuse and Alcoholism (NIAAA) [6,9,10]. Second, we used a single measurement of laboratory parameters to calculate the FIB-4 scores which precluded examining the evolution of fibrosis over time. Furthermore, nearly half of the patients had normal aminotransferases values, as has been previously described for IDUs [34]; despite the lack of correlation between liver enzyme alterations and liver damage, it is possible that FIB-4 scores are affected by normal liver enzymes [20]. Third, the HAART status of the HIV-positive patients was represented by a qualitative covariate, which hindered an analysis of the effect of antiretroviral treatment on FIB-4.

In summary, this study shows that unhealthy alcohol use strongly influence FIB-4 in HCV- monoinfected patients, whereas in the context of HCV/HIV coinfection, HIV-related immune depression exerts a major negative role on FIB-4 results, with no significant worsening by alcohol intake.

Author Contributions

Conceived and designed the experiments: RM AM. Performed the experiments: RM JT DF. Analyzed the data: AM AS SPH EM. Contributed reagents/materials/analysis tools: AS. Wrote the paper: RM AM DF.

References

1. Thomas DL, Seeff LB (2005) Natural history of hepatitis C. Clin Liver Dis 9: 383,98, vi DOI:10.1016/j.cld.2005.05.003.
2. Massard J, Ratziu V, Thabut D, Moussalli J, Lebray P, et al. (2006) Natural history and predictors of disease severity in chronic hepatitis C. J Hepatol 44: S19–S24 DOI:10.1016/j.jhep.2005.11.009.
3. Davis GL, Lau JY (1997) Factors predictive of a beneficial response to therapy of hepatitis C. Hepatology 26: 122S–127S DOI:10.1002/hep.510260721.
4. Poynard T, Ratziu V, Charlotte F, Goodman Z, McHutchison J, et al. (2001) Rates and risk factors of liver fibrosis progression in patients with chronic hepatitis c. J Hepatol 34: 730–739.
5. Sulkowski MS, Thomas DL (2003) Hepatitis C in the HIV-Infected Person. Ann Intern Med 138: 197–207.
6. Benhamou Y, Bochet M, Di Martino V, Charlotte F, Azria F, et al. (1999) Liver fibrosis progression in human immunodeficiency virus and hepatitis C virus coinfected patients. The Multivirc Group. Hepatology 30: 1054–1058 DOI:10.1002/hep.510300409.
7. Benhamou Y, Di Martino V, Bochet M, Colombet G, Thibault V, et al. (2001) Factors affecting liver fibrosis in human immunodeficiency virus-and hepatitis C virus-coinfected patients: impact of protease inhibitor therapy. Hepatology 34: 283–287 DOI:10.1053/jhep.2001.26517.
8. Qurishi N, Kreuzberg C, Luchters G, Effenberger W, Kupfer B, et al. (2003) Effect of antiretroviral therapy on liver-related mortality in patients with HIV and hepatitis C virus coinfection. Lancet 362: 1708–1713 DOI:10.1016/S0140-6736(03)14844-1.
9. Blackard JT, Welge JA, Taylor LE, Mayer KH, Klein RS, et al. (2011) HIV mono-infection is associated with FIB-4 - A noninvasive index of liver fibrosis - in women. Clin Infect Dis 52: 674–680 DOI:10.1093/cid/ciq199.
10. Chaudhry AA, Sulkowski MS, Chander G, Moore RD (2009) Hazardous drinking is associated with an elevated aspartate aminotransferase to platelet ratio index in an urban HIV-infected clinical cohort. HIV Med 10: 133–142 DOI:10.1111/j.1468-1293.2008.00662.x.
11. Gebo KA, Herlong HF, Torbenson MS, Jenckes MW, Chander G, et al. (2002) Role of liver biopsy in management of chronic hepatitis C: a systematic review. Hepatology 36: S161–S172 DOI:10.1053/jhep.2002.36989.
12. Sulkowski MS, Thomas DL (2005) Epidemiology and natural history of hepatitis C virus infection in injection drug users: implications for treatment. Clin Infect Dis 40 Suppl 5: S263–S269 DOI:10.1086/427440.
13. Fleming CA, Craven DE, Thornton D, Tumilty S, Nunes D (2003) Hepatitis C virus and human immunodeficiency virus coinfection in an urban population: low eligibility for interferon treatment. Clin Infect Dis 36: 97–100 DOI:10.1086/344907.
14. Zinkernagel AS, von Wyl V, Ledergerber B, Rickenbach M, Furrer H, et al. (2006) Eligibility for and outcome of hepatitis C treatment of HIV-coinfected individuals in clinical practice: the Swiss HIV cohort study. Antivir Ther 11: 131–142.
15. Leroy V, Monier F, Bottari S, Trocme C, Sturm N, et al. (2004) Circulating matrix metalloproteinases 1, 2, 9 and their inhibitors TIMP-1 and TIMP-2 as serum markers of liver fibrosis in patients with chronic hepatitis C: comparison with PIIINP and hyaluronic acid. Am J Gastroenterol 99: 271–279.
16. Sanvisens A, Serra I, Tural C, Tor J, Ojanguren I, et al. (2009) Hyaluronic acid, transforming growth factor-beta1 and hepatic fibrosis in patients with chronic hepatitis C virus and human immunodeficiency virus co-infection. J Viral Hepat 16: 513–518 DOI:10.1111/j.1365-2893.2009.01103.x.
17. Pohl A, Behling C, Oliver D, Kilani M, Monson P, et al. (2001) Serum aminotransferase levels and platelet counts as predictors of degree of fibrosis in chronic hepatitis C virus infection. Am J Gastroenterol 96: 3142–3146 DOI:10.1111/j.1572-0241.2001.05268.x.
18. Sterling RK, Lissen E, Clumeck N, Sola R, Correa MC, et al. (2006) Development of a simple noninvasive index to predict significant fibrosis in patients with HIV/HCV coinfection. Hepatology 43: 1317–1325 DOI:10.1002/hep.21178.
19. Vallet-Pichard A, Mallet V, Nalpas B, Verkarre V, Nalpas A, et al. (2007) FIB-4: an inexpensive and accurate marker of fibrosis in HCV infection. comparison with liver biopsy and fibrotest. Hepatology 46: 32–36 DOI:10.1002/hep.21669.

20. Sebastiani G, Vario A, Guido M, Alberti A (2008) Performance of noninvasive markers for liver fibrosis is reduced in chronic hepatitis C with normal transaminases. J Viral Hepat 15: 212–218 DOI:10.1111/j.1365-2893.2007.00932.x.
21. Vallet-Pichard A (2008) Predictive value of FIB-4 versus Fibrotest, APRI, FIBROINDEX and FORNS to noninvasively estimate fibrosis in hepatitis C. Hepatology 47: 763.
22. Nunes D, Fleming C, Offner G, Craven D, Fix O, et al. (2010) Noninvasive markers of liver fibrosis are highly predictive of liver-related death in a cohort of HCV-infected individuals with and without HIV infection. Am J Gastroenterol 105: 1346–1353 DOI:10.1038/ajg.2009.746.
23. Sanvisens A, Fuster D, Serra I, Tor J, Tural C, et al. (2011) Estimated Liver Fibrosis and its Impact on All-Cause Mortality of HCV-Monoinfected and HCV/HIV-Coinfected Drug Users. Curr HIV Res 9:256–262.
24. Saitz R (2005) Clinical practice. Unhealthy alcohol use. N Engl J Med 352: 596–607 DOI:10.1056/NEJMcp042262.
25. National Institute in Alcohol Abuse and Alcoholism (1995) The Physician's guide to helping patients with alcohol problems. *USDHHS NIH Publ* 95–3769.
26. Muga R, Roca J, Egea JM, Tor J, Sirera G, et al. (2000) Mortality of HIV-positive and HIV-negative heroin abusers as a function of duration of injecting drug use. J Acquir Immune Defic Syndr 2000; 23: 332–338.
27. Hutchinson SJ, Bird SM, Goldberg DJ (2005) Influence of alcohol on the progression of hepatitis C virus infection: a meta-analysis. Clin Gastroenterol Hepatol 3: 1150–1159.
28. Siu L, Foont J, Wands JR (2009) Hepatitis C virus and alcohol. Semin Liver Dis 29: 188–199 DOI:10.1055/s-0029-1214374.
29. Tural C, Fuster D, Tor J, Ojanguren I, Sirera G, et al. (2003) Time on antiretroviral therapy is a protective factor for liver fibrosis in HIV and hepatitis C virus (HCV) co-infected patients. J Viral Hepat 10: 118–125.
30. Merchante N, Giron-Gonzalez JA, Gonzalez-Serrano M, Torre-Cisneros J, Garcia-Garcia JA, et al. (2006) Survival and prognostic factors of HIV-infected patients with HCV-related end-stage liver disease. AIDS 20: 49–57.
31. Sulkowski MS, Thomas DL, Chaisson RE, Moore RD (2000) Hepatotoxicity associated with antiretroviral therapy in adults infected with human immunodeficiency virus and the role of hepatitis C or B virus infection. JAMA 283: 74–80.
32. Thomas DL, Astemborski J, Rai RM, Anania FA, Schaeffer M, et al. (2000) The natural history of hepatitis C virus infection: host, viral, and environmental factors. JAMA 284: 450–456.
33. Corey KE, Kane E, Munroe C, Barlow LL, Zheng H, et al (2009) Hepatitis C virus infection and its clearance alter circulating lipids: implications for long-term follow-up. Hepatology 50: 1030–7 DOI:10.1002/hep.23219.
34. Inglesby TV, Rai R, Astemborski J, Gruskin L, Nelson KE, et al (1999) A prospective, community-based evaluation of liver enzymes in individuals with hepatitis C after drug use. Hepatology 29: 590–596 DOI:10.1002/hep.510290219.

8

Ribavirin Exerts Differential Effects on Functions of Cd4+ Th1, Th2, and Regulatory T Cell Clones in Hepatitis C

Bettina Langhans*, Hans Dieter Nischalke, Simone Arndt, Ingrid Braunschweiger, Jacob Nattermann, Tilman Sauerbruch, Ulrich Spengler

Department of Internal Medicine I, University of Bonn, Bonn, Germany

Abstract

Ribavirin improves outcomes of therapy in chronic hepatitis C but its mode of action has still remained unclear. Since ribavirin has been proposed to modulate the host's T cell responses, we studied its direct effects on $CD4^+$ T cell clones with diverse functional polarization which had been generated from patients with chronic hepatitis C. We analysed in vitro proliferation ([^{3}H] thymidine uptake) and cytokine responses (IL-10, IFN-gamma) at varying concentrations of ribavirin (0–10µg/ml) in 8, 9 and 7 $CD4^+$ TH1, TH2 and regulatory T cell (Treg) clones, respectively. In co-culture experiments, we further determined effects of ribarivin on inhibition of TH1 and TH2 effector cells by Treg clones. All clones had been generated from peripheral blood of patients with chronic hepatitis C in the presence of HCV core protein. Ribavirin enhanced proliferation of T effector cells and increased production of IFN-gamma in TH1 clones, but had only little effect on IL-10 secretion in TH2 clones. However, ribavirin markedly inhibited IL-10 release in Treg clones in a dose dependent fashion. These Treg clones suppressed proliferation of T effector clones by their IL-10 secretion, and in co-culture assays ribavirin reversed Treg-mediated suppression of T effector cells. Our *in vitro* data suggest that - in addition to its immunostimulatory effects on TH1 cells - ribavirin can inhibit functions of HCV-specific Tregs and thus reverses Treg-mediated suppression of T effector cells in chronic hepatitis C.

Editor: Golo Ahlenstiel, University of Sydney, Australia

Funding: Work has been supported by a grant from the Deutsche Forschungsgemeinschaft (SP 483/4-1, SP483/4-2 and SFB/TRR57), the Wilhelm Sander Stiftung (2009.045.1) and the H.W. and J. Hector Foundation (M42). The funders had no role in study design, data collection and analysis, decision to publish, or preparation of the manuscript.

Competing Interests: The authors have declared that no competing interests exist.

* E-mail: bettina.langhans@ukb.uni-bonn.de

Introduction

Hepatitis C virus (HCV) infection is a major gobal cause of liver cirrhosis and liver cancer [1], which is treated with interferon-based combination therapies. Adding the nucleoside analogue ribavirin to pegylated interferon (PEG-IFN) markedly improves outcomes of antiviral therapy [2]. Nevertheless its mode of action has remained elusive. At present, four hypotheses have been proposed comprising 1) inhibition of the host enzyme IMPDH, 2) inhibition of the NS5B-encoded RNA-dependent RNA polymerase (RdRp), 3) action of ribavirin as a putative RNA mutagene, and 4) improved HCV clearance by the immune system due to a ribavirin-induced switch of T cell polarization towards the more antiviral TH1 profile [3].

Although data have remained controversial, resolution of HCV infection appears to be linked to strong HCV-specific T cell responses [4]. In particular, HCV elimination under PEG-IFN/ribavirin combination therapy seems to be associated with improved HCV-specific T helper (TH) cell responses, which, however, peak either late during treatment or after achieving a therapeutic response [5–6]. Several lines of evidence indicate that the host antiviral response may be compromised during chronic HCV infection: high serum levels of IL-4 and IL-10 have been observed in patients with chronic hepatitis C [7–8], and a favourable clinical response to interferon therapy appeared to be associated with a reduction of TH2 cytokine levels and promotion of TH1-mediated immune responses [9–10].

Ribavirin is a nucleoside analogue, which reduces hepatic inflammation but exerts only little effect on HCV RNA levels [11]. An immunodulatory role of ribavirin has been deduced from studies in mice and from in vitro stimulation experiments with human $CD4^+$ and $CD8^+$ T cells using either mitogen or superantigen for stimulation [12–14]. Whereas these studies suggested simultaneous down-regulation of TH2 cytokines and up-regulation of TH1 cytokines, a recent in vitro stimulation study of PBMC with HCV antigens confirmed IL10 down-regulation but failed to detect up-regulated production of IFN-gamma [15]. Likewise, ex vivo studies in patients under treatment did not uniformly confirm up-regulation of interferon-gamma [5,9]. In summary, the putative immunomodulatory functions of ribavirin have remained controversial but reduced production of IL-10 seems to be a key difference between responders and non-responders to IFN/ribavirin combination therapy.

HCV-specific T effector cells appear to be impaired by a variety of diffent mechanisms also comprising activation of CD4+ regulatory T cells (Tregs) [16–18]. Tregs express Foxp3 (forkhead transcription factor box3), produce IL-10, and can suppress cytokine-production and proliferation of virus-specific T effector cells in a contact-dependent manner [16–18]. Thus, Tregs may contribute importantly to HCV persistence and resistance to immune-based antiviral therapy. Recently we succeeded in establishing HCV core-specific CD25+CD4+ T cells clones from patients with chronic hepatitis C, which to some extent seem to reflect functions and phenotype of HCV-specific adaptive CD4+ Tregs [19].

To clarify the effect of ribavirin on functions of Tregs we compared its direct in vitro action on our adaptive Treg clones to that of autologous TH1 and TH2 polarized T effector cell clones obtained from the same patient with chronic hepatitis C.

Materials and Methods

Ethics Statement

The reported studies were approved by the Institutional Review Boards of the Bonn University Ethics Committee. Written informed consent was obtained from the patients prior to sample collection. Samples were coded and data stored anonymously.

Study Groups

T cell clones were established from the peripheral blood of treatment-naïve, non-cirrhotic patients with chronic hepatitis C genotype 1 (8 males and 4 females; age: 45 (30–68) years, median (range)).

Reagents

Recombinant HCV core protein (genotype 1, amino acids (aa) 1–115; <4.0 pg/µg LPS) was purchased from Mikrogen GmbH (Martinsried, Germany). Human recombinant IL-2 (rIL-2) and OKT-3 (human anti-CD3) were obtained from R&D Systems (Wiesbaden, Germany), anti-CD28 from BD Biosciences (Heidelberg, Germany) and cytomegalovirus (CMV) glycoprotein p65 from AUSTRAL Biologicals (San Ramon, California, USA).

OpTmizer™ T-Cell Expansion SFM medium and Dynabeads® Human Treg Expander (Invitrogen, Karlsruhe, Germany) were used for cell culture. Synthetic ribavirin was purchased from Sigma-Aldrich Chemie GmbH (Taufkirchen, Germany).

Generation of HCV-specific T Cell Clones

Peripheral blood mononuclear cells (PBMC) were isolated by Ficoll-Paque gradient centrifugation (PAA Laboratories GmbH, Linz, Austria) from heparinized blood of patients with chronic hepatitis C. Freshly isolated PBMC ($5x10^5$cells/ml) were stimulated with recombinant HCV core protein (10 µg/ml) in the presence of rIL-2 (100 U/ml). After 10 days, cells were re-stimulated with core protein and supplemented with irradiated autologous feeder cells ($5x10^5$ PBMC/ml). After 20 days, cells were seeded in Terasaki plates (Greiner bio-one, Frickenhausen, Germany) under conditions of limiting dilution (0.1, 0.3, and 0.5 cells/well). After 10 days, clones were picked from plates with less than 10% positive wells and re-stimulated at 10–14 day intervals in the presence of IL-2 and Treg Expander beads. Clones were classified into TH1, TH2 cells and Tregs by analyzing cytokine secretion and proliferation after stimulation with anti-CD3/anti-CD28 (1 and 2.5 µg/ml) (table 1). Overall we obtained 8, 9, and 7 TH1, TH2 and Treg clones from the 12 HCV-infected patients of this study, respectively. TH1 cells were IFN-gamma^{high}, IL-4^{low} and IL-10^{negative}. TH2 cells were IFN-gamma^{negative}, IL-4^{high} and produced variable amounts of IL-10. The antigen-specificity of TH1 and TH2 clones was undetermined. Tregs were IFN-gamma^{negative}, IL-4^{negative}, IL-10^{positive} and did not proliferate after stimulation with anti-CD3/anti-CD28. All Treg clones expressed a typical Treg phenotype ($CD25^+$, $Foxp3^+$, $CD127^-$, $CTLA\text{-}4^+$) and in addition showed HLA-DR-restricted specificity for HCV. Of note, they could be induced to release IL-10 in response to recombinant HCV core - but not to a CMV control protein - as described in great detail elsewhere [19].

Table 1. Cytokine profiles and proliferation of Treg, TH2 and TH1 clones from patients with chronic hepatitis C.

	IL-4 (pg/ml)	IL-10 (pg/ml)	IFN-gamma (pg/ml)	poliferation (SI)
Treg clones				
#1	7	178	1	0
#2	29	730	5	1
#3	25	96	5	1
#4	15	69	1	1
#5	1	957	1	1
#6	33	194	27	2
#7	0	474	1	2
TH2 clones				
#8	671	519	4	21
#9	719	81	10	23
#10	1514	157	1	15
#11	661	219	6	10
#12	999	352	10	13
#13	901	254	8	19
#14	1283	615	20	21
#15	642	286	1	15
#16	640	54	0	31
TH1 clones				
#17	40	3	9648	35
#18	36	1	5085	15
#19	16	21	2512	42
#20	13	2	8010	36
#21	6	0	4100	7
#22	0	0	2523	15
#23	6	3	1206	15
#24	20	23	893	19

Based on the stimulation of control cells, cytokine values equal or greater 50 pg/ml were considered positive.
doi:10.1371/journal.pone.0042094.t001

Effect of Ribavirin on Functions and Phenotype of T Cell Clones

We stimulated TH1, TH2 and Treg clones with anti-CD3/anti-CD28 in the absence or presence of ribavirin various concentrations of (0, 1, 5 and 10 µg/ml) and measured their proliferative responses and cytokine production. Proliferation was studied via [^{3}H] thymidine up-take assays on day 5, as described previously [19]. Stimulation indices (SI) were calculated as the ratio of [^{3}H] thymidine uptake relative to the medium controls. SIs>4 were considered positive.

72 h after stimulation anti-CD3/anti-CD28 IFN-gamma was measured in the supernatants of TH1 clones, and IL-10 was measured in the supernatants of TH2 and Treg clones. IL-10 and IFN-gamma were captured with primary antibodies JES3-9D7 and NIB42, and bound cytokines detected with the corresponding biotin-labeled antibodies JES3-268 and S.B3 (all BD Biosciences), respectively. Cytokine/antibody complexes were revealed by horseradish peroxidise-conjugated streptavidin using TMB (tetra-

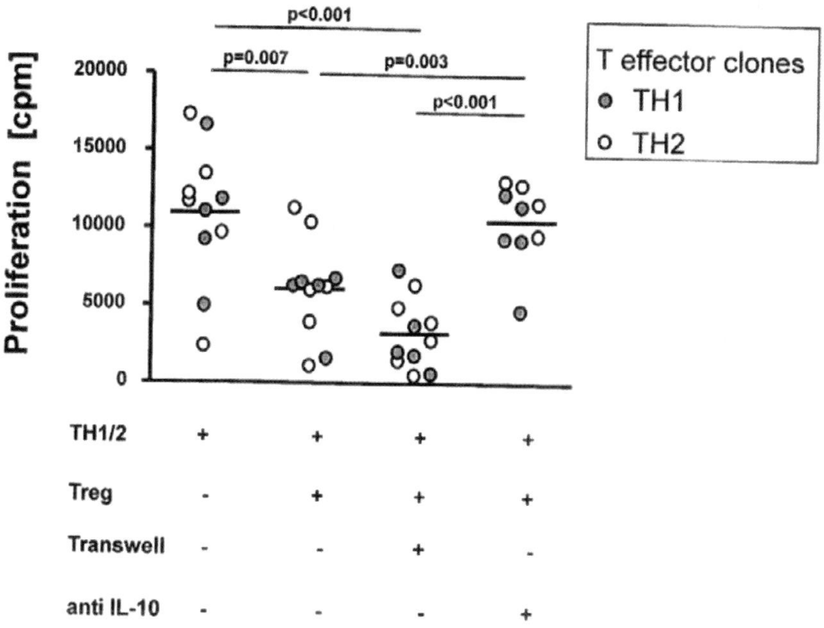

Figure 1. Inhibition of TH cell proliferation by CD4+ Treg clones. This figure illustrates that Treg clones generated from patients with chronic hepatitis C inhibit proliferation of autologous anti-CD3/anti-CD28 stimulated TH1 and TH2 clones. Inhibition of TH1 and TH2 clones was not altered when direct cell-contact was prevented by co-culture in a semipermeable transwell system. Co-culture experiments with a neutralising IL-10 antibody (10 µg/ml; clone 23738) prevented Treg-mediated suppression of TH1 and TH2 clones indicating that inhibition of TH1 and TH2 clones by Treg clones involved IL-10 production as a major soluble inhibitor. Proliferative responses were studied via [^{3}H] thymidine assays. The figures present mean±SEM of experiments with TH1 (filled circles) and TH2 clones (open circles), respectively.

methylbenzidine) as a substrate. Plates were read in an ELISA reader (Tecan, Crailsheim, Germany) at 450 nm.

Using flow cytometry (CANTO II, BD Bioscience) and antibodies APC anti-human CD152 (clone L3D10) and FITC anti-human CD39 (clone A1) (both Biolegend, Germany) we analysed expression in Treg clones at ribavirin concentrations of 0, 1, 5, 10 µg/ml.

To study potential effects of ribavirin on the expansion phase of Tregs we studied if ribavirin (1, 5, 10 µg/ml) affected the proliferation of anti-CD3/anti-CD28 stimulated Tregs in the presence of high amounts of recombinant IL-2 (100 IU/ml).

Ribavirin is frequently used in combination with IFN-alpha, which also regulates the dynamic balance in T cell subsets [20]. Typical concentrations under treatment of hepatitis C are 1–5 µg/ml for ribavirin [21,22] and 10–100 IU/ml for IFN-alpha, respectively [21,23]. Therefore, we analysed the effects of ribavirin on IL-10 secretion in Tregs in the presence of 100 IU/ml Interferon alfa-2a (Roferon-A, Roche; kindly provided by Dr. S. Zahn, Department of Dermatology, University of Bonn).

Influence of Ribavirin on mRNA Levels of Transcription Factors in T Cell Clones

To check if ribavirin alters mRNA expression levels of transcription factors T-bet and GATA-3 in TH1 and TH2 clones we also measured changes of T-bet and GATA-3 upon stimulation with ribavirin by quantitative real time PCR on a Light Cycler® instrument (Roche, Germany).

First, total RNA was extracted using the RNeasy Mini Kit (Qiagen, Germany) according to the manufacturer's instructions. Elimination of genomic DNA and reverse transcription was carried out using the QuantiTect Reverse Transcription Kit (Qiagen, Germany) according to the manufacturer's standard protocol.

For each PCR run 1 µL of the obtained cDNA was used as template. PCR was carried out in a final volume of 10 µL on a LightCycler instrument using the LightCycler FastStart DNA-Master SYBR Green I kit (Roche Molecular Diagnostics, Mannheim, Germany). Primers of the house-keeping gene ß-actin were purchased from TibMolbiol (Berlin, Germany): sense 5′-TGGCATCGTGATGGACTCC-3′, antisense 5′ AATGT-CACGCACGATTTCCC-3′. Analysis of T-bet and GATA-3 mRNA expression was conducted with commercially available QuantiTect Primer Assays following the instructions of the manufacturer (T-bet: Hs_TBX21_1_SG, GATA-3: Hs_GA-TA3_1_SG; Qiagen). The amplification protocol consisted of an initial denaturation step at 95°C for 10 min, followed by 40 cycles (denaturation at 95°C for 2 sec, annealing at 60°C for 5 sec, extension at 72°C for 15 sec) and fluorescence acquisition at 72°C. PCR products were identified by melting curve analysis (95°C for 10 sec, 65°C for 15 sec and a slow ramp (0.2°C/sec) to 95°C with continuous fluorescent acquisition). The LightCycler® software version 3.5 was used in all PCR experiments.

Changes of transcription factor mRNA under ribavirin were calculated as follows: Ct (threshold cycle) values were normalized in a first step by subtracting the Ct value of the housekeeping gene ß-actin control ($\Delta Ct = Ct$, target – Ct, control) [24]. Expression of gene-specific mRNA upon ribavirin stimulation was calculated by subtracting the normalized median ΔCt of cells in the presence of ribavirin versus cells without ribavirin ($\Delta\Delta Ct =$ median ΔCt, ribavirin – median ΔCt, without ribaviri). Changes in transcription factor mRNA expression are given as $2^{-\Delta\Delta Ct}$ ratios [25].

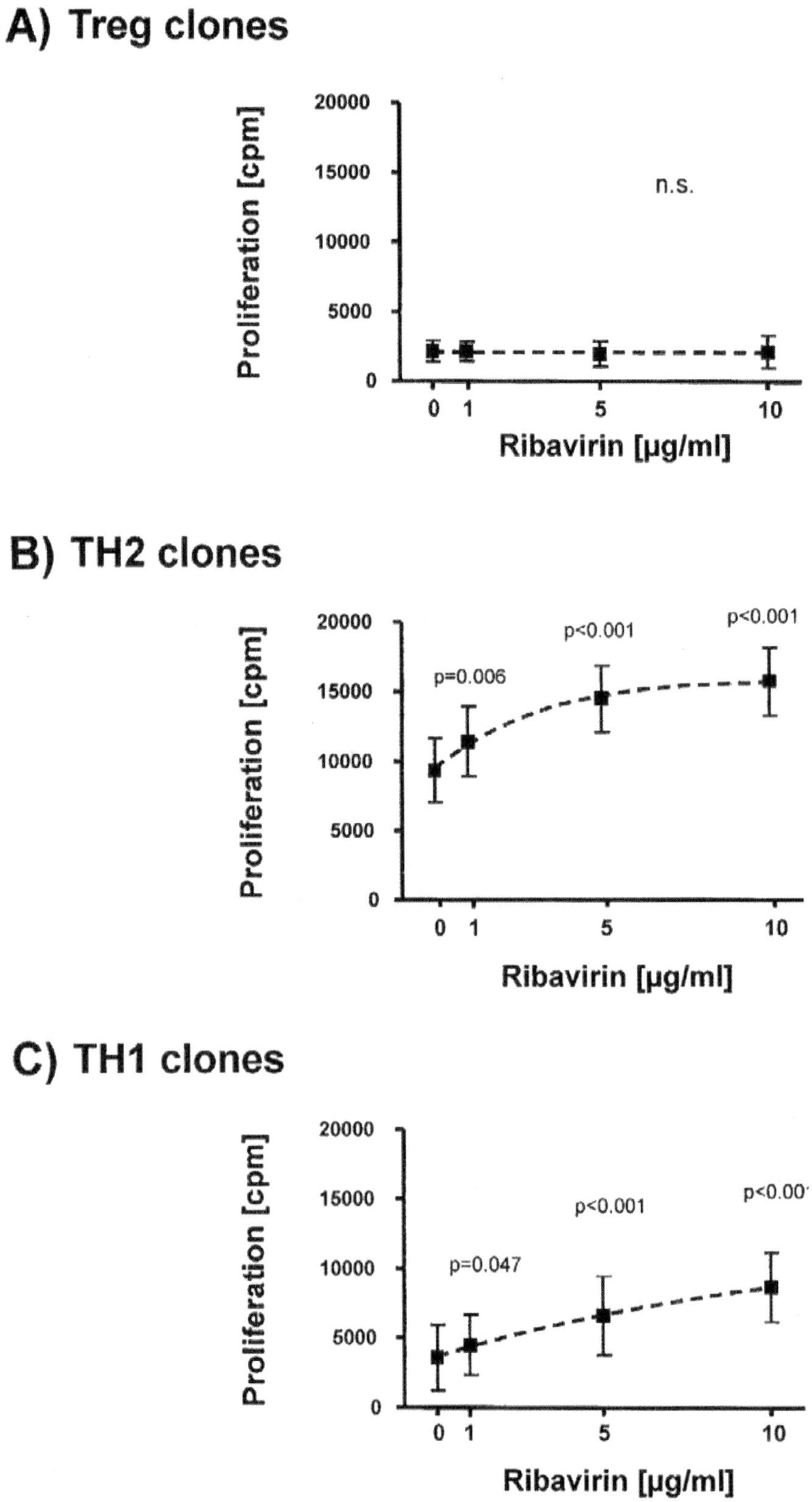

Figure 2. Effect of ribavirin on proliferation of differentially polarized CD4$^+$ T cell clones. Figure 2 shows dose response curves of proliferation ([^{3}H] thymidine uptake, cpm = counts per minute; mean ± SEM) versus ribavirin concentrations (0, 1, 5 and 10 μg/ml) in anti-CD3/anti-CD28-activated Treg clones (A; n = 7), TH2 clones (B; n = 8) and TH1 clones (C; n = 7). Response curves were obtained by a non-linear curve fit with the GraphPad Prism Response Curve module (GraphPad Prism 4 Software, San Diego California, USA). Statistical significance was calculated by 1-way ANOVA with correction for repeated measurements.

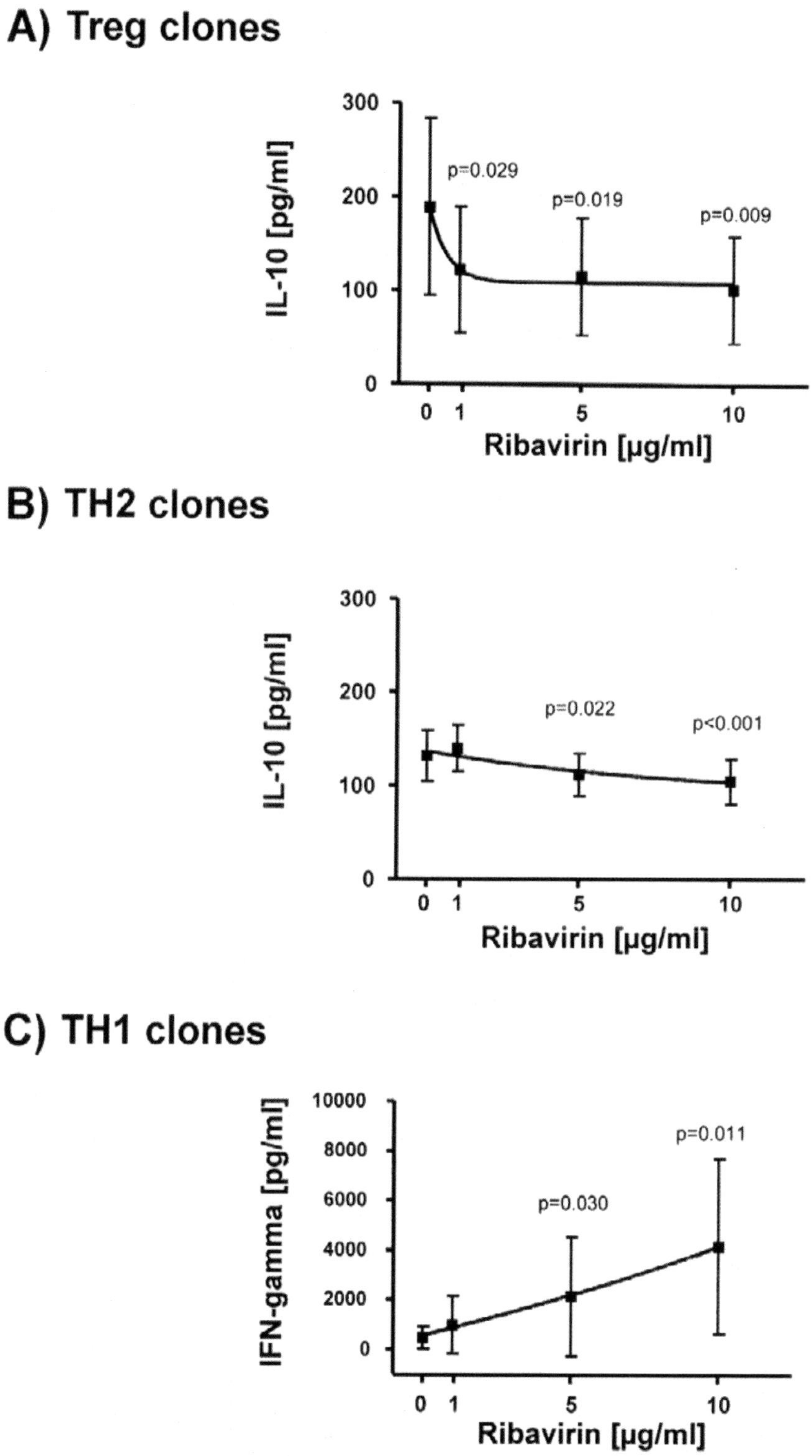

Figure 3. Effect of ribavirin on cytokine secretion in differentially polarized CD4^{+} **T cell clones.** Figure 3 illustrates dose response curves of cytokine release (pg/ml) versus ribavirin concentrations (0, 1, 5 and 10 µg/ml) in anti-CD3/anti-CD28-activated Treg clones (A; n = 7), TH2 clones (B; n = 9) and TH1 clones (C; n = 8). Dose response curves were calculated analogous to figure 2.

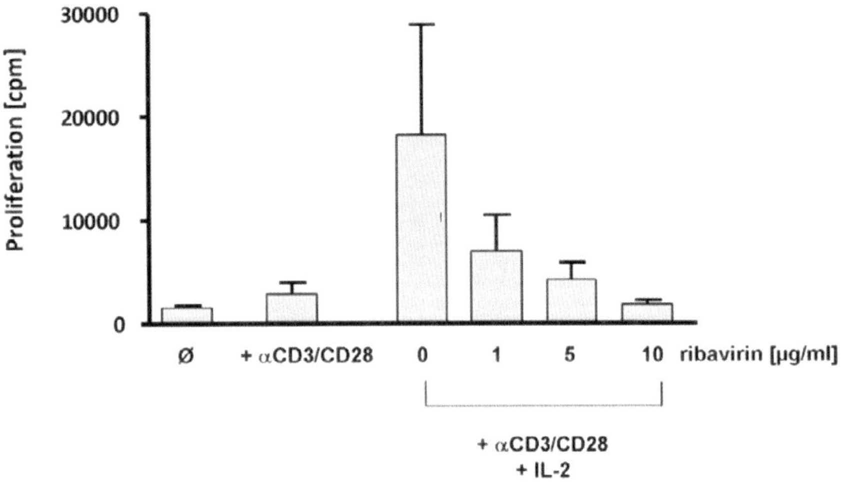

Figure 4. Influence of ribavirin on the proliferation of Treg clones in the presence of IL-2. Figure 4 demonstrates that anti-CD3/anti-CD28-stimulated Tregs markedly proliferate in the presence of high amounts of recombinant IL-2 (100 IU/ml). Adding ribavirin at various concentrations (0, 1, 5 10 μg/ml) proliferation of Tregs was significantly reduced under these experimental conditions.

Assessment of Treg Suppressor Function Against Autologous TH1 and TH2 Reporter Clones in Co-culture Experiments

Inhibitory capacity of Treg clones was analyzed in co-culture assays with stimulated autologous TH1 or TH2 clones. Effector T cells (5×10^4 cells/well) were stimulated with anti-CD3/anti-CD28. Treg clones were added at 1:1 ratio. After 5 days, proliferation was measured via [^{3}H] thymidine incorporation.

In addition, we performed co-culture experiments of TH1 and TH2 effector clones with Treg clones in the presence of varied concentrations of ribavirin (0, 1, 2.5, 5 μg/ml). To clarify the role of Treg-produced IL-10 for inhibition of TH1 and TH2 cells, we also studied co-cultures using transwells, which disrupt direct cell-cell contacts (tissue culture inserts, 0.2 μm Nanopore® Membrane, Nunc). In addition, we performed blocking experiments using a neutralising antibody to IL-10 (clone 23738, 10 μg/ml; R&D Systems, Germany).

To clarify the relationship of the ribavirin effect to hepatitis C we also performed co-culture assays using freshly isolated Tregs and $CD4^+$ TH cells from healthy donors ($CD4^+$ $CD25^+$ $CD127^{dim/-}$ Regulatory T Cell Isolation Kit II, Miltenyi, Germany) at various concentrations of ribavirin (0, 2.5, 5 μg/ml).

Statistics

Dose response curves were constructed by non-linear curve fit using an uphill and downhill model with variable slopes as appropriate. Differences between experiments were compared by paired t tests and 1-way ANOVA with correction for repeated measurements. To assess over-all inhbition in the co-culture assays, we plotted proliferation of TH cells in the presence of Tregs versus proliferation without Tregs for each concentration of ribavirin (0–5 μg/ml). Then, Treg-mediated inhibition was calculated from the slope obtained by a linear regression analysis.

All calculations and curve fittings were performed using the GraphPad Prism software package 4.0 (GraphPad Prism, San Diego California, USA). $P<0.05$ was considered as statistically significant.

Results

With our cloning strategy we obtained 24 $CD4^+$ T cell clones from 12 patients with chronic hepatitis C, which - based on their cytokine profiles and proliferative responses - could definitely be classified as Tregs, TH2 cells or TH1 cells, respectively (table 1). Details on the characteristics of the distinct subtypes of T cell clones have been reported previously [19].

To confirm the regulatory function of our 7 Treg clones from chronic hepatitis C, we performed co-culture assays to determine their inhibitory capacity against autologous TH1 and TH2 clones after anti-CD3/anti-CD28 stimulation (figure 1). These co-culture inhibition assays demonstrated that our Treg clones could substantially suppress proliferation of TH1 and TH2 clones (figure 1). Co-culture in semipermeable transwells, which disrupt direct cell-cell contacts but still permit the exchange of soluble factors, indicated that inhibition of TH1 and TH2 clones was mediated by a soluble molecule, which could be identified as IL-10 in blocking experiments with a neutralizing IL-10 antibody (figure 1).

To determine the direct influence of ribavirin on differentially polarized $CD4^+$ T cells from chronic hepatitis C, we stimulated our Treg, TH1 and TH2 clones with anti-CD3/anti-CD28 in the presence of variable concentrations of ribavirin and measured their proliferation (figure 2) and cytokine responses (figure 3). Ribavirin did not alter expression of surface markers in Tregs which are considered to be involved Treg-mediated suppression (CTLA-4 ΔMFI: 1.7±3.1%; CD39 ΔMFI: 1.4±2.6%). Furthermore, ribavirin had no effect on the proliferation of Treg clones under normal tissue culture conditions (figure 2A). However, proliferation of both TH2 clones (figures 2B) and TH1 clones (figure 2C) was enhanced in a dose-dependent fashion.

Concerning Treg and TH2 clones, we observed that adding ribavirin to Tregs dose-dependently resulted in reduced IL-10 responses (figure 3A), while its addition to TH2 clones had only minor effects on IL-10 production (figure 3B). On the other hand, addition of ribavirin to TH1 clones, which do not produce IL-10 but IFN-gamma, markedly augmented their cytokine production (figure 3C). However, ribavirin did not significantly alter expression of transcription factors T-bet and GATA-3 in TH1

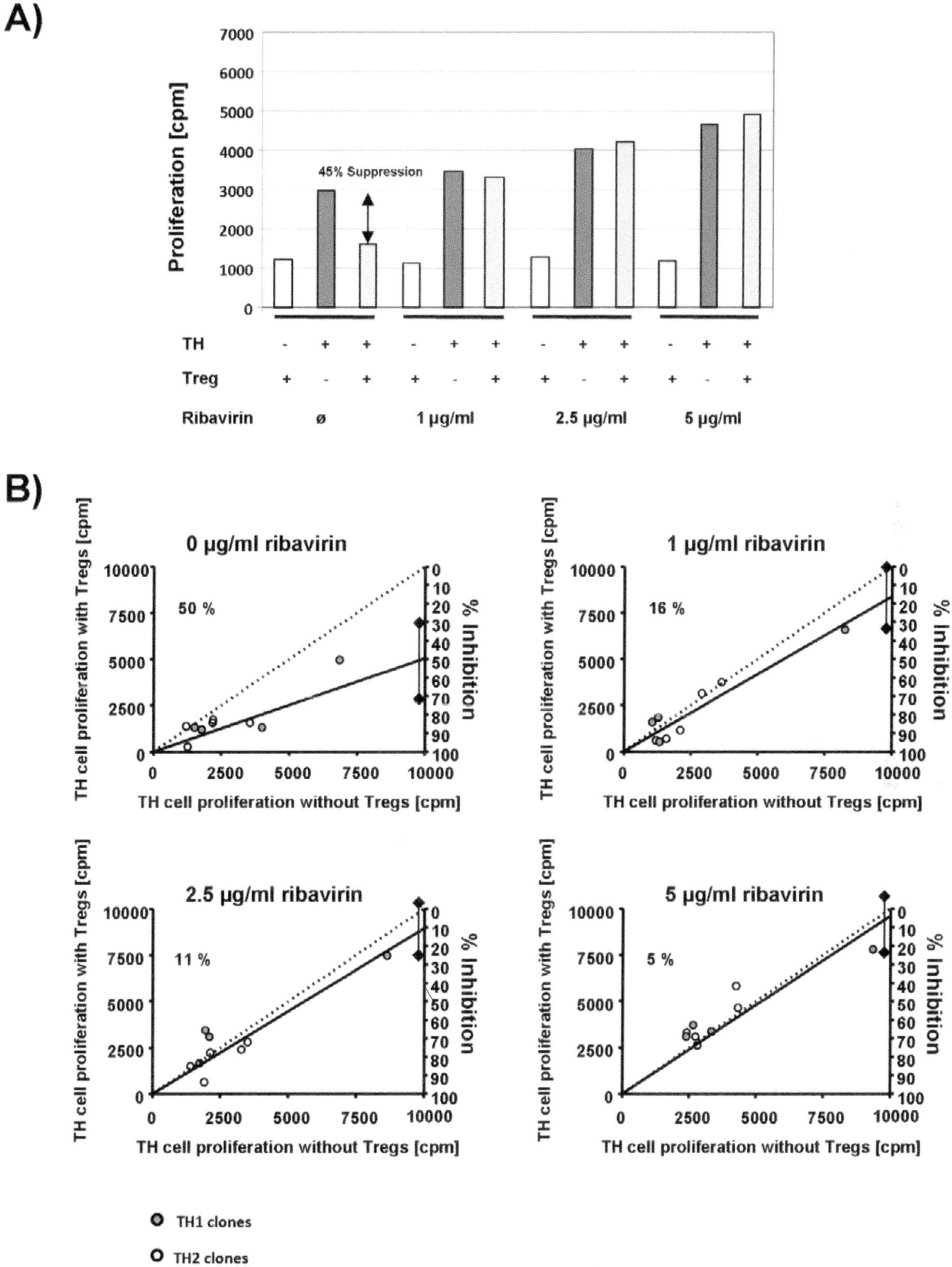

Figure 5. Reversal of Treg-mediated inhibition of T effector cell proliferation by ribavirin. Figure 4A illustrates a representative co-culture experiment of TH1 clone #18 and Treg clone #4 in the presence of varied concentrations of ribavirin (0–5 µg/ml). Figure 4B provides a summary of

all co-culture experiments of TH1 and TH2 effector clones with autologous Treg clones in the presence of varied concentrations of ribavirin (0–5 μg/ml). Each plot summarizes the effects for a defined concentration of ribavirin. The x-coordinate of each plot indicates proliferation (cpm = counts per minute) of a T effector clone without Tregs. The coordinate on the left y-axis shows the corresponding proliferation in the presence of autologous Treg clones (1:1 ratio). Dots below the dotted line illustrate Treg-mediated inhibition of T effector cell proliferation. The straight line represents the linear regression line of all co-culture experiments. Intersection of this line with the right y-axis shows overall percent inhibition and its 95% confidence interval.

and TH2 clones (T-bet: 1.34±0.78, GATA-3: 1.55±0.82; $2^{-\Delta\Delta Ct}$ ± SD).

Tregs which do not proliferate under normal culture conditions can be expanded in vitro by adding high amounts of recombinant IL-2. To find out if ribavirin affects proliferation of Tregs during IL-2 induced expansion, we also studied proliferation of anti-CD3/anti-CD28 stimulated Tregs in the presence of 100 IU/ml recombinant IL-2. As it is shown in figure 4, adding ribavirin inhibited IL-2 driven Treg expansion in a dose-dependent fashion.

Ribavirin is frequently used in combination with IFN-alpha. Therefore, we also studied whether the ribavirin-associated effects were detectable in the presence of IFN-alpha. Of note, ribavirin still inhibited IL-10 secretion in Tregs in the presence of 100 IU/ml IFN-alpha (57% inhibition of IL-10 production at 5 μg/ml ribavirin in the presence of 100 IFN-alpha).

To clarify the relationship between HCV infection and effects of ribavirin on Treg functions we also studied Treg clones from individuals with spontaneous recovery from HCV-infection. Of note, adding ribavirin to Treg clones from self-limited HCV infection did not alter IL-10 production (0 μg/ml ribavirin: 176±66; 1 μg/ml: 172±89; 5 μg/ml: 151±82; 10 μg/ml: 143±83, pg/ml IL-10; MW ± SD).

Finally, we performed co-culture inhibition assays in the absence and presense of various ribavirin concentrations. Adding ribavirin to co-culture assays using freshly isolated $CD4^+$ $CD25^+$ Tregs and autologous $CD4^+$ TH cells from healthy donors did not result in abrogation of Treg-mediated suppression (2.5 μg/ml ribavirin: 27±22% inhibition; 5 μg/ml ribavirin: 37±17% inhibition). In contrast, adding ribavirin to co-culture assays of Treg clones from patients with chronic hepatitis C resulted in a dose-dependent reversal of Treg-mediated inhibition of T effector cell proliferation (figure 5).

Discussion

Ribavirin was initially designed as a direct antiviral agent for the treatment of distinct viral disease, and later on proved to be a pivotal combination partner to enhance efficacy of IFN-based therapy and probably also of direct antiviral agents in chronic hepatitis C [2,26]. When inhibition of HCV replication could not be confirmed later on, it was proposed that ribavirin might exert effects on host immunity in chronic hepatitis C.

This study used differently polarized $CD4^+$ T cell clones from patients with chronic hepatitis C to analyse the effects of ribavirin on T cell functions in vitro. Our experiments revealed directly enhanced proliferation of T effector cells independently from their TH1/TH2 polarization. Furthermore, TH1 cells produce more IFN-gamma, while only little effect on IL-10 production was noted in TH2 cells. Our data largely correspond to similar in vitro studies in mice and human T cells [10,12–14]. Taken together these in vitro findings have been considered to reflect a ribavirin-induced shift in the overall immune balance towards improved antiviral immunity. Nevertheless, ex vivo data remained controversial in this respect [5,9,15], but lower production of IL-10 remained the key difference between responders and non-responders to PEG-IFN/ribavirin combination therapy.

Of note, previous studies had been done in preparation of peripheral blood mononuclear cells and thus could not attribute changes in cytokine production to individually polarized T cells. In line with these previous reports our study in $CD4^+$ T cell clones confirmed a conspicuous direct effect of ribavirin on TH1 cells, which may be linked to altered expression of interferon regulatory factors [27–29]. On the other hand, our data suggest that changes in TH2 functions are unlikely to contribute much to the overall anti-HCV effect of ribavirin, because we observed only slightly reduced production of IL-10 in our TH2 clones.

$CD4^+$ Tregs are an alternative source of immunomodulatory cytokines such as IL-10. Thus far, however, frequencies of Tregs in liver and blood have not shown a clear pattern to treatment outcomes [30–33]. In two recent studies numbers of Tregs remained unchanged in peripheral blood, whereas exposure to PEG-IFN/ribavirin resulted in increased frequencies of Tregs in the liver [30,32]. None of the previous studies, however, has studied functions of single Tregs and specifically addressed the potential role of ribavirin.

Here, our in vitro analysis of Treg clones revealed the novel finding that ribavirin markedly reduced production of IL-10 in Tregs, but did not affect their overall low proliferative capacity.

Beyond that, our co-culture assays showed that ribavirin-mediated inhibition of IL-10 production of Treg clones clearly resulted in improved proliferation of T effector cells irrespective from their antigen-specificity and functional polarization.

Our data suggest that ribavirin specifically affects Tregs in patients with chronic hepatitis C, because we observed only negligible effects in Treg clones from patients with self-limited HCV infection and Tregs from healthy controls. Nevertheless we did not check explicitly antigen-specificity of the T cell clones in the current experiments. However, we have shown previously that our Treg clones recognize epitopes on HCV core in an antigen-specific, HLA-DR-restricted fasion [19]. Thus, it is quite likely that the newly discovered action of ribavirin on Tregs holds also true for Tregs in patients with chronic hepatitis C. Moreover, we demonstrated inhibitory activity of ribavirin on Treg function at concentration levels which are typically achieved in vivo during ribavirin treatment (1–5 μg/ml) [21,22]. Moreover, the ribavirin effect could also be demonstrated at therapeutic concentrations of IFN-alpha (100 IU/ml) suggesting that our in vitro findings might have relevance for the in vivo situation under interferon/ribavirin combination therapy.

Overall, we did not find that ribavirin modulate transcription factors regulating TH1/TH2 cell responses. However, Brenndörfer et al. recently demonstrated that ribavirin can reverse the HCV NS3/4A-mediated impairment of antiviral signalling pathways in vivo [34].

In summary our analysis of T cell clones supports the concept of immune-mediated activity of ribavirin and suggests that this compound affects the T cell balance by two supplementary mechanisms: ribavirin directly enhances proliferation and cytokine production of TH1 cells, and importantly also reverses Treg-mediated inhibition of T effector cells by inhibiting IL-10 release of HCV-specific Tregs. Beyond that, in vivo reduced IL-10 production under ribavirin may also result in down-regulated expression of ICOS, altered costimulatory signalling and increased priming of T cells towards TH1 differentiation [35].

Thus, in chronic hepatitis C ribavirin is likely to shift the functional balance in the immune system between Tregs and T effector cells towards more efficous effector responses, thus strengthening the antiviral activity of PEG-IFN/ribavirin combination therapy.

Author Contributions

Conceived and designed the experiments: BL US. Performed the experiments: BL SA IB. Analyzed the data: BL US. Contributed reagents/materials/analysis tools: BL HDN JN TS US. Wrote the paper: BL US.

References

1. Shepard CW, Finelli L, Alter MJ (2005) Global epidemiology of hepatitis C virus infection. Lancet Infect Dis 5: 558–567.
2. Aghemo A, Rumi MG, Colombo M (2009) Pegylated IFN-alpha2a and ribavirin in the treatment of hepatitis C. Expert Rev Anti Infect Ther 7: 925–935.
3. Lau JYN, Tam RC, Liang TJ, Hong Z (2002) Mechanism of action of ribavirin in the combination treatment of chronic HCV infection. Hepatology 35: 1002–1009.
4. Spengler U, Nattermann J (2007) Immunopathogenesis in hepatitis C virus cirrhosis. Clin Sci 112: 141–155.
5. Barnes E, Harcourt G, Brown D, Lucas M, Phillips R, et al. (2002) The dynamics of T-lymphocyte responses during combination therapy for chronic hepatitis C virus infection. Hepatology 36: 743–754.
6. Rahman F, Heller T, Sobao Y, Mizukoshi E, Nascimbeni M, et al. (2004) Effects of antiviral therapy on the cellular immune response in acute hepatitis C. Hepatology 40 (1): 87–97.
7. Reiser M, Marousis CG, Nelson DR, Lauer G, González-Peralta RP, et al. (1997) Serum interleukin 4 and interleukin 10 levels in patients with chronic hepatitis C virus infection. J Hepatol 26: 471–478.
8. Cacciarelli TV, Martinez OM, Gish RG, Villanueva JC, Krams SM (1996) Immunoregulatory cytokines in chronic hepatitis C virus infection: pre- and posttreatment with interferon alfa. Hepatology 24: 6–9.
9. Cramp ME, Rossol S, Chokshi S, Carucci P, Williams R, et al. (2000) Hepatitis C virus-specific T-cell reactivity during interferon and ribavirin treatment in chronic hepatitis C. Gastroenterology 118: 346–355.
10. Fang SH, Lai MY, Hwang LH, Yang PM, Chen PJ, et al. (2001) Ribavirin enhances interferon-gamma levels in patients with chronic hepatitis C treated with interferon-alpha. Biomed Sci 8: 484–491.
11. Dusheiko G, Main J, Thomas H, Reichard O, Lee C, et al. (1996) Ribavirin treatment for patients with chronic hepatitis C: results of a placebo-controlled study. J Hepatol 25: 591–598.
12. Hultgren C, Milich DR, Weiland O, Sällberg M (1998) The antiviral compound ribavirin modulates the T helper (Th) 1/Th2 subset balance in hepatitis B and C virus-specific immune responses. Gen Virol 79: 2381–2391.
13. Fang SH, Hwang LH, Chen DS, Chiang BL (2000) Ribavirin enhancement of hepatitis C virus core antigen-specific type 1 T helper cell response correlates with the increased IL-12 level. J Hepatol 33: 791–798.
14. Tam RC, Pai B, Bard J, Lim C, Averett DR, et al. (1999) Ribavirin polarizes human T cell responses towards a Type 1 cytokine profile. J Hepatol 30: 376–382.
15. Rigopoulou EI, Abbott WG, Williams R, Naoumov NV (2007) Direct evidence for immunomodulatory properties of ribavirin on T-cell reactivity to hepatitis C virus. Antiviral Res 75: 36–42.
16. Manigold T, Racanelli V (2007) T-cell regulation by CD4 regulatory T cells during hepatitis B and C virus infections: facts and controversies. Lancet Infect Dis 7: 804–813.
17. Dolganiuc A, Szabo G (2008) T cells with regulatory activity in hepatitis C virus infection: what we know and what we don't. J Leukoc Biol 84: 614–622.
18. Alatrakchi N, Koziel M (2009) Regulatory T cells and viral liver disease. J Viral Hepat 16: 223–229.
19. Langhans B, Braunschweiger I, Arndt, S Schulte W, Satoguina J, et al. (2010) Core-specific adaptive regulatory T-cells in different outcomes of hepatitis C. Clin Sci 119: 97–109.
20. Golding A, Rosen A, Petri M, Akhter E, Andrade F (2010) Interferon-alpha regulates the dynamic balance between human activated regulatory and effector T cells: implications for antiviral and autoimmune responses. Immunology 131: 107–117.
21. Khakoo S, Glue P, Grellier L, Wells B, Bell A, et al. (1998) Ribavirin and interferon alfa-2b in chronic hepatitis C: assessment of possible pharmacokinetic and pharmacodynamic interactions Br J Clin Pharmacol 46: 563–570.
22. Slavenburg S, Huntjens-Fleuren HWHA, Dofferhoff TSN, Richter C, Koopmans PP, et al. (2011) Ribavirin plasma concentration measurements in patients with hepatitis C. Early ribavirin concentrations predict steady-state concentrations. Ther Drug Monit 33: 40–44.
23. Nicot F, Legrand-Abravanel F, Lafont T, Dubois M, Sauné K, et al. (2008) Serum concentrations of ribavirin and pegylated interferon and virla responses in patients infected with HIV and HCV. J Med Virol 80: 1523–1529.
24. Mori R, Wang Q, Danenberg KD, Pinski JK, Danenberg PV (2008) Both beta-actin and GAPDH are useful reference genes for normalization of quantitative RT-PCR in human FFPE tissue samples of prostate cancer. Prostate 68: 1555–1560.
25. Weglarz L, Molin I, Orchel A, Parfiniewicz B, Dzierzewicz Z (2006) Quantitative analysis of the level of p53 and p21(WAF1) mRNA in human colon cancer HT-29 cells treated with inositol hexaphosphate. Acta Biochim Pol 53: 349–356.
26. Clark V, Nelson DR (2012) The role of ribavirin in direct acting antiviral drug regimens for chronic hepatitis C. Liver Int Feb 32 Suppl 1: 103–7.
27. Feld JJ, Lutchman GA, Heller T, Hara K, Pfeiffer JK, et al. (2010) Ribavirin improves early responses to peginterferon through improved interferon signaling Gastroenterology139: 154–62.e4.
28. Thomas E, Feld JJ, Li Q, Hu Z, Fried MW, et al. (2011) Ribavirin potentiates interferon action by augmenting interferon-stimulated gene induction in hepatitis C virus cell culture models. Hepatology 53: 32–41.
29. Stevenson NJ, Murphy AG, Bourke NM, Keogh CA, Hegarty JE, et al. (2011) Ribavirin enhances IFN-α signalling and MxA expression: a novel immune modulation mechanism during treatment of HCV. PLoS One 6(11): e27866–e27866.
30. Burton JR Jr, Klarquist J, Im K, Smyk-Pearson S, Golden-Mason L, et al. (2008) Prospective analysis of effector and regulatory $CD4^+$ T cells in chronic HCV patients undergoing combination antiviral therapy. J Hepatol 49: 329–338.
31. Akiyama M, Ichikawa T, Miyaaki H, Motoyoshi Y, Takeshita S, et al. (2010) Relationship between regulatory T cells and the combination of pegylated interferon and ribavirin for the treatment of chronic hepatitis type C. Intervirology 53: 154–160.
32. Claassen MA, de Knegt RJ, Janssen HL, Boonstra A (2011) Retention of $CD4^+$ $CD25^+$ $FoxP3^+$ regulatory T cells in the liver after therapy-induced hepatitis C virus eradication in humans. J Virol 85: 5323–5330.
33. Westin J, Hellstrand K, Dhillon AP, Lagging M, DITTO-HCV Study Group (2011) Are FoxP3(+) cells involved in hyporesponsiveness to interferon/ribavirin therapy in chronic hepatitis C? J Viral Hepat 18: 149–151.
34. Brenndörfer ED, Brass A, Söderholm J, Frelin L, Bode JG, Sählber M (2012) The HCV NS3/4A-mediated impairment of the hepatic antiviral immune response is reversed by protease inhibition or ribavirin in vivo. EASL: abstract #1234.
35. Atsukawa M, Nakatsuka K, Kobayashi T, Shimizu M, Tamura H, et al. (2012) Ribavirin downmodulates inducible costimulator on CD4+ T cells and their interleukin-10 secretion to assist in hepatitis C virus clearance. J Gastroenterol Hepatol 27: 823–831.

9

Positive Association Between Hepatitis C Infection and Oral Cavity Cancer: A Nationwide Population-Based Cohort Study in Taiwan

Fu-Hsiung Su[1,2], Shih-Ni Chang[3,4,5], Pei-Chun Chen[5,6], Fung-Chang Sung[5,7], Shiang-Fu Huang[8], Hung-Yi Chiou[1,9], Chien-Tien Su[1,2], Cheng-Chieh Lin[10,11,12], Chih-Ching Yeh[1,7]*

1 School of Public Health, College of Public Health and Nutrition, Taipei Medical University, Taipei, Taiwan, **2** Department of Family Medicine, Taipei Medical University Hospital, Taipei, Taiwan, **3** The Ph.D. Program for Cancer Biology and Drug Discovery, China Medical University, Taichung, Taiwan, **4** Institute of Biomedical Sciences, Academia Sinica, Taipei, Taiwan, **5** Management Office for Health Data, China Medical University Hospital, Taichung, Taiwan, **6** Graduate Institute of Epidemiology and Preventive Medicine, National Taiwan University College of Public Health, Taipei, Taiwan, **7** Department of Public Health, China Medical University, Taichung, Taiwan, **8** Department of Otolaryngology, Head and Neck Surgery, Chang Gung Memorial Hospital, Chang Gung University, Tao-Yuan, Taiwan, **9** Center of Excellence for Cancer Research, Taipei Medical University, Taipei, Taiwan, **10** Department of Family Medicine, China Medical University Hospital, Taichung, Taiwan, **11** School of Medicine, College of Medicine, China Medical University, Taichung, Taiwan, **12** Department of Healthcare Administration, College of Health Science, Asia University, Taichung, Taiwan

Abstract

Objectives: The association between viral hepatitis (B and C) and oral cavity cancer has been widely debated. This nationwide, population-based cohort study assessed the subsequent risk of oral cavity cancer among patients with chronic viral hepatitis infection.

Materials and Methods: Data were retrieved from insurance claims data of 1,000,000 randomly sampled individuals covered under the Taiwan National Health Insurance system. We identified a total of 21,199 adults with chronic viral hepatitis infection (12,369 with HBV alone, 5,311 with HCV alone, and 3,519 with HBV/HCV dual infections) from 2000–2005. Comparison group comprised 84,796 sex- and age-matched subjects without viral hepatitis during the same study period. Incidence and risk of subsequent oral cavity cancer were measured until 2008.

Results: The incidence of oral cavity cancers was 2.28-fold higher among patients with HCV alone than non-viral hepatitis group (6.15 versus 2.69 per 10,000 person-years). After adjusting for sociodemographic covariates, HCV alone was significantly associated with an increased risk for oral cavity cancer (hazard ratio (HR) = 1.90, 95% confidence interval (CI) = 1.20–3.02). This positive association was highest among individuals in the 40–49-year age group (HR = 2.57, 95% CI = 1.21–5.46). However, there were no significant associations between HBV alone or HBV/HCV dual infections and risk for oral cavity cancer.

Conclusion: Our data suggest that HCV but not HBV infection is a risk factor for oral cavity cancer. In addition, subjects with HCV infection tend to be at early onset risk for oral cavity cancer. This finding needs to be replicated in further studies.

Editor: Xiao-Ping Miao, MOE Key Laboratory of Environment and Health, School of Public Health, Tongji Medical College, Huazhong University of Science and Technology, China

Funding: This study was supported by the National Sciences Council, Executive Yuan (grant numbers DOH 97-HP-1101, 2008–2010), China Medical University Hospital (grant number 1MS1, DMR-94-080), Taiwan Department of Health Clinical Trial and Research Center (grant number DOH 100-TD-B-111-004), Taiwan Department of Health Cancer Research Center for Excellence (DOH100-TD-C-111-005), and Taiwan Department of Health Center of Excellence for Cancer Research in Taipei Medical University (DOH101-TD-C-111-008). The funders had no role in study design, data collection and analysis, decision to publish, or preparation of the manuscript.

Competing Interests: The authors have declared that no competing interests exist.

* E-mail: ccyeh@tmu.edu.tw

Introduction

Oral cavity cancer comprises of 2% to 3% of all malignancies (reviewed in Kademani) [1]. Oral squamous cell carcinoma (OSCC) is the most common type of oral carcinoma and accounts for approximately one ninth of oral malignancies. The identified risk factors of oral cavity cancer include tobacco use, alcohol consumption, race, chewing of betel leaves and areca nuts, and low socioeconomic status (SES). Recently, the role that viruses play in the development of oral cavity cancer has also received tremendous interest [1,2,3].

Overall, 12% of the global cancer burden is conservatively estimated to be virus-attributable [4]. Currently, six human viruses have been classified by the International Agency for Research on Cancer (IARC) as being carcinogenic to humans based on sufficient evidence supporting their etiologic association with human cancers, namely Epstein-Barr virus, hepatitis B virus

(HBV), several types of human papilloma virus (HPV), human T-cell lymphotropic virus type 1, hepatitis C virus (HCV), and Kaposi's sarcoma-associated herpesvirus [5].

In addition to the association with hepatocellular carcinoma, HCV infection has been associated with other neoplasms including smoking and alcohol-related cancers, such as cancers of the pancreas, lung, and kidney, and the oropharygeal cancer [6] and non-Hodgkin lymphoma [7]. HBV infection also has been associated with intrahepatic cholangiocaricinoma and non-Hodgkin lymphoma [8,9] as well as pancreas cancer [10].

Previous studies have provided evidence that HCV infection is associated with the development of oral cavity cancer [11,12,13]. In 1995, Nagao et al. demonstrated an increased prevalence of HCV antibody and RNA in OSCC patients [11]. A study conducted at a veterans administration medical center in New Orleans reported that 21.2% of 99 patients with squamous cell carcinoma of the head and neck (SCCHN) were coinfected with HCV, which was significantly higher than previously published data (9.9%) ($P<0.004$) [12]. In another study from Japan that evaluated the prevalence of HCV in 4,402 inpatients requiring oral surgery, Takata et al. found that HCV antibody was more prevalent in patients with oral cavity cancer than in those with impacted teeth before adjustment for age (odds ratio (OR) = 2.433; $P<0.05$); however, this difference was reversed after age adjustment (OR = 0.443; $P<0.05$) [13]. They also suggested that HBV surface antigen was more prevalent in patients with benign oral tumors than in healthy subjects. Thus, there seems to be controversy with respect to the relationship between HCV and HBV infections and oral cavity cancer. Whether there is a potential link between chronic HCV and/or HBV infection and the risk of developing oral cavity cancer, namely OSCC, has yet to be investigated.

In Taiwan, oral cavity cancer ranked as the fifth most prevalent cancer in 2008 and approximately 93% of those patients were men with OSCC [14]. In addition, Taiwan is a region in which HBV infection is endemic and with a high prevalence of HCV infection [15]. Therefore, Taiwan provides a unique setting in which to study the association between hepatitis and oral cavity cancer. In the present study, we used a nationwide population-based insurance dataset to assess the possible association between chronic viral hepatitis infection and oral cavity cancer.

Materials and Methods

Data Sources

Data analyzed in this study were retrieved from the Taiwan National Health Insurance Research Database (NHIRD), which is managed by the Taiwan National Health Research Institute (NHRI). In 1995, Taiwan commenced its state-run National Health Insurance (NHI) program [16]. By the end of 1996, this insurance program covered approximately 96% of the total population, and contracted with 97% of the hospitals and 90% of the clinics on the island [17]. The Taiwan NHIRD comprises claims data of 1,000,000 individuals randomly selected from all insured enrollees. This sample represents the original medical claims for all islanders under the NHI program. With approval from the NHRI, we used data for ambulatory care claims, all inpatient claims, and updated registries for beneficiaries from the year 2000 to the year 2005 in this study. Diagnoses were coded according to the *International Classification of Disease, Ninth revision, clinical Modification* (ICD-9-CM). The database used in this study can be interlinked by the scrambled unique individual's personal identification number (PIN). The NHRI safeguards the privacy and confidentiality of all beneficiaries and transfers the health insurance data to health researchers after ethical approval has been obtained. In this analysis, access of the NHIRD has been approved by the NHRI Ethics Review Committee.

Study Sample

Our data consisted of NHIRD data during the period 1996 to 2008. In order to limit our study sample to the adult population, we only selected patients older than 18 years of age. In this study, we identified patients with newly identified HBV (ICD-9-CM: 070.2, 070.3, V02.61) and HCV (ICD-9-CM: 070.41, 070.44, 070.51, 070.54, V02.62) infections during the period of 2000–2005 as the exposure group. The index date for the patients with HBV and HCV was the date of their first medical visit. We excluded subjects with a diagnosis of HIV (ICD-9-CM: 042, 043, 044, V08 and 795.8). Subjects with a diagnosis of malignant neoplasm (ICD-9-CM: 140–230) that had been established before the index date and subjects with missing information on age or sex were excluded. After excluding 20 cases of HIV, 466 cases of cancer diagnosed before index date, and 838 subjects under 18 years of age, 12,369, 5,311, and 3,519 subjects with HBV, HCV and HBV/HCV dual infections were enrolled in this study. For the comparison group, we used a systematic random sampling method to select 4 insured people without viral hepatitis for every insured person with viral hepatitis during the same period. Patients and comparison subjects were age- and sex-matched. To avoid the comparison group being mixed up with new-identified HBV and HCV groups, patients in whom HBV and HCV identified during the follow-up period were excluded. Originally, 939,971 subjects were retrieved from the NHIRD after excluding any type of chronic hepatitis (including diagnoses of HBV and HCV and chronic hepatitis (ICD-9-CM: 070.9, 571.4, 571.8, and 571.9)) or missing information on age and sex. A total of 84,796 non-viral hepatitis subjects were finally enrolled in this study with same exclusion criteria of the exposure group (Fig. 1).

Statistical Analysis

We first compared the distribution of sociodemographic factors (sex, age, occupation, monthly income, and the geographical location, and the urbanization level of the community in which the patient resided) and the proportions of comorbidities between the cohorts with and those without viral hepatitis (HBV and HCV). Potential baseline comorbidities, including diabetes mellitus (DM) (ICD-9-CM: 250), coronary artery disease (CAD) (ICD-9-CM: 410–414), hyperlipidemia (ICD-9-CM: 272), and hypertension (ICD-9-CM: 401–405), were also ascertained in patients with and without chronic viral hepatitis by searching for the presence of diagnostic codes at any time starting in fiscal year 2000.

The incidence rates of oral cavity cancer in the three groups of patients with viral hepatitis (HBV alone, HCV alone, and HBV/HCV dual infections) were calculated in the follow-up period until the end of 2008. Follow-up time (in person-years) was calculated for each person until oral cavity cancer was diagnosed or censored for death, migration, or discontinued enrolment in the NHI database. The rate ratio was determined under the Poisson assumption. Crude and adjusted hazard ratio (HR) and 95% confidence interval (CI) for factors associated with risk of oral cavity cancer were estimated using univariate and multivariate Cox proportion hazard regression models. To address the hypothesis of the presence of an association between viral hepatitis and oral cavity cancer, interaction between viral hepatitis status and sex as well as the age of developing oral cavity cancer was tested in the Cox models. All analyses were performed by SAS statistical software for Windows (Version 9.1; SAS Institute, Inc., Cary, NC, USA), and the significance level was set to be 0.05.

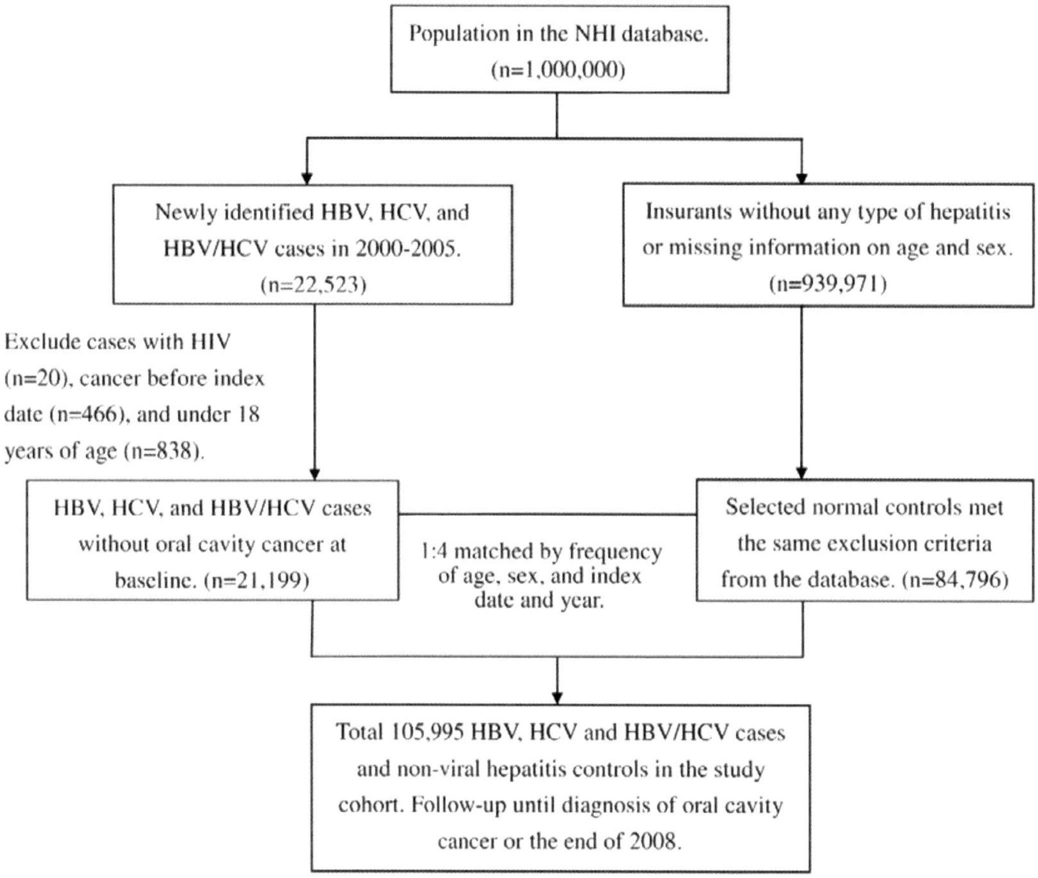

Figure 1. Study flow chart showing the selection of subjects. Footnotes: NHI, National Health Insurance.

Results

Baseline Characteristics and Comorbidities of the Study Subjects

In our study, the patients with HCV infection were more likely to be older, blue collar workers, living in lower urbanization level areas in southern Taiwan, as well as to have lower income levels than the 84,769 non-viral hepatitis comparison subjects (Table 1). They also were more likely to have DM, hypertension, and hyperlipidemia. On the contrary, patients with HBV tended to be younger and to have a lower prevalence of CAD and hypertension than subjects in the non-viral hepatitis comparison group.

Incidence Densities and HR of Oral Cancer among Viral Hepatitis

In total, we observed 198 cases of oral cavity cancer (174 males and 24 females) among 682,647 person-years, with an incidence density of 2.90 per 10,000 person-years (Table 2). The univariate Cox proportional hazard regression analysis revealed that the risk of developing oral cavity cancer among men with hepatitis was more than 5-fold higher than among women with hepatitis (HR = 5.88, 95% CI = 3.84–9.01). The highest age-specific HR was observed in the 50–59-year age group (HR = 15.9, 95% CI = 6.36–39.5). People residing in eastern Taiwan and those residing on offshore islands had 2.99-fold higher risk (95% CI = 1.88–4.75) of developing oral cavity cancer than individuals living in northern Taiwan. Blue collar workers tended to have a significantly higher risk of developing oral cavity cancer than white collar workers (HR = 1.65, 95% CI = 1.20–2.27). Subjects with a monthly income ranging from 1–15841 NT dollars were at the highest of developing oral cavity cancer (HR = 2.49, 95% CI = 1.45–4.27) among the income groups. The incidence of oral cavity cancer was approximately 2.3-fold higher in the cohort of patients with HCV infection than subjects in the non-viral hepatitis group (6.15 versus 2.69 per 10,000 person-years) (HR = 2.28, 95% CI = 1.44–3.60). There was no significant association between patients with HBV alone or patients with HBV+HCV dual infections and risk of developing oral cavity cancer. In addition, baseline comorbidities, including DM, CAD, hyperlipidemia, and hypertension were not significant risk factors for developing oral cavity cancer.

Significant predictors in the univariate analysis were included in a multivariate Cox hazard model to identify the most important risk factors for oral cavity cancer (Table 2). Because occupation and monthly income were highly correlated, we selected monthly income for multivariate analysis. In the multivariate Cox hazard model, we found that men had a 6.7-fold greater risk of developing oral cavity cancer than women (HR = 6.70, 95% CI = 4.34–10.3). The highest age-specific HR still remained in the 50–59-year age group (HR = 17.9, 95% CI = 7.11–45.0). Individuals living in eastern Taiwan and islands had significantly highest risk of developing oral cavity cancer (HR = 2.52, 95% CI = 1.58–4.03), whereas monthly income levels were not related to the disease risk. The multivariate Cox model also showed that the risk of developing oral cavity cancer was significantly higher among subjects with HCV infection than among individuals with no

Table 1. Baseline characteristics and comorbidities between viral hepatitis and non-viral hepatitis adult groups identified in 2000–2005.

	Viral hepatitis								
	No		HBV alone		HCV alone		HBV+HCV		
	N = 84796		N = 12369		N = 5311		N = 3519		
Variables	n	(%)	n	(%)	n	(%)	n	(%)	p-value[†]
Sex									<0.0001
Women	37444	(44.2)	5145	(41.6)	2653	(50.0)	1563	(44.4)	
Men	47352	(55.8)	7224	(58.4)	2658	(50.1)	1956	(55.6)	
Age, years									<0.0001
18–29	18200	(21.5)	3472	(28.1)	527	(9.9)	551	(15.7)	
30–39	17556	(20.7)	3113	(25.2)	668	(12.6)	608	(17.3)	
40–49	19068	(22.5)	2842	(23.0)	1120	(21.1)	805	(22.9)	
50–59	13760	(16.2)	1619	(13.1)	1113	(21.0)	708	(20.1)	
60–69	10316	(12.2)	883	(7.1)	1105	(20.8)	591	(16.8)	
70–79	5032	(5.9)	380	(3.1)	660	(12.4)	218	(6.2)	
≥80	864	(1.0)	60	(0.5)	118	(2.2)	38	(1.1)	
Geographic region									<0.0001
Northern	40020	(47.2)	5468	(44.2)	1540	(29.0)	1126	(32.0)	
Central	16791	(19.8)	2672	(21.6)	1153	(21.7)	729	(20.7)	
Southern	21349	(25.2)	3297	(26.7)	2196	(41.4)	1401	(39.8)	
Eastern and Islands	6635	(7.8)	932	(7.5)	422	(8.0)	263	(7.5)	
Occupation									<0.0001
Public	8132	(9.6)	1490	(12.1)	419	(7.9)	339	(9.6)	
Labor	27421	(32.3)	3671	(29.7)	2522	(47.5)	1488	(42.3)	
Business	37891	(44.7)	5802	(46.9)	1611	(30.3)	1268	(36.0)	
Low income	371	(0.4)	46	(0.4)	49	(0.9)	19	(0.5)	
Retired and others	10981	(13.0)	1360	(11.0)	710	(13.4)	405	(11.5)	
Urbanization level									<0.0001
1	25896	(30.5)	3627	(29.3)	1069	(20.1)	804	(22.9)	
2	24648	(29.1)	3712	(30.0)	1530	(28.8)	1001	(28.5)	
3	15623	(18.4)	2327	(18.8)	888	(16.7)	625	(17.8)	
4	18621	(22.0)	2702	(21.9)	1823	(34.3)	1089	(31.0)	
Monthly income, NT$									<0.0001
0	18817	(22.2)	2560	(20.7)	1147	(21.6)	722	(20.5)	
1–15840	10378	(12.2)	1280	(10.4)	637	(12.0)	353	(10.0)	
15841–25000	36597	(43.2)	5043	(40.8)	2743	(51.7)	1752	(49.8)	
>25000	19004	(22.4)	3486	(28.2)	784	(14.8)	692	(19.7)	
Diabetes mellitus									<0.0001
No	78312	(92.4)	11364	(91.9)	4320	(81.3)	2991	(85.0)	
Yes	6484	(7.7)	1005	(8.1)	991	(18.7)	528	(15.0)	
Coronary artery disease									<0.0001
No	37983	(44.8)	6495	(52.5)	2468	(46.5)	1757	(49.9)	
Yes	46813	(55.2)	5874	(47.5)	2843	(53.5)	1762	(50.1)	
Hypertension									<0.0001
No	69159	(81.6)	10479	(84.7)	3463	(65.2)	2575	(73.2)	
Yes	15637	(18.4)	1890	(15.3)	1848	(34.8)	944	(26.8)	
Hyperlipidemia									<0.0001
No	76023	(89.7)	10797	(87.3)	4289	(80.8)	2905	(82.6)	
Yes	8773	(10.4)	1572	(12.7)	1022	(19.2)	614	(17.5)	

Urbanization level: 1 indicate the highest level of urbanization and 4 the lowest.
[†]Chi-square test.

Table 2. Incidence density of oral cavity cancer for viral hepatitis and non-viral hepatitis adult cohorts identified in 2000–2005.

				Univariate		Multivariate	
	Cases	PY	I[a]	HR	(95% CI)	HR	(95% CI)
Sex							
Women	24	305111	0.79	1.00	(reference)	1.00	(reference)
Men	174	377536	4.61	5.88	(3.84–9.01)***	6.70	(4.34–10.3)***
Age, years							
18–29	5	150172	0.33	1.00	(reference)	1.00	(reference)
30–39	33	143684	2.30	6.91	(2.70–17.7)***	7.43	(2.88–19.2)***
40–49	65	155956	4.17	12.5	(5.05–31.2)***	13.7	(5.47–34.5)***
50–59	58	110782	5.24	15.9	(6.36–39.5)***	17.9	(7.11–45.0)***
60–69	28	81639	3.43	10.4	(4.01–26.9)***	10.6	(4.08–27.6)***
70–79	8	35840	2.23	6.92	(2.26–21.1)**	6.25	(2.03–19.2)***
≥80	1	4572	2.19	7.24	(0.85–62.0)	6.59	(0.77–56.6)
Geographic region							
Northern	53	309978	1.71	1.00	(reference)	1.00	(reference)
Central	45	137697	3.27	1.91	(1.28–2.84)**	1.68	(1.12–2.51)*
Southern	73	182033	4.01	2.34	(1.64–3.34)***	1.98	(1.38–2.84)**
Eastern and island	27	52932	5.10	2.99	(1.88–4.75)***	2.52	(1.58–4.03)***
Occupation							
Public	17	67960	2.50	1.10	(0.65–1.87)		
Labor	85	226777	3.75	1.65	(1.20–2.27)**		
Business	68	299509	2.27	1.00	(reference)		
Low income	1	2916	3.43	1.53	(0.21–11.0)		
Retired and others	27	85484	3.16	1.39	(0.89–2.18)		
Monthly income, NT$							
0	23	146869	1.57	1.00	(reference)	1.00	(reference)
1–15840	31	79023	3.92	2.49	(1.45–4.27)**	1.37	(0.79–2.37)
15841–25000	107	298236	3.59	2.27	(1.45–3.56)**	1.13	(0.71–1.79)
>25000	37	158519	2.33	1.47	(0.88–2.48)	0.65	(0.38–1.12)
Viral hepatitis							
No	147	546846	2.69	1.00	(reference)	1.00	(reference)
HBV alone	21	78803	2.66	1.00	(0.63–1.58)	1.11	(0.70–1.75)
HCV alone	21	34150	6.15	2.28	(1.44–3.60)**	1.90	(1.20–3.02)**
HBV+HCV	9	22848	3.94	1.46	(0.75–2.86)	1.21	(0.62–2.38)

PY, person-years; I, incidence; HR, hazard ratio; CI, confidence interval.
a: incidence rate (per 10,000 person-years).
*$P<0.05$, ** $P<0.01$, *** $P<0.0001$.

hepatitis group (HR = 1.90, 95% CI = 1.20–3.02). Further data analysis showed that HCV was a significant risk factor for oral cavity cancer even after excluding individuals with diagnoses of smoking-related cancers (including ICD-9-CM: 146–150, 157, 160–162, and 189) during the follow-up period (HR = 1.92, 95% CI = 1.21–3.04) (not shown in the tables).

Adjusted HRs of Oral Cavity Cancer with Viral Hepatitis by Age and Sex Stratification

Table 3 shows the age-specific and sex-specific HRs of oral cavity cancer for hepatitis cohorts compared to the comparison cohort. The adjusted HRs of oral cavity cancer among subjects infected with HCV alone were highest in those aged 40–49 years (HR = 2.57, 95% CI = 1.21–5.46) followed by those <40 years old (HR = 2.48, 95% CI = 0.75–8.19). However, no significant associations appeared for those with HBV alone or those with HCV/HBV dual infections. Furthermore, the sex-specific adjusted HRs of oral cavity cancer associated with HCV were 1.69 (95% CI = 0.49–5.83) for women and 1.88 (95% CI = 1.14–3.09) for men. On the contrary, there were no significant risks of oral cavity cancer in those with sole HBV infection or those with HBV/HCV dual infections. The interaction between HCV status and age of developing oral cavity cancer was moderately significant ($P = 0.078$). In the contrast, the interaction between HCV status and sex was not statistically significant ($P = 0.97$).

Table 3. Adjusted HRs and 95% CIs of oral cavity cancer associated with viral hepatitis compared with non-viral hepatitis by age and sex stratification.

	Viral hepatitis					
	HBV alone		HCV alone		HBV + HCV	
	aHR	(95% CI)	aHR	(95% CI)	aHR	(95% CI)
Age, years[a]						
<40	1.01	(0.39–2.63)	2.48	(0.75–8.19)	1.86	(0.44–7.84)
40–49	0.85	(0.36–1.98)	2.57	(1.21–5.46)*	0.93	(0.22–3.82)
50–59	1.24	(0.53–2.92)	1.67	(0.70–3.95)	1.55	(0.55–4.34)
≥60	1.86	(0.65–5.33)	1.20	(0.42–3.45)	0.65	(0.09–4.76)
Interaction		p = 0.16		p = 0.078		p = 0.61
Sex[b]						
Women	1.18	(0.27–5.12)	1.69	(0.49–5.83)	1.18	(0.16–8.92)
Men	1.08	(0.66–1.75)	1.88	(1.14–3.09)*	1.28	(0.63–2.62)
Interaction		p = 0.83		p = 0.97		p = 0.90

aHR: adjusted hazard ratio.
a: adjusted for sex, region, and income.
b: adjusted for age, region, and income.
*$P<0.05$, ** $P<0.01$.

Discussion

In this nationwide, population-based cohort study conducted in an area where both viral hepatitis and oral cavity cancer are endemic, significant risk of developing oral cavity cancer was observed in patients with HCV but not HBV infection. We also found that, in the general Taiwanese population, male subjects tended to have a 6.7-fold higher risk of developing oral cavity cancer than female counterparts. This finding is compatible with the finding reported in the Taiwan government cancer registry report [14]. The age of developing oral cavity cancer among HCV carriers (peak age group: 40–49 years) also tended to be younger than that of the general population (peak age group: 50–59 years). We also observed that subjects residing in the eastern Taiwan and islands had significantly highest risk of developing oral cavity cancer, followed by those living in the southern part of Taiwan.

HCV infection predisposes patients to extrahepatic disorders involving renal, dermatologic, hematologic, and rheumatologic systems as well as autoimmune abnormalities [18,19]. Extrahepatic manifestations may result from immunologic trigger mechanisms as well as viral invasion and replication that affect extrahepatic tissues and organs [20].

The association between HCV infection and oral cavity cancer is still controversial [11,12,13]. HCV is a virus with triple tissue tropism – hepatotropism, lymphotropism, and sialotropism [21]. HCV RNA has been detected in saliva and salivary tissue in patients with chronic salivary gland disorders, a finding that suggests that HCV, a sialotropic virus, can reside within salivary gland cells [22]. Other studies, however, have shown that HCV detection in saliva and in salivary glands is not related to oral health conditions [23,24,25]. Grossmann et al. suggest that HCV might play an indirect role in causing diseases of the oral cavity and salivary glands by stimulating an immune response [21]. In addition, one of the most frequently reported oral extrahepatic manifestations of HCV infection is lichen planus [26,27,28]. This premalignant condition is associated with the development of OSCC [29]. In a Brazilian cross-sectional study, there was a significant association between oral lichen planus and hepatitis C in their cohort of 215 patients with chronic HCV infection [21]. The progression of lichen planus into OSCC in patients with hepatitis C has been described in two case reports [29,30]. Several studies have shown that the transformation rate of oral lichen planus to OSCC is approximately 0.04% to 1.74% [31,32]. Interestingly, Nobles et al. demonstrated no predilection for the development of oral cavity cancers in patients infected with HCV [12]. Therefore, the role that HCV and its viral proteins play in the pathogenesis of oral diseases remains unclear.

Furthermore, Nagao et al. reported a higher prevalence of HCV antibody and RNA in patients with oral cavity cancer [11]. However, in 2002, Takata et al. reported, after age adjustment, a significantly decreased prevalence of HCV antibody in their patients with oral cavity cancer [13]. Using logistic regression analysis to eliminate the influence of age, Takata and colleagues suggested that the increased prevalence of HCV antibody in oral cavity cancer patients is more likely due to age differences rather than to carcinogenic action of HCV [11,27,28]. In addition, Nobles et al. observed that HCV patients present with an earlier age of onset of squamous cell carcinoma of the head and neck (SCCHN) than controls [12]. The age difference between these two groups may reflect differences in risk factors for the development of hepatitis C. The increased prevalence of intravenous drug abuse among younger populations, and socio-economic differences between young and old age groups may also explain the age difference. Nobles and his colleagues also suggested HCV is considered a cofactor instead of a comorbid condition in relation to the development of head and neck cancer [12]. The localization of HCV RNA in oral lichen planus and OSCC tissue derived from patients with hepatitis C may provide one possible explanation to oral carcinogenesis of HCV [28]. In this prospective cohort study, we demonstrated that HCV is a risk factor for the development of oral cavity cancer (HR = 2.57, 95% CI = 1.21–5.46 in the 40–49 year age group). The risk of developing oral cavity caner among patients with HCV is 10 years earlier than the general population. This finding is unlike the finding reported in the retrospective case study by Takata and his colleagues [13]. In addition, multivariate Cox regression analysis revealed that males had a 6.7-fold greater risk of developing oral cavity cancer than females. The discrepancy between men and women in the general population can be explained by the fact that men tend to be engaged in riskier lifestyle behaviors than women, such as cigarette smoking (46.8% vs. 4.3%), frequent alcohol consumption (15.1% vs. 2.6%), and betel quid chewing (14.4% vs. 1.5%) [33,34,35]. However, among the HCV infected subjects, female carriers are at similar risk of developing oral cavity cancer to their male counterparts (HRs were 1.69 and 1.88, respectively). Cacoub et al. suggested that female sex is one of the risk factors associated with developing extrahepatic manifestations of HCV infection [36]. Although another possibility to explain the stronger association of HCV with oral cancer for females compared to males might be due to the small number of female oral cancer subjects in our cohort, this finding provided an interesting observation. Further studies with larger female samples are needed to verify this observation.

In this study, infection with HBV alone and HBV/HCV coinfection were not correlated with oral cavity cancer. Our finding is consistent with that reported in a Japanese study, which showed that high levels of HBV surface antigen were observed in patients with benign oral tumors but not in patients with oral cavity cancer requiring dental surgery [13]. Their finding suggests that HBV infection is unlikely to play a major role in oral tumor formation. A study by Bokor-Bratic also suggested that oral leukoplakia was not associated with HBV infection in Serbia [37]. In addition, only HCV has the lymphatrophic character that is assumed to be the cause of HCV-associated extrahepatic manifestations [38]. Therefore, this HCV's lymphatrophic character may explain why we found that HCV, but not HBV, was associated with oral cavity cancer. HBV and HCV are both hepatrophic viruses. Their coinfection is associated with clinically and histologically more severe liver disease and higher risk for the development of hepatocellular carcinoma [15,39]. Cho et al. have recently demonstrated in a meta-analysis study that co-infection of HBV and HCV has a subadditive risk for HCC [40]. Other clinical studies suggested a reciprocal interference of one virus on the replication of the other or both [41,42]. Some other clinical studies also showed co-infected cases with the phenomenon of HBV dominant or HCV dominant effect [43,44]. This reciprocal interference between HBV and HCV may also explain the lack of increasing incidence of oral cavity cancer among our HBV+HCV infected population as one or both viruses were inhibited for their replication. Further prospective cohort studies are required to verify this finding.

This study has 2 main strengths. First, our study is the very first one used complete nationwide population-based data to assess the association between chronic viral hepatitis infection and oral cavity cancer. The sample size is large to differentiate risk difference between those with HBV and HCV infections. Second, selection and nonresponse biases may have been minimized by the comprehensive coverage of the NHI system (>96% of the islanders) and the large sample size.

This study had several limitations. First, some patients with hepatitis infection do not have obvious clinical symptoms and, therefore, might not seek medical attention. Claims for medical services would, therefore, not be available for those patients. As a result, some patients with asymptomatic hepatitis infection were most likely included in the comparison group. However, if viral hepatitis infection is associated causally with oral cavity cancer, this misclassification may lead the estimated HRs toward the null and further strengthen our findings. In addition, the overall seroprevalence of antibody to HCV (anti-HCV) in Taiwan has been estimated approximately <3% [45,46]. The prevalence of chronic HCV infection identified in our cohort was approximately 2.2%. Therefore, the positive association between HCV and oral cavity cancer in our cohort is accountable. Second, some oral cavity cancer risk factors, such as chewing of betel nut, smoking, and alcohol consumption were unavailable in the insurance claims database. Therefore, we cannot rule out some of the potential confounding effects associated with these factors. Ko et al. suggested that betel quid chewing is the most potent risk factor for oral cavity cancer in Taiwan, followed by cigarette smoking and alcohol drinking [47]. In Taiwan, the prevalence of cigarette smoking and betel quid chewing is highest in the eastern region, followed by the southern region [33]. Betel nut chewers in Taiwan are who tend to be poorly educated, low income earners, and blue collar workers [33]. We, hence, included monthly income and geographical regions in our multivariate Cox hazard model to reduce confounding effects caused by betel quid chewing, cigarette smoking, and alcohol consumption. In addition, in Taiwan, almost all betel quid chewers are smokers [33]. After excluding smoking-related cancers among our subjects, we found that the HR of oral cavity cancer for HCV alone infection increased from 1.90 to 1.92. Therefore, these lifestyle factors may not significantly confound our results as we thought. Third, the diagnoses of oral cavity cancer, HBV infection, HCV infection, and other comorbidities based on International Classification of Disease codes may be less accurate than those obtained through a standardized procedure. However, the NHI Bureau of Taiwan randomly samples a fixed percentage of claims from every hospital and randomly interviews patients and reviews charts each year to verify the diagnosis validity and quality of care [48]. Patients with confirmed oral cavity cancer deserve medical cares as the "Catastrophic Illness" with minimum co-payment under the Taiwan NHI plan. All cancers are histology confirmed. The diagnoses of oral cavity cancer are likely accurate and are representative of all oral cavity cancer in Taiwan. Fourth, the vast majority of the residents in Taiwan are of Chinese ethnicity. Hence, the ability to generalize the results to other racial/ethnic groups is unclear given that the transmission route of viral hepatitis infection in Chinese might not be the same as that in other ethnic groups. Fifth, there is some plausibility for the association of lichen planus (one of the most frequently reported oral extrahepatic manifestations of HCV infection) and oral cavity cancer [29]. However, the incidence of lichen planus in our subjects was not indexed on the insurance records.

In summary, in this nationwide population-based cohort study conducted in a country in which both viral hepatitis and oral cavity cancer are endemic, we found a positive association between oral cavity cancer and HCV infection. Male subjects were at higher risk of developing oral cavity cancer than their female counterparts. Patients with HCV presented at an earlier age of onset of oral cavity cancer than subjects in the viral hepatitis-free control group. More perspective cohort studies are needed to determine the association between oral cavity cancer and HCV infection.

Acknowledgments

This study is based in part on data from the National Health Insurance Research Database provided by the Bureau of National Health Insurance, Department of Health, Taiwan and managed by the National Health Research Institutes. The interpretations and conclusions contained herein do not represent those of the Bureau of National Health Insurance, Department of Health, or the National Health Research Institutes.

Author Contributions

Conceived and designed the experiments: FHS SFH FCS HYC CCY. Performed the experiments: FHS CCY CTS PCC SNC. Analyzed the data: SNC PCC FCS HYC. Contributed reagents/materials/analysis tools: CCL SFH. Wrote the paper: FHS FCS CCY.

References

1. Kademani D (2007) Oral cancer. Mayo Clin Proc 82: 878–887.
2. Lin WJ, Jiang RS, Wu SH, Chen FJ, Liu SA (2011) Smoking, alcohol, and betel quid and oral cancer: a prospective cohort study. J Oncol 2011: 525976.
3. Conway DI, Petticrew M, Marlborough H, Berthiller J, Hashibe M, et al. (2008) Socioeconomic inequalities and oral cancer risk: a systematic review and meta-analysis of case-control studies. Int J Cancer 122: 2811–2819.
4. Parkin DM (2006) The global health burden of infection-associated cancers in the year 2002. Int J Cancer 118: 3030–3044.
5. Sarid R, Gao SJ (2011) Viruses and human cancer: from detection to causality. Cancer Lett 305: 218–227.
6. Omland LH, Farkas DK, Jepsen P, Obel N, Pedersen L (2010) Hepatitis C virus infection and risk of cancer: a population-based cohort study. Clin epidemiol 2: 179–186.
7. Giordano TP, Henderson L, Landgren O, Chiao EY, Kramer JR, et al. (2007) Risk of non-Hodgkin lymphoma and lymphoproliferative precursor diseases in US veterans with hepatitis C virus. JAMA 297: 2010–2017.
8. Engels EA, Cho ER, Jee SH (2010) Hepatitis B virus infection and risk of non-Hodgkin lymphoma in South Korea: a cohort study. Lancet Oncol 11: 827–834.
9. Fwu CW, Chien YC, You SL, Nelson KE, Kirk GD, et al. (2011) Hepatitis B virus infection and risk of intrahepatic cholangiocarcinoma and non-Hodgkin

lymphoma: a cohort study of parous women in Taiwan. Hepatology 53: 1217–1225.

10. Iloeje UH, Yang HI, Jen CL, Su J, Wang LY, et al. (2010) Risk of pancreatic cancer in chronic hepatitis B virus infection: data from the REVEAL-HBV cohort study. Liver Int 30: 423–429.
11. Nagao Y, Sata M, Tanikawa K, Itoh K, Kameyama T (1995) High prevalence of hepatitis C virus antibody and RNA in patients with oral cancer. J Oral Pathol Med 24: 354–360.
12. Nobles J, Wold C, Fazekas-May M, Gilbert J, Friedlander PL (2004) Prevalence and epidemiology of hepatitis C virus in patients with squamous cell carcinoma of the head and neck. Laryngoscope 114: 2119–2122.
13. Takata Y, Takahashi T, Fukuda J (2002) Prevalence of hepatitis virus infection in association with oral diseases requiring surgery. Oral Dis 8: 95–99.
14. Bureau of Health Promotion, Department of Health, Taiwan, ROC. Cancer Registry Annual Report, 1995–2008. Taipei: Department of Health, Executive Yuan, Taiwan, ROC.
15. Tsai MC, Kee KM, Chen YD, Lin LC, Tsai LS, et al. (2007) Excess mortality of hepatocellular carcinoma and morbidity of liver cirrhosis and hepatitis in HCV-endemic areas in an HBV-endemic country: geographic variations among 502 villages in southern Taiwan. J Gastroenterol Hepatol 22: 92–98.
16. Lu JF, Hsiao WC (2003) Does universal health insurance make health care unaffordable? Lessons from Taiwan. Health Aff (Millwood) 22: 77–88.
17. Chiang TL (1997) Taiwan's 1995 health care reform. Health Policy 39: 225–239.
18. Gumber SC, Chopra S (1995) Hepatitis C: a multifaceted disease. Review of extrahepatic manifestations. Ann Intern Med 123: 615–620.
19. Zignego AL, Ferri C, Pileri SA, Caini P, Bianchi FB (2007) Extrahepatic manifestations of Hepatitis C Virus infection: a general overview and guidelines for a clinical approach. Dig Liver Dis 39: 2–17.
20. Hadziyannis SJ (1996) Nonhepatic manifestations and combined diseases in HCV infection. Dig Dis Sci 41: 63S–74S.
21. Grossmann Sde M, Teixeira R, de Aguiar MC, de Moura MD, do Carmo MA (2009) Oral mucosal conditions in chronic hepatitis C Brazilian patients: a cross-sectional study. J Public Health Dent 69: 168–175.
22. Grossmann Sde M, Teixeira R, Oliveira GC, Gleber-Netto FO, Araujo FM, et al. (2010) Xerostomia, hyposalivation and sialadenitis in patients with chronic hepatitis C are not associated with the detection of HCV RNA in saliva or salivary glands. J Clin Pathol 63: 1002–1007.
23. Lins L, Almeida H, Vitvisk L, Carmo T, Parana R, et al. (2005) Detection of hepatitis C virus RNA in saliva is not related to oral health status or viral load. J Med Virol 77: 216–220.
24. Maticic M, Poljak M, Kramar B, Seme K, Brinovec V, et al. (2001) Detection of hepatitis C virus RNA from gingival crevicular fluid and its relation to virus presence in saliva. J Periodontol 72: 11–16.
25. Liou TC, Chang TT, Young KC, Lin XZ, Lin CY, et al. (1992) Detection of HCV RNA in saliva, urine, seminal fluid, and ascites. J Med Virol 37: 197–202.
26. Lodi G, Giuliani M, Majorana A, Sardella A, Bez C, et al. (2004) Lichen planus and hepatitis C virus: a multicentre study of patients with oral lesions and a systematic review. Br J Dermatol 151: 1172–1181.
27. Nagao Y, Tanaka J, Nakanishi T, Moriya T, Katayama K, et al. (2002) High incidence of extrahepatic manifestations in an HCV hyperendemic area. Hepatol Res 22: 27–36.
28. Nagao Y, Sata M, Noguchi S, Seno'o T, Kinoshita M, et al. (2000) Detection of hepatitis C virus RNA in oral lichen planus and oral cancer tissues. J Oral Pathol Med 29: 259–266.
29. Porter SR, Lodi G, Chandler K, Kumar N (1997) Development of squamous cell carcinoma in hepatitis C virus-associated lichen planus. Oral Oncol 33: 58–59.
30. Carrozzo M, Carbone M, Gandolfo S, Valente G, Colombatto P, et al. (1997) An atypical verrucous carcinoma of the tongue arising in a patient with oral lichen planus associated with hepatitis C virus infection. Oral Oncol 33: 220–225.
31. Bouquot JE, Gorlin RJ (1986) Leukoplakia, lichen planus, and other oral keratoses in 23,616 white Americans over the age of 35 years. Oral Surg Oral Med Oral Pathol 61: 373–381.
32. Barnard NA, Scully C, Eveson JW, Cunningham S, Porter SR (1993) Oral cancer development in patients with oral lichen planus. J Oral Pathol Med 22: 421–424.
33. Wen CP, Tsai SP, Cheng TY, Chen CJ, Levy DT, et al. (2005) Uncovering the relation between betel quid chewing and cigarette smoking in Taiwan. Tob Control 14 Suppl 1: i16–22.
34. Wen CP, Levy DT, Cheng TY, Hsu CC, Tsai SP (2005) Smoking behaviour in Taiwan, 2001. Tob Control 14 Suppl 1: i51–55.
35. Chuang YC, Chuang KY (2008) Gender differences in relationships between social capital and individual smoking and drinking behavior in Taiwan. Soc Sci Med 67: 1321–1330.
36. Cacoub P, Renou C, Rosenthal E, Cohen P, Loury I, et al. (2000) Extrahepatic manifestations associated with hepatitis C virus infection. A prospective multicenter study of 321 patients. The GERMIVIC. Groupe d'Etude et de Recherche en Medecine Interne et Maladies Infectieuses sur le Virus de l'Hepatite C. Medicine 79: 47–56.
37. Bokor-Bratic M (2006) No evidence of hepatitis C virus infection in Serbian patients with oral leukoplakia. J Oral Pathol Med 35: 626–629.
38. Agnello V, De Rosa FG (2004) Extrahepatic disease manifestations of HCV infection: some current issues. J Hepatol 40: 341–352.
39. Shepard CW, Finelli L, Alter MJ (2005) Global epidemiology of hepatitis C virus infection. Lancet Infect Dis 5: 558–567.
40. Cho LY, Yang JJ, Ko KP, Park B, Shin A, et al. (2011) Coinfection of hepatitis B and C viruses and risk of hepatocellular carcinoma: systematic review and meta-analysis. Int J Cancer 128: 176–184.
41. Chu CM, Yeh CT, Liaw YF (1998) Low-level viremia and intracellular expression of hepatitis B surface antigen (HBsAg) in HBsAg carriers with concurrent hepatitis C virus infection. J Clin Microbiol 36: 2084–2086.
42. Sheen IS, Liaw YF, Chu CM, Pao CC (1992) Role of hepatitis C virus infection in spontaneous hepatitis B surface antigen clearance during chronic hepatitis B virus infection. J Infect Dis 165: 831–834.
43. Ohkawa K, Hayashi N, Yuki N, Masuzawa M, Kato M, et al. (1995) Long-term follow-up of hepatitis B virus and hepatitis C virus replicative levels in chronic hepatitis patients coinfected with both viruses. J Med Virol 46: 258–264.
44. Zarski JP, Bohn B, Bastie A, Pawlotsky JM, Baud M, et al. (1998) Characteristics of patients with dual infection by hepatitis B and C viruses. J Hepatol 28: 27–33.
45. Lee SD, Chan CY, Wang YJ, Wu JC, Lai KH, et al. (1991) Seroepidemiology of hepatitis C virus infection in Taiwan. Hepatology 13: 830–833.
46. Chen DS, Kuo GC, Sung JL, Lai MY, Sheu JC, et al. (1990) Hepatitis C virus infection in an area hyperendemic for hepatitis B and chronic liver disease: the Taiwan experience. J Infect Dis 162: 817–822.
47. Ko YC, Huang YL, Lee CH, Chen MJ, Lin LM, et al. (1995) Betel quid chewing, cigarette smoking and alcohol consumption related to oral cancer in Taiwan. J Oral Pathol Med 24: 450–453.
48. Bureau of National Health Insurance. Available: http://www.nhi.gov.tw/information/bulle-tin_file/421_0890036465–19.doc. Accessed: 2012 Feb 1.

Aflatoxin-Induced *TP53 R249S* Mutation in HepatoCellular Carcinoma in Thailand: Association with Tumors Developing in the Absence of Liver Cirrhosis

Stephanie Villar[1]¶, Sandra Ortiz-Cuaran[1]¶, Behnoush Abedi-Ardekani[1], Doriane Gouas[1], Andre Nogueira da Costa[1], Amelie Plymoth[2], Thiravud Khuhaprema[3], Anant Kalalak[3], Suleeporn Sangrajrang[3], Marlin D. Friesen[4], John D. Groopman[4], Pierre Hainaut[1,5]*

1 International Agency for Research on Cancer, Lyon, France, **2** Karolinska Institute, Stockholm, Sweden, **3** National Cancer Institute, Bangkok, Thailand, **4** Bloomberg School of Public Health, Johns Hopkins University, Baltimore, Maryland, United States of America, **5** International Prevention Research Institute, Lyon, France

Abstract

Primary Liver Cancer (PLC) is the leading cause of death by cancer among males in Thailand and the 3rd among females. Most cases are hepatocellular carcinoma (HCC) but cholangiocarcinomas represent between 4 and 80% of liver cancers depending upon geographic area. Most HCC are associated with chronic infection by Hepatitis B Virus while a G→T mutation at codon 249 of the *TP53* gene, *R249S*, specific for exposure to aflatoxin, is detected in tumors for up to 30% of cases. We have used Short Oligonucleotide Mass Analysis (SOMA) to quantify free circulating *R249S*-mutated DNA in plasma using blood specimens collected in a hospital case:control study. Plasma *R249S*-mutated DNA was detectable at low concentrations (≥67 copies/mL) in 53 to 64% of patients with primary liver cancer or chronic liver disease and in 19% of controls. 44% of patients with HCC and no evidence of cirrhosis had plasma concentrations of *R249S*-mutated DNA ≥150 copies/mL, compared to 21% in patients with both HCC and cirrhosis, 22% in patients with cholangiocarcinoma, 12% in patients with non-cancer chronic liver disease and 3% of subjects in the reference group. Thus, plasma concentrations of *R249S*-mutated DNA ≥150 copies/mL tended to be more common in patients with HCC developing without pre-existing cirrhosis ($p = 0.027$). Overall, these results support the preferential occurrence of *R249S*-mutated DNA in HCC developing in the absence of cirrhosis in a context of HBV chronic infection.

Editor: Michael Bouchard, Drexel University College of Medicine, United States of America

Funding: This work was supported by funds from IARC and from Ligue Contre le Cancer, Département du Rhône, France. The funders had no role in study design, data collection and analysis, decision to publish, or preparation of the manuscript.

Competing Interests: The authors have declared that no competing interests exist.

* E-mail: pierre.hainaut@i-pri.org

¶ These authors contributed equally to this work.

Introduction

Liver cancer accounts for approximately 6% of all new cancer cases diagnosed worldwide; it is the fifth most common cancer in men and the eighth most common in females worldwide [1,2]. The majority of primary liver cancers in adults are hepatocellular carcinoma (HCC; 90%) whereas cholangiocarcinomas (CC) account for about 9% of the cases, with peaks in incidence in parts of South-East Asia. Approximately 80% of HCCs and the resulting deaths occur in low and middle income countries of Eastern Asia, Sub-Saharan Africa and South America, where high incidences of Hepatitis B Virus (HBV) and/or Hepatitis C Virus (HCV) are endemic and where aflatoxin-contaminated staple foods are consumed [3]. CC develops in intra-hepatic billiary epithelial cells and is caused by the chronic infection of billiary ducts by liver flukes *Opisthorchis viverrini* and *Clonorchis Sinesis*. These liver flukes are endemic mainly in Eastern Asia, notably in Thailand, Laos, Vietnam and South-Eastern China [4]. According to a recent evaluation of the carcinogenic risk to humans by the International Agency for Research on Cancer Monographs, there is only limited evidence for association chronic HBV/HCV with risk of CC and no evidence for association with aflatoxin exposure [5,6].

In Thailand, liver cancer is the leading cause of death from cancer among men (age-standardized incidence rates, world standard, ASR = 35.1) and the third leading cause in women (ASR = 16.6) [1]. The geographical distribution of cholangiocarcinoma matches the prevalence of chronic infection by *O. viverrini*, which is endemic in the north-east and rare in southern Thailand. In males, the age-standardized incidence rates (ASR, world standard) for HCC and CC, respectively, are 11.6 and 7.2 for Chiang Mai, 11.0 and 10.4 for Lampang, 12.5 and 67.5 for Khon Kaen, 8.3 and 2.2 for Bangkok and 5.9 and 0.4 for Songkhla [7]. In Thailand, nationwide infant vaccination against HBV began in 1992 [8,9].

Aflatoxin exposure is a major risk factor for HCC in particular in regions where exposure to HBV is endemic. Aflatoxins are fungal toxins produced by *Aspergillus flavus* and *Aspergillus parasiticus*, which contaminate staple foods including groundnuts. Storage of crops in hot humid conditions can promote growth of the aflatoxin-producing fungi and results in increased accumulation of the toxin [10,11]. Aflatoxin B_1 (AFB_1), the most abundant form, is metabolized by P450 enzymes in the liver to generate an epoxide which is highly reactive with DNA, forming adducts at N7 position of Guanine. Lack of repair of this lesion may lead to permanent DNA mutations, preferentially G to T transversions. A hotspot for mutation by AFB_1 has been identified at codon 249 in the *TP53* suppressor gene (AGG to AGT, Arginine to Serine, *R249S*). Recent evidence confirms that this position is a preferential site for AFB_1 adduct formation [12]. There is a remarkable ecological concordance between AFB_1 exposure, chronic HBV infection and presence of *R249S* in HCC [13,14]. However, how the mutant protein p.R249S contributes to hepatocarcinogenesis and co-operates with HBV in this process is still a matter of debate.

In Thailand, the main dietary sources of exposure to AFB_1 are maize and groundnuts (peanuts). Individual exposure to AFB_1 has been estimated to vary between 53 and 73 ng/kg/day, although this figure is likely to differ widely among geographic areas and ecological zones [11]. A recent estimate of the risk of HCC attributable to aflatoxin for Thailand has provided figures of 0.53–0.73 and 15.9–21.9/10^5 person years, in HBsAg-negative and positive subjects, respectively [11]. In a recent study on a small group of surgically resected HCC patients at the National Cancer Institute, Bangkok, we reported *R249S* mutation in 7/26 (27%) cases, suggesting that the contribution of AFB_1 to the burden of HCC in Thailand is far from negligible [15]. However, an earlier epidemiological study in Thailand using a albumin-adduct bio-marker to assess aflatoxin exposure, failed to identify an aflatoxin-associated risk for HCC [16].

In previous studies, we and others have shown that circulating free DNA (CFDNA) from plasma is a suitable surrogate source of liver-derived DNA for detection of *R249S* mutations. Overall levels of CFDNA are higher in patients with liver cancer than controls (for review see [17]). In the Gambia and in the Qidong area of People's Republic of China, two regions of high HBV prevalence and widespread AFB_1 exposure, high plasma concentrations of *R249S*-mutated DNA were found to be strongly associated with HCC [18,19]. In the Gambia, the use of a highly sensitive mass spectrometric technique (Short Oligonucleotide Mass Analysis, SOMA) has allowed detection of low levels *R249S*-mutated DNA in the plasma of asymptomatic HBV carriers, suggested to occur as a result of ongoing AFB_1 exposure [20]. In Thailand, a previous study comparing HCC cases and controls has reported the SOMA detection of *R249S*-mutated DNA in 9/34 HCC cases (26%) and in 10/68 (14.7%) controls [21]. In this study, we have used plasma collected in a case-referent design at National Cancer Institute, Bangkok, to evaluate the association of *R249S*-mutated DNA plasma concentrations with the occurrence of HCC, CC or chronic liver disease. Our results suggest a preferential association between *R249S* and HCC developing in the absence of documented previous history of liver cirrhosis.

Methods

Ethics Statement

Written consent was obtained from all participants in the Thailand case-referent study and this study was approved by the Institutional Review Boards of the Thailand National Cancer Institute and the International Agency for Research on Cancer.

Study Participants

This study has been carried out using protocols, specimens and data from the International Liver Cancer Study (ILCS), an international initiative that aims to contribute to intervention, prevention, early diagnosis and control of liver cancer through the understanding of its causes and mechanisms in different populations. ILCS Thailand is a case – referent study in which subjects were recruited from fifty five provinces all around the country from April 2008 to December 2009. Diagnosis of hepatocellular carcinoma and cholangiocarcinoma was based on concordant clinical examination and abdominal imaging. Individuals assigned to the reference group presented no clinical evidence of liver disease and were selected among the group of patients that came to the Institute for their annual check-up.

Quantitation of *TP53 R249S* Mutation in CFDNA

Circulating free DNA was extracted from 1 mL of plasma using QiAmp circulating nucleic acid kit (Qiagen, Hilden, Germany) according to the manufacturer's protocol for purification of Circulating DNA from 1 mL, 2 mL or 3 mL serum or plasma. Purified DNA was eluted from the QiAmp Silica column with water (2×50 µL) (PCR-grade, Sigma, St Louis, MO, USA). Quantitation of extracted DNA was performed by fluorimetry using picogreen (Molecular Probes, Eugene, OR, USA). *R249S*-mutated DNA was detected and quantified in reference to an internal standard plasmid by SOMA as described previously [20,22]. Plasma concentrations were expressed as copies of *R249S*-mutated DNA per mL of plasma. The limit of determination for the method was 67 copies of *R249S*-mutated DNA/mL plasma.

Statistical Analyses

Odds ratios (ORs), χ^2 and p-values were calculated using STATA 11.1 (College Station, Texas). Odds ratios were adjusted for sex and age as well as for HBsAg and HCV-Ab.

Results

Characteristics of Study Population

Demographic information and hepatitis infection status of cases of HCC without cirrhosis (HCC/no cirrhosis; n = 50), HCC with cirrhosis (HCC/cirrhosis; n = 34), cholangiocarcinoma (CC; n = 36), chronic liver disease (CLD; n = 56) and of the reference group (R; n = 133) are presented in Table 1. Median age was 55 years (range 42–74) for HCC/cirrhosis, 52 (33–71) for HCC/no cirrhosis, 57 (37–72) for CC and 53 (35–72) for CLD. Of note, 38% (19/50) of HCC/no cirrhosis were under 50 years of age, compared to 18% for HCC/cirrhosis. (p = 0.045). Male to female ratio was 4:1 for HCC/no cirrhosis, 3:1 for HCC/cirrhosis, 2:1 for CC and 1.5:1 for CLD. Figure 1 shows the geographic distribution of the place of residence of the cases at the time of diagnosis. Patients originated from all around the country, but were mainly from the North-East and the Central-South regions. HCC/cirrhosis cases tended to cluster in the Central-South region (mainly larger Bangkok area), as compared to HCC/no cirrhosis (predominantly rural) and to CC (predominantly originating from north-eastern Thailand).

HBV carriage, as assessed by detection of HBsAg, was significantly more frequent in HCC/no cirrhosis (62%; OR: 11.7, 95%CI [5.0–21.3]); HCC/cirrhosis (50%; OR: 12.3, 95%CI [4.4–34.3]) and CLD (52%; OR: 9.6, 95%CI [4.3–21.6]) as compared to R (14%; Reference; $p = <0.001$). Of note, the proportion of HBsAg-positive subjects in the R group was higher than expected based on current WHO health statistics for the Thai population [9]. Conversely, CC were less associated with HBsAg positivity than the R group (2.8%; OR: 0.2, 95%CI [0.02–1.04]). HCV seropositivity was confirmed in 14% of HCC/no cirrhosis and in 32.3% of HCC/cirrhosis (X_2, $p = 0.044$). As for HBV, the lowest proportion of HCV positive patients was observed in CC (5.6%).

Table 1. Characteristics of the study participants.

		Status n (%)				
		Hepatocellular carcinoma without cirrhosis	Hepatocellular carcinoma with cirrhosis	Cholangicarginoma	Chronic liver disease	Reference group
N		**50**	**34**	**36**	**56**	**133**
	<40	5 (10)	0 (0)	1 (2.8)	5 (8.9)	5 (3.8)
Age, years	40–49	14 (28)	6 (17.6)	6 (16.7)	12 (21.4)	28 (21)
	50–59	18 (36)	19 (55.9)	13 (36.1)	26 (46.5)	51 (38.4)
	≥60	13 (26)	9 (26.5)	16 (44.4)	13 (23.2)	49 (36.8)
Sex	Men	41 (82)	26 (76.5)	23 (63.9)	34 (60.7)	77 (57.9)
	Women	9 (18)	8 (23.5)	13 (36.1)	22 (39.3)	56 (42.1)
	Negative	19 (38)	16 (47)	34 (94.4)	27 (48.2)	112 (84.2)
HBsAg	Positive	31 (62)	17 (50)	1 (2.8)	29 (51.8)	19 (14.3)
	N/A	0 (0)	1 (3)	1 (2.8)	0 (0)	2 (1.5)
	OR [95% CI][§]	11.67 [4.99–21.3]	12.32 [4.43–34.27]	0.18 [0.02–1.04]	9.64 [4.31–21.57]	1.00
Hepatitis C	Negative	43 (86)*	23 (67.7)	34 (94.4)	43 (76.8)	133 (100)
	Positive	7 (14)*	11 (32.3)	2 (5.6)	13 (23.2)	0 (0)

[§]OR for HBsAg positivity calculated in relation to the R group. * X_2 test when compared HCC/no cirrhosis Vs HCC/cirrhosis (p value = 0.044).

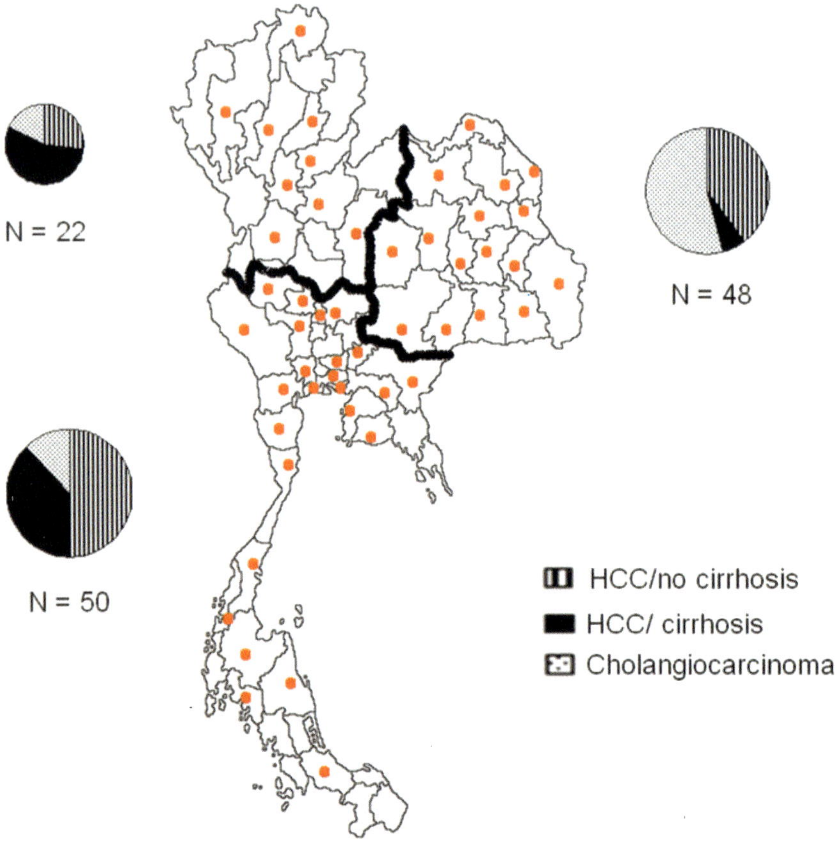

Figure 1. Geographic distribution of liver cancer cases. Dots represent the distribution by province. Pie charts describe the distribution of HCC/no cirrhosis (lines), HCC/cirrhosis (full black) and CC (small dots) among the Northwest, Northeast and Central-south parts of the country.

TP53 R249S-mutated DNA Plasma Concentrations

Figure 2 shows the proportions of subjects for each study group with detectable *R249S*-mutated DNA at 6 cutoff concentrations from 67 to 160 copies/mL plasma). At the method's limit of determination (67 copies/mL), the 4 liver disease groups had similar proportions of patients positive for *R249S*-mutated DNA (53–64%), clearly separated from the R group, for which only 19% of subjects were positive. Increasing the cutoff concentration better resolved the 5 study groups. We thus selected a lower cutoff concentration of 150 copies/mL for further comparisons of *R249S*-mutated DNA concentrations between the 4 liver disease groups and the reference group (Figure 3).

Median plasma concentrations of *R249S*-mutated DNA were higher for the HCC/no cirrhosis group (328 copies/mL) than HCC/cirrhosis group (273 copies/mL) with wide concentration ranges for both groups (154–11,576 copies/mL and 152–8,675 copies/mL, respectively). Of note, although the medians for the two HCC groups are similar, the number of individuals in the 70% percentile is higher for HCC/no cirrhosis (n = 11) than for HCC/cirrhosis (n = 3).In contrast, for the CC, CLD and R groups, median plasma concentrations of *R249S*-mutated DNA were lower (252, 256 and 20 copies/mL), respectively, and concentration ranges smaller ([170–446], [150–352] and [155–216]). Taken together, data in Figures 2 and 3 show that (1) high copy numbers of *R249S* were associated with HCC (with or without cirrhosis), whereas CC, CLD and R groups had similarly low *R249S* copy numbers; (2) the proportion of patients with measurable plasma concentrations of *R249S*-mutated DNA was highest in the HCC/no cirrhosis group (44%). Strikingly, this proportion was lower for the HCC/cirrhosis (21%) and CC (22%) groups, which were both higher than CLD (12%) and R (3%) groups. These results indicate that plasma concentrations of *R249S*-mutated DNA occurred most often and at highest concentrations in the HCC/no cirrhosis group, although measurable lower concentrations were observed in the other disease groups.

Association between Plasma *R249S*-mutated DNA, Chronic Hepatitis Virus Infection and Alpha-fetoprotein Levels

We next examined associations between plasma *R249S*-mutated DNA positivity (>150 copies/mL) and markers of chronic HBV and HCV infections (Table 2) and levels of alpha-fetoprotein (AFP) (Table 3). Table 2 shows that HCC with or without cirrhosis was strongly associated with HBsAg positivity in patients with both high and low plasma concentrations of *R249S*-mutated DNA. However, the strongest association was observed in patients with HCC/no cirrhosis and high plasma concentrations of *R249S*-mutated DNA. In the latter group, the proportion of HBsAg-positive patients (73%) was higher than in patients with HCC/cirrhosis at either high or low plasma concentrations of *R249S*-mutated DNA (43% and 52%, respectively) or patients with HCC/no cirrhosis with low plasma concentrations of *R249S*-mutated DNA (54%). With HCV, a significant association was observed between HCV infection and HCC/cirrhosis, irrespective of plasma concentration of *R249S*-mutated DNA ($p = 0.03$). Of note, only HCC/cirrhosis was significantly associated with HCV infection when compared to non-HCC subjects (CC, CLD and reference group) (Table 2). Table 3 shows that the distribution of patients with levels of AFP>100 ng/mL was similar between HCC/no cirrhosis and HCC/cirrhosis. However, in the latter group, there was a larger proportion of patients with undetectable or low levels of AFP among HCC/cirrhosis with low plasma concentrations of *R249S*-mutated DNA (56% vs 0%, $p = 0.025$).

Discussion

In this study, we have used a highly sensitive and quantitative mass spectrometric method, SOMA, to investigate the relation-

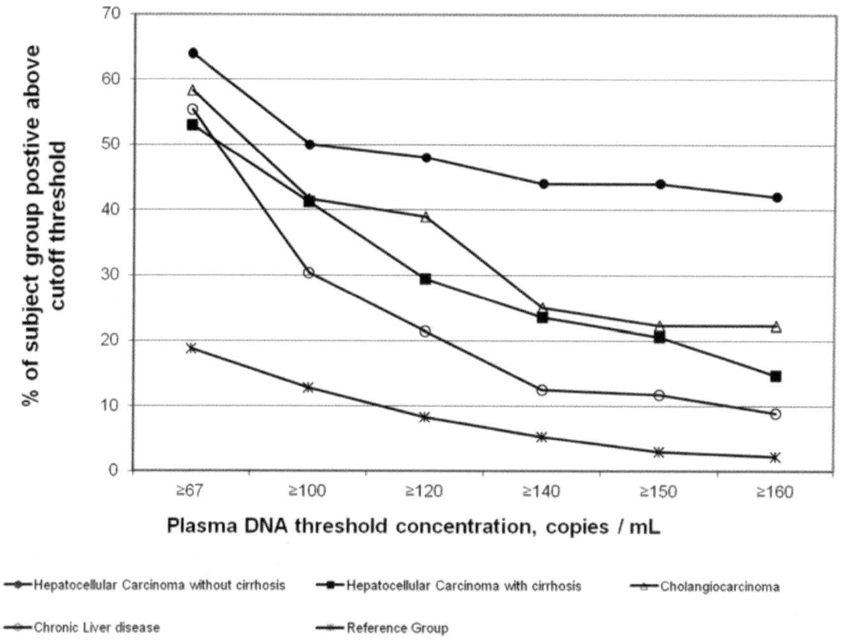

Figure 2. Distribution of the liver disease and reference groups at different cutoffs of positivity of *TP53 R249S* mutation. At 150 copies/mL there is a clear distinction among the three liver cancer groups the chronic liver disease subjects and the reference group. The proportion of patients at this cut-off is higher in HCC/no cirrhosis (44%) than in all other groups (HCC/cirrhosis (21%), CC (22%), CLD (12%) and R (3)).

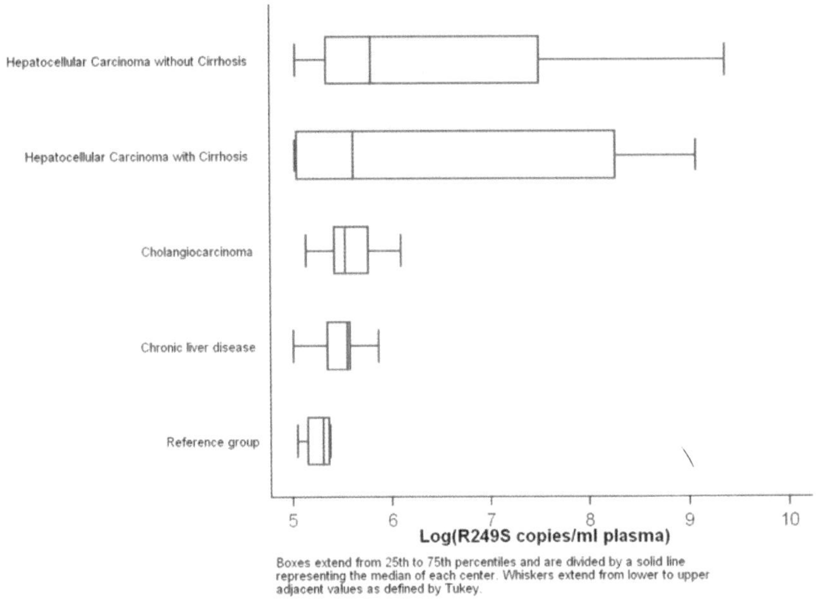

Figure 3. Box and whisker distributions of *TP53 R249S-mutated DNA plasma concentrations* (≥150 copies/mL) for the different groups. Boxes extend from 25th to 75th percentiles and are divided by a solid line representing the median of each centre. The median levels for the different groups are: 328 in HCC/no cirrhosis, 273 in HCC/cirrhosis, 252 in CC, 256 in CLD and 202 in R.

ships between liver cancer and aflatoxin-related plasma *TP53 R249S*-mutated DNA concentrations in free circulating DNA using blood specimens collected in a hospital case: control design. We show that plasma *R249S*-mutated DNA was detected at >67 copies/mL in over 53% of patients with liver cancer or chronic liver disease, and only in 19% of control subjects (including 8% of HBsAg positive subjects). However, when considering only subjects with *R249S*-mutated DNA concentrations >150 copies/mL, a clear distinction could be made between the different liver disease statuses. While 44% of HCC/no cirrhosis patients had plasma *R249S*-mutated DNA concentrations greater than 150 copies/mL, this proportion dropped to 21% in patients with HCC/cirrhosis, 22% in CC patients, 12% in CLD patients and 3% in the reference group. This observation indicates that *R249S*-mutated DNA plasma concentrations greater than 150 copies/mL are associated with HCC preferentially developing without

Table 2. Relation between Plasma *R249S*-mutated *DNA* and HBs-antigen (HBsAg) and HCV-antibody (HCV-ab).

	Status n (%)				
	Hepatocellular carcinoma without cirrhosis	**Hepatocellular carcinoma with cirrhosis**	**Cholangicarginoma**	**Chronic liver disease**	**Reference group**
R249S+	22 (44)	7 (21)	8 (22)	6 (11)	4 (3)
HBsAg+	16 (73) ***	3 (43) *	0	1 (17)	1 (25)
HBsAg−	6 (27)	3 (43)	8 (100)	5 (83)	3 (75)
HBsAg NA		1 (14)			
R249S−	28 (56)	27 (79)	28 (78)	50 (89)	129 (97)
HBsAg+	15 (54) ***	14 (52) ***	1 (3.5)	28 (56)	18 (14)
HBsAg−	13 (46)	13 (48)	26 (93)	22 (44)	109 (84)
HBsAg NA			1 (3.5)		2 (2)
R249S+	22 (44)	7 (21)	8 (22)	6 (11)	4 (3)
HCV+	3 (14) ns	4 (57) *	1 (13)	1 (1.8)	0
HCV−	19 (86)	3 (43)	7 (87)	5 (8.9)	4 (100)
R249S−	28 (56)	27 (79)	28 (78)	50 (89)	129 (97)
HCV+	4 (14) ns	7 (26) ***	1 (2.8)	12 (24)	0
HCV−	24 (86)	20 (74)	27 (75)	38 (76)	129 (100)

X_2 test when compared to cholangiocarcinoma, chronic liver disease and reference group all together (*: p value <0.05; ***: p value <0.001; NA: Not Available; ns: non significant).

Table 3. Relation between Plasma *R249S-mutated DNA* and AFP.

	Status n(%)				
	Hepatocellular carcinoma without cirrhosis	**Hepatocellular carcinoma with cirrhosis**	**Cholangicarginoma**	**Chronic liver disease**	**Reference group**
R249S+	22 (44)	7 (21)	8 (22)	6 (11)	4 (3)
AFP<100	7 (32)	0	7 (87)	6 (100)	4 (100)
AFP>=100	3 (14)	1 (14)	1 (13)	0	0
AFP>=400	12 (54)	6 (86)	0	0	0
R249S -	28 (56)	27 (79)	28 (78)	50 (89)	129 (97)
AFP<100	9 (32)	15 (56)	28 (100)	48 (96)	129 (100)
AFP>=100	3 (11)	3 (11)	0	2 (4)	0
AFP>=400	16 (57)	9 (33)	0	0	0
X_2 **test (*p* value)***	0.950	0.025*			

*X_2 test comparing individuals with *R249S* >=150 copies/mL against individuals with *R249S* <150 copies/mL.

cirrhosis. Strikingly, there was no difference in *R249S*-mutated DNA plasma concentrations between HCC developing in a context of cirrhosis and CC, a pathology that originates from non-hepatocyte liver cells and has not been shown to be associated with exposure to aflatoxin. Patients with HCC/no cirrhosis and with high *R249S*-mutated DNA plasma concentrations tended to be more frequently HBsAg positive (73%) than patients with HCC/no cirrhosis with low or undetectable concentrations. Furthermore, in patients with HCC/cirrhosis, the proportion of HBsAg positive subjects was similar, irrespective of *R249S*-mutated DNA plasma concentration. Overall, these results highlight the preferential occurrence of *R249S*-mutated DNA in the plasma of subjects developing HCC in the absence of cirrhosis and/or in subjects who are chronic carriers of HBV.

In a previous study on HCC tissues collected at the NCI, Bangkok, we have detected plasma *R249S*-mutated DNA in 7/26 HCC cases (27%) [15]. Although case: control studies conducted in the early nineties employing biomarkers of aflatoxin exposure have concluded that levels of aflatoxin exposure were low in the Thai population [16], a recent assessment of aflatoxin contamination in two dietary staples in Thailand, peanuts and maize, has reported mean aflatoxin levels which are 3 to 5 times higher than the Thailand regulation limit (20 µg/kg) [23]. Thus levels of dietary exposure to aflatoxin are far from negligible in Thailand and the presence of the mutated DNA in plasma is consistent with the notion that this toxin, together with HBV chronic carriage, remains a major etiological factor for HCC in Thailand. The apparent discrepancy between our detection of plasma *R249S*-mutated DNA and the low levels of aflatoxin biomarkers detected by case: control study in a similar population may be due to the fact that such biomarkers are short-lived in comparison with *TP53 R249S* mutation in liver cells. Thus, in controls, the exposure biomarker is present in only a small proportion of the subjects, whereas in cases, the biomarker is no longer detectable as exposure leading to mutation might have taken place months or years ahead of diagnosis.

In a study on asymptomatic chronic HBV carriers in The Gambia, West Africa, we have found that *R249S*-mutated DNA could be detected at relatively low levels in the plasma of subjects with dietary exposure to aflatoxin, with a seasonal variation that may reflect the dynamics of exposure, mutation formation, elimination of mutated cells and shedding of cell debris into the bloodstream [20]. In the present study, we show that low plasma levels of *R249S*-mutated DNA (>67 copies/mL plasma, compatible with the lower detection limit in asymptomatic subjects from the Gambia) are detectable in a variable proportion of controls, of subjects with chronic liver disease and of liver cancer patients, independently of liver cancer histological type and pathological profile. This low concentration of *R249S*-mutated DNA may occur as the consequence of ongoing exposure to aflatoxin (in controls) and of ongoing destruction of non-cancer cells having acquired a mutation (in patients with CLD, CC, HCC/cirrhosis or HCC/no cirrhosis). However, when only plasma concentrations above a higher cutoff are considered (>150 copies/mL), plasma *R249S*-mutated DNA may essentially, but not exclusively occur as the result of shedding of cellular material by cancer cells containing the mutation. Thus, the high proportion (44%) of patients with HCC/no cirrhosis that are positive above this level may correspond to patients who actually have a liver tumour that contains the mutation. In patients with HCC/cirrhosis or with CC, the proportion of positive subjects above the 150 copies/mL threshold is similar (21 to 22%) but the actual copy numbers are much higher in HCC/cirrhosis patients (up to 8,675 copies/mL) than in CC patients (up to 446 copies/mL) (Figure 3). In patients with CC or CLD, plasma *R249S*-mutated DNA concentrations are actually very low and similar to those observed in the reference group. In the latter group, presence of *R249S* at levels ≥150 copies/mL may correspond to patients with particularly high, ongoing levels of exposure to aflatoxin or who harbor small populations of cells having acquired the mutation. Of the 5 control subjects with plasma *R249S*-mutated DNA concentrations ≥150 copies/mL, only one was positive for HBsAg, indicating that positivity for plasma *R249S*-mutated DNA in control subjects was not restricted to HBV chronic carriers.

In conclusion, the present study provides evidence that acquisition and persistence of the *TP53* mutation *R249S* occurs preferentially in HCC that develops in a context of chronic infection by HBV and without clear clinical evidence of prior or concomitant liver cirrhosis. Although pre-existing cirrhosis is detected in the vast majority (90%) of HCC cases in Western Europe and in the US, it is actually a less frequent phenomenon in HCC occurring in a context of high HBV endemicity/high exposure to aflatoxin although its exact rate of occurrence is poorly documented. In The Gambia, we have observed that cirrhosis was detectable in 62% of patients at the time of HCC diagnosis and this proportion was 59% in patients with plasma

R249S-mutated DNA [24]. In Thailand, the prospective follow-up of a group of 1810 males HBV carriers aged over 30 over 7 years led to the detection of 36 cases of HCC, 18 (50%) of which developed without any prior evidence of cirrhosis (P.Srivatanakul, unpublished observations). Overall, our results suggest that the development of HCC without pre-existing cirrhosis is enhanced or accelerated in a context of HBV chronic infection and of aflatoxin-induced *TP53 R249S* mutation, suggesting that these two factors cooperate in a distinct pathway of development of hepatocellular carcinoma.

Acknowledgments

Gilles Ferro for his support with the statistical analyses.

Author Contributions

Conceived and designed the experiments: PH MDF JDG. Performed the experiments: SV SOC DG MDF. Analyzed the data: SOC SV BAA DG ANdC MDF PH. Contributed reagents/materials/analysis tools: AP MDF JDG PH BAA ANdC. Wrote the paper: SOC SV PH MDF. Designed the study and acquired the data: SS AP TK AK. Critically revised the manuscript for important intellectual content: SS AP TK AK.

References

1. Ferlay J, Shin H, Bray F, Forman D, Mathers C, et al. (2010) GLOBOCAN 2008: Cancer Incidence and Mortality Worldwide. IARC Lyon, France.
2. International Agency for Research on Cancer (2008) World Cancer Report. IARC Lyon, France.
3. Feitelson MA, Sun B, Satiroglu Tufan NL, Liu J, Pan J, et al. (2002) Genetic mechanisms of hepatocarcinogenesis. Oncogene 21: 2593–2604.
4. Shin HR, Oh JK, Masuyer E, Curado MP, Bouvard V, et al. (2010) Epidemiology of cholangiocarcinoma: an update focusing on risk factors. Cancer Sci 101: 579–585.
5. International Agency for Research on Cancer (2002) Some traditional herbal medicines, some mycotoxins, naphthalene and styrene.IARC Lyon, France.
6. International Agency for Research on Cancer (2009) A review of human carcinogens. Part B: biological agents. IARC Lyon, France.
7. Srivatanakul P, Sriplung H, Deerasamee S (2004) Epidemiology of liver cancer: an overview. Asian Pac J Cancer Prev 5: 118–125.
8. Poovorawan Y, Theamboonlers A, Vimolket T, Sinlaparatsamee S, Chaiear K, et al. (2000) Impact of hepatitis B immunisation as part of the EPI. Vaccine 19: 943–949.
9. Poovorawan Y, Chongsrisawat V, Theamboonlers A, Leroux-Roels G, Kuriyakose S, et al. (2011) Evidence of protection against clinical and chronic hepatitis B infection 20 years after infant vaccination in a high endemicity region. J Viral Hepat 18: 369–375.
10. Strosnider H, Azziz-Baumgartner E, Banziger M, Bhat RV, Breiman R, et al. (2006) Workgroup report: public health strategies for reducing aflatoxin exposure in developing countries. Environ Health Perspect 114: 1898–1903.
11. Liu Y, Wu F (2010) Global burden of aflatoxin-induced hepatocellular carcinoma: a risk assessment. Environ Health Perspect 118: 818–824.
12. Besaratinia A, Kim SI, Hainaut P, Pfeifer GP (2009) In vitro recapitulating of TP53 mutagenesis in hepatocellular carcinoma associated with dietary aflatoxin B1 exposure. Gastroenterology 137: 1127–37, 1137.
13. Gouas D, Shi H, Hainaut P (2009) The aflatoxin-induced TP53 mutation at codon 249 (R249S): biomarker of exposure, early detection and target for therapy. Cancer Lett 286: 29–37.
14. Wild CP, Gong YY (2010) Mycotoxins and human disease: a largely ignored global health issue. Carcinogenesis 31: 71–82.
15. Galy O, Chemin I, Le RE, Villar S, Le Calvez-Kelm F, et al. (2011) Mutations in TP53 and CTNNB1 in Relation to Hepatitis B and C Infections in Hepatocellular Carcinomas from Thailand. Hepat Res Treat 2011: 697162. 697162 p.
16. Srivatanakul P, Parkin DM, Khlat M, Chenvidhya D, Chotiwan P, et al. (1991) Liver cancer in Thailand. II. A case-control study of hepatocellular carcinoma. Int J Cancer 48: 329–332.
17. Gormally E, Caboux E, Vineis P, Hainaut P (2007) Circulating free DNA in plasma or serum as biomarker of carcinogenesis: practical aspects and biological significance. Mutat Res 635: 105–117.
18. Kirk GD, Camus-Randon AM, Mendy M, Goedert JJ, Merle P, et al. (2000) Ser-249 p53 mutations in plasma DNA of patients with hepatocellular carcinoma from The Gambia. J Natl Cancer Inst 92: 148–153.
19. Groopman JD, Johnson D, Kensler TW (2005) Aflatoxin and hepatitis B virus biomarkers: a paradigm for complex environmental exposures and cancer risk. Cancer Biomark 1: 5–14.
20. Villar S, Le Roux-Goglin E, Gouas DA, Plymoth A, Ferro G, et al. (2011) Seasonal Variation in TP53 R249S-mutated Serum DNA With Aflatoxin Exposure And Hepatitis B Virus Infection. Environ Health Perspect.
21. Kuang SY, Lekawanvijit S, Maneekarn N, Thongsawat S, Brodovicz K, et al. (2005) Hepatitis B 1762T/1764A mutations, hepatitis C infection, and codon 249 p53 mutations in hepatocellular carcinomas from Thailand. Cancer Epidemiol Biomarkers Prev 14: 380–384.
22. Lleonart ME, Kirk GD, Villar S, Lesi OA, Dasgupta A, et al. (2005) Quantitative analysis of plasma TP53 249Ser-mutated DNA by electrospray ionization mass spectrometry. Cancer Epidemiol Biomarkers Prev 14: 2956–2962.
23. Lipigorngoson S, Limtrakul P, Suttajit M, Yoshizawa T (2003) In-house direct cELISA for determining aflatoxin B1 in Thai corn and peanuts. Food Addit Contam 20: 838–845.
24. Umoh NJ, Lesi OA, Mendy M, Bah E, Akano A, et al. (2011) Aetiological differences in demographical, clinical and pathological characteristics of hepatocellular carcinoma in The Gambia. Liver Int 31: 215–221.

11

SPF Rabbits Infected with Rabbit Hepatitis E Virus Isolate Experimentally Showing the Chronicity of Hepatitis

Jian Han, Yaxin Lei, Lin Liu, Peng Liu, Junke Xia, Yulin Zhang, Hang Zeng, Lin Wang, Ling Wang*, Hui Zhuang

Department of Microbiology, School of Basic Medical Sciences, Peking University Health Science Center, Beijing, China

Abstract

This study focused on investigating the pathogenesis seen in specific-pathogen-free (SPF) rabbits following infection with a homologous rabbit HEV isolate (CHN-BJ-rb14) and comparing it to that seen following infection with a heterologous swine genotype 4 HEV isolate (CHN-XJ-SW13). Three of the four animals inoculated with the homologous rabbit HEV became infected, exhibiting an intermittent viremia, obvious fluctuations of liver function biomarkers alanine aminotransferase (ALT) and aspartate aminotransferase (AST), and persistent fecal virus shedding throughout the nine month study. In addition, liver histopathology showed both chronic inflammation and some degree of fibrosis. Both positive and negative-stranded HEV RNA and HEV antigen expression were detected in liver, brain, stomach, duodenum and kidney from the necropsied rabbits. Inflammation of extrahepatic tissue (duodenum and kidney) was also observed. Three of the four rabbits inoculated with the heterologous genotype 4 swine HEV also became infected, showing similar levels of anti-HEV antibody to that generated following infection with the homologous virus isolate. The duration of both viremia and fecal shedding of virus was however shorter following infection with the heterologous virus and there was no significant elevation of liver function biomarkers. These results suggest that rabbit HEV infection may cause more severe hepatitis and prolong the course of the disease, with a possible chronic trend of hepatitis in SPF rabbits.

Editor: Xiang-Jin Meng, Virginia Polytechnic Institute and State University, United States of America

Funding: This work was partially supported by the National Science Foundation of China (Grant No. 81271827, http://www.nsfc.gov.cn/Portal0/default152.htm) and Specialized Research Fund for the Doctoral Program of Higher Education (Grant No.20120001110098, http://www.cutech.edu.cn/cn/kyjj/gdxxbsdkyjj/A010301Index_1.htm). The funders had no role in study design, data collection and analysis, decision to publish, or preparation of the manuscript.

Competing Interests: The authors have declared that no competing interests exist.

* Email: lingwang@bjmu.edu.cn

Introduction

Hepatitis E virus (HEV), the cause of hepatitis E, appears to be transmitted primarily by the fecal-oral route. In common with Hepatitis A virus with which it shares a number of molecular characteristics, it was initially assumed that HEV only caused acute self-limited disease [1]. However, in the recent years, it has been shown that HEV infection can lead to chronic hepatitis in immune-compromised individuals, such as solid-organ transplant (SOT) patients [2], HIV-positive patients [3] and leukemia patients receiving chemotherapy [4]. The mortality rate associated with HEV infection is generally low (<1%), but it can reach as high as 25–30% in infected pregnant women [5].

HEV is a non-enveloped virus with a positive-sense, single-stranded RNA genome of approximately 7.2 kb, in which the 5′ non-coding region is followed by three partially overlapping open reading frames (ORFs) and a polyadenylated 3′ non-coding region. It is the sole member of the family Hepeviridae [6]. Four genotypes of HEV have been recognized to-date. Genotypes 1 and 2 are restricted to humans, are most commonly found in the developing countries of Asia, Africa and South America [7] and appear to be transmitted mainly via contaminated water. Genotypes 3 and 4 have a more extended host range which includes humans, pigs and other mammals and are responsible for sporadic cases of disease in both developing and industrialized countries either through direct contact with infected animals, or through the consumption of contaminated animal meat and viscera [8].

The first non-human strain of HEV was isolated from a pig in the United States in 1997 and consequently designated swine HEV [9]. The virus has been isolated from various animal species, including chickens, deer, mongooses, foxes, ferrets, rats, bats, wild boars and trout [10–18]. In 2009, a new HEV was isolated from farmed rabbits in China [19]. The rabbit HEV strains isolated to-date show 73–77%, 70–76%, 75–82%, 71–77% identity to the genotypes 1, 2, 3, 4 respectively at the nucleotide level and 53–65% identity to avian HEV isolates [20]. Phylogenetically, rabbit HEV isolates are most closely related to genotype 3 [21,22], although some have suggested that they represent a novel genotype [19,23]. Under experimental conditions, rabbit HEV has been shown to be able to give cross-species infections in the monkeys and pigs [24,25]. Swine HEV isolates have also been shown to be able to infect rabbits [26], indicating rabbits may serve as a non-primate small animal model for HEV infection. However, the pathogenesis profile of HEV infection of rabbits has not been clearly defined. Therefore, the aim of this study was to investigate the pathogenesis of rabbit HEV in its

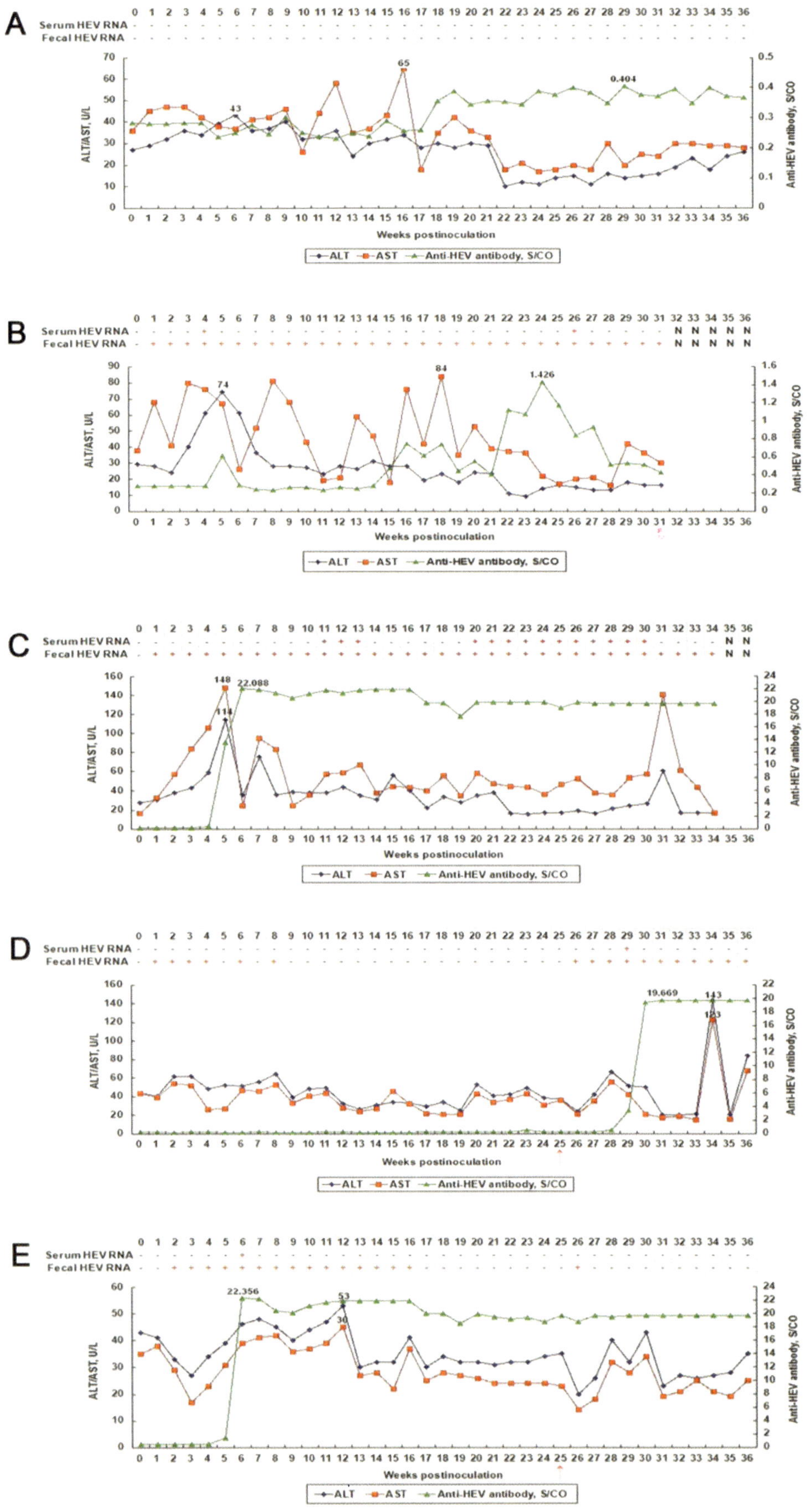
A
Serum HEV RNA
Fecal HEV RNA
ALT/AST, U/L
Anti-HEV antibody, S/CO
43
65
0.404
Weeks postinoculation
ALT AST Anti-HEV antibody, S/CO
B
Serum HEV RNA
Fecal HEV RNA
74
84
1.426
ALT/AST, U/L
Anti-HEV antibody, S/CO
Weeks postinoculation
ALT AST Anti-HEV antibody, S/CO
C
Serum HEV RNA
Fecal HEV RNA
148
22.088
114
ALT/AST, U/L
Anti-HEV antibody, S/CO
Weeks postinoculation
ALT AST Anti-HEV antibody, S/CO
D
Serum HEV RNA
Fecal HEV RNA
19.669
143
ALT/AST, U/L
Anti-HEV antibody, S/CO
Weeks postinoculation
ALT AST Anti-HEV antibody, S/CO
E
Serum HEV RNA
Fecal HEV RNA
22.356
53
ALT/AST, U/L
Anti-HEV antibody, S/CO
Weeks postinoculation
ALT AST Anti-HEV antibody, S/CO

Figure 1. Dynamic seroconversion of anti-HEV, HEV RNA,ALT and AST observed in rabbits. (**A**) Rabbit C1 in group 1 inoculated with sterile PBS. (**B**) Rabbit R1 in group 2 inoculated with rabbit HEV strain. (**C**) Rabbit R3 in group 2 1inoculated with rabbit HEV strain. (**D**) Rabbit S2 in group 3 inoculated with a genotype 4 swine HEV at 0wpi, and rabbit HEV at 25wpi. (**E**) Rabbit S4 in group 3 inoculated with a genotype 4 swine HEV at 0wpi, and rabbit HEV at 25wpi. Note: ↑ indicates group 3 rabbits were inoculated with rabbit HEV strain at 25wpi (when recovered from initial infection).

natural host and compare it to that given by a genotype 4 swine HEV isolate.

Materials and Methods

Ethics Statement

The animal experiments were approved by the Committee of Laboratory Animal Welfare and Ethics, Peking University Health Science Center. This study was performed in strict accordance with the Principles of Laboratory Animal Care (NIH publication no.85Y23, revised 1996).

Virus Inocula

The rabbit HEV strain CHN-BJ-rb14 (JQ768461) used in this study was recovered from a rabbit fecal sample [24]. The swine HEV strain CHN-XJ-SW13 (GU119961) used was from fecal samples of a pig taken in Xinjiang, China [27]. The fecal samples were diluted in phosphate-buffered saline (PBS; pH 7.4) to make a 10% (wt/vol) suspension, clarified by centrifugation at 5000 rpm at 4°C for 30 min and filtered sequentially through 0.45 μM and 0.22 μM filters. The resulting suspensions were stored at −80°C. The titers of the CHN-BJ-rb14 and CHN-XJ-SW13 inocula used were both adjusted 10^4 genome equivalents (GE) per milliliter (mL) as determined by semi-quantitative nested reverse transcription PCR (RT-nPCR) [20].

Animals

3-month old SPF New Zealand white rabbits (2–2.50 kg) were obtained from the Department of Laboratory Animal Science of Peking University Health Science Center. Prior to being infected with HEV, all animals were tested for ALT and AST to establish the baseline and were confirmed negative for anti-HEV antibody by an enzyme-linked immunosorbent assay (ELISA) and negative for HEV RNA in fecal/serum by RT-nPCR.

Experimental Design

Ten SPF rabbits were divided at random into 3 groups. Group 1 consisted of two rabbits (C1 and C2), which were inoculated intravenously (i.v.) with 1 mL of sterile PBS as negative controls. Group 2 consisted of four rabbits (R1, R2, R3 and R4) and these were inoculated i.v. with 1 m L of the rabbit HEV (strain CHN-BJ-rb14). Group 3 consisted of four rabbits (S1, S2, S3 and S4) which were inoculated i.v. initially with 1 mL of the genotype 4 swine HEV (strain CHN-XJ-SW13). Following their recovery from this initial infection they were inoculated i.v. at 25 wpi with 1 mL the rabbit HEV (strain CHN-BJ-rb14). Each animal was housed in a separate cage and allowed access to food and drinking water *ad libitum*.

Sample Collection and Processing

Serum and fecal samples were collected at weekly intervals post-inoculation (wpi) and stored at −80°C. Serum samples were tested for levels of ALT, AST and anti-HEV antibody using standard methods [24]. Serum and fecal samples were tested weekly for HEV RNA by nRT-PCR [24]. In addition, bile and a number of different types of tissue and organs including liver, brain, stomach, duodenum, kidney, lung, bladder, and spleen were collected either from animals that died as a result of accidents during the course of the study or those euthanized. One rabbit R1 died as a result of accidents during the course of the study and nine rabbits (C1-C2, R2-R4, S1-S4) survived until euthanasia. Approximately 100 mg of the tissue or organs collected was homogenized in 1 mL of TRIzol reagent (Invitrogen, Burlington, ON, Canada) and clarified by centrifugation at 12,000 rpm for 15 min at 4°C. The supernatants from this centrifugation were harvested and stored at −80°C for later by nRT-PCR. The tissue and organs samples were also processed for histopathology and immunohistochemistry by first being fixed in 10% neutral buffered formalin immediately following sampling. To prevent cross-contamination during necropsy, individually wrapped, sterile disposable materials and new sterile scalpel blades were used for each sample. The organs containing excreta (feces and bile), that can harbor high titres of HEV were sampled last to reduce the potential for cross- contamination.

Histopathology and Immunohistochemistry

Tissue and organ samples were fixed in 10% neutral buffered formalin, embedded in paraffin and cut into 5 μM serial sections. Slides were stained with hematoxylin and eosin (H&E) and Masson's Trichrome. The samples were photographed and analyzed using a microscope (Olympus CX31, Japan) equipped with a digital camera with the assistance of Motic Images Plus 2.0 software.

For immunohistochemistry, tissue and organs sections were deparaffinised, hydrated, water-bath heated for antigen retrieval and blocked with the addition of 3% hydrogen peroxide. Sections were then incubated overnight with a 1:20 dilution of monoclonal antibody (mouse-anti-genotype 1 HEV'S ORF2 antibody, Wantai, Biopharmaceutical, Beijing, China), washed with PBS and stained for visualization using the 2-step plus Poly-HRP Anti-Mouse/Rabbits IgG Detection System (PV-9000, K123307E, ZSGB) combined with DAB substrate (ZLI-9018, K125905A, ZSGB), according to the supplier's instructions.

Determination of ALT and AST Concentrations

All rabbits were monitored weekly for 36 weeks following virus challenge. ALT and AST concentrations in serum were measured on the day of collection by using standard methods on a SmartSpec 3000 spectrophotometer (BioRad, CA) [24]. Animals were considered to be suffering from hepatitis when the serum ALT concentration exceeded the pre-challenge ALT level by more than two-fold [28].

ELISA for Anti-HEV Antibody

All serum samples were tested for anti-HEV antibody using a commercial HEV specific sandwich ELISA assay, based on the E2 protein of genotype 1 HEV (amino acids 394–606 of HEV ORF2), according to the manufacturer's instructions (Wantai, Biopharmaceutical, Beijing, China). Sample/cutoff (S/CO) values were calculated and values >1 were considered positive [29].

Table 1. Detection of HEV RNA in fecal/serum samples collected weekly from rabbits.

Group	Rabbit ID	Positive (+) or Negative (-) in Fecal/Serum Samples at Indicated Wpi																																		
		0	1	2	3	4	5	6	7	8	9	10	11	12	13	14	15	16	17	18	19	20	21	22	23	24	25	26	27	28	29	30	31	32	33	34	35	36
1[a]	C1	−/−	−/−	−/−	−/−	−/−	−/−	−/−	−/−	−/−	−/−	−/−	−/−	−/−	−/−	−/−	−/−	−/−	−/−	−/−	−/−	−/−	−/−	−/−	−/−	−/−	−/−	−/−	−/−	−/−	−/−	−/−	−/−	−/−	−/−	−/−	−/−	−/−
	C2	−/−	−/−	−/−	−/−	−/−	−/−	−/−	−/−	−/−	−/−	−/−	−/−	−/−	−/−	−/−	−/−	−/−	−/−	−/−	−/−	−/−	−/−	−/−	−/−	−/−	−/−	−/−	−/−	−/−	−/−	−/−	−/−	−/−	−/−	−/−	−/−	−/−
2[b]	R1	−/−	+/−	+/−	+/−	+/+	+/−	+/−	+/−	+/−	+/−	+/−	+/−	+/−	+/−	+/−	+/−	+/−	+/−	+/−	+/−	−/−	−/−	+/−	+/−	+/−	+/−	+/+	−/−	+/−	+/−	+/−	+/−	N/N	N/N	N/N	N/N	N/N
	R2	−/−	+/−	+/−	+/−	+/−	+/−	+/−	+/+	+/−	+/−	+/−	+/−	+/−	+/−	+/+	+/−	+/−	+/−	+/−	+/−	+/−	+/−	+/−	+/−	+/−	+/−	+/−	+/−	+/+	+/−	+/+	+/−	+/+	+/+	+/−	+/−	N/N
	R3	−/−	+/−	+/−	+/−	+/−	+/−	+/−	+/−	+/−	+/−	+/−	+/+	+/+	+/+	+/−	+/−	+/−	+/−	+/−	+/−	+/+	+/+	+/+	+/+	+/+	+/+	+/+	+/+	+/+	+/+	+/+	+/−	+/−	+/−	+/−	N/N	N/N
	R4	−/−	+/−	+/+	+/−	+/−	+/−	+/−	+/−	+/−	+/−	+/−	+/−	+/−	+/−	+/−	+/−	−/−	+/−	−/−	+/−	−/−	+/−	+/−	+/−	+/−	+/−	+/−	+/−	+/−	+/−	+/−	+/−	+/+	+/+	+/−	+/−	+/−
3[c]	S1	−/−	−/−	+/−	+/−	+/−	+/−	+/−	+/−	+/−	+/−	+/−	+/−	−/−	−/−	+/−	+/−	−/−	+/−	+/−	−/−	−/−	−/−	−/−	−/−	−/−	−/−	−/−	+/−	−/−	−/−	−/−	−/−	−/−	−/−	−/−	−/−	−/−
	S2	−/−	+/−	−/−	+/−	−/−	+/−	−/−	+/−	+/−	−/−	−/−	−/−	−/−	−/−	−/−	−/−	−/−	−/−	−/−	−/−	−/−	−/−	−/−	−/−	−/−	−/−	+/−	+/−	+/−	+/+	+/−	+/−	+/−	+/−	+/−	+/−	+/−
	S3	−/−	+/+	+/−	+/−	+/−	−/−	+/−	−/−	+/−	+/−	−/−	+/−	+/−	+/−	+/−	+/−	−/−	+/−	−/−	+/−	−/−	−/−	−/−	−/−	−/−	−/−	+/−	+/−	−/−	−/−	−/−	−/−	−/−	−/−	−/−	−/−	−/−
	S4	−/−	−/−	+/−	+/−	+/−	+/−	+/+	+/−	+/−	+/−	+/−	+/−	−/−	+/−	+/−	−/−	+/−	−/−	−/−	−/−	−/−	−/−	−/−	−/−	−/−	−/−	+/−	−/−	−/−	−/−	−/−	−/−	−/−	−/−	−/−	−/−	−/−

[a]Inoculated with sterile PBS (negative controls).
[b]Inoculated with a rabbit HEV strain CHN-BJ-rb14(JQ768461) (experimental group).
[c]Inoculated with a genotype 4 swine HEV strain CHN-XJ-SW13(GU119961) at 0wpi and at 25wpi (when recovered from initial infection) inoculated with a rabbit HEV strain CHN-BJ-rb14(JQ768461) (experimental group).
N No samples were collected due to accidental death or being necropsied.

Detection and Analysis of Positive/Negative-stranded HEV RNA

HEV RNA was extracted from 100 μL of serum/fecal samples or from 500 μL supernatants of tissue homogenates using TRIzol reagent (Invitrogen, Burlington, ON, Canada) according to the instructions. RT-nPCR for detecting positive/negative-stranded HEV RNA was carried out as previously described [24]. Two sets of specific external and internal primer pairs for partial fragments of ORF1 (129–373 nt) and ORF2 (5,983–6,349 nt) were used [24]. Negative and positive controls were included in all assays. RNA extraction and other pre-PCR amplification steps were performed in a separate clean room to avoid cross-contamination. The final amplicons were analyzed by 1% (w/v) agarose gel electrophoresis and visualized by ethidium bromide staining [24]. Selected amplicons of positive/negative-stranded HEV RNA were sequenced to confirm the specific virus inocula used for animal infections.

Results

Profile of HEV Infection in the Rabbit

The profile of HEV infection in the rabbit was monitored through the assay of two liver specific enzymes, ALT and AST; through the detection of HEV RNA in feces and by following the level of anti-HEV antibodies in sera. Prior to virus inoculation, all rabbits were negative for anti-HEV antibody and HEV RNA in serum/fecal samples, and had normal levels of ALT and AST (data not shown).

The control rabbits C1 and C2 were negative for anti-HEV antibody, fecal/serum HEV RNA and had normal ALT and AST levels throughout the study (Fig. 1A, Table 1).

However, an interesting and unexpected result was observed in the rabbits in group 2 inoculated with rabbit HEV. First, persistent fecal shedding of HEV RNA was detected in all rabbits of group 2 from 1 wpi till 36 wpi or to the end of this study (lasting for 9 months). In this group, the peak levels of ALT were at least 3–4 fold higher than baseline values, and peak levels of AST were elevated by approximately 2-fold above baseline levels. Focusing on one of the animals (R3) in this group, it seroconverted for anti-HEV antibodies at 5 wpi and the S/CO values jumped to a peak value of 22 at 6 wpi and maintained at 18–20 level thereafter. In this animal the peak levels of ALT reached was 114 U/L at 5wpi, and a dramatic elevation of AST (148 U/L at 5 wpi) to more than 8-fold above the baseline value of 17 U/L was also seen. Although fecal shedding of virus was detected in R3 throughout the post infection period, viremia was only evident during 11–13 wpi and 20–30 wpi (Fig. 1C, Table 1). The other animals in this group showed a similar disease profile to R3, with the exception that positive sero-conversion was only detected at 22–25 wpi for R1 and the S/CO values were only weakly positive, ranging from 1.072–1.426 (Fig. 1B, Table 1).

In contrast to group 2, the animals in group 3 showed no obvious elevations for ALT and AST following inoculation with inoculated with swine HEV. Rabbit S4 in this group seroconverted for anti-HEV antibodies at 5 wpi, with the S/CO values of anti-HEV jumping to a peak value of 22 at 6 wpi and being maintained at 18–20 thereafter (Fig. 1E, Table 1). Persistent fecal HEV RNA excretion was seen for animal S4 from 2 wpi to 16 wpi, but was not detected thereafter until 25 wpi. All the rabbits in this group were inoculated with the rabbit HEV at 25 wpi. Following this second virus challenge, fecal HEV RNA was detected only once at 26 wpi (Fig. 1E, Table 1). The other animals in this group had a similar disease profile with the exception of rabbit S2, which remained

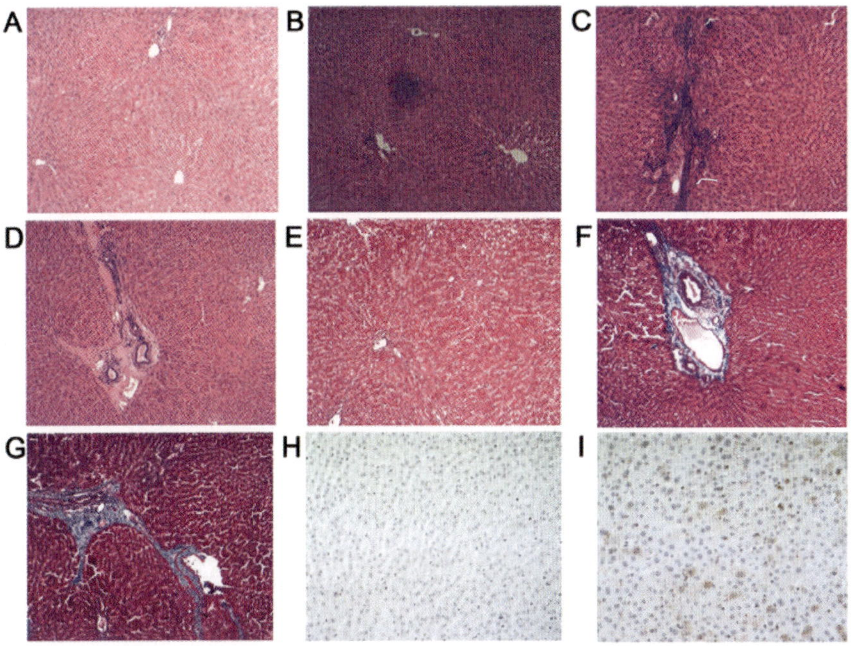

Figure 2. Liver histology. A–D (H & E stain, original magnification, ×10), E–G (Masson's trichrome stain, original magnification, ×10), H–I (Immunohistochemistry, original magnification, ×40). (**A**) Liver section from a control rabbit with no visible pathological signs of HEV infection. (**B**)-(**C**) Lymphocytes distributed focal or scattered in hepatic lobule, the inflammatory cells gathered along blood vessel walls. (**D**) Chronic inflammatory cells infiltrate the portal area, blood vessel walls thickening associated with fibrosis, local hyaline degeneration. (**E**) No histopathological changes with minimal staining limited to areas immediately adjacent to portal structures. (**F**) Artery wall thickening associated with moderate to severe fibrosis. (**G**) More advanced portal and periportal fibrosis with short fibrous septa. (**H**) Negative immunohistochemistry result for HEV antigen in liver sections from the control rabbits. (**I**) Positive results for HEV antigen in liver sections of experimental groups.

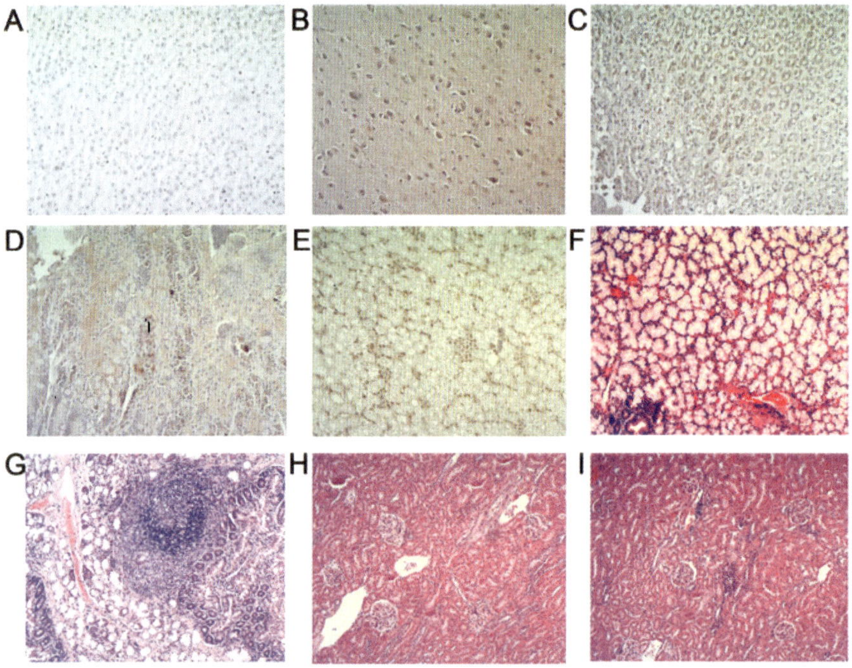

Figure 3. Extrahepatic tissue histology. A–E (Immunohistochemistry, original magnification, ×40), F–J (H & E stain, original magnification, ×10). (**A**) Negative immunohistochemistry result for HEV antigen in extrahepatic tissue sections from the control rabbits. (**B**)–(**E**) Positive results for HEV antigen in brain, stomach, duodenum and kidney. (**F**) Duodenum section from a control rabbit with no visible pathological signs of inflammation. (**G**) A large number of lymphocytes infiltrate mucosal interstitial, focal lymph follicles formed in duodenum sections. (**H**) Kidney section from a control rabbit with no visible pathological signs of HEV infection. (**I**) Multifocal lymphocytes and mononuclear cells infiltrate in renal interstitial.

seronegative for anti-HEV antibody until 4 weeks after the second virus inoculation with rabbit HEV at 25 wpi. Following seroconversion of this animal, S/CO values peaked at 20 and were maintained at this level for the 6 weeks until the end of the study. (Fig. 1D, Table 1).

Liver Histopathology and Immunohistochemistry (IHC)

No gross histopathology lesions, no histopathological chronic inflammation or HEV antigens of were observed in liver sections of control group (Group 1) animals (Fig. 2A, 2E and 2H). Histopathology done on animals from Group 2 also showed no gross histopathological lesions, but chronic inflammatory cell infiltrations were observed (Fig. 2B and 2C) and portal fibrosis was obvious (Fig. 2D, 2F and 2G). In addition, HEV antigens were observed in the liver sections of all animals from groups 2 and 3 (Fig. 2I).

HEV Replication in Extrahepatic Tissue of Infected Rabbits

Positive and negative strand HEV RNA, indicative of active virus replication, was detected in a range of extrahepatic tissues (brain, stomach, duodenum, kidney, bile, lung and bladder) taken from Group 2 infected animals. The positive staining for HEV antigens seen on carrying out IHC staining of brain, stomach, duodenum and kidney sections made from Group 2 infected animals served to provide confirmatory evidence of extrahepatic virus replication (Fig. 3B, 3C, 3D and 3E). Extrahepatic tissue sections made from control group (Group 1) animals were as expected negative for HEV antigen expression (Fig. 3A, 3F and 3H). Interestingly, histological staining of both duodenal and kidney tissues from HEV infected animals (Group 2) showed clear evidence of infiltration with inflammatory cells (Fig. 3G and 3I).

Discussion

HEV is a well-known pathogen classically associated with acute viral hepatitis [1]. However, a number of more recent studies have shown that infection with genotype 3 HEV can lead to the development of chronic hepatitis in immunocompromised patients [2–4]. HEV infection has also been linked to a number of extra-hepatic conditions, including involvement in neurologically based symptomologies [30]. This association of HEV with a range of disease pathologies [31–33], coupled to a clear need to establish a tractable small animal model for this pathogen of growing medical importance has stimulated studies of HEV pathogenesis. There have been previous studies that suggested rabbits could be a possible small animal model for HEV infection [26,34], but none has focused on defining the pathogenic profile of the virus. The most interesting result obtained in the current study focusing on this aspect of HEV biology was that infection of the SPF rabbits used with a homologous rabbit HEV isolate lead in some cases to the development of chronic hepatitis and an associated liver fibrosis. Interestingly this chronic disease pathology was not seen when rabbits were infected with the heterologous genotype 4 swine HEV. Chronic HEV infection has been defined previously as the presence of persistently elevated liver enzyme levels and detectable HEV RNA in the serum and/or stool for at least 6 months [35], and in this study, the rabbits inoculated with rabbit HEV conformed to this definition with persistent fecal shedding and elevated liver enzymes being evident for more than six months after infection. The detection of both the positive/negative-stranded HEV and HEV antigen in brain, stomach, duodenum and kidney, together with the histopathologic changes seen in the duodenum and kidney of HEV infected animals, raises the possibility that the replication of virus in extrahepatic tissues may be responsible some of the clinical symptoms that have been reported. Furthermore, the detection of HEV replication in brain tissue via PCR and immunohistochemistry, provides some evidence based explanation of the neurological signs and symptoms that have been associated with HEV infection [36]. It also indicates that clinicians should consider the possibility of HEV infection in patients with neurologic disorders of unknown etiology.

However, the mechanism of this chronic trend caused by rabbit HEV was unclear. The reported chronic HEV infections occurred mostly in immunocompromised patients and were caused by genotype 3 HEV [2–4]. Recently, cases of chronic hepatitis E in immunocompetent patients were reported [37,38]. Whether the acute viral infection developed to chronic course or not mainly depends on both factors of virus and host. For the interprets of the chronicity of rabbit HEV infection, we thought that phylogenetically the rabbit HEV genome is most closely related to that of genotype 3 HEV isolates, which is considered to be related to developing chronic hepatitis [2–4,37,38]. Moreover, rabbit HEV was characterized by an insertion of 31 aa in X domain of ORF1 (929–959 aa) [20]. Whether the insertions leading to the chronic trend is unclear and need further study. Besides, long period of nine months persistent fecal virus shedding together with high titer anti-HEV antibody for group 2 rabbits during the disease progress was observed. This result was contradicted with previous study that the neutralizing antibody anti-HEV could neutralize the HEV and therefore the virus should be cleared by high titer anti-HEV antibody [39]. A new report stated that the 'non-enveloped' virus HEV in blood can derive the host's membranes, therefore can escape from the neutralizing antibodies of HEV [40]. This may be another factor responsible for the chronicity of HEV infection.

In summary, this study has provided the first experimental evidence that SPF rabbits experimentally infected with a homologous rabbit HEV isolate develop signs of chronic hepatitis. Given the increasing medical importance of HEV infections and their association with chronic symptomology in some patient groups, the underlying mechanisms responsible for the chronic pattern of pathogenesis seen in this study deserves further study.

Acknowledgments

We are grateful to Professor Malcolm A. McCrae of University Warwick, UK for proofreading the manuscript.

Author Contributions

Conceived and designed the experiments: JH LingW. Performed the experiments: JH. Analyzed the data: JH YL LL PL JX YZ H. Zeng LinW. LingW. H. Zhuang. Contributed reagents/materials/analysis tools: LingW. Contributed to the writing of the manuscript: JH.

References

1. Kamar N, Bendall R, Legrand-Abravanel F, Xia NS, Ijaz S, et al. (2012) Hepatitis E. Lancet 379: 2477–2488.
2. Kamar N, Selves J, Mansuy JM, Ouezzani L, Peron JM, et al. (2008) Hepatitis E virus and chronic hepatitis in organ-transplant recipients. N Engl J Med 358: 811–817.
3. Dalton HR, Bendall RP, Keane FE, Tedder RS, Ijaz S (2009) Persistent carriage of hepatitis E virus in patients with HIV infection. N Engl J Med 361: 1025–1027.
4. Tavitian S, Peron JM, Huynh A, Mansuy JM, Ysebaert L, et al. (2010) Hepatitis E virus excretion can be prolonged in patients with hematological malignancies. J Clin Virol 49: 141–144.
5. Khuroo MS (1980) Study of an epidemic of non-A, non-B hepatitis. Possibility of another human hepatitis virus distinct from post-transfusion non-A, non-B type. Am J Med 68: 818–824.
6. Emerson SU, Anderson D, Arankalle A, Meng XJ, Purdy M, et al. (2004) Hepevirus. In: Fauquet CM, Mayo MA, Maniloff J, Desselberger U, Ball LA (Eds.), Virus Taxonomy, VIIIth Report of the ICTV. Elsevier/Academic Press, London, pp. 851–855.
7. Aggarwal R (2010) Hepatitis E virus and person-to-person transmission. Clin Infect Dis 51: 477–479.
8. Hoofnagle JH, Nelson KE, Purcell RH (2012) Hepatitis E. N Engl J Med 367: 1237–1244.
9. Meng XJ, Purcell RH, Halbur PG, Lehman JR, Webb DM, et al. (1997) A novel virus in swine is closely related to the human hepatitis E virus. Proc Natl Acad Sci U S A 94: 9860–9865.
10. Haqshenas G, Shivaprasad HL, Woolcock PR, Read DH, Meng XJ (2001) Genetic identification and characterization of a novel virus related to human hepatitis E virus from chickens with hepatitis-splenomegaly syndrome in the United States. J Gen Virol 82: 2449–2462.
11. Tomiyama D, Inoue E, Osawa Y, Okazaki K (2009) Serological evidence of infection with hepatitis E virus among wild Yezo-deer, Cervus nippon yesoensis, in Hokkaido, Japan. J Viral Hepat 16: 524–528.
12. Nakamura M, Takahashi K, Taira K, Taira M, Ohno A, et al. (2006) Hepatitis E virus infection in wild mongooses of Okinawa, Japan: Demonstration of anti-HEV antibodies and a full-genome nucleotide sequence. Hepatol Res 34: 137–140.
13. Bodewes R, van der Giessen J, Haagmans BL, Osterhaus AD, Smits SL (2013) Identification of multiple novel viruses, including a parvovirus and a hepevirus, in feces of red foxes. J Virol 87: 7758–7764.
14. Raj VS, Smits SL, Pas SD, Provacia LB, Moorman-Roest H, et al. (2012) Novel hepatitis E virus in ferrets, the Netherlands. Emerg Infect Dis 18: 1369–1370.
15. Johne R, Plenge-Bonig A, Hess M, Ulrich RG, Reetz J, et al. (2010) Detection of a novel hepatitis E-like virus in faeces of wild rats using a nested broad-spectrum RT-PCR. J Gen Virol 91: 750–758.
16. Drexler JF, Seelen A, Corman VM, Fumie TA, Cottontail V, et al. (2012) Bats worldwide carry hepatitis E virus-related viruses that form a putative novel genus within the family Hepeviridae. J Virol 86: 9134–9147.
17. Takahashi M, Nishizawa T, Sato H, Sato Y, Jirintai, et al. (2011) Analysis of the full-length genome of a hepatitis E virus isolate obtained from a wild boar in Japan that is classifiable into a novel genotype. J Gen Virol 92: 902–908.
18. Batts W, Yun S, Hedrick R, Winton J (2011) A novel member of the family Hepeviridae from cutthroat trout (Oncorhynchus clarkii). Virus Res 158: 116–123.
19. Zhao C, Ma Z, Harrison TJ, Feng R, Zhang C, et al. (2009) A novel genotype of hepatitis E virus prevalent among farmed rabbits in China. J Med Virol 81: 1371–1379.
20. Geng J, Fu H, Wang L, Bu Q, Liu P, et al. (2011) Phylogenetic analysis of the full genome of rabbit hepatitis E virus (rbHEV) and molecular biologic study on the possibility of cross species transmission of rbHEV. Infect Genet Evol 11: 2020–2025.
21. Purdy MA, Khudyakov YE (2010) Evolutionary history and population dynamics of hepatitis E virus. PLoS One 5: e14376.
22. Cossaboom CM, Cordoba L, Dryman BA, Meng XJ. 2011. Hepatitis E virus in rabbits, Virginia, USA. Emerg Infect Dis 17: 2047–2049.
23. Geng J, Wang L, Wang X, Fu H, Bu Q, et al. (2011) Study on prevalence and genotype of hepatitis E virus isolated from Rex Rabbits in Beijing, China. J Viral Hepat 18: 661–667.
24. Liu P, Bu QN, Wang L, Han J, Du RJ, et al. (2013) Transmission of hepatitis E virus from rabbits to cynomolgus macaques. Emerg Infect Dis 19: 559–565.
25. Cossaboom CM, Cordoba L, Sanford BJ, Pineyro P, Kenney SP, et al. (2012) Cross-species infection of pigs with a novel rabbit, but not rat, strain of hepatitis E virus isolated in the United States. J Gen Virol 93: 1687–1695.
26. Ma H, Zheng L, Liu Y, Zhao C, Harrison TJ, et al. (2010) Experimental infection of rabbits with rabbit and genotypes 1 and 4 hepatitis E viruses. PLoS One 5: e9160.
27. Fu H, Wang L, Zhu Y, Geng J, Li L, et al. (2011) Analysing complete genome sequence of swine hepatitis E virus (HEV), strain CHN-XJ-SW13 isolated from Xinjiang, China: putative host range, and disease severity determinants in HEV. Infect Genet Evol 11: 618–623.
28. Zhang J, Ge SX, Huang GY, Li SW, He ZQ, et al. (2003) Evaluation of antibody-based and nucleic acid-based assays for diagnosis of hepatitis E virus infection in a rhesus monkey model. J Med Virol 71: 518–526.
29. Wang YC, Zhang HY, Xia NS, Peng G, Lan HY, et al. (2002) Prevalence, isolation, and partial sequence analysis of hepatitis E virus from domestic animals in China. J Med Virol 67: 516–521.
30. Kamar N, Izopet J, Cintas P, Garrouste C, Uro-Coste E, et al. (2010) Hepatitis E virus-induced neurological symptoms in a kidney-transplant patient with chronic hepatitis. Am J Transplant 10: 1321–1324.
31. Purcell RH, Emerson SU (2008) Hepatitis E: an emerging awareness of an old disease. J Hepatol 48: 494–503.
32. Takahashi M, Nishizawa T, Yoshikawa A, Sato S, Isoda N, et al. (2002) Identification of two distinct genotypes of hepatitis E virus in a Japanese patient with acute hepatitis who had not travelled abroad. J Gen Virol 83: 1931–1940.
33. Pujhari SK, Kumar S, Ratho RK, Chawla YK, Chakraborti A (2010) Phylogenetic analysis and subtyping of acute and fulminant strains of hepatitis

E virus isolates of North India with reference to disease severity. Arch Virol 155: 1483–1486.
34. Cheng X, Wang S, Dai X, Shi C, Wen Y, et al. (2012) Rabbit as a novel animal model for hepatitis E virus infection and vaccine evaluation. PLoS One 7: e51616.
35. Kaba M, Richet H, Ravaux I, Moreau J, Poizot-Martin I, et al. (2011) Hepatitis E virus infection in patients infected with the human immunodeficiency virus. J Med Virol 83: 1704–1716.
36. Kamar N, Bendall RP, Peron JM, Cintas P, Prudhomme L, et al. (2011) Hepatitis E virus and neurologic disorders. Emerg Infect Dis 17: 173–179.
37. Gonzalez TA, Moreira VV, Mateos LM, Achecar JL (2011) Chronic hepatitis E in an immunocompetent patient. Gastroenterol Hepatol 34: 398–400.
38. Grewal P, Kamili S, Motamed D (2014) Chronic hepatitis E in an immunocompetent patient: A case report. Hepatology 59: 347–348.
39. Shrestha MP, Scott RM, Joshi DM, Mammen MJ, Thapa GB, et al. (2007) Safety and efficacy of a recombinant hepatitis E vaccine. N Engl J Med 356: 895–903.
40. Feng Z, Lemon SM (2013) Peek-a-boo: membrane hijacking and the pathogenesis of viral hepatitis. Trends Microbiol. pii: S0966-842X (13)00203-5. doi:10.1016/j.tim.2013.10.005. [Epub ahead of print].

12

None of the Six SNPs of IL28B Could Predict Treatment Responses in Genotype 2 Chronic HCV Infected Patients by Propensity Score Matching Analysis

Wen-Juei Jeng[1,4], Chun-Yen Lin[1,2], Ji-Yih Chen[2,3], Chang-Wen Huang[1], Chien-Hao Huang[1], I-Shyan Sheen[1,2]*

1 Division of Hepatology, Department of Gastroenterology and Hepatology, Linkou Medical Center, Chang Gung Memorial Hospital, Taoyuan, Taiwan, **2** College of Medicine, Chang Gung University, Taoyuan, Taiwan, **3** Department of Rheumatology, Allergy and Immunology, Linkou Medical Center, Chang Gung Memorial Hospital, Taoyuan, Taiwan, **4** Institute of Clinical Medicine, National Yang-Ming University, Taipei, Taiwan

Abstract

Background & Aims: A combination of pegylated interferon-alpha and ribavirin (PR) is the standard therapy for patients with chronic hepatitis C. The impact of polymorphism of interleukin-28B *(IL28B)* on sustained virological response (SVR) to PR has been well documented in patients with CHC genotype-1 (GT1), but it is controversial in genotype-2 (GT2) CHC patients. This study investigated the predictability of six single nucleotide polymorphisms (SNP) of *IL28B* on the treatment responses of PR in patients with CHC GT2.

Method: 197 CHC GT2 consecutive patients who received PR treatment in our prospective cohort were enrolled. Hepatitis C virus (HCV) genotyping, quantification of HCV-RNA and genotyping of the ten SNPs of *IL28B* were performed. Six SNPs of *IL28B* were chosen for analysis. The propensity score matching (PSM) analysis was applied using patients with CHC GT1 in another prospective cohort as a positive comparison to avoid covariate bias.

Results: The distribution of the six SNPs was similar in GT1 and GT2 patients. Five of these SNPs had strong association with treatment responses in GT1 but not in GT2 patients. After PSM analysis, these five SNPs still showed strong association with rapid virological response (RVR), cEVR and SVR in GT1 and had no influence in GT2 patients. Furthermore, rs12979860 and baseline viral load were the predictors for both RVR and SVR in GT1 patients. However, only baseline viral load could predict RVR and SVR in GT2 patients. In addition, in patients without RVR, rs12979860 was the only predictor for SVR in GT1 but no predictor for SVR was found in GT2.

Conclusions: The genetic polymorphisms of *IL28B* had no impact on treatment responses in GT2 patients.

Editor: Golo Ahlenstiel, University of Sydney, Australia

Funding: This work was supported by NMRP: 98-3112-B-182A-003 and NMRP: 360021 from the National Science Council, Taiwan, and CMRPG 390682, 37542, 360463 from Chang Gung Memorial Hospital. The funders had no role in study design, data collection and analysis, decision to publish or preparation of the manuscript.

Competing Interests: The authors have declared that no competing interests exist.

* E-mail: issheen.jks@gmail.com

Introduction

Chronic hepatitis C (CHC) is a worldwide health issue affecting around 180 million people. The persistent inflammation caused by this virus may result in cirrhosis and hepatocellular carcinoma. A combination therapy of pegylated interferon-α (PegIFN) and ribavirin (PR) is a standard of care for chronic hepatitis C virus infection [1]. Current treatment strategy for CHC is to tailor the treatment guided by genotypes and on treatment viral response according to the roadmap concept [1,2]. With these recommended strategies, a sustained virological response (SVR) rate could reach around 76–84% among patients with HCV genotype 2/3 (GT2/3) chronic infection, significantly better than the 42–52% in patients with HCV genotype 1 (GT1) [2].

Host genetic factors on the treatment efficacy for CHC have been proposed for a long time due to the ethnic differences in the treatment outcome. Better SVR rates, with 61–80% for GT1 and 80–95% for GT2/3 in Asian patients, were the main supporting evidence [3–12]. Recent genome-wide associated studies demonstrated strong evidence that single nucleotide polymorphisms (SNPs) of *Interluekin-28B (IL28B)* correlated significantly with SVR in GT1 patients when treated with PR [13–17]. Notably, the frequency of advantageous genotype of *IL28B* is highest in Asians and lowest in African-Americans, and it parallels the SVR rate in each population [13]. Furthermore, these genotypes of *IL28B* are also correlated with the spontaneous clearance of hepatitis C virus [14] and with viral kinetics during treatment in GT1 patients [17]. However, the results of the influences of these genetic variances on the treatment responses in GT2 patients were conflicting [18–22].

The aim of the present study was to use the propensity score matching (PSM) analysis to extend our understanding of genetic association in a cohort of patients with HCV GT2 chronic infection.

Materials and Methods

Patients

We conducted a retrospective analysis of our prospective cohort of consecutive adult Taiwanese patients with CHC GT1 and GT2 who visited the HCV team of the Department of Gastroenterology and Hepatology, Linkou Medical Center, Chang Gung Memorial Hospital. A universal 24-week regimen of PR (pegylated interferon alfa-α 2a 180 mcg/week or pegylated interferon alfa-α 2b 1.5 mcg/Kg/week, ribavirin 1000 mg-1200 mg/day) was reimbursed by the Bureau of National Health Insurance of Taiwan between February 2002 and December 2008. A total of 388 patients who provided written informed consent for this study, including genomic analysis, were enrolled. Patients with decompensated liver disease, hepatoma, co-infection with hepatitis B virus or with human immunodeficiency virus, or with apparent autoimmune hepatitis and alcoholic liver disease, were excluded from this cohort. Twenty-six percent of our patients had a history of blood transfusion, tattooing on skin or eyebrows, patterning of eyes, or piercing of earlobes. The remaining patients had no clear infection routes. Further, the distribution of infection routes in the GT1 and GT2 groups was similar.

Table 1. Baseline characteristics of chronic hepatitis C patients with genotype 1 and 2.

Variable	Total (N = 388)	GT 1 (N = 191)	GT 2 (N = 197)	P value
Gender, n (%)				0.128
male	235 (60.6)	123 (64.4)	112 (56.9)	
female	153 (39.4)	68 (35.6)	85 (43.1)	
Viral load, n (%)				0.044
$<0.4\times10^6$ IU/ml	205 (52.8)	91(47.6)	114 (57.9)	
$\geq0.4\times10^6$ IU/ml	183 (47.2)	100 (52.4)	83 (42.1)	
Fibrosis stage, n (%)				0.410
F0-2	201 (51.8)	103 (53.9)	98 (49.7)	
F3-4	187 (48.2)	88 (46.1)	99 (50.3)	
Age, *y*	51.2±10.6	51.4±11.1	51.1±10.0	0.838
BMI, *Kg/m²*	24.5±3.3	24.5±3.3	24.6±3.2	0.603
HbA1c, %	5.7±1.1	5.6±1.0	5.7±1.1	0.430
ALB, *g/dL*	4.5±0.4	4.5±0.4	4.5±0.5	0.894
AST, *IU/L*	95±54	92±52	97±57	0.407
ALT, *IU/L*	153±106	149±107	157±106	0.256
GGT, *IU/L*	47±48	43±48	51±47	0.188
ALP, *IU/L*	82±44	80±25	85±57	0.668
Bilirubin, *mg/dL*	0.9±0.4	0.9±0.3	0.9±0.5	0.330
RVR, n (%)	293 (75.5)	133 (69.6)	160 (81.2)	0.008
cEVR, n (%)	316 (81.4)	147 (77.0)	169 (85.8)	0.025
SVR, n (%)	311 (80.2)	131 (68.6)	180 (91.4)	<0.001

Continuous variables were expressed as mean ± standard deviation; BMI: body mass index; HbA1c: glycohemoglobin; ALB: albumin; AST: aspartate transaminase; ALT: alanine transaminase; GGT: gamma-glutamyl transpeptidase; ALP: alkaline phosphatase; RVR: rapid virologic response; cEVR: complete early virologic response; SVR: sustained virologic response.

All patients received pre-treatment liver biopsies that were evaluated by one liver-specialized pathologist using the Metavir scoring system. HCV genotypes were determined by a genotype-specific probe-based assay in the 5′ untranslated region (LiPA; Innogenetics, Ghent, Belgium).

For analysis of the responses to treatment, subjects with SVR were defined as undetectable serum HCV-RNA 24 weeks after cessation of treatment. The subjects with rapid virological response (RVR) were defined as undetectable serum HCV-RNA 4 weeks after starting treatment. Complete early virological response (cEVR) was defined as undetectable serum HCV-RNA at week 12 after treatment.

The HCV antibody was tested by the Architect anti-HCV (Abbott Diagnostics, Irving, TX, USA). The HCV-RNA was quantitated by the VERSANT HCV RNA 3.0 Assay (bDNA) (Bayer Diagnostics, Tarrytown, NY, USA; lower limit of detection at 3200 copies/ml) or COBAS TaqMan HCV Test (TaqMan HCV; Roche Molecular Systems Inc., Branchburg, NJ, USA; lower limit of detection at concentrations of 15 IU/ml). Those with undetectable RNA by bDNA were reassayed by Cobas Amplicor HCV v2.0 kit (Roche Molecular Systems, Pleasanton, CA, USA; lower limit of detection at concentrations of 100 copies/ml).

Genomic DNA Extraction and *IL28 B* Genotyping

Nucleic acid isolation. Anti-coagulated peripheral blood was obtained from patients with CHC GT1. Genomic DNA was isolated from EDTA anti-coagulated peripheral blood using the Pure gene DNA isolation kit (Gentra Systems, Minneapolis, MN) as previously described [23].

Taqman-based assay for the genotyping of SNPs. The oligonucleotide sequence flanking ten *IL28B* polymorphisms were designed as primer for Taqman allelic discrimination assays. Both allele specific primers were labeled with a fluorescent dye (FAM and VIC) and used in the PCR reaction. Aliquots of the PCR product were genotyping with allele specific probe of SNPs using real time PCR (ABI) [24]. IL28B variants rs12979860 C>T, rs8099917 T>G, rs12980275 A>G, rs8105790 T>C, rs7248668 G>A, rs10853728 C>G were diagnosed from whole blood samples using validated pyrosequencing™ assays. We used these six SNPs from ten of our previous report [23] because of significant deviations from the Hardy-Weinberg equilibrium in two SNPs and used one as the representative of the haplotype (three SNPs).

Ethics Statements

All patients in this study had provided written informed consent. This study protocol conformed to the ethical guidelines of the 1975 Declaration of Helsinki and was approved by the ethical committees of Chang Gung Memorial Hospital.

Statistical Analysis

Chi-square test or Fisher's exact probability test was used to compare the categorical variables where appropriate. Continuous variables were compared using Mann-Whitney U test or Student's *t*-test. Univariate and multivariate logistic regression analyses for the significant independent predictors of virological responses were conducted using patients' demographics, clinical variables and *IL28B* SNPs. Variables that achieved statistical *P* value<0.10 on univariate analysis were entered into multivariate logistic regression analysis. The propensity score matching (PSM) analysis [24–26] was applied for bias reduction in the investigation of the association between SNPs and the treatment outcomes in GT1 and GT2 patients. Variables possibly influencing the treatment

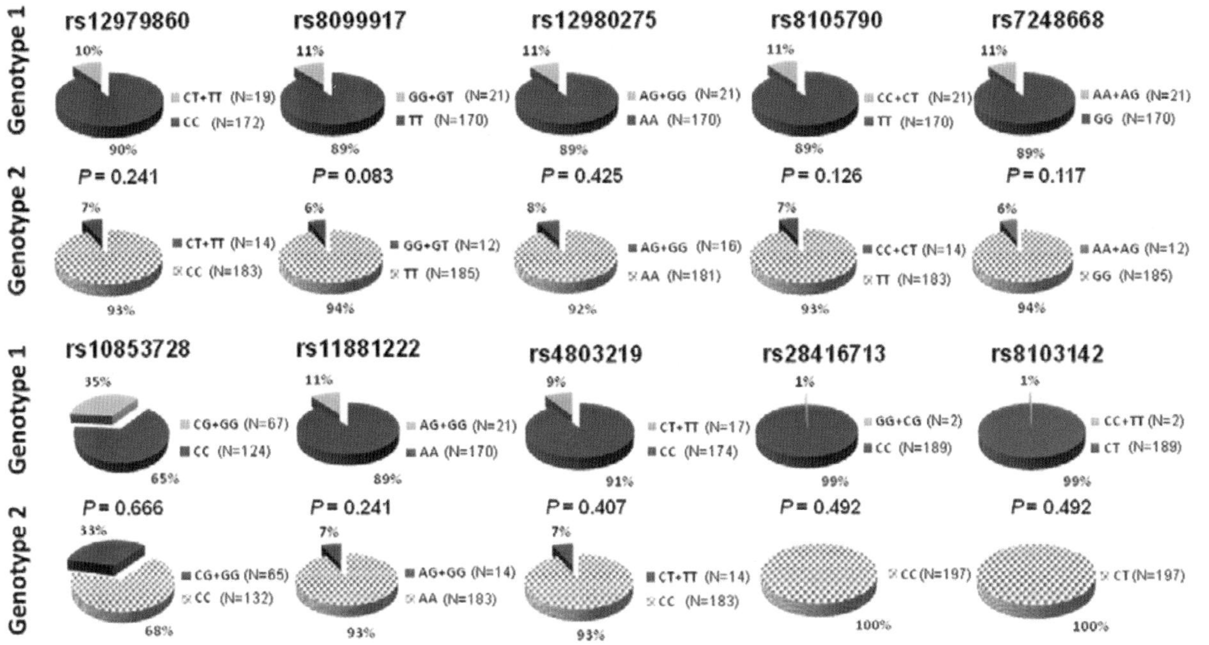

Figure 1. The distribution of the ten SNPs of IL 28B between GT1 and GT2. The genotypic distributions of the 10 SNPs of IL28B were similar in GT1 and GT2 patients (p>0.05).

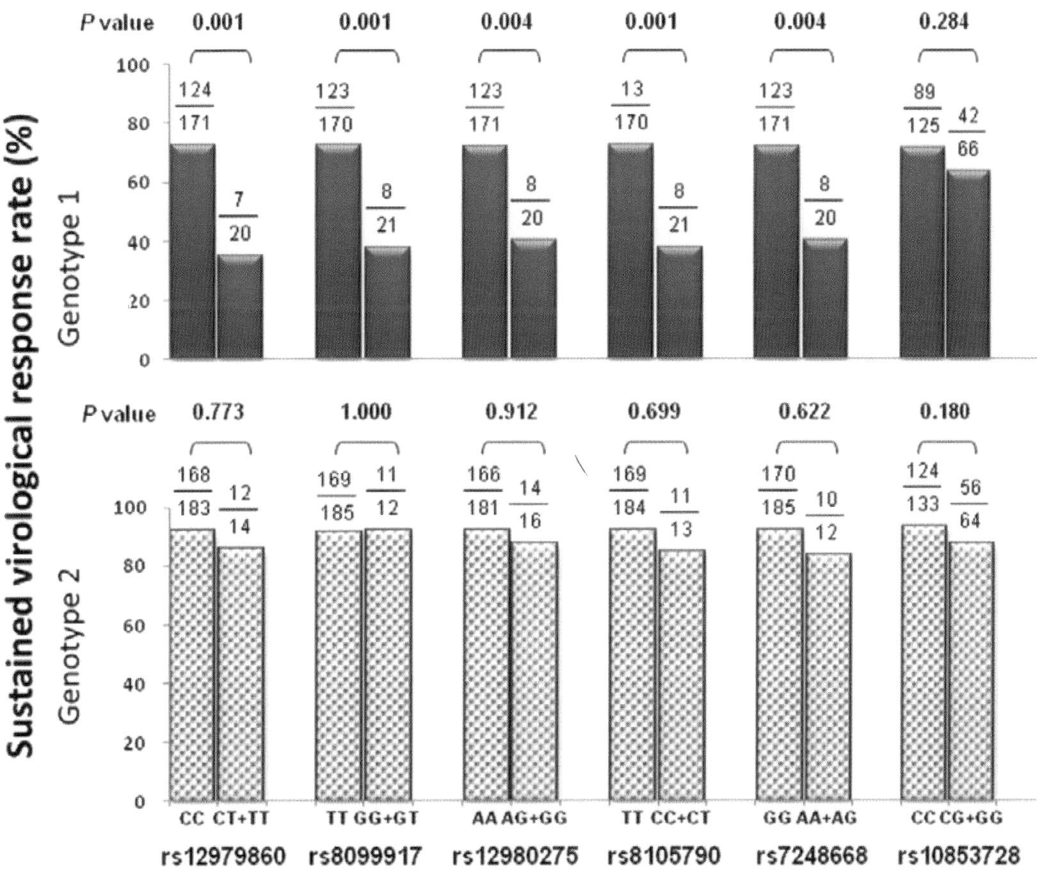

Figure 2. The correlation of SNPs with SVR in GT1 and GT2 patients. Six SNPs were chosen for analysis (rs12979860, rs8099917, rs12980275, rs8105790, rs7248668, 10853728). Five (rs12979860, rs8099917, rs12980275, rs8105790, and rs7248668) of these six SNPs revealed significant association with SVR in GT1 patients while none of them revealed any relationship between these SNPs and the SVR in GT2 patients.

Table 2. Baseline characteristics of chronic hepatitis C patients with genotype 1 and 2 after PSM.

Variable	Total (N = 290)	GT 1 (N = 145)	GT 2 (N = 145)	P value
Male, n (%)	180 (62.1)	90 (62.1)	90 (62.1)	1.000
RNA≥0.4×10^6 IU/ml, n (%)	134 (46.2)	67 (46.2)	67 (46.2)	1.000
Fibrosis stage 3–4, n (%)	118 (40.7)	59 (40.7)	59 (40.7)	1.000
Age, *y*	50.3±10.7	50.0±11.4	50.7±10.1	0.597
BMI, *Kg/m²*	24.4±3.0	24.5±3.2	24.4±2.9	0.678
HbA1c, *%*	5.7±1.2	5.7±1.1	5.7±1.2	0.699
ALB, *g/dL*	4.5±0.4	4.5±0.4	4.5±0.4	0.278
AST, *IU/L*	93±55	92±54	94±56	0.976
ALT, *IU/L*	156±116	153±117	159±116	0.557
GGT, *IU/L*	46±50	44±54	47±46	0.802
ALP, *IU/L*	79±25	78±25	79±26	0.574
Bilirubin, *mg/dL*	1.0±0.4	1.0±0.3	0.9±0.5	0.164
RVR, n (%)	208 (71.7)	89 (61.4)	119 (82.1)	<0.001
cEVR, n (%)	228 (78.6)	102 (70.3)	126 (86.9)	0.001
SVR, n (%)	229 (79.0)	99 (68.3)	130 (89.7)	<0.001

outcomes, including gender, baseline HCV-RNA viral load, fibrosis stage, glycohemoglobin (HbA1c) and basal metabolic index (BMI) were used to generate a propensity score ranging from 0 to 1 by logistic regression. Nearest available matching on the estimated propensity score was used to select the GT1 and find the GT2 subject with the closest propensity score. One hundred and forty-five well-matched pairs of GT1 and GT2 patients were obtained. All *P* values less than 0.05 by the two-tailed test were considered statistically significant. All statistical analyses were performed with the SPSS statistical software for Windows (version 16, SPSS. Inc., Chicago, IL, USA).

Results

None of the SNPs of *IL28B* were Associated with SVR in GT2 Patients, though they were in GT1 Patients

The demographic characteristics of these patients are shown in Table 1. There were 191 GT1 and 197 GT2 patients. More patients of GT1 had high viral load (HCV-RNA≥0.4×10^6 IU/ml) than GT2 patients (GT1 vs. GT2:52.4% vs. 42.1%, $p=0.044$). Other demographic data were comparable between these two groups. Similar to previous literature, the rates of RVR, cEVR and SVR were significantly lower in GT1 patients than GT2 patients (Table 1). The genotypic distributions of the six SNPs of IL28B were similar in GT1 and GT2 patients (Figure 1). Five (rs12979860, rs8099917, rs12980275, rs8105790, and rs7248668) of these six SNPs revealed significant association with SVR in GT1 patients. These SNPs had no influence on the SVR in GT2 patients (Figure 2).

After balancing the covariates in GT1 and GT2 patients to reduce the bias possibility by the PSM (Table 2), all the treatment responses of GT1 were significantly lower than GT2 (SVR: 68.3% vs. 89.7%, $P<0.001$; RVR: 61.4% vs. 82.1%, $P<0.001$; cEVR: 70.3% vs. 86.9%, $P=0.001$). As for the relationship between the SNPs of *IL28B* and the treatment responses (Figure 3), five out of the six SNPs showed significant association with RVR, cEVR and SVR in GT1 patients, but none of these SNPs had any relationship with treatment responses in GT2 patients.

Different Predictors for RVR, cEVR and SVR in GT1 and GT2 Patients

Because the SNPs of *IL28B* had different impacts on the treatment responses in GT1 and GT2 patients, we therefore analyzed the possible predictors for treatment responses in these two PSM adjusted patient groups. In the prediction of RVR, rs12979860 and baseline HCV RNA viral load were the independent predictors in GT1 patients, while baseline HCV-RNA viral load was the only predictor in GT2. In the cEVR prediction analysis, only RVR was the predictor in both GT1 and GT2 patients. As for the SVR, rs12979860, age, baseline viral load and RVR were the predictors in GT1 patients, while BMI, gender and baseline viral load were the predictors in GT2 patients (Table 3).

In our previous report [27], we found that in GT1 patients with RVR, only baseline viral load could predict the SVR. As for GT1 patients without RVR, rs12979860 became the predictor for SVR. Similar observation was found in GT1 patients in this PSM analysis. However, in GT2 patients with RVR, baseline RNA, fibrosis and ALT levels were the predictors for SVR. Interestingly, none of these factors including SNPs of *IL28B* were associated with SVR in GT2 patients without RVR (Table 4).

Discussion

The treatment of CHC has evolved rapidly. Response to tailored treatment planning has been emphasized after a roadmap concept is established [2]. The discovery of the host genome factors of *IL-28B* was a milestone since it demonstrated and explained the influence of genetic variations and ethnicity on the efficacy of interferon-based therapy for patients with GT1 CHC [28,29]. In our previous report, by genotyping six SNPs of *IL28B*, we had shown a significant correlation of genetic polymorphisms of *IL28B* with SVR in GT1 Asian patients [27]. The present study revealed that none of the six SNPs had association with either RVR or SVR in Asian GT2 patients, even by PSM approach.

Though the impact of polymorphisms of *IL28B* on the treatment responses of GT1 patients is very clear, the impact of this genetic polymorphism on the treatment responses in GT2

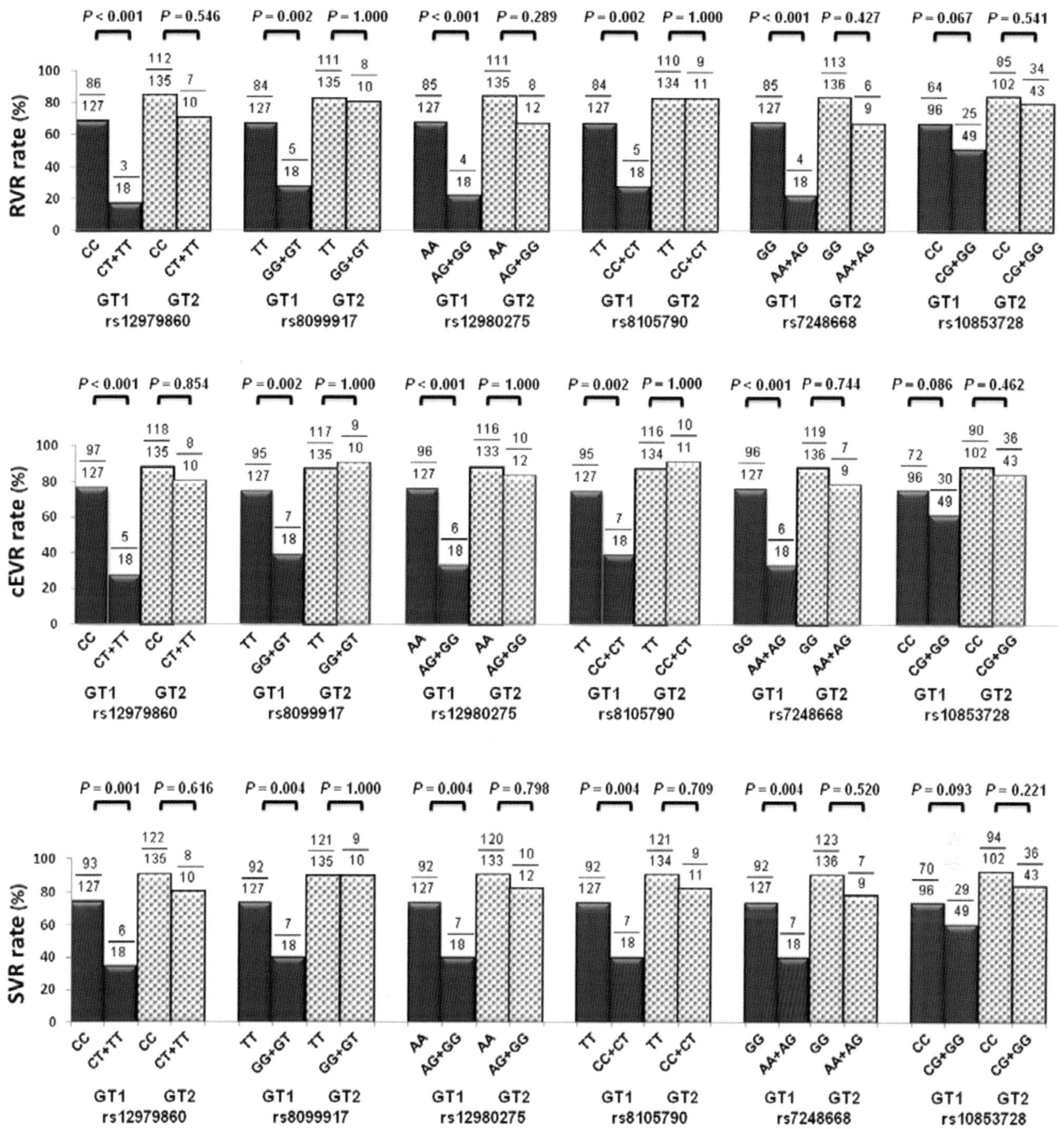

Figure 3. The role of SNPs in RVR (3A), EVR (3B) and SVR (3C) between GT1 and GT2 after PSM analysis. Five out of these SNPs (rs12979860, rs8099917, rs12980275, rs8105790, rs7248668) showed significant association with RVR, cEVR and SVR in GT1 patients but none of these SNPs had relationship with treatment responses in GT2 patients.

patients is still controversial [18–22]. Rauch et al. had reported that genotype of *rs8099917* had no significant impact on the SVR in Swiss patients infected with HCV GT2 or 3 [15]. Yu et al. [19] found no influence of *rs8099917* on SVR of Asian HCV GT2 patients, but a higher RVR rate in those with *TT rs8099917*. On the other hand, in Italian patients, Mangia [18], Lindh [20] and Sarrazin [21] reported that the genotype of *rs12979860* had significant association with SVR in patients with HCV GT2 or GT3 infection. Kawaoka [22] found that the initial viral load and *rs8099917* genotype are significantly independent predictors of SVR in genotype 2 patients in Japan.

The three reports [18,20,21] about the impact of IL28B on the treatment outcomes of chronic hepatitis C GT2 or GT3 patients showed IL28B polymorphism was associated with SVR in the 24-week treatment and the effect was only observed in the non-RVR patients. In one of them, Sarrazin et al. [21] claimed only GT3 but not GT2 patients had a significantly higher SVR rate in the patients with advantageous allele. The other two did not further

Table 3. Predictors for RVR, cEVR and SVR in both GT1 and GT2 patients after PSM.

	Variables	UV		MV		
		OR	P value	OR	95% CI	P value
RVR	GT1					
	rs12979860	10.49	<0.001	13.0	3.3–51.0	<0.001
	rs8099917	5.08	0.004			
	rs12980275	7.08	0.001			
	rs8105790	5.08	0.004			
	rs7248668	7.08	0.001			
	rs10853728	1.92	0.069			
	HbA1c	0.81	0.161			
	Viral load	3.83	<0.001	4.5	2.1–9.7	<0.001
	GT2					
	HbA1c	0.99	0.995			
	Viral load	2.61	0.034	2.6	1.1–6.3	0.034
cEVR	GT1					
	rs12979860	8.41	<0.001			
	rs8099917	4.67	0.003			
	rs12980275	6.19	0.001			
	rs8105790	4.67	0.003			
	rs7248668	6.19	0.001			
	rs10853728	1.90	0.088			
	BMI	0.89	0.039			
	GGT	0.99	0.068			
	ALP	0.99	0.058			
	RVR	264.00	<0.001	264.0	33.6–2075.0	<0.001
	Viral load	4.05	<0.001			
	GT2					
	BMI	0.82	0.032			
	GGT	1.01	0.214			
	ALP	0.98	0.068			
	RVR	265.50	<0.001	265.5	31.3–2250.3	<0.001
	Viral load	1.72	0.277			
SVR	GT1					
	rs12979860	5.47	0.002	4.4	1.2–16.8	0.028
	rs8099917	4.13	0.007			
	rs12980275	4.13	0.007			
	rs8105790	4.13	0.007			
	rs7248668	4.13	0.007			
	rs10853728	1.86	0.095			
	Age	0.97	0.044	0.96	0.9–0.99	0.033
	BMI	0.86	0.010			
	Gender	2.09	0.043			
	Viral load	4.85	<0.001	4.2	1.7–10.3	0.002
	Fibrosis stage	2.28	0.024			
	RVR	7.14	<0.001	3.8	1.6–9.1	0.003
	cEVR	5.36	<0.001			
	GPT	1.00	0.127			
	ALB	2.13	0.140			
	GT2					
	Age	0.99	0.822			
	BMI	0.78	0.015	0.8	0.7–1.0	0.049

Table 3. Cont.

Variables	UV		MV		
	OR	P value	OR	95% CI	P value
Gender	5.38	0.006	0.2	0.1–0.7	0.009
Viral load	9.15	0.005	7.4	1.5–35.7	0.013
Fibrosis stage	4.70	0.011			
RVR	2.60	0.110			
cEVR	2.79	0.112			
GPT	1.01	0.030			
ALB	4.08	0.044			

UV: Univariate analysis; MV: Multivariate analysis.

divide their patients into GT2 and GT3 groups [18,20]. However, genotype 2 and 3 are not really the same [30,31]. Here, our patients are all GT2 HCV infections, and no associations between treatment outcomes (SVR or RVR) and rs12979860 polymorphism were found. In our study, the polymorphism of IL28B SNPs influences the RVR in GT1 patients rather than GT2 patients.

In addition, the distribution of the homozygous responding allele was around 40% in Caucasians but it is the dominant pattern (about 90%) in our patients. Furthermore, the dosage of pegylated interferon and ribavirin varied among Western studies (PEG-INTRON: 1.0 or 1.5 mcg/kg/week; ribavirin: 600–1400 mg/day), and treatment duration varied from 12 weeks to 24 weeks. In the present study, we used a fixed dosage of PegIFN and RBV (PEG-INTRON: 1.5 mcg/kg/week or pegasys 180 mcg/week; ribavirin: 1000–1200 mg/day), and a fixed duration (24 weeks). These factors may also contribute to the different conclusions in different studies.

To investigate the association between SNPs and treatment outcome in an observational database rather than a randomized control trial, a propensity score matching analysis was an

Table 4. Predictors for SVR in both GT1 and GT2 patients with or without RVR after PSM.

Variables	With RVR					Without RVR				
	UV		MV			UV		MV		
	OR	P value	OR	95% CI	P value	OR	P value	OR	95% CI	P value
GT-1										
rs12979860	1.02	0.989				4.20	0.045	4.2	1.0–17.1	0.045
rs8099917	1.37	0.788				3.18	0.111			
rs12980275	1.55	0.708				3.67	0.071			
rs8105790	1.37	0.788				3.18	0.111			
rs7248668	1.85	0.607				2.27	0.219			
rs10853728	1.03	0.965				2.00	0.215			
Age	0.98	0.359				0.96	0.094			
Gender	3.83	0.028	0.3	0.1–1.0	0.054	1.56	0.431			
BMI	0.883	0.137				0.85	0.109			
Viral Load	4.63	0.013	4.2	1.2–14.3	0.024	2.54	0.107			
Fibrosis stage	2.83	0.080				1.59	0.397			
GPT	1.01	0.089				1.00	0.939			
GGT	1.02	0.312				0.99	0.544			
GT-2								No significant variable		
Age	1.01	0.838				0.95	0.350			
Gender	3.04	0.100				1.48	0.220			
BMI	0.77	0.048				0.86	0.369			
Viral Load	6.38	0.023	8.8	1.5–50.8	0.015	9.00	0.065			
Fibrosis stage	3.58	0.075	5.3	1.1–26.7	0.043	12.80	0.038			
GPT	1.01	0.039	1.0	1.0–1.1	0.010	1.01	0.466			
GGT	1.01	0.540				1.00	0.902			

important method used to reduce patient selection bias [24–26] and to avoid imbalance covariates between groups. Through PSM, we used GT1 patients as a comparison group to match covariates that had been reported to influence treatment responses between GT1 and GT2 patient groups. The results still demonstrated the SNPs (rs12979860, rs8099917, rs12980275, rs8105790, and rs7248668) had no relationship with SVR in GT2 patients, though they had significant impact on SVR in GT1 patients. Therefore, it is fair to claim that the genotype of *IL28B* had great impact on the treatment response only in GT1 patients but not GT2 patients. In addition, till now only two SNPs of *IL28B*, rs8809917 and rs12979860, had been investigated in GT2 patients. We studied six SNPs of *IL28B* that had been published before [13–16] and found that none of these SNPs had any relationship with the treatment responses in GT2 patients.

In previous studies [7,32,33] and ours focusing on GT1 patients [27], the genetic variants of IL28B SNP had a more significant impact on SVR in patients without RVR rather than those with RVR. However, in the present studies, the genetic variants of IL28B SNP did not influence the treatment outcome in both the RVR group and non-RVR group in GT2 patients using propensity score matching analysis. Similar results were found by Yu [19], also done in an Asian population, that the SNP of *IL28B* had no impact on SVR in GT2 patients, whether RVR had been achieved or not.

Much better response rates (RVR, cEVR and SVR) have been demonstrated in GT2 patients than GT1 patients. The stronger sensitivity of HCV GT2 to PR might offset the increasing response to PR by *IL28B*, even for those GT2 patients with no RVR, though two reports from Europe [18,20] showed that the SNP of *IL28B* had a significant impact on SVR in GT2 or GT3 patients who did not achieve RVR. The majority of their patients were genotype 3 and the response to PR treatment was not as good in genotype 3 as it was in genotype 2. Therefore, further studies on the association of IL28B and SVR in only genotype 2 Caucasian patients are needed.

The limitation of this study is that the sample size was not big enough. Further external validation in larger populations as well as in Western countries is necessary. In addition, hidden bias may remain even after PSM because of matching only the controls for observed variables (to the extent that they are perfectly measured).

In conclusion, our data demonstrated that none of the six SNPs of *IL28B* had any relationship with SVR in GT2 patients, irrespective of the overall number of patients, or in those with or without RVR.

Acknowledgments

We greatly appreciated the secretarial and clerical help from Hui-Chuan Cheng, Mon-Tzy Lu and Pei-Ling Lin.

Author Contributions

Conceived and designed the experiments: CYL ISS JYC. Performed the experiments: CYL ISS JYC. Analyzed the data: CWH. Contributed reagents/materials/analysis tools: ISS CYL JYC. Wrote the paper: WJJ. Revised the manuscript for important intellectual content: WJJ CHH.

References

1. Davis GL, Albright JE, Cook SF, Rosenberg DM (2003) Projecting future complications of chronic hepatitis C in the United States. Liver Transpl 9: 331–338.
2. Ghany MG, Strader DB, Thomas DL, Seeff LB (2009) Diagnosis, management, and treatment of hepatitis C: an update. Hepatology 49: 1335–1374.
3. Manns MP, McHutchison JG, Gordon SC, Rustgi VK, Shiffman M, et al. (2001) Peginterferon alfa-2b plus ribavirin compared with interferon alfa-2b plus ribavirin for initial treatment of chronic hepatitis C: a randomised trial. Lancet 358: 958–965.
4. Fried MW, Shiffman ML, Reddy KR, Smith C, Marinos G, et al. (2002) Peginterferon alfa-2a plus ribavirin for chronic hepatitis C virus infection. N Engl J Med 347: 975–982.
5. Bruno S, Camma C, Di Marco V, Rumi M, Vinci M, et al. (2004) Peginterferon alfa-2b plus ribavirin for naive patients with genotype 1 chronic hepatitis C: a randomized controlled trial. J Hepatol 41: 474–481.
6. Hadziyannis SJ, Sette H, Jr., Morgan TR, Balan V, Diago M, et al. (2004) Peginterferon-alpha2a and ribavirin combination therapy in chronic hepatitis C: a randomized study of treatment duration and ribavirin dose. Ann Intern Med 140: 346–355.
7. Mangia A, Santoro R, Minerva N, Ricci GL, Carretta V, et al. (2005) Peginterferon alfa-2b and ribavirin for 12 vs. 24 weeks in HCV genotype 2 or 3. N Engl J Med 352: 2609–2617.
8. von Wagner M, Huber M, Berg T, Hinrichsen H, Rasenack J, et al. (2005) Peginterferon-alpha-2a (40KD) and ribavirin for 16 or 24 weeks in patients with genotype 2 or 3 chronic hepatitis C. Gastroenterology 129: 522–527.
9. Shiffman ML, Suter F, Bacon BR, Nelson D, Harley H, et al. (2007) Peginterferon alfa-2a and ribavirin for 16 or 24 weeks in HCV genotype 2 or 3. N Engl J Med 357: 124–134.
10. Yu ML, Dai CY, Huang JF, Hou NJ, Lee LP, et al. (2007) A randomised study of peginterferon and ribavirin for 16 versus 24 weeks in patients with genotype 2 chronic hepatitis C. Gut 56: 553–559.
11. McHutchison JG, Lawitz EJ, Shiffman ML, Muir AJ, Galler GW, et al. (2009) Peginterferon alfa-2b or alfa-2a with ribavirin for treatment of hepatitis C infection. N Engl J Med 361: 580–593.
12. Rumi MG, Aghemo A, Prati GM, D'Ambrosio R, Donato MF, et al. (2010) Randomized study of peginterferon-alpha2a plus ribavirin vs peginterferon-alpha2b plus ribavirin in chronic hepatitis C. Gastroenterology 138: 108–115.
13. Ge D, Fellay J, Thompson AJ, Simon JS, Shianna KV, et al. (2009) Genetic variation in IL28B predicts hepatitis C treatment-induced viral clearance. Nature 461: 399–401.
14. Thomas DL, Thio CL, Martin MP, Qi Y, Ge D, et al. (2009) Genetic variation in IL28B and spontaneous clearance of hepatitis C virus. Nature 461: 798–801.
15. Tanaka Y, Nishida N, Sugiyama M, Kurosaki M, Matsuura K, et al. (2009) Genome-wide association of IL28B with response to pegylated interferon-alpha and ribavirin therapy for chronic hepatitis C. Nat Genet 41: 1105–1109.
16. Suppiah V, Moldovan M, Ahlenstiel G, Berg T, Weltman M, et al. (2009) IL28B is associated with response to chronic hepatitis C interferon-alpha and ribavirin therapy. Nat Genet 41: 1100–1104.
17. Thompson AJ, Muir AJ, Sulkowski MS, Ge D, Fellay J, et al. (2010) Interleukin-28B polymorphism improves viral kinetics and is the strongest pretreatment predictor of sustained virologic response in genotype 1 hepatitis C virus. Gastroenterology 139: 120–129 e118.
18. Mangia A, Thompson AJ, Santoro R, Piazzolla V, Tillmann HL, et al. (2010) An IL28B polymorphism determines treatment response of hepatitis C virus genotype 2 or 3 patients who do not achieve a rapid virologic response. Gastroenterology 139: 821–827, 827 e821.
19. Yu ML, Huang CF, Huang JF, Chang NC, Yang JF, et al. (2011) Role of interleukin-28B polymorphisms in the treatment of hepatitis C virus genotype 2 infection in Asian patients. Hepatology 53: 7–13.
20. Lindh M, Lagging M, Farkkila M, Langeland N, Morch K, et al. (2011) Interleukin 28B gene variation at rs12979860 determines early viral kinetics during treatment in patients carrying genotypes 2 or 3 of hepatitis C virus. J Infect Dis 203: 1748–1752.
21. Sarrazin C, Susser S, Doehring A, Lange CM, Muller T, et al. (2011) Importance of IL28B gene polymorphisms in hepatitis C virus genotype 2 and 3 infected patients. J Hepatol 54: 415–421.
22. Kawaoka T, Hayes CN, Ohishi W, Ochi H, Maekawa T, et al. (2011) Predictive value of the IL28B polymorphism on the effect of interferon therapy in chronic hepatitis C patients with genotypes 2a and 2b. J Hepatol 54: 408–414.
23. Chen JY, Lin CY, Wang CM, Lin YT, Kuo SN, et al. (2011) IL28B genetic variations are associated with high sustained virological response (SVR) of interferon-alpha plus ribavirin therapy in Taiwanese chronic HCV infection. Genes Immun 12: 300–309.
24. Hung HH, Chiou YY, Hsia CY, Su CW, Chou YH, et al. (2011) Survival rates are comparable after radiofrequency ablation or surgery in patients with small hepatocellular carcinomas. Clin Gastroenterol Hepatol 9: 79–86.
25. Pearl J (2009) Understanding propensity scores. Causality: models, reasoning, and inference, 2nd ed. Cambridge university press, Cambridge.
26. D'Agostino RB Jr (1998) Propensity score methods for bias reduction in the comparison of a treatment to a non-randomized control group. Stat Med 17: 2265–2281.
27. Lin CY, Chen JY, Lin TN, Jeng WJ, Huang CH, et al. (2011) IL28B SNP rs12979860 is a critical predictor for on-treatment and sustained virologic response in patients with hepatitis C virus genotype-1 infection. PLoS One 6: e18322.

28. Afdhal NH, McHutchison JG, Zeuzem S, Mangia A, Pawlotsky JM, et al. (2011) Hepatitis C pharmacogenetics: state of the art in 2010. Hepatology 53: 336–345.
29. Rauch A, Kutalik Z, Descombes P, Cai T, Di Iulio J, et al. (2010) Genetic variation in IL28B is associated with chronic hepatitis C and treatment failure: a genome-wide association study. Gastroenterology 138: 1338–1345, 1345 e1331–1337.
30. Rizzetto M HS, Ackrill AM (2004) Sustained virological response (SVR) to Peginterferon Alfa-2A (40KD) (PEGASYS) plus ribavirin (Copegus): comparison of outcomes in patients infected with HCV genotype 2 and 3. Hepatology 40: 252A.
31. Zeuzem S, Hultcrantz R, Bourliere M, Goeser T, Marcellin P, et al. (2004) Peginterferon alfa-2b plus ribavirin for treatment of chronic hepatitis C in previously untreated patients infected with HCV genotypes 2 or 3. J Hepatol 40: 993–999.
32. Yu ML, Dai CY, Huang JF, Chiu CF, Yang YH, et al. (2008) Rapid virological response and treatment duration for chronic hepatitis C genotype 1 patients: a randomized trial. Hepatology 47: 1884–1893.
33. Kamal SM, Ismail A, Graham CS, He Q, Rasenack JW, et al. (2004) Pegylated interferon alpha therapy in acute hepatitis C: relation to hepatitis C virus-specific T cell response kinetics. Hepatology 39: 1721–1731.

13

Relation of *IL28B* Gene Polymorphism with Biochemical and Histological Features in Hepatitis C Virus-Induced Liver Disease

José A. Agúndez[1], Elena García-Martin[2], María L. Maestro[3], Francisca Cuenca[4], Carmen Martínez[1], Luis Ortega[5], Miguel Carballo[6], Marta Vidaurreta[3], Marta Agreda[4], Gabriela Díaz-Zelaya[5], Avelina Suárez[7], Manuel Díaz-Rubio[8], José M. Ladero[8]*

1 Department of Pharmacology, University of Extremadura, Cáceres, Spain, **2** Department of Biochemistry & Molecular Biology, University of Extremadura, Cáceres, Spain, **3** Genomics Unit, Service of Clinical Biochemistry, Hospital Clínico San Carlos, Instituto de Investigación Sanitaria del Hospital Clínico San Carlos (IdISSC), Madrid, Spain, **4** Liver Unit, Service of Gastroenterology, Hospital Clínico San Carlos, Instituto de Investigación Sanitaria del Hospital Clínico San Carlos (IdISSC), Madrid, Spain, **5** Service of Pathology, Hospital Clínico San Carlos, Instituto de Investigación Sanitaria del Hospital Clínico San Carlos (IdISSC), Madrid, Spain, **6** Laboratory of Molecular Genetics, Hospital de Terrassa, Terrassa (Barcelona), Spain, **7** Service of Clinical Microbiology, Hospital Clínico San Carlos (IdISCC), Madrid, Spain, **8** Liver Unit, Service of Gastroenterology, Hospital Clínico San Carlos, Department of Medicine, Medical School, Universidad Complutense, Instituto de Investigación Sanitaria del Hospital Clínico San Carlos (IdISSC), Madrid, Spain

Abstract

Background/Aims: Polymorphism at the *IL28B* gene may modify the course of hepatitis C virus (HCV) chronic infection. Our aim was to study the influence of *IL28B* rs12979860 gene polymorphism on the biochemistry and pathology of HCV-induced disease in the clinical course from mild chronic hepatitis C to hepatocellular carcinoma.

Methods: We have determined the rs12979860 single nucleotide polymorphism (SNP) upstream *IL28B* gene in two groups of patients with HCV-induced chronic liver disease: 1) 268 patients (159 men) with biopsy-proven chronic hepatitis C, to analyse its relation with biochemical, virological and histological features; and 2) 134 patients (97 men) with HCV-related hepatocellular carcinoma. The distribution of the analysed SNP in hepatocellular carcinoma patients was compared with that found in untreated chronic hepatitis C patients. All patients were white and most were Spaniards.

Results: In multivariate analysis ALT values were higher ($P = 0.001$) and GGT values were lower ($P < 0.001$) in chronic hepatitis C patients homozygotes for the major rs12979860C allele as compared with carriers of the mutated rs12979860T allele. Steatosis was more frequent (Odds ratio = 1.764, 95% C.I. 1.053–2.955) and severe ($P = 0.026$) in carriers of the rs12979860T allele. No relation was found between the analysed SNP and METAVIR scores for necroinflammation and fibrosis, and there were no differences in the distribution of the analysed SNP between hepatocellular carcinoma and untreated chronic hepatitis C patients.

Conclusion: The *IL28B* rs12979860 polymorphism correlates with the biochemical activity and the presence and severity of liver steatosis in chronic hepatitis C.

Editor: Gulam Waris, Rosalind Franklin University of Medicine and Science, United States of America

Funding: Financial support: FIS PS09/00943, PS09/00469, and RETICS RD07/0064 from Fondo de Investigación Sanitaria, Instituto de Salud Carlos III, Spain GR10068 from Junta de Extremadura, Spain. Financed in part with FEDER funds from the European Union. The funders had no role in study design, data collection and analysis, decision to publish, or preparation of the manuscript.

Competing Interests: The authors have declared that no competing interests exist.

* E-mail: jladero.hcsc@salud.madrid.org

Introduction

The natural history of the infection with hepatitis C virus (HCV) is variable and difficult to define. Firstly, the proportion of infected patients that clear the virus in the acute phase of the infection broadly oscillates between 14% and 46% of cases [1]. Long-term follow up studies in patients with chronic hepatitis C have shown a great variability in the rate of progression of the liver disease, although after 2 or more decades many infected persons develop progressive hepatic fibrosis and cirrhosis, that is related to a high risk of suffering from hepatocellular carcinoma (HCC). There are some well-known host-related factors that are clearly associated with a more rapid and severe progression of the liver disease, as when it is acquired at an older age [2], and the metabolic syndrome complex (non-alcoholic liver steatosis, obesity and type II diabetes mellitus) [3]. Data on a more benign course in female gender are controversial [4,5]. There are some reports on host genetic factors related to the risk of acute HCV infection becoming chronic [6] and to the rate of progression in the chronic phase, as are some human leukocyte antigen class II antigens [7,8] and polymorphisms in the genes of transforming growth factor-β_1 [9] and angiotensin II [10].

A genome wide association study (GWAS) has identified a non-coding single nucleotide polymorphism (SNP), rs12979860, that resides 3 kb upstream of the *IL28B* gene, located in the long arm of chromosome 19, which encodes IFN-λ3 [11]. Two other GWAS identified a second non-coding SNP, rs8099917, located 7.5 kb upstream of the *IL28B* start codón [12,13]. Both SNPs are in partial linkage disequilibrium and are part of an *IL28B* haplotype that shows ethnic variations and is a strong determinant of response (or lack of response) to therapy for HCV chronic infection [14,15].

The mechanisms that regulate the influence of *IL28B* polymorphisms on the success rate of therapy in chronic hepatitis C remain unknown. These genetic traits are not related with levels of intrahepatic *IL28B* gene expression but the baseline expression of interferon stimulated genes (ISGs) is significantly higher in patients carrying the minor rs8099917G allele [16,17], that is in linkage disequilibrium with the minor rs12979860T allele, thus letting a narrower margin of response when HCV acutely infects the liver or when interferon-based therapy is instituted in chronically infected patients [18]. These findings may explain why the spontaneous clearance of HCV virus is more frequent in subjects with the rs12979860CC genotype [19–21] and that this genotype and the linked rs8099917TT genotype are predictors of SVR, as unanimously confirm several studies [11–13,16,22–28].

In spite of the high number of studies mentioned above, data on the influence of the *IL28B* gene polymorphism on the natural history of untreated chronic HCV infection are scarce. Abe *et al.* [29] found that Japanese patients carrying the rs8099917TT genotype had lower plasma levels of gamma glutamyl transferase (GGT) and showed more severe necro-inflammation and fibrosis scores in liver biopsies as compared to carriers of the minor G allele, but the weak ($0.01<p<0.05$) association of the histological scores with the *IL28B* polymorphism needs independent confirmation.

IL28B polymorphism-related differences in the baseline immune response to HCV infection may influence the severity of liver necro-inflammation, the main stimulus for fibrogenesis that is the hallmark of an unfavourable course of chronic hepatitis C.

The aim of this study was to investigate the distribution of the rs12979860 SNP upstream of the *IL28B* gene in a well-phenotyped population of chronically HCV-infected patients covering the whole spectrum of disease severity, from null-mild fibrosis to hepatocellular carcinoma, to elucidate whether this polymorphic trait may be related with the course of chronic HCV infection.

Materials and Methods

Starting by October 1997 we collected and stored peripheral blood for DNA extraction from all HCV-infected patients referred to our Liver Unit who gave informed consent according with the Declaration of Helsinki. The study was approved by the local ethics committee of the Hospital Clínico San Carlos, Madrid, Spain. The study design included two series of patients: 1) patients with a diagnosis of chronic hepatitis C and positive HCV viremia who were scheduled for their first liver biopsy and naïve for antiviral therapy; and 2) patients with a diagnosis of hepatocellular carcinoma (HCC) on HCV-induced liver cirrhosis in accordance with current criteria [30]. All HCC patients were considered as cirrhotic because most of them were diagnosed with liver cirrhosis before the diagnosis of CHC and the clinical study of the remaining ones was consistent with cirrhosis. Moreover, hepatocellular carcinoma is exceptional in HCV-induced non-cirrhotic chronic liver disease [1]. A blood sample was taken for standard laboratory tests and DNA extraction on the same day of the liver biopsy in patients of the group 1, and when a definite HCC diagnosis was established in patients of the group 2. Patients with HIV or active HBV infections were excluded. A database was created to include clinical and demographical data, and baseline biochemical, virological and histological results.

Ethics Statement

All patients provided informed consent according with the Declaration of Helsinki. The study was approved by the local ethics committee of the Hospital Clínico San Carlos, Madrid, Spain. This consent was verbal, after providing to patients with full explanation of the objectives and methods of the study, guarantying them absolute privacity in accordance with the Spanish legal rules, that are more strict than those in other European countries. This circumstance was communicated to the Ethics Commmittee before obtaining its authorization. In addition, the determination of the IL28B polymorphism is a routine method at the clinical laboratory of our centre since april2011.

Laboratory Methods

Quantitative analysis of HCV-RNA was performed with the Cobas Amplicor HCV Monitor version 2.0 (Roche Molecular Diagnostic). The detection range was 600 IU/mL to 8.5×10^5 IU/mL. Starting from July 2005, viral RNA was extracted automatically using Cobas AmpliPrep, and the viral load was detected using Real-Time polymerase chain reaction (PCR) using Cobas TaqMan (Roche Diagnostics) which has a detection range of between 10 IU/mL and 2×10^8 IU/mL [31]. Viral load was classified as low (<400000 IU/ml) or high (≥400000 IU/ml), according with Witthöft *et al.* [32] HCV genotypes were determined by a reverse hybridization assay (INNO-LiPA; Innogenetics). The genotypes are assigned on the basis of sequence variations in the 5′untranslated region of HCV following gene amplification using reverse transcription polymerase chain reaction (RT-PCR).

Liver biopsy specimens obtained from patients of group 1 were examined by the same pathologist. Necroinflammation grade and fibrosis stage were scored using the METAVIR system [33]. To perform some analysis, necroinflammation was classified as null-significant (0–2) versus severe (3). Fibrosis was coded as non-mild fibrosis (F0–F1) versus moderate-advanced fibrosis (F2–F4). Steatosis of the liver was evaluated according with the Brunt score [34]: absent or grade 0 (<5% of hepatocytes affected), grade 1 (5–33% of hepatocytes affected), grade 2 (33–66% of hepatocytes affected); and grade 3 (>66% of hepatocytes affected).

IL28B genotyping was carried out by means of custom TaqMan Assay (Applied Biosciences Hispania, Alcobendas, Madrid, Spain) designed to detect the rs12979860 SNP. The detection was carried out by qPCR in an Eppendorf realplex thermocycler by using fluorescent probes. The amplification conditions were as follows: After a denaturation time of 10 min at 96°C, 45 cycles of 92°C 15 sec 60°C 90 sec were carried out and fluorescence was measured at the end of every cycle and at endpoint. All samples were determined by triplicate and genotypes were assigned both, by the gene identification software (RealPlex 2.0, Eppendorf) and by analysis of the reference cycle number for each fluorescence curve, calculated by the use of CalQPlex algorithm (Eppendorf). For technical validation purposes, the amplified fragments for twenty individuals carrying the rs12979860 C/C and C/T genotypes and eleven individuals with the T/T genotype were sequenced, and in all cases the genotypes fully corresponded with those detected with fluorescent probes.

Statistical Analysis

Continuous variables, expressed as mean (SD), were compared with the Student' *t* test or the Mann-Whitney *U* test, each when adequate, depending on their Gaussian distribution. A p value <0.05 was considered significant. Categorical variables were compared with the χ^2 or the Fisher exact tests, each when appropriate, and the effect of differences was established by calculating the odds ratio with the 95% confidence interval.

The variables different at a p value <0.05 in the univariate analysis were included in a multivariate analysis based on a logistic regression model to identify which ones were independently related to the determined SNP in the vicinity of the *IL28B* gene.

Results

Group 1 (Chronic Hepatitis C)

Two hundred and sixty eight patients were included. Patient profiles are shown in Table 1. Most patients were men (59.3%). All patients were Caucasian, mostly Spaniards. One hundred and seven (39.9%) carried the rs12979860CC homozygous genotype, whereas the remaining 161 were homo- (33 patients, 12.3%) or heterozygotes (128 patients, 47.8%) for the T allele. The studied polymorphism was in Hardy-Weinberg equilibrium.

Biochemical baseline data that showed differences at a p value <0.05 when comparing carriers of the rs12979860CC genotype with carriers of the rs12979860CT/TT genotypes were ALT (0.012), AST/ALT ratio (p = 0.002), GGT (p<0.001), and serum cholesterol (p = 0.022). In the multivariate analysis only lower values for GGT (p<0.001) and higher values for ALT (p = 0.001) were related with the 12979860CC genotype. (Table 1)

Necroinflammatory grade and fibrosis stage were not related with the rs12979860 genotype. (Table 2).

Liver steatosis was present in a greater percentage of carriers of the T allele than in CC homozygotes (44.0% *vs.* 30.8%, Odds ratio = 1.764, 95% C.I. = 1.053–2.955) and there was a significant trend towards higher grades of steatosis in carriers of the T allele (Chi^2 for trend = 4.946, *P* = 0.026). (Table 2). When the analysis was restricted to patients infected by HCV genotype 1, similar results were obtained (45.1% *vs.* 32.9%, Odds ratio = 1.618, 95% C.I. = 0.925–2.834, and Chi^2 for trend = 3.934, *P* = 0.047).

METAVIR necroinflammatory grade was significantly correlated at a *P*<0.001 for Spearman's *rho* test with serum ALT (alanine amino transferase) and GGT values, but not with the remaining biochemical variables included in the analysis. METAVIR fibrosis stage correlated at the same level of significance with the inverse of platelet count and with serum AST (aspartate amino transferase), ALT, GGT and ferritin values.

Group 2 (HCV-related Hepatocellular Carcinoma)

One hundred and thirty four patients (97 males, mean age at diagnosis 67.4 years, SD 9.4, range 41–88) were included in this group. All were white Spaniards. The diagnosis of HCC was based on the pathological exam of surgical biopsy or cytological aspirate in 73 patients, and according with current imaging criteria [30] in the remaining 61. All patients in this group had detectable titers of anti-HCV antibodies in serum. Only two patients had been previously treated with interferon-ribavirin before developing HCC.

Fifty two patients (38.8%) carried the rs12979860CC homozygous genotype, whereas the remaining 82 were homo- (16 patients, 11.9%) or heterozygotes (66 patients, 49.3%) for the T allele. (Table 3).

Former ethanol use ≥ 40 g/day was reported by 52 patients (50 men). The distribution of the analyzed SNP was very similar as comparing these patients with moderate drinkers or teetotallers (*P*>0.80 for each comparison, data not shown).

Table 1. Analysis of biochemical and virological parameters in relation with the rs12979860 genotype in 268 patients with chronic hepatitis C.

Parameter	All patients (268 cases)	CC genotype (107 cases)	T allele carriers (161 cases)	*P* (univariate)	*P* (multivariate)
Age (yrs.)	47.2 (10.5)	45.9 (10.4)	48.3 (10.5)	0.076	
Gender (M/F)	159/109	66/41	93/68	OR = 1.177 95% C.I. = 0.714–.940	
Viral load ≤/>400.000 IU/mL/n.a.	48/213/7	20/83/4	28/130/3	OR = 1.118 95% C.I. = 0.592–2.114	
Viral genotype 1/non 1/n.a.	225/40/3	84/20/3	141/20/0	OR = 0.596 95% C.I. = 0.303–1.171	
Hb (g/dL)	15.1 (1.4)	15.0 (1.4)	15.2 (1.4)	0.399	
Platelets (10^9/L)	202 (59)	202 (57)	203 (61)	0.830	
Bilirubin (mg/dL)	0.83 (0.45)	0.78 (0.36)	0.87 (0.50)	0.135	
AST (IU)	67 (48)	71 (47)	64 (48)	0.224	
ALT (IU)	112 (94)	130 (103)	99 (85)	**0.012**	**0.001**
AST/ALT	0.69 (0.28)	0.64 (0.24)	0.73 (0.30)	**0.002**	0.593
GGT (IU)	79 (118)	47 (42)	100 (146)	**<0.001**	**<0.001**
Alkaline phosphatase (IU)	111 (59)	111 (54)	111 (62)	0.986	
Cholesterol (mg/dL)	178 (36)	184 (40)	173 (31)	**0.022**	0.102

Major allele: C. Minor allele: T.
n.a.: not available.

Table 2. Analysis of histological features in relation with the rs12979860 genotype in 268 patients with chronic hepatitis C.

Feature	CC genotype (107 cases)	T allele carriers (161 cases)	Statistics CC *vs.* T carriers	CT genotype (128 cases)	TT genotype (33 cases)	Statistics CT *vs.* TT
METAVIR necroinflammatory grade (0/1/2/3)	1/16/40/50	3/30/68/60	Chi $^{2\ LT}$ = 2.409 (P = 0.121)	2/21/57/48	1/9/11/12	Chi $^{2\ LT}$ = 0.952 (P = 0.329)
METAVIR fibrosis stage (0/1/2/3/4)	21/33/17/28/8	28/56/27/35/15	Chi $^{2\ LT}$ = 0.0002 (P = 0.989)	20/46/22/27/13	8/10/5/8/2	Chi $^{2\ LT}$ = 0.466 (P = 0.495)
Steatosis (Brunt score 0/1/2/3/n.a.)	74/27/6/0/0	89/56/10/4/2	Chi $^{2\ LT}$ = 4.946 (P = 0.026)	71/43/9/4/1	14/13/1/0/1	Chi $^{2\ LT}$ = 0.066 (P = 0.798)
Steatosis (Brunt score) 0/>0/n.a.	74/33/0	89/70/2	O.R. = 1.764 95% C.I. = 1.053–2.955	71/56/1	14/14/1	O.R. = 1.268 95% C.I. = 0.559–2.877

Major allele: C. Minor allele: T.
n.a. = not available.
Chi^{2LT}: Chi square for linear trend.

Comparative Analysis of HCV-infected Patients with and without HCC

To evaluate the possible relation between the analyzed *IL28B* SNP and the stage of the HCV-induced liver disease, the CHC patients in the chronic hepatitis group who had not received antiviral therapy after performing the liver biopsy were compared with the group of patients with hepatocellular carcinoma. No significant differences were found between both groups in the distribution of the studied *IL28B* gene SNP (Table 3).

Discussion

The relation between genetic polymorphisms in the vicinity of the *IL28* gene and the response to pegylated interferon and ribavirin combined therapy for hepatitis C has been clearly demonstrated since the rs12979860 SNP was identified. Several GWAS studies independently disclosed that the possession of any of the homozygous genotypes rs12979860CC or rs8099917TT, which are in strong linkage disequilibrium, greatly increases the probability to obtain sustained viral response after antiviral treatment. [11–13,16,22–28].

However, information on the possible influence of these polymorphisms on the course of hepatitis C infection is presently very limited and incomplete. It has been shown that the carriers of the favourable genotypes have a higher rate of spontaneous clearance of HCV during the acute phase of the infection [19–21]. In this study we have shown that GGT levels are lower in patients with chronic hepatitis C that carry the rs12979860CC genotype than in homo- or heterozygotes for the T mutated allele. Abe *et al.* [29], in a cohort of 364 adult Japanese patients with chronic HCV infection, reported a similar and highly significant ($p = 0.001$) association between the rs8099917TT genotype and GGT lower values, a link that could be explained because both traits are predictive of a favourable response to therapy.

Table 3. Distribution of the *IL28B* gene rs12979860 genotype in untreated patients with chronic hepatitis C (CHC) and in patients with HCV-related hepatocellular carcinoma (HCC).

IL28B genotype	Group		Statistics
	CHC 98 patients (%)	HCC 134 patients (%)	
CC	37 (37.8)	52 (38.8)	
CT	49 (50.0)	66 (49.3)	$\chi^2 = 0.041$
TT	11 (11.2)	16 (11.9)	$P = 0.979$
T allele frequency	0.386	0.366	O.R. = 0.985 95% C.I. = 0.672–1.445

In addition, we have found that rs12979860CC genotype is associated with higher serum ALT than the remaining genotypes, a finding that is in agreement with data of Thompson *et al.* [35] obtained from a GWAS study that disclosed that only the rs12979860 SNP was significantly associated with baseline ALT levels. Serum ALT is considered as a marker of necroinflammatory activity in the liver as confirms the analysis of our data that shows a linear increase of ALT levels related to METAVIR activity score. These findings are contradictory with those reported by Abe *et al.* [29] who found that ALT and AST levels were lower in carrier of the rs8099917TT genotype, although these authors do not provide the level of significance for this association.

However, our results do not confirm the suggested relation between the *IL28B* gene polymorphism and the histological necroinflammatory activity reported by Abe *et al.* [29] and Thompson *et al.* [35]. Most patients included in the present study were infected with HCV genotype 1. Hence, we have not been able to confirm the interesting results reported by Bochud et al. [36] linking the rs8099917G allele, that is associated with poor response to therapy, with lower necroinflammatory activity ($p = 0.04$) and milder fibrosis ($p = 0.02$) in patients infected with non-1 HCV genotypes.

The relation between *IL28B* polymorphism and the stage of fibrosis is controversial. Abe *et al.* [29] found higher fibrosis METAVIR scores among carriers of the rs8099917TT genotype. However, Di Marco et al. [37] in a group of 131 patients with thalassemia major and chronic HCV infection who underwent a liver biopsy reported that older age and the carrier state of the minor alleles at rs12979860 and rs8099917 sites were associated with more severe liver fibrosis ($p < 0.001$ and $p < 0.005$, respectively). Falleti et al. [38] in a group of 629 HCV-positive patients, disclosed that subjects with the rs12979860TT homozygous genotype had a mean fibrosis score higher than the remaining CC or CT genotypes ($p < 0.05$). Nevertheless, Thompson *et al.* [39] reported that the rs12979860 polymorphism was not associated with advanced hepatic fibrosis in CHC, a finding that is in agreement with our results that are far from the statistical significance for the determined SNP.

Fabris *et al.* [40] analysed the distribution of rs12979860 C and T alleles in a miscellaneous group of Italian patients with chronic liver diseases, most HCV-related, including patients with mild hepatitis (Ishak staging score ≤ 2), cirrhosis and HCC. They concluded that the T allele is more prevalent in HCV-induced cirrhosis than in cirrhosis from other causes ($p<0.005$) but not when comparing HCV-induced cirrhosis with milder hepatitis C ($p = 0.09$).

Hepatic steatosis is a frequent finding in chronic hepatitis C, as a probable consequence of a disturbance of lipid metabolism [41]. Our study shows that steatosis is significantly more frequent in CHC patients carrying the mutated T allele, in agreement with two previous studies. Tillmann et al [42] analysed two independent cohorts of patients with a global size of 325 patients with chronic hepatitis C; steatosis was present in 28 of 88 rs12979860CC genotype patients (31.8%) and in 139 of 237 patients carrying the rs12979860T allele (58.6%). These differences were highly significant when each group was analysed separately (as did the authors) or when considering them as a unique group (Odds ratio = 3.04, 95% C.I. = 1.81–5.10). In the second study [43] that included 153 Japanese patients, the analysis of the rs8099917 genotype yielded similar results. A new aspect disclosed in our study is that steatosis is not only more frequent, but also more severe in patients carrying the mutated T allele.

Hepatocellular carcinoma (CHC) represents the most advanced step in the natural course of chronic hepatitis C infection that fortunately is reached only by a minority of patients. If the hypothesis of the existence of any relationship between the *IL28B* genetic polymorphism and the severity of HCV-induced liver disease holds true, the most logical finding should be the existence of differences in the genotype frequencies among the different stages of the disease. We have found no differences in the frequencies of the *IL28B* genotypes as comparing a group of HCV-induced HCC patients with a group of 98 untreated patients with CHC. Our results are coincidental with those reported by other groups, both in Caucasian [36] and in Japanese [44,45] populations. However, Asahina *et al.* [46] reported that carriers of the rs8099917 TT genotype had a higher rate of sustained viral response to interferon-based therapy (as expected) and that this genotype was associated with a lower incidence of HCC, both in sustained viral responders and in non-responders. A direct effect of the *IL28B* polymorphism on the risk of HCC may not be inferred from these results, as SVR clearly improves the natural course of chronic HCV infection [47,48] and, among non-responders, the effect of the *IL28B* polymorphism was indirect and associated with slightly lower levels of ALT and alpha-feto protein. Eurich et al. [49], in a study of patients who received a liver graft due to severe HCV-induced liver disease, found that the 12979860TT genotype was more frequent in the 61 patients with HCC on the explanted liver than in the 106 patients without HCC ($p = 0.041$), suggesting that the major C allele plays a protective role against the development of HCC. In addition, Ren *et al.* [50] found that the rs12979860 T allele was related to the susceptibility of both chronic hepatitis B virus (HBV) infection and HBV-related HCC in a group of Chinese patients. Thus, controversy remains about the possible relation between the *IL28B* gene polymorphism and the risk of developing HCC.

We conclude that the *IL28B* rs12979860CC genotype in patients with chronic hepatitis C is related with higher serum ALT, that is considered as a marker of hepatic necroinflammation, and with lower values of GGT, which increase is a surrogate marker of liver fibrosis and a negative predictive factor of response to therapy [51]. In addition, the carrier state of the rs12979860 T allele is associated with greater frequency and severity of hepatic steatosis in chronic hepatitis C. However, we have not found any relation among this polymorphism and necroinflammatory grade and fibrosis stage directly shown by the liver biopsy, neither with the risk of developing HCV-related hepatocellular carcinoma.

Acknowledgments

We thank Ms. Gara Esguevillas, Ms. Isabel Salas and Ms. Debbie Benn for their technical assistance.

Author Contributions

Conceived and designed the experiments: JML JAA. Performed the experiments: EG-M MLM CM MC MV. Analyzed the data: JML. Contributed reagents/materials/analysis tools: FC LO MA AS GD-Z MD-R. Wrote the paper: JML JAA.

References

1. Seeff LB (2002) Natural history of chronic hepatitis C. Hepatology 36: S35–S46. [PMID: 12407575].
2. Chen SL, Morgan TR (2006) The natural history of hepatitis C virus (HCV) infection. Int J Med Sci 3: 47–52. [PMID: 16614742].
3. Seeff LB (2009) The history of the "natural history" of hepatitis C (1968–2009) Liver Int 29 Suppl 1: 89–99. [PMID: 19207971].
4. Bissell DM (1999) Sex and hepatic fibrosis. Hepatology 29: 988–989. [PMID: 10551508].
5. Williams MJ, Lang-Lenton M, Trent HCV study group (2011) Progression of initially mild hepatic fibrosis in patients with chronic hepatitis C infection. J Viral Hepat 18: 17–22. [PMID: 20088889].
6. Martínez C, García-Martín E, Ladero JM, Herráez O, Ortega L, et al. (2007) GSTT1 and GSTM1 null genotypes may facilitate hepatitis C virus infection becoming chronic. J Infect Dis 195: 1320–1323. [PMID: 17397002].
7. Minton EJ, Smillie D, Neil KR, Irving WL, Underwood JC, et al. (1998) Association between MHC class II alleles and clearance of circulating hepatitis C virus. J Infect Dis 178: 39–44.[PMID: 9652421].
8. Singh R, Kaul R, Kaul A, Khan K (2007) A comparative review of HLA associations with hepatitis B and C viral infections across global populations. World J Gastroenterol 13: 1770–1787. [PMID: 17465466].
9. Wang H, Mengsteab S, Tag CG, Gao CF, Hellerbrand C, et al. (2005) Transforming growth factor-beta1 gene polymorphisms are associated with progression of liver fibrosis in Caucasians with chronic hepatitis C infection. World J Gastroenterol 11: 1929–1936. [PMID: 15800982].
10. Kunzler S, Baumann M, Schirmacher F, Dries V, Bayer E, et al. (2001) Prediction of progressive liver fibrosis in hepatitis C infection by serum and tissue levels of transforming growth factor-β. J Virol 8: 430–437. [PMID: 11703574].
11. Ge D, Fellay J, Thompson AJ, Simon JS, Shianna KV, et al. (2009) Genetic variation in IL28B predicts hepatitis C treatment-induced viral clearance. Nature 461: 399–401. [PMID: 19684573].
12. Suppiah V, Moldovan M, Ahlenstiel G, Berg T, Weltman M, et al. (2009) IL28B is associated with response to chronic hepatitis C interferon-α and ribavirin therapy. Nature Genetics 41: 1100–1104. [PMID: 19749758].
13. Tanaka Y, Nishida N, Sugiyama M, Kurosaki M, Matsuura K, et al. (2009) Genome-wide association of IL28B with response to pegylated interferon-α and ribavirin therapy for chronic hepatitis C. Nature Genetics 41: 1105–1109. [PMID: 19749757].
14. Balagopal A, Thomas DL, Thio CL (2010) IL28B and the control of hepatitis C virus infection. Gastroenterology 139: 1865–1876. [PMID: 20950615].
15. Afdhal NH, McHutchison JG, Zeuzem S, Mangia A, Pawlotsky JM, et al. (2010) Hepatitis C pharmacogenetics: State of the art in 2010. Hepatology 53: 336–345. [PMID: 21254181].
16. Honda M, Sakai A, Yamashita T, Nakamoto Y, Mizukoshi E, et al. (2010) Hokuriku Liver Study Group. Hepatic ISG expression is associated with genetic variation in interleukin 28B and the outcome of IFN therapy for chronic hepatitis C. Gastroenterology 139: 499–509. [PMID: 20434452].
17. Urban TJ, Thompson AJ, Bradrick SS, Fellay J, Schuppan D, et al. (2010) IL28B genotype is associated with differential expression of intrahepatic interferon-stimulated genes in patients with chronic hepatitis C. Hepatology 52: 1888–1896. [PMID: 20931559].
18. Ahlenstiel G, Booth DR, George J (2010) IL28B in hepatitis C virus infection: translating pharmacogenomics into clinical practice. J Gastroenterol 45: 903–910. [PMID: 20635099].

19. Thomas DL, Thio CL, Martin MP, Qi Y, Ge D, et al. (2009) Genetic variation on IL28B and spontaneous clearance of hepatitis C virus. Nature 461: 798–801. [PMID: 19759533].
20. Montes-Cano MA, García-Lozano JR, Abad-Molina C, Romero-Gómez M, Barroso N, et al. (2010) Interleukin-28B genetic variants and hepatitis virus infection by different viral genotypes. Hepatology 52: 33–37. [PMID: 20578254].
21. Tillmann HL, Thompson AJ, Patel K, Wiese M, Tenckhoff H, et al. (2010) German Anti-D Study Group. A polymorphism near IL28B is associated with spontaneous clearance of acute hepatitis C virus and jaundice. Gastroenterology 189: 1586–1592. [PMID: 20637200].
22. McCarthy JJ, Li JH, Thompson A, Suchindran S, Lao XQ, et al. (2010) Replicated association between IL28B gene variant and a sustained response to pegylated interferon and ribavirin. Gastroenterology; 138: 2307–2314. [PMID: 20176026].
23. Thompson AJ, Muir AJ, Sulkowski MS, Ge D, Fellay J, et al. (2010) Interleukin-28B polymorphism improves viral kinetics and is the strongest pre-treatment predictor of sustained virologic response in genotype 1 hepatitis C virus. Gastroenterology 139: 120–129. [PMID: 20399780].
24. Stättermayer AF, Stauber R, Hofer H, Rutter K, Beinhardt S, et al. (2011) Impact of IL28B genotype on the early and sustained virologic response in treatment-naïve patients with chronic hepatitis C. Clin Gastroenterol Hepatol 9: 344–350. [PMID: 20728570].
25. Hayes CN, Kobayashi M, Akuta N, Suzuki F, Kumada H, et al. (2011) HCV substitutions and IL28B polymorphisms on outcome of peg-interferon plus ribavirin combination therapy. GUT 60: 261–267. [PMID: 21068134].
26. Rauch A, Kutalik Z, Descombes P, Cai T, Di Iulio J, et al. (2010) Swiss Hepatitis C Cohort Study; Swiss HIV Cohort Study. Genetic variation in IL28B is associated with chronic hepatitis C and treatment failure: a genome-wide association study. Gastroenterology 138: 1338–1345. [PMID: 20060832].
27. Kurosaki M, Tanaka Y, Nishida N, Sakamoto N, Enomoto N, et al. (2011) Pre-treatment prediction of response to pegylated-interferon plus ribavirin for chronic hepatitis C using genetic polymorphism in IL28B and viral factors. J Hepatol 54: 439–448. [PMID: 21129805].
28. Ladero JM, García-Martín E, Fernández C, Carballo M, Devesa MJ, et al. (2012) Predicting response to therapy in chronic hepatitis C: An approach combining interleukin-28B gene polymorphisms and clinical data. J Gastroenterol Hepatol 27: 279–285. [PMID: 21722179].
29. Abe H, Ochi H, Maekawa T, Hayes CN, Tsuge M, et al. (2010) Common variation of IL28 affects gamma-GTP levels and inflammation of the liver in chronically infected hepatitis C virus patients. J Hepatol 53: 439–443. [PMID: 21145800].
30. Lencioni R (2011) Evolving strategies in the diagnosis of hepatocellular carcinoma. J Hepatol 54: 184–186. [PMID: 20950887].
31. Heid CA, Stevens J, Livak KJ, Williams PM (1996) Real time quantitative PCR. Genome Res 6: 989–994. [PMID: 8908518].
32. Witthöft TH, Möller B, Wiedmann KH, Mauss S, Link R, et al. (2007) Safety, tolerability and efficacy of peginterferon alpha-2a and ribavirin in chronic hepatitis C in clinical practice: The German Open Safety Trial. J Viral Hepat 14: 788–796. [PMID: 17927615].
33. The French METAVIR Cooperative Study Group (1994) Intraobserver and interobserver variations in liver biopsy interpretation in patients with chronic hepatitis C. Hepatology 20: 15–20. [PMID: 8020885].
34. Brunt E, Janney C, Di Bisceglie A, Neuschwander-Tetri B, Bacon B (1999) Nonalcoholic steatohepatitis: a proposal for grading and staging the histological lesions. Am J Gastroenterol 94: 2467–2474.[PMID: 10484010].
35. Thompson AJ, Clark PJ, Zhu M, Zhu Q, Ge D, et al. (2010) Genome wide-association study identifies IL28B polymorphism to be associated with baseline ALT and hepatic necro-inflammatory activity in chronic hepatitis C patients enrolled in the IDEAL study. Hepatology 52 (Suppl). pp 1220A–1221A.
36. Bochud P-Y, Bibert S, Kutalik Z, Patin E, Guergnon J, et al. (2012) IL28B alleles associated with poor hepatitis C virus (HCV) clearance protect against inflammation and fibrosis in patients infected with non-1 HCV genotypes. Hepatology 55: 384–94. [PMID: 22180014].
37. Di Marco V, Bronte F, Calvaruso V, Capra M, Borsellino Z, et al. (2011) IL28B polymorphisms influence stage of liver fibrosis and spontaneous or interferon-induced viral clearance in thamassemia patients with hepatitis C virus infection. Haematologica [Epub ahead of print] [PMID: 22180419].
38. Falleti E, Bitetto D, Fabris C, Cussigh A, Fornasiere E, et al. (2011) Role of interleukin 28B rs12979860 C/T polymorphism on the histological outcome of chronic hepatitis C: relationship with gender and viral genotype. J Clin Immunol 31: 891–899. [PMID: 21747799].
39. Thompson AJ, Clark PJ, Fellay J, Muir AJ, Tillmann HL, et al. (2010) IL28B genotype is not associated with advanced hepatic fibrosis in chronic hepatitis C patients enrolled in the IDEAL study. Hepatology 52 (Suppl). pp 437A–438A.
40. Fabris C, Falleti E, Cussigh A, Bitetto D, Fontanini E, et al. (2011) IL-28B re12979060 C/T allele distribution in patients with liver cirrhosis: Role in the course of chronic viral hepatitis and the development of HCC. J Hepatol 54: 716–722. [PMID: 21146242].
41. Li JH, Lao XQ, Tillmann HL, Rowell J, Patel K, et al. (2010) Interferon-lambda genotype and low serum low-density lipoprotein cholesterol levels in patients with chronic hepatitis C infection. Hepatology 51: 1904–1911. [PMID: 20235331].
42. Tillmann HL, Patel K, Muir AJ, Guy CD, Li JH, et al. (2011) Beneficial IL28B genotype associated with lower frequency of hepatic steatosis in patients with chronic hepatitis C. J Hepatol 55: 1195–2000. [PMID: 21703198].
43. Ohnishi M, Tsuge M, Kohno T, Zhang Y, Abe H, et al. (2012) IL28B polymorphism is associated with fatty change in the liver of chronic hepatitis C patients. J Gastroenterol [Epub ahead of print].[PMID: 22350701].
44. Miura M, Maekawa S, Kadokura M, Sueki R, Komase K, et al. (2011) Analysis of viral amino acids sequences and the IL28B SNP influencing the development of hepatocellular carcinoma in chronic hepatitis C. Hepatol Int [Epub ahead of print]. [PMID: 22022823].
45. Joshita S, Umemura T, Katsuyama Y, Ichikawa Y, Kimura T, et al. (2011) Association of IL28B gene polymorphism with development of hepatocellular carcinoma in Japanese patients with chronic hepatitis C virus infection. Hum Immunol 73; 298–300. [PMID 22245236].
46. Asahina Y, Tanaka K, Suzuki Y, Tamaki N, Hoshioka T, et al. (2011) Association between IL28B gene variation and development of hepatocellular carcinoma after interferon therapy in patients with chronic hepatitis C. J Hepatol 54 (Suppl 1): S37.
47. Trapero-Marugán M, Mendoza J, Chaparro M, González-Moreno L, Moreno-Monteagudo JA, et al. (2011) Long-term outcome of chronic hepatitis C patients with sustained virological response to interferon plus ribavirin. World J Gastroenterol 17: 493–498. [PMID: 21274379].
48. Maruoca D, Imazeki F, Arai M, Kanda T, Fujiwara K, et al. (2012) Long-term cohort study of chronic hepatitis C according to interferon efficacy. J Gastroentrol Hepatol 27: 291–299. [PMID: 21793911].
49. Eurich D, Boas-Knoop S, Bahra M, Neuhaus R, Somasundaram R, et al. (2012) Role of IL28B polymorphism in the development of hepatitis C virus-induced hepatocelular carcinoma, graft fibrosis, and posttransplant activiral therapy. Transplantation 93: 644–649 [PMID: 22411462].
50. Ren S, Lu J, Du X, Huang Y, Ma L, et al. (2012) Genetic variation in IL28B is associated with the development of hepatitis B-related hepatocellular carcinoma. Cancer Immunol Immunother [Epub ahead of print]. [PMID: 22310928].
51. Cuenca F, Fernández C, Devesa MJ, López-Alonso G, Mayol J, et al. (2010) Predictive baseline criteria of primary therapeutic failure in chronic hepatitis C genotype 1. Rev Esp Enferm Dig 102: 234–238. [PMID 20486745].

14

Micro-RNA Profiling in Human Serum Reveals Compartment-Specific Roles of miR-571 and miR-652 in Liver Cirrhosis

Christoph Roderburg[1], Tobias Mollnow[1], Brenda Bongaerts[2], Natalia Elfimova[3], David Vargas Cardenas[1], Katharina Berger[1], Henning Zimmermann[1], Alexander Koch[1], Mihael Vucur[1], Mark Luedde[4], Claus Hellerbrand[5], Margarete Odenthal[3], Christian Trautwein[1], Frank Tacke[1], Tom Luedde[1]*

1 Department of Medicine III, University Hospital RWTH Aachen, Aachen, Germany, **2** Department of Pathology, Maastricht University Medical Center, Maastricht, The Netherlands, **3** Institute for Pathology, University Hospital Cologne, Cologne, Germany, **4** Department of Cardiology and Angiology, University of Kiel, Kiel, Germany, **5** Department of Internal Medicine I, University of Regensburg, Regensburg, Germany

Abstract

Background and Aims: Micro-RNAs (miRNAs) have recently emerged as crucial modulators of molecular processes involved in chronic liver diseases. The few miRNAs with previously proposed roles in liver cirrhosis were identified in screening approaches on liver parenchyma, mostly in rodent models. Therefore, in the present study we performed a systematic screening approach in order to identify miRNAs with altered levels in the serum of patients with chronic liver disease and liver cirrhosis.

Methods: We performed a systematic, array-based miRNA expression analysis on serum samples from patients with liver cirrhosis. In functional experiments we evaluated the relationship between alterations of miRNA serum levels and their role in distinct cellular compartments involved in hepatic cirrhosis.

Results: The array analysis and the subsequent confirmation by qPCR in a larger patient cohort identified significant alterations in serum levels of miR-513-3p, miR-571 and miR-652, three previously uncharacterized miRNAs, in patients with alcoholic or hepatitis C induced liver cirrhosis. Of these, miR-571 serum levels closely correlated with disease stages, thus revealing potential as a novel biomarker for hepatic cirrhosis. Further analysis revealed that up-regulation of miR-571 in serum reflected a concordant regulation in cirrhotic liver tissue. In isolated primary human liver cells, miR-571 was up-regulated in human hepatocytes and hepatic stellate cells in response to the pro-fibrogenic cytokine TGF-β. In contrast, alterations in serum levels of miR-652 were stage-independent, reflecting a concordant down-regulation of this miRNA in circulating monocytes of patients with liver cirrhosis, which was inducible by proinflammatory stimuli like bacterial lipopolysaccharide.

Conclusion: Alterations of miR571 and miR-652 serum levels in patients with chronic liver disease reflect their putative roles in the mediation of fibrogenic and inflammatory processes in distinct cellular compartments involved in the pathogenesis of liver cirrhosis.

Editor: Robert Lafrenie, Sudbury Regional Hospital, Canada

Funding: This work was supported by the German Research Foundation (SFB-TRR57 P06 and P09, Ta434/2-1), a starting grant of the European Research Council within the FP 7 (ERC-2007-Stg/208237-Luedde-Med3-Aachen), the Interdisciplinary Centre for Clinical Research (IZKF) "BIOMAT" and a grant from the START-program of the medical faculty Aachen to C.R. The funders had no role in study design, data collection and analysis, decision to publish, or preparation of the manuscript.

Competing Interests: The authors have declared that no competing interests exist.

* E-mail: tluedde@ukaachen.de

Introduction

Many chronic liver diseases are still not sufficiently treatable and often progress to liver cirrhosis representing the major risk factor for the development of hepatocellular carcinoma (HCC) [1]. Despite recent advances e.g. in the treatment of viral hepatitis, pharmacological strategies to prevent fibrogenesis, to facilitate the reversal of fibrosis/cirrhosis or to prevent the complications of advanced hepatic cirrhosis are still limited [2], underlining the need to establish a better understanding of the molecular mechanisms underlying the pathogenesis of hepatic cirrhosis.

Micro-RNAs (miRNAs) are small, non-coding, 21–23 nucleotide long RNAs that negatively regulate gene expression by base pairing with the 3′-untranslated region (UTR) of their target mRNAs [3]. miRNAs are involved in highly regulated processes such as cell injury, proliferation or carcinogenesis [4,5]. In the liver, previous studies have shown that miRNAs play a fundamental role in acute liver injury, viral hepatitis or hepatocarcinogenesis [6,7,8,9]. In addition, systematic array approaches on liver tissue from mice and primary hepatic stellate cells (HSCs) recently revealed important functional roles of certain miRNAs in hepatic fibrogenesis. As such, it was shown that members of the miR-29 family integrate pro-fibrogenic and pro-inflammatory signals in hepatic stellate cells and control expression of various extracellular matrix genes during hepatic fibrogenesis [10,11,12]. Since miRNAs control networks of target genes and are thus promising therapeutic targets, such findings are of high potential for the establishment of miRNA-based antifibrotic therapies, which have already been tested in other organs like the heart [13].

Previous studies on the role of miRNAs in chronic liver disease have focused on certain miRNAs identified in screening approaches on rodent liver samples or hepatic stellate cell cultures [10,11,12,14]. However, some members of the broad spectrum of human miRNAs are not yet established in rodent array systems. Moreover, chronic liver disease and liver cirrhosis represent systemic diseases with regulatory processes not only occurring in the liver but also in other cellular compartments like immune cells [15]. Therefore, alternative experimental approaches are needed, which employ primary human specimen and acknowledge chronic liver disease as a systemic disorder influenced by distinct cellular compartments.

It has recently become evident that certain disease conditions are associated with alterations in serum levels of miRNAs [16]. Despite the potential of these findings for the establishment of novel biomarkers, serum-level alterations of miRNAs might reflect important regulatory processes occurring in distinct cellular compartments involved in disease pathogenesis. In line with this hypothesis, we recently demonstrated that the functional role of miR-29 in liver fibrosis correlated with a significant decrease of miR-29 serum levels [10]. Therefore, in the present study we performed a comprehensive, unbiased array approach on serum samples from patients and healthy controls in order to identify novel miRNAs that play a role in chronic liver disease and liver cirrhosis.

Materials and Methods

Patients and controls

The study protocol was approved by the local ethics committee (ethics committee of University Hospital Aachen, RWTH Aachen), and written informed consent was obtained from each patient. The study was conducted according to the principles expressed in the Declaration of Helsinki.

We studied 67 patients with chronic liver diseases [15]. Characteristics of the study cohort are summarized in table 1. Importantly, patients were excluded in case of systemic inflammatory response syndrome (SIRS) or sepsis, HIV-infection, systemic steroid medication (prednisolone >7.5 mg/d or equivalent doses) and malignant tumor(s) except for hepatocellular carcinoma. As a control group, 17 matched healthy volunteers were recruited from the local blood transfusion institute that had normal aminotransferase activities, no history of liver disease or alcohol abuse and were tested negative for HBV, HCV and HIV infections.

All blood samples were taken by one physician, and strictly the same protocol was applied to all samples (centrifugation time, materials, etc.). Furthermore a "needle to freezer time" of less than 30 min was defined for all samples. All samples were handled at 4°C until storing them for final analysis at −80°C. RNA extraction and cDNA transcription was performed simultaneously for all samples.

For tissue-specific miRNA-regulation analysis, samples were taken from explanted cirrhotic livers (n = 13) from patients that underwent liver transplantation with different disease etiologies (Data S1) [15]. As controls, liver tissues were obtained from patients undergoing partial liver resection for hepatic metastases of colorectal cancer. Only liver tissues judged as non-cancerous by local pathologists and without histological evidence for both liver fibrosis and inflammation were used to serve as control tissue [15].

miRNA isolation from serum

Total RNA, including miRNA, was extracted from serum samples using Phenol-Chloroform extraction as previously described [10,11,12]. In short, 400 µl serum was spiked with 20 nM miScript miRNA mimic SV40 (Qiagen) for sample normalization according to references [6,17,18,19,20] (Figure S1). 800 µl Phenol (Qiazol, Qiagen, Hilden; Germany) and 200 µl Chloroform were added to the sample and mixed vigorously for 15 sec followed by incubation at room temperature for 10 min. Samples were centrifuged for 15 min at 12,000 g until complete phase separation. The aqueous phase, containing total RNA, was

Table 1. Clinical data of patients with liver cirrhosis.

				Child-Pugh stages of liver cirrhosis		
	Controls	**All patients**	**no cirrhosis**	**Child A**	**Child B**	**Child C**
[n(%)]	17	67	6 (9%)	25 (37.3%)	10 (14.9%)	26 (38.8%)
Gender (m/f) [n(%)]	12/5	43/24	2/4	16/9	6/4	19/7
Age (years)	46 (23–68)	58 (29–82)	39 (29–56)	62 (37–82)	57 (40–77)	55 (38–81)
Etiology [n(%)]						
Viral Hepatitis		18 (26.9%)	2 (33.3%)	9 (36%)	5 (50%)	2 (7.7%)
Biliary		5 (7.5%)	0 (0%)	2 (8%)	2 (20%)	1 (3.8%)
Alcohol		43 (64.2%)	4 (66.7%)	13 (52%)	3 (30%)	23 (88.5%)
Cryptogenic		1 (1.5%)	0 (0%)	1 (4%)	0 (0%)	0 (0%)
Complications [n(%)]						
Ascites		28 (41.8%)	1 (1.6%)	4 (16%)	6 (60%)	17 (65.4%)
Esophageal varices		35 (52.2%)	0 (0%)	10 (40%)	6 (60%)	19 (73.1%)
Encephalopathy		10 (14.9%)	0 (0%)	0 (0%)	1 (10%)	9 (34.6%)

precipitated with 500 µl 100% Isopropanol and 20 µg Glykogen (Fermentas, St. Leonroth; Germany) over night at −20°C. After centrifugation at 4°C for 15 min (12,000 g) the pellets were washed once with 70% ethanol. Precipitated RNA was resuspended in 30 µl RNase free water (Ambion, Austin, TX). To assess the quantity and quality of RNA, the samples were measured using a NanoDrop spectrophotometer (NanoDrop, Wilmington, DE) and by microfluidic electrophoresis using a Small RNA Chip for Agilent's Bioanalyzer (Agilent Technologies, Waldbronn).

Microarray

Total RNA was extracted as described above. For cDNA synthesis, 1,5 ng of total RNA was transcribed in a 10-µL volume with the TaqMan microRNA RT kit (Applied Biosystems, Foster City, CA) according to the manufacturer's recommendations. Because of generally low RNA concentrations in serum, an additional pre-amplification step for miRNAs was performed using the MegaPlex RT & PreAmp Human Pool Set (Applied Biosystems). 2,5 µl cDNA was used for the pre-amplification reaction and the pre-amplification product was diluted for further analysis according to the manufacturer's recommendations. For the miRNA screening, quantitative real-time PCR was performed with the TaqMan human miRNA array pool A and B v2.0 (Applied Biosystems). 9 µL of the diluted pre-amplification product was used in each of the real-time PCR arrays. P-value adjustment was performed using the Bejamini-Hochberg method. All analysis have been performed MIAME-compliant and raw data were deposited in a MIAME- compliant database (ArrayExpress), as detailed on the MGED Society website http://www.mged.org/Workgroups/MIAME/miame.html. The accession number will be received during the review.

Isolation of HSC and hepatocytes from human livers

Primary human HSC were isolated from tissue samples obtained from patients undergoing partial liver resection. Experimental procedures were performed according to guidelines of the local ethics committee with patient's informed consent. Primary HSC were isolated using EGTA/collagenase perfusion and pronase incubation, and seperation from nonparenchymal liver cells was attained by arabinogalactan gradient ultracentrifugation as described previously [17]. HSC were cultured in Dulbecco's modified Eagle's medium supplemented with 10% fetal calf serum and 100 U/ml penicillin/streptomycin. Stimulation of the HSC was carried out on 6-well-plates with 10 ng/mL recombinant human TGF-β1 (R&D Systems) and as control, cells were left untreated.

Primary human hepatocytes were isolated and cultivated in serum-free medium (DMEM supplemented with 4.5 g/l glucose, 0.4 ng/ml hydrocortisone, 0.415 mU/ml insulin, 2 mM glutamine, and 100 U/ml penicillin/streptomycin) as previously described [21].

Isolation of monocytes and lymphocytes from human blood

Blood of healthy donors was collected in EDTA tubes and directly applied to PBMC isolation by Ficoll Density Gradient (LSM-1077, PAA) and further $CD14^{+}CD16^{-}$ and $CD14^{+}CD16^{+}$ monocytes were selectively purified by MACS methodology using 'Monocyte-isolation-Kit-II' and '$CD16^{+}$-monocytes-isolation-kit', respectively (Miltenyi). Lymphocytes serving as control cells were isolated from PBMC after depletion of monocytes with anti-CD14 microbeads.

For further materials and methods please see Data S1.

Results

Systematic profiling of serum miRNA levels in patients with distinct entities of liver cirrhosis

We performed a systematic array analysis on miRNA-serum levels of patients with liver cirrhosis from different entities and compared them to expression profiles of healthy controls (Figure 1 A). The screening cohort consisted of four age- and sex-matched patients with histologically and clinically confirmed compensated alcoholic liver cirrhosis (Child-Pugh class A), four patients with decompensated alcoholic cirrhosis (Child-Pugh class C), four patients with compensated hepatitis C-related cirrhosis (Child-Pugh class A) and four healthy volunteers as controls (Data S1). While several miRNAs with high-fold-changes were detected, only three of the individual miRNAs represented on the microarray showed significantly diverging levels between healthy controls and liver cirrhosis patients. Of these three miRNAs, levels of miR-513-3p and miR-571 were significantly increased while levels of miR-652 were significantly decreased (Figure 1 A). Array results for these latter three as well as three other representative miRNAs (miR-10a, mir-29a and miR-221) were confirmed by qPCR (Figure S2 A, B). Furthermore, a hierarchical cluster analysis for miR-513-3p, miR-571 and miR-652 revealed two distinct subsets, one containing the control samples and the other containing all cirrhosis patients included into the array analysis (Figure 1 B), thus confirming the different abundance between patients and controls.

Apart from these three significantly regulated miRNAs, we identified a panel of miRNAs with divergent pattern between patients and controls in our array analysis, of which a striking number had been previously studied in the context of liver disease and organ fibrosis, including miR-99 (up) [22], miR-30e (down) [23], miR-132 (up) [24], miR-196b (down) [25] and miR-221 (up) [26] (Figure 1 A). However, only miR-513-3p, miR-571 and miR-652 reached statistical significance (Figure 1 B). Thus, by applying a systematic array approach, we identified a subset of miRNAs differentially regulated in sera of patients with liver cirrhosis of hepatitis C and alcoholic etiology.

Next, we analyzed serum levels of miR-513-3p, miR-571 and miR-652 in a cohort of 17 healthy controls and 67 patients with chronic liver diseases by qPCR analysis (Table 1). In this larger collective, we observed a significant alteration for miR-513-3p, miR-571 and miR-652 in patients with liver cirrhosis, which was concordant to the previous findings in the array analysis (Figure 2 A). In addition, three other miRNAs (miR-10a, miR-29a, miR-221), which were strongly but not significantly altered or unaltered in the array, showed a concordant and significant regulation in the larger collective (Figure S2 C). Of note these results could be confirmed in a second, independent collective of patients with liver cirrhosis that were compared with a collective of patients treated for non-hepatic diseases (Figure S3). Moreover, we validated our results by analyzing serum levels of certain miRNAs that were previously shown to be altered in cirrhotics (miR-21, miR-34a, miR-122) [17,27,28]. In line with these previous findings, qPCR analysis revealed an up-regulation of miR-34a and miR-122 in our larger qPCR-cohort, while levels of miR-21 were unchanged (Figure S4).

Finally, ROC curve analysis showed that miR-513-3p, miR-571 and miR-652 were highly predictive for the presence of liver disease/cirrhosis (Figure 2 B). Their diagnostic accuracy could even be increased, when miRNA serum levels were combined (Figure 2 C) and were dramatically superior to that of classical markers such as platelets, INR or albumin (AUROC about 0.6),

A

miRNA differentially expressed between controls and patients with liver cirrhosis

Up-regulated in cirrhosis			Down-regulated in cirrhosis		
miRNA	**ΔΔCt (Normal-Cirrhosis**	**Adj. P-value**	**miRNA**	**ΔΔCt (Normal - Cirrhosis)**	**Adj. P-value**
miR-135a*	8.66	0.137	miR-370	-4.70	0.302
miR-564	7.93	0.144	miR-196b	-4.80	0.137
miR-571	**7.80**	**0.048**	miR-330-3p	-4.84	0.148
miR-801	6.81	0.154	miR-148b	-4.84	0.185
miR-513-3p	**6.61**	**0.039**	miR-339-3p	-5.00	0.209
miR-138	6.58	0.144	miR-744	-5.04	0.179
miR-99b*	6.48	0.137	miR-132	-5.06	0.137
miR-643	6.22	0.309	miR-886-5p	-5.06	0.172
miR-923	6.0	0.267	miR-454	-5.32	0.221
miR-188-5p	5.92	0.144	miR-486-5p	-5.35	0.351
miR-760	5.63	0.144	miR-221	-5.46	0.338
miR-30e	5.55	0.172	miR-139-3p	-5.61	0.255
miR-610	5.32	0.154	miR-491-5p	-5.78	0.144
miR-573	5.23	0.221	**miR-652**	**-6.60**	**0.027**
miR-509-3p	5.03	0.154	miR-425	-7.70	0.195

B

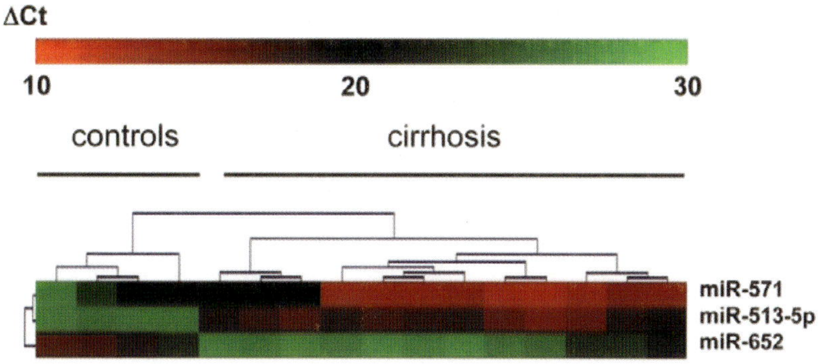

Figure 1. Systematic profiling of serum miRNA levels in patients with distinct entities of liver cirrhosis. (A) Microarray analysis for miRNA levels was performed using RNA extracts from serum of four healthy subjects as control and patients with liver cirrhosis of different etiologies and stages of disease (for detailed clinical parameters see Data S1). The fifteen miRNAs with strongest up- or down-regulation are depicted. Significantly regulated miRNAs are highlighted in bold type. (B) Hierarchical cluster analysis of the significantly regulated miRNAs miR-513-3p; miR-571; miR-652; bright green: under-expression; black: no change; bright red: over-expression.

when used in the same setting. Thus, the confirmation of our array results in a large cohort of liver disease patients by qPCR indicated an involvement of miR-513-3p, miR-571 and miR-652 in the pathogenesis of liver cirrhosis.

Association of miRNA-serum-patterns with etiology and stage of cirrhosis

We next analyzed our array data with respect to miRNA regulations in serum between either different stages of liver cirrhosis or different etiologies in order to identify more specific stage- or etiology-dependent miRNAs, with a focus on the regulation of miR-652, miR-571 and miR-513-3p. By using hierarchical cluster analysis of all miRNAs comparing Child A and C cirrhosis due to alcoholic disease, the samples split into two defined clusters, differentiating patients with compensated from patients with decompensated cirrhosis (Figure 3 A). However, when we tried to define specific single miRNAs distinguishing early and late stages of cirrhosis, only miR-140 and miR-340 were significantly regulated on the array level between both groups (Figure 3 B). The subsequent qPCR analysis from the total cohort of patients confirmed a trend for a differential regulation of miR-140 and miR-340, but did not reach statistical significance (Figure S5). On the other hand, among the previously identified miR-652, miR-571 and miR-513-3p, only serum levels of miR-571 were significantly elevated in patients with Child C compared to Child A cirrhosis (Figure 3 C). Interestingly, serum levels of miR-571 were significantly correlated with biomarkers of liver synthesis capacity such as pseudocholinesterase (PCHE), prothrombin time, international normalized ratio (INR) or coagulation factor V activity (Data S1), raising the possibility that this distinct miRNAs could serve as a novel serum biomarker reflecting disease severity in liver cirrhosis.

To evaluate if serum miRNA patterns are also dysregulated in an etiology-specific way we next compared serum miRNA expression patterns between patients with alcoholic and hepatitis C cirrhosis at the same stage of liver disease (Child-Pugh class A).

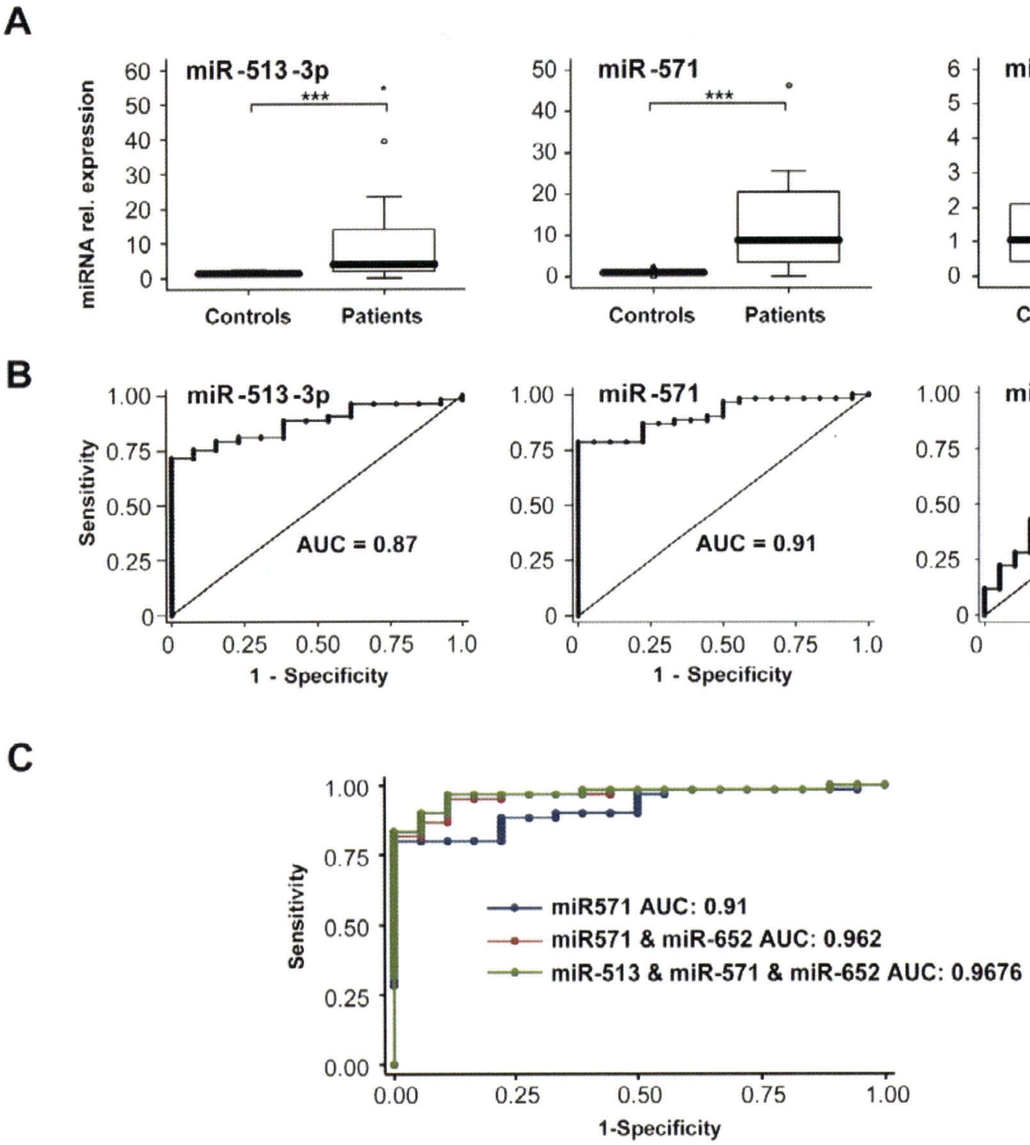

Figure 2. Serum levels of miR-513-3p, miR-571 and miR-652 are significantly altered in the serum of patients with chronic liver disease and liver cirrhosis. (A) Serum levels of the three significantly regulated miRNAs (miR-513-3p; miR-571; miR-652) were analyzed by qPCR in a collective of 17 healthy controls and 67 patients with chronic liver disease and liver cirrhosis. Results are depicted as box plot. The thick line represents the median of relative expression. (B) Receiver operating characteristic (ROC) curve analysis displaying the diagnostic power in predicting cirrhosis of these miRNAs when analyzed as single markers (area under the curve (AUC) 0.87; 0.91; 0.75). (C) ROC curve analysis displaying the diagnostic power in predicting cirrhosis of different combinations of these miRNAs (AUC 0.91; 0.962; 0.9676). $^{**}P<0.001$.

Again, hierarchical cluster analysis on the array-data revealed distinct clustering between alcoholic and hepatitis C cirrhosis (Figure 3 D). Seven miRNAs in the array analysis collective were regulated significantly different between these two groups (Figure 3 E), but significance was lost when the larger cohort was analyzed by qPCR. Importantly, miR-652, miR-571 and miR-513-3p did not differ dependent on disease etiology (Figure 3 F). Furthermore, to exclude a bias in regulation of these miRNA by co-morbidities or demographic differences, we correlated miR-652, miR-571 and miR-513-3p levels with age, gender, body mass index and serum creatinine concentration. None of these single parameters correlated with these miRNAs (Data S1). Therefore, in line with our initial hypothesis, the gene array approach indeed allowed us to identify three etiology-independent miRNAs specifically regulated in serum of liver disease patients, with miR-571 being a previously unrecognized miRNA that is also closely associated with the stage of liver cirrhosis.

Serum levels of miR-571 and miR-652 reflect their specific regulation in distinct cellular compartments involved in the pathogenesis of liver cirrhosis

It is presently unclear and controversially debated which molecular mechanisms are responsible for alterations in serum miRNA levels in certain disease conditions. Especially, it is not known if changes in serum levels reflect a passive release of miRNAs during cell death or if they are actively secreted and might play a functional role as "messengers" [29,30]. We thus aimed at assessing if divergent patterns of the identified set of serum miRNAs correlated with their regulation in the cellular compartments that are most likely involved in the initiation and

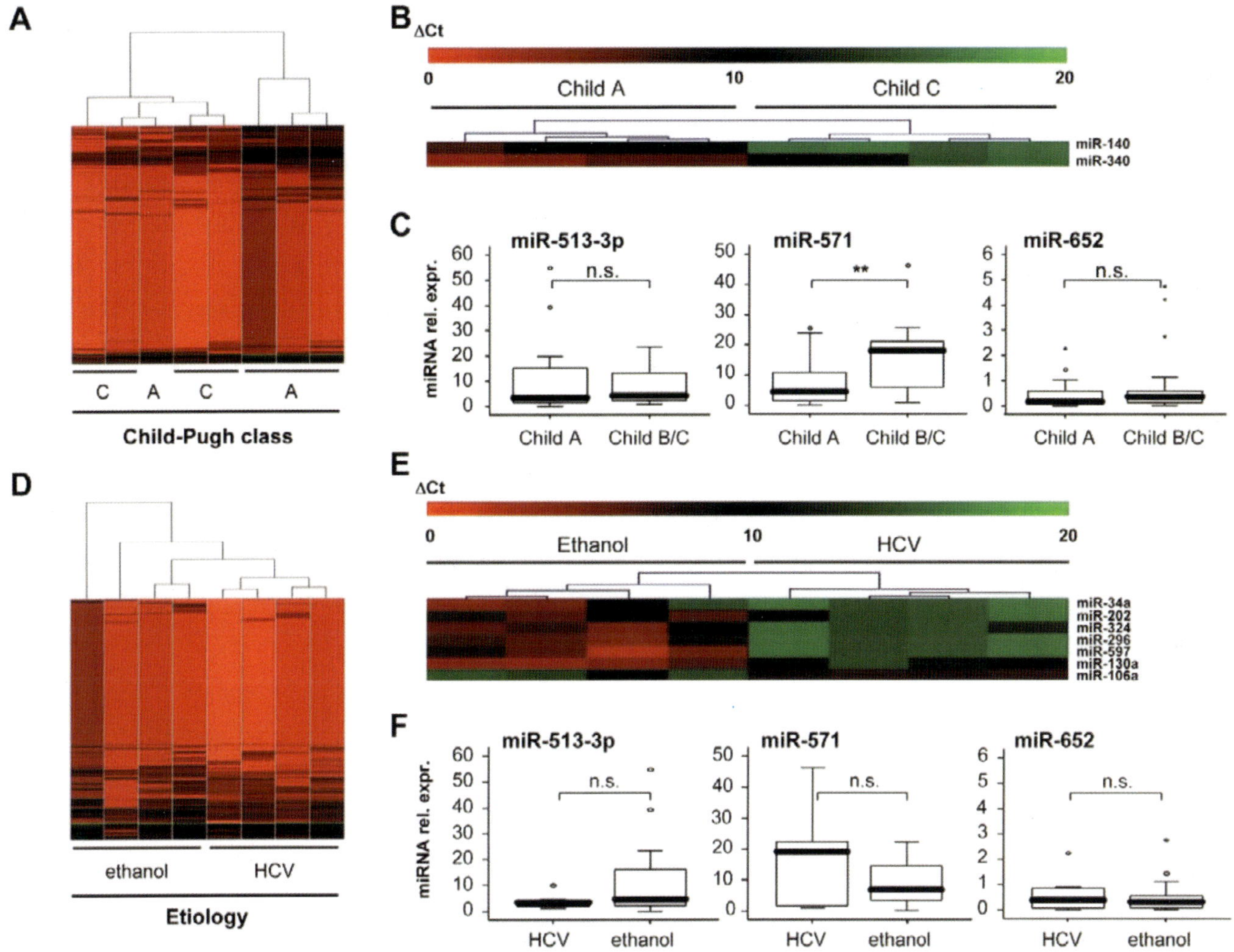

Figure 3. Correlation of miRNA serum levels with Child-Pugh class and etiology of liver disease. (A) Microarray data of the serum of eight patients with alcoholic liver cirrhosis at different stages of disease (Child-Pugh A and Child-Pugh C) in a hierarchical cluster analysis; bright green: under-expression; black: no change; bright red: over-expression. (B) Hierarchical cluster analysis of the significantly regulated miRNAs; bright green: under-expression; black: no change; bright red: over-expression. (C) Serum levels of miR-513-3p, miR-571 and miR-652 in the patients with alcoholic liver cirrhosis were analyzed by qPCR. Results are depicted as box plot. The thick line represents median of relative expression. (D) Microarray data of serum of the serum of four patients with ethanol-toxic liver cirrhosis (Child-Pugh A) and the four hepatitis C related cirrhosis (Child-Pugh A) in a hierarchical-cluster-analysis; bright green: under-expression; black: no change; bright red: over-expression. (E) Hierarchical cluster analysis of the significantly regulated miRNAs; bright green: under-expression; black: no change; bright red: over-expression. (F) Serum levels of miR-513-3p, miR-571 and miR-652 in the patients with alcoholic liver cirrhosis (Child-Pugh A) and hepatitis C related cirrhosis (Child-Pugh A) were analyzed by qPCR. Results are depicted as box plot. The thick line represents median of relative expression. $^{**}P<0.01$.

promotion of liver cirrhosis, namely liver tissue as well as circulating immune cells such as monocytes or lymphocytes [15,31].

To test the hypothesis that these miRNAs are differentially regulated within distinct compartments, we analyzed primary human liver tissue from cirrhotic patients (Data S1) and also isolated primary circulating monocytes as well as lymphocytes from patients with liver cirrhosis and healthy controls at high purities using magnetic bead separation techniques (Data S1). Interestingly, only levels of miR-571, but not of miR-652 or miR-513-3p, were concordantly regulated between serum and liver tissue from cirrhosis patients compared to healthy controls (Figure 4 A), suggesting that the liver is the primary source of serum miR-571 in cirrhosis patients. In contrast and concordant with its serum-specific regulation, miR-652 was significantly down-regulated in circulating monocytes isolated from patients compared to controls (Figure 4 B), while none of the three miRNAs were significantly dysregulated in the lymphocyte compartment (Figure 4 C).

In order to elucidate which hepatic cell population involved in liver cirrhosis likely contributes to miR-571 regulation in liver and serum of cirrhotic patients, we compared cell type-specific expression levels of these miRNAs in isolated primary human hepatocytes, hepatic stellate cells and monocytes/macrophages (Figure 4 D). Interestingly, miR-571 was expressed at similar levels in all of these cell compartments. In contrast, expression of miR-652 was restricted to monocytes/macrophages, indicating primary functions in regulating innate immune responses. Altogether, these data indicate that alterations of serum levels of miR-571 and miR-652 in liver cirrhosis patients reflect distinct regulatory mechanisms in different cell compartments involved in this disease, namely the liver and monocytes.

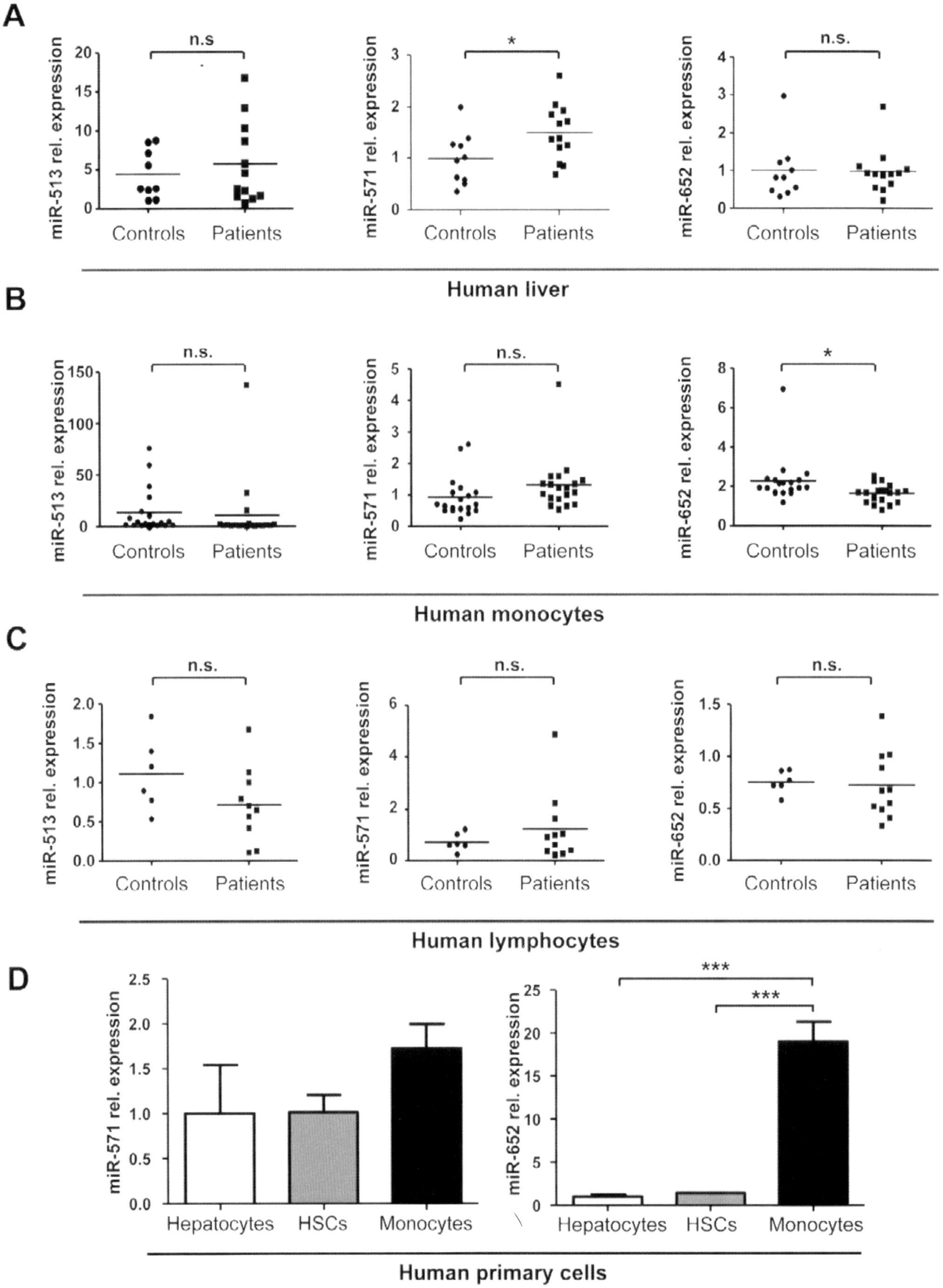
A
n.s
*
n.s.
miR-513 rel. expression
miR-571 rel. expression
miR-652 rel. expression
Controls
Patients
Human liver
B
n.s.
n.s.
*
Controls
Patients
Human monocytes
C
n.s.
n.s.
n.s.
Controls
Patients
Human lymphocytes
D
***
***
miR-571 rel. expression
miR-652 rel. expression
Hepatocytes
HSCs
Monocytes
Human primary cells

Figure 4. Serum levels of miR-571 and miR-652 reflect their specific regulation in distinct organs and cell compartments involved in the pathogenesis of liver cirrhosis. (A) Expression of miR-513-3p, miR-571 and miR-652 was analyzed by qPCR in liver samples of patients with liver cirrhosis (n = 13) and livers from patients without chronic liver disease (n = 10) as control. (B) Expression of miR-513-3p, miR-571 and miR-652 was analyzed by qPCR in MACS-sorted monocytes of patients with liver cirrhosis (n = 19) and healthy donors (n = 19) as control. (C) Expression of miR-513-3p, miR-571 and miR-652 was analyzed by qPCR in lymphocytes of patients with liver cirrhosis (n = 11) and healthy donors (n = 6) as control. Results are depicted as dot plot with each dot representing one individual patient. The line represents the mean of relative expression. (D) qPCR analysis of miR-571 and miR-652 expression in human primary hepatocytes, HSCs and monocytes, respectively. Results are depicted as mean, error bars denote SEM. *$P<0.05$, ***$P<0.001$.

miR-571 and miR-652 integrate pro-fibrotic and inflammatory signals in human HSCs and monocytes

Based on the prominent up-regulation of hepatic and circulating miR-571 in cirrhotic patients, we hypothesized that miR-571 might be centrally involved in cellular responses to profibrogenic signals. The most relevant collagen-producing cell types in liver fibrosis are HSCs, and the cytokine TGF-β is one of the key profibrogenic mediators [32,33]. When primary human HSCs, isolated from cirrhotic liver explants, were stimulated with TGF-β, miR-571 was significantly up-regulated (Figure 5 A). On the other hand, miR-652 did not show a specific regulation upon TGF-β stimulation. However, stimulation of monocytic U937 cells with the proinflammatory ligand bacterial lipopolysaccharide (LPS) led to a significant down-regulation of miR-652, while miR-571 remained unaffected (Figure 5 B). These data support that miR-571 is involved in the regulation of hepatic fibrogenesis, while

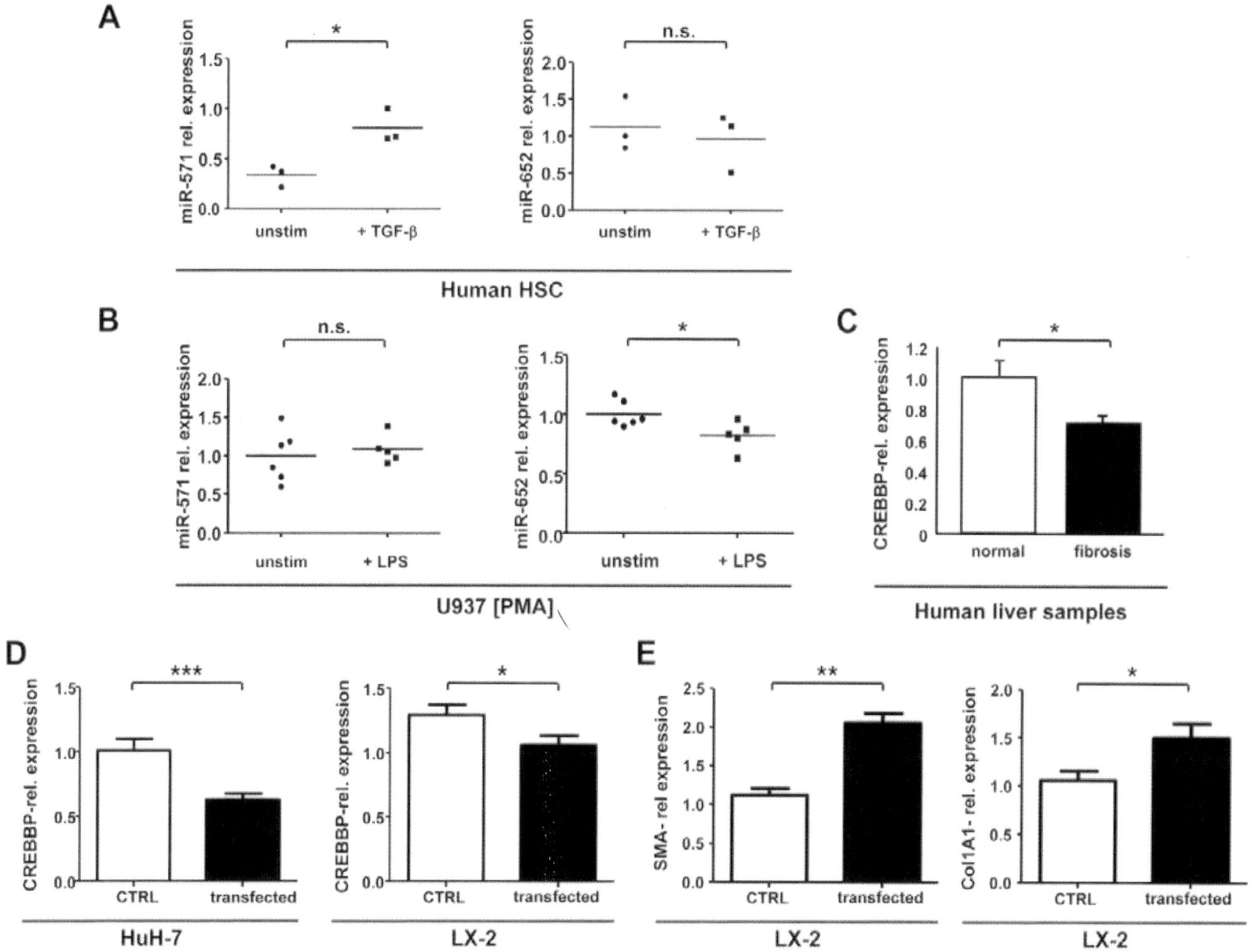

Figure 5. miR-571 and miR-652 integrate pro-fibrotic and inflammatory signals in human HSCs and monocytes. (A) Expression of miR-571 and miR-652 in primary human HSCs in response to stimulation with TGF-β for 48 h was measured by qPCR. Results are depicted as dot plot with each dot representing one individual patient. The line represents the mean of relative expression. (B) We stimulated U937 cells with PMA into a monocytic differentiation. miR-571 and miR-652 expression levels in response to stimulation with LPS for 48 h were measured by qPCR. Results are depicted as dot plot with each dot representing one individual patient. The line represents the mean of relative expression. (C) Expression of CREBBP was analyzed by qPCR in liver samples of patients with liver cirrhosis (n = 13) and non-liver diseased donors (n = 10) as control. Results are depicted as mean, error bars denote SEM. (D) HuH-7 cells and LX-2 cells were transfected with indicated amounts of miR-571 mimic. Expression of CREBBP was determined after two days of transfection by qPCR. Results are depicted as mean, error bars denote SEM. (E) Activation of stellate cells was determined by qPCR-based analysis of SMA- and Col1A1-expression in LX-2 cells. **$P<0.01$, ***$P<0.001$.

miR-652 is part of an inflammatory signaling network accompanying the pathophysiological processes during liver cirrhosis in monocytes/macrophages.

To our knowledge, there is currently no published information on possible functions and putative target genes of these respective miRNAs available. To get a first insight into their function, we performed a broad *in silico*- target screen for putative miR-571 targets, the miRNA with the most prominent regulation in our analysis, by using two different miRNA-target prediction algorithms. Among others, we identified CREB-binding protein (CREBBP) as a possible target gene for miR-571 (Data S1), a gene involved in general transcriptional regulation previously associated with the regulation and pathogenesis of liver fibrosis [34,35]. In line with up-regulation of miR-571, CREBBP was down-regulated in liver tissue from cirrhosis patients compared with healthy controls (Figure 5 C). Moreover, transfection of HuH-7 and LX-2 cells, cell lines representing human hepatocytes or HSC, respectively, with miR-571 led to a moderate, but significant down-regulation of CREBBP on RNA level (Figure 5 D), suggesting that CREBBP might be one possible target gene mediating miR-571-dependent effects in the regulation of liver cirrhosis. Finally, up-regulation of miR-571 leads to a moderate up-regulation of SMA and Col1A1 in LX-2 cells, indicating that miR-571 might be involved in activation of stellate cells during fibrogenesis (Figure 5 E).

Discussion

While previous screening approaches to study the role of miRNAs in liver fibrosis/cirrhosis focused on their regulation in liver tissue or hepatic stellate cells [10,11,12], in the present study we performed a systematic array approach on serum samples from liver cirrhosis patients. By this approach, we identified a set of three miRNAs, miR-513-3p, miR-571 and miR-652, which to our knowledge have previously not been characterized in liver cirrhosis nor in any other physiological or pathological condition in humans or rodents. The key prerequisite for their identification was the significant alteration in serum even in the relatively small collective of samples included in the array analysis, which was then confirmed within the larger cohort of chronic liver disease patients. To our opinion, this approach thus represents a successful methodological alternative to previous studies, which mainly addressed regulations of pre-defined, single miRNAs in serum [10]. Moreover, our array approach included patients with alcoholic and hepatitis C-related liver disease, enabling us to identify miRNAs with putative etiology-independent roles in hepatic cirrhosis. From these three miRNAs, miR-571 not only identified most reliably patients with chronic liver diseases, but was also closely associated with cirrhosis progression, underlining its potential as a novel serum biomarker. Therefore, further evaluation in larger prospective trials is warranted to assess its potential diagnostic or prognostic value in patients with hepatic fibrosis or cirrhosis.

Serum parameters in general can show certain variability, and the reproducibility of serum tests depends on the nature of the marker itself as well as the standardized handling and preparation of the sample. While protein based markers are more or less prone to degradation [20], it has been consistently shown that serum miRNAs remain stable after being subjected to severe conditions that would normally degrade most RNAs, such as boiling, very low or high pH levels, extended storage, and 10 freeze–thaw cycles [36]. Moreover, specimen collection, processing, and purification of miRNA were strictly standardized in the present study in order to avoid any bias (see Materials and Methods). In line with numerous previously published studies [6,17,19,20], we used spiked-in RNAs that were added into the serum sample before miRNA extraction for normalization of miRNA serum levels. This method is preferred by many groups to other normalization methods. As such, it was suggested that frequently used reference genes like U6 small nuclear RNA (RNU6B) and 5S ribosomal RNA show a less stable expression than others and are easily degraded in serum samples [37,38]. Furthermore, levels of certain miRNAs (miR-142-3p and miR-16) that were claimed to be evenly expressed in patient and control serum samples in some studies were found to be significantly altered in others [17,39]. The fact that by using spiked-in RNA for normalization we could show a similar regulation of certain miRNAs (miR-21, miR-34a, miR-122) [17,27,28] as demonstrated previously in other cohorts of cirrhotics (Figure S4) as well as our confirmatory experiments in a second, independent cohort of liver cirrhosis patients (Figure S4) strongly support the robustness of the de-regulation of the newly identified miRNAs in chronic liver disease.

The key finding of this study was a striking concordance between miRNA-levels in the serum and their specific regulations in different cellular compartments involved in the pathogenesis of chronic liver disease, raising the yet unanswered question which molecular processes underlie regulation of miRNA serum levels and if serum-miRNAs might withhold a specific function. On one hand, increased levels of miRNAs such as miR-513-3p or miR-571 might reflect an epiphenomenon resulting from increased hepatic cell death in chronic liver disease, a hypothesis that cannot be ruled out on basis of our data. However, some recent data have provided evidence that some miRNAs are not only passively released but in turn actively secreted from cells and integrated into vesicles, potentially serving as messengers to influence gene transcription in other cells [29,30]. The specific up-regulation of miR-571 in HSC, the main matrix-producing cell compartment activated during fibrogenesis, in response to TGF-β, the most prominent pro-fibrogenic cytokine [32], supports a contribution of these cells to changes in miR-571 serum levels. Given the vast amount of potential miR-571-target genes, among those CREBBP, a general modulator of gene transcription [40], it is conceivable that miR-571 is released from certain hepatic cells in an active process to modulate transcriptional programs in other cells or cell compartments involved in liver cirrhosis. Interestingly, we previously demonstrated a similarly concordant regulation between liver tissue and serum levels in liver cirrhosis for miR-29 [10]. In contrast, miR-221, which is up-regulated in livers of cirrhosis patients [26], showed a down-regulation in the serum in our array analysis (see Figure 1 A), which was confirmed as significant by qPCR in our large collective (Figure S2). These data suggest that different molecular processes are connecting serum levels of distinct miRNA with their tissue-specific regulation in the liver. However, the quantitative relations between alterations in intracellular miRNA concentrations and serum miRNA levels are not known.

miR-652 represented another strongly regulated miRNA in patients with chronic liver disease, on which further experiments revealed interesting differences to miR-571. Most strikingly, miR-652 showed a significant down-regulation in patients with chronic liver disease, correlating with its regulation in circulating monocytes rather than parenchymal or resident liver cells. The selective expression of miR-652 in innate immune cells supports the hypothesis that indeed this cellular down-regulation played a causative role for decreased serum levels in the patient group. The finding that miR-652 levels integrated proinflammatory stimuli like LPS suggests that this miRNA is involved in the mediation of inflammatory signals in immune cells. These mechanisms are likely not liver-specific, but might represent a general innate immune response mechanism present in many chronic inflammatory conditions such as hepatic fibrosis. In line with this hypothesis, miR-652 showed a high predictive value for the presence of chronic liver disease but did not correlate with the stage of cirrhosis. Therefore, next to further functional characterizations in monocytes/macrophages, it might be interesting to test serum levels and the predictive value of miR-652 in other acute and chronic inflammatory disease states, e.g. rheumatoid arthritis, inflammatory bowel disease or sepsis.

In conclusion, using a systematic array approach on serum samples from patients with chronic liver disease, we identified etiology-independent alterations of serum levels of miR-513-3p, miR-571 and miR-652, three previously uncharacterized miRNAs. Moreover, we demonstrated that miR571- and miR-652-serum levels in patients with chronic liver disease reflect their putative roles in the mediation of fibrogenic and inflammatory processes in distinct cellular compartments involved in the pathogenesis of liver cirrhosis. These results might lead to the identification of novel regulatory networks in different cellular compartments as a basis for future miRNA-based therapeutic strategies for the treatment of chronic liver disease and liver cirrhosis.

Supporting Information

Data S1 Overview of supplementary data and supplementary tables.

Figure S1 SV40 and U6 were used for normalization of PCR based analysis. (A) SV40 levels, used for normalization in further experiments, were determined by qPCR in sera of patients with liver cirrhosis and controls. (B) U6 expression, used for normalization in further experiments, were determined by qPCR in livers samples of patients with liver cirrhosis and controls.

Figure S2 Confirmation of the array based results by using qPCR. (A) Levels of miR-513-3p, miR-571 and miR-652 were analyzed by qPCR in the samples used for the initial array analysis in order to confirm the array based results. (B) miR-29a, miR-221 and miR-10a were analyzed by qPCR in the samples used for the initial array analysis in order to further confirm the array based results by extending this analysis on other miRNAs. (C) Serum levels of miR-29a, miR-221 and miR-10a were analyzed in the large collective of patients with liver cirrhosis and controls, revealing comparable results to the analysis in the smaller collective used for array analysis. $^{*}P<0.05$, $^{***}P<0.001$.

Figure S3 Confirmation of alterations of serum levels of miR-513-3p, miR-571 and miR-652 in a second cohort of patients. Serum level of miR-513-3p, miR-571 and miR-652 were analyzed in a second collective of patients with chronic liver disease and patients without chronic liver disease (n = 13 each) in order to confirm that the alterations remain stable when patients instead of healthy individuals were used as control. $^{*}P<0.05$.

Figure S4 Validation of the array- and qPCR based data. (A) Microarray analysis for miRNA levels was performed using RNA extracts from serum of four healthy subjects as control and patients with liver cirrhosis of different etiologies and stages of disease (for detailed clinical parameters see Data S1). Three miRNAs previously published in the context of liver cirrhosis are depicted to confirm the reliability of the array based results. (B) Serum levels of miR-21, miR-34a and miR-122 were analyzed in the large collective of patients with liver cirrhosis and controls, revealing comparable alterations to previously published results. $^{**}P<0.01$, $^{***}P<0.001$.

Figure S5 Analysis of miR-140 and miR-340 in the serum of patients with liver cirrhosis. (A) Serum levels of miR-140 and miR-340 in the patients with alcoholic liver cirrhosis (Child-Pugh A and Child-Pugh C) were analyzed by qPCR. Results are depicted as box plot. The thick line represents median of relative expression. (B) ROC curve analysis displaying the diagnostic power of selected miRNAs in predicting advanced stage of liver cirrhosis.

Acknowledgments

The authors would like to thank Michaela Roderburg-Goor and members of the Luedde-lab for helpful discussions. This paper is dedicated to Prof. Dr. M.P. Manns on the occasion of his 60th birthday.

Author Contributions

Conceived and designed the experiments: CR TL BB FT. Performed the experiments: CR BB DVC KB MV HZ TM NE ML. Analyzed the data: CR BB TL FT CT TM KB FT AK ML MO. Contributed reagents/materials/analysis tools: HZ FT CH MO NE. Wrote the paper: CR TL FT CT.

References

1. Schuppan D, Afdhal NH (2008) Liver cirrhosis. Lancet 371: 838–851.
2. Gieling RG, Burt AD, Mann DA (2008) Fibrosis and cirrhosis reversibility - molecular mechanisms. Clin Liver Dis 12: 915–937, xi.
3. Kloosterman WP, Plasterk RH (2006) The diverse functions of microRNAs in animal development and disease. Dev Cell 11: 441–450.
4. Huang Y, Shen XJ, Zou Q, Wang SP, Tang SM, et al. (2011) Biological functions of microRNAs: a review. J Physiol Biochem 67: 129–139.
5. Ha TY (2011) MicroRNAs in Human Diseases: From Cancer to Cardiovascular Disease. Immune Netw 11: 135–154.
6. Wang K, Zhang S, Marzolf B, Troisch P, Brightman A, et al. (2009) Circulating microRNAs, potential biomarkers for drug-induced liver injury. Proc Natl Acad Sci U S A 106: 4402–4407.
7. Li YP, Gottwein JM, Scheel TK, Jensen TB, Bukh J (2011) MicroRNA-122 antagonism against hepatitis C virus genotypes 1–6 and reduced efficacy by host RNA insertion or mutations in the HCV 5′ UTR. Proc Natl Acad Sci U S A 108: 4991–4996.
8. Ding J, Huang S, Wu S, Zhao Y, Liang L, et al. (2010) Gain of miR-151 on chromosome 8q24.3 facilitates tumour cell migration and spreading through downregulating RhoGDIA. Nat Cell Biol 12: 390–399.
9. Hou J, Lin L, Zhou W, Wang Z, Ding G, et al. (2011) Identification of miRNomes in human liver and hepatocellular carcinoma reveals miR-199a/b-3p as therapeutic target for hepatocellular carcinoma. Cancer Cell 19: 232–243.
10. Roderburg C, Urban GW, Bettermann K, Vucur M, Zimmermann H, et al. (2011) Micro-RNA profiling reveals a role for miR-29 in human and murine liver fibrosis. Hepatology 53: 209–218.
11. Bandyopadhyay S, Friedman RC, Marquez RT, Keck K, Kong B, et al. (2011) Hepatitis C virus infection and hepatic stellate cell activation downregulate miR-29: miR-29 overexpression reduces hepatitis C viral abundance in culture. J Infect Dis 203: 1753–1762.
12. Sekiya Y, Ogawa T, Yoshizato K, Ikeda K, Kawada N (2011) Suppression of hepatic stellate cell activation by microRNA-29b. Biochem Biophys Res Commun 412: 74–79.
13. Thum T, Gross C, Fiedler J, Fischer T, Kissler S, et al. (2008) MicroRNA-21 contributes to myocardial disease by stimulating MAP kinase signalling in fibroblasts. Nature 456: 980–984.
14. Varnholt H, Drebber U, Schulze F, Wedemeyer I, Schirmacher P, et al. (2008) MicroRNA gene expression profile of hepatitis C virus-associated hepatocellular carcinoma. Hepatology 47: 1223–1232.
15. Zimmermann HW, Seidler S, Nattermann J, Gassler N, Hellerbrand C, et al. (2010) Functional contribution of elevated circulating and hepatic non-classical CD14CD16 monocytes to inflammation and human liver fibrosis. PLoS One 5: e11049.

16. Mendrick DL (2011) Transcriptional profiling to identify biomarkers of disease and drug response. Pharmacogenomics 12: 235–249.
17. Cermelli S, Ruggieri A, Marrero JA, Ioannou GN, Beretta L (2011) Circulating microRNAs in patients with chronic hepatitis C and non-alcoholic fatty liver disease. PLoS One 6: e23937.
18. Cortez MA, Bueso-Ramos C, Ferdin J, Lopez-Berestein G, Sood AK, et al. (2011) MicroRNAs in body fluids–the mix of hormones and biomarkers. Nat Rev Clin Oncol 8: 467–477.
19. Jungebluth P, Alici E, Baiguera S, Le Blanc K, Blomberg P, et al. (2011) Tracheobronchial transplantation with a stem-cell-seeded bioartificial nanocomposite: a proof-of-concept study. Lancet 378: 1997–2004.
20. Mitchell PS, Parkin RK, Kroh EM, Fritz BR, Wyman SK, et al. (2008) Circulating microRNAs as stable blood-based markers for cancer detection. Proc Natl Acad Sci U S A 105: 10513–10518.
21. Wanninger J, Neumeier M, Bauer S, Weiss TS, Eisinger K, et al. (2011) Adiponectin induces the transforming growth factor decoy receptor BAMBI in human hepatocytes. FEBS Lett 585: 1338–1344.
22. Estep M, Armistead D, Hossain N, Elarainy H, Goodman Z, et al. (2010) Differential expression of miRNAs in the visceral adipose tissue of patients with non-alcoholic fatty liver disease. Aliment Pharmacol Ther 32: 487–497.
23. Duisters RF, Tijsen AJ, Schroen B, Leenders JJ, Lentink V, et al. (2009) miR-133 and miR-30 regulate connective tissue growth factor: implications for a role of microRNAs in myocardial matrix remodeling. Circ Res 104: 170–178, 176p following 178.
24. Estep M, Armistead D, Hossain N, Elarainy H, Goodman Z, et al. (2010) Differential expression of miRNAs in the visceral adipose tissue of patients with non-alcoholic fatty liver disease. Aliment Pharmacol Ther 32: 487–497.
25. Xie T, Liang J, Guo R, Liu N, Noble PW, et al. (2011) Comprehensive microRNA analysis in bleomycin-induced pulmonary fibrosis identifies multiple sites of molecular regulation. Physiol Genomics 43: 479–487.
26. Pineau P, Volinia S, McJunkin K, Marchio A, Battiston C, et al. (2010) miR-221 overexpression contributes to liver tumorigenesis. Proc Natl Acad Sci U S A 107: 264–269.
27. Bihrer V, Friedrich-Rust M, Kronenberger B, Forestier N, Haupenthal J, et al. (2011) Serum miR-122 as a biomarker of necroinflammation in patients with chronic hepatitis C virus infection. Am J Gastroenterol 106: 1663–1669.
28. Bihrer V, Waidmann O, Friedrich-Rust M, Forestier N, Susser S, et al. (2011) Serum microRNA-21 as marker for necroinflammation in hepatitis C patients with and without hepatocellular carcinoma. PLoS One 6: e26971.
29. Valadi H, Ekstrom K, Bossios A, Sjostrand M, Lee JJ, et al. (2007) Exosome-mediated transfer of mRNAs and microRNAs is a novel mechanism of genetic exchange between cells. Nat Cell Biol 9: 654–659.
30. Vickers KC, Palmisano BT, Shoucri BM, Shamburek RD, Remaley AT (2011) MicroRNAs are transported in plasma and delivered to recipient cells by high-density lipoproteins. Nat Cell Biol 13: 423–433.
31. Zimmermann HW, Seidler S, Gassler N, Nattermann J, Luedde T, et al. (2011) Interleukin-8 is activated in patients with chronic liver diseases and associated with hepatic macrophage accumulation in human liver fibrosis. PLoS One 6: e21381.
32. Bataller R, Brenner DA (2005) Liver fibrosis. J Clin Invest 115: 209–218.
33. Luedde T, Schwabe RF (2011) NF-kappaB in the liver linking injury, fibrosis and hepatocellular carcinoma. Nat Rev Gastroenterol Hepatol 8: 108–118.
34. Gressner OA, Lahme B, Rehbein K, Siluschek M, Weiskirchen R, et al. (2008) Pharmacological application of caffeine inhibits TGF-beta-stimulated connective tissue growth factor expression in hepatocytes via PPARgamma and SMAD2/3-dependent pathways. J Hepatol 49: 758–767.
35. Wu XL, Zeng WZ, Jiang MD, Qin JP, Xu H (2008) Effect of Oxymatrine on the TGFbeta-Smad signaling pathway in rats with CCl4-induced hepatic fibrosis. World J Gastroenterol 14: 2100–2105.
36. Chen X, Ba Y, Ma L, Cai X, Yin Y, et al. (2008) Characterization of microRNAs in serum: a novel class of biomarkers for diagnosis of cancer and other diseases. Cell Res 18: 997–1006.
37. Peltier HJ, Latham GJ (2008) Normalization of microRNA expression levels in quantitative RT-PCR assays: identification of suitable reference RNA targets in normal and cancerous human solid tissues. RNA 14: 844–852.
38. Hummel R, Hussey DJ, Haier J (2010) MicroRNAs: predictors and modifiers of chemo- and radiotherapy in different tumour types. Eur J Cancer 46: 298–311.
39. Resnick KE, Alder H, Hagan JP, Richardson DL, Croce CM, et al. (2009) The detection of differentially expressed microRNAs from the serum of ovarian cancer patients using a novel real-time PCR platform. Gynecol Oncol 112: 55–59.
40. Fuller-Pace FV (2006) DExD/H box RNA helicases: multifunctional proteins with important roles in transcriptional regulation. Nucleic Acids Res 34: 4206–4215.

Table 2. Diagnostic performances of LS and FT and their suggested optimal cutoff values.

Method	Fibrosis stage	AUROC (95% CI)	Cutoffs	Sensitivity (%)	Specificity (%)	NPV (%)	PPV (%)
LS	F≥2	0.873 (0.802–0.944)	8.8 kPa	78.0	86.7	41.9	97.0
	F≥3	0.897 (0.846–0.949)	10.2 kPa	86.3	90.4	86.3	90.4
	F = 4	0.910 (0.867–0.953)	14.1 kPa	84.0	84.9	89.4	77.8
FT	F≥2	0.903 (0.838–0.968)	0.32	79.3	93.3	45.2	98.5
	F≥3	0.907 (0.862–0.952)	0.52	86.0	90.0	81.8	92.5
	F = 4	0.866 (0.815–0.918)	0.68	80.0	84.0	87.0	75.9

LS, liver stiffness; FT, FibroTest; AUROC, area under the receiver operating characteristics curve; CI, confidence interval; NPV, negative predictive value; PPV, positive predictive value.

Then, sections 4 μm thick were stained with hematoxylin and eosin (H&E) and Masson's trichrome. All liver tissue samples were evaluated by an experienced hepatopathologist (YN Park) who was blinded to the patients' clinical histories. Specimens that were shorter than 20 mm and considered by the pathologists to be unsuitable for fibrosis assessment were excluded from the analysis. Liver histology was evaluated semiquantitatively according to the Batts and Ludwig scoring system [28]. Fibrosis was staged on a 0–4 scale: F0, no fibrosis; F1, portal fibrosis; F2, periportal fibrosis; F3, septal fibrosis; and F4, cirrhosis. Significant fibrosis was defined as F2 or more, advanced fibrosis as F3 or more, and cirrhosis as F4.

5. Statistical analyses

The major goals of this study were to prospectively validate the diagnostic performance of FT for detection of the presence of histological significant fibrosis, advanced fibrosis, and cirrhosis in comparison with LS and to suggest optimal cutoff values in patients with CHB. To assess the diagnostic performance of each noninvasive index, receiver operating characteristic (ROC) curves were constructed and the areas under the ROC curves (AUROCs) were calculated. Then, to evaluate the usefulness of the noninvasive method, the sensitivity, specificity, positive predictive value (PPV), and negative predictive value (NPV) were determined from the ROC curves. Furthermore, we evaluated the usefulness of combined use of FT and LS as a surrogate marker for liver biopsy.

Statistical analyses were performed using SAS software version 9.1.3 (SAS, Cary, NC). In all analyses, $p<0.05$ was taken to indicate statistical significance.

Results

1. Patients baseline characteristics

A total of 350 consecutive patients were screened for possible inclusion in the study. Based on the exclusion criteria, a total of 194 patients (mean age 46.7 years, 119 male) were analyzed (Figure 1).

The patients' characteristics are summarized in Table 1. The mean ALT level was 58.4 IU/L, while the mean AST level was 44.1 IU/L. The mean LS and FT were 14.2 kPa and 0.53, respectively. The mean length and the median number of fragments of liver biopsy samples were 21.3 mm and 2, respectively. The fibrosis stages were F0 in 0 (0%) patients, F1 in 30 (15.5%), F2 in 50 (25.7%), F3 in 39 (20.1%), and F4 in 75 (38.7%). All patients had well-preserved liver functions.

2. Diagnostic performances of LS and FT

As shown in Figure 2, the overall mean values of LS (Fig. 2A) and FT (Fig. 2B) increased in parallel with the increase in fibrosis stage (all $p<0.05$). As the fibrosis stage increased from F1 to F4, the mean value of LS increased from 6.9±4.2 kPa in F1, 9.7±5.7 kPa in F2, 12.1±2.97 kPa in F3, and 21.1±10.1 kPa in F4, while that of FT also increased from 0.16±0.17 in F1, 0.34±0.18 in F2, 0.6±0.23 in F3, and 0.76±0.19 in F4. LS and FT were significantly different between F1 and F2 ($p=0.035$ and $p<0.001$), F2 vs. F3 ($p=0.034$ and $p<0.001$), and F3 vs. F4 ($p<0.001$ and $p<0.001$), respectively.

With regard to the diagnostic performances of LS and FT in the prediction of histological liver fibrosis, the AUROCs of LS and FT were 0.873 (95% confidence interval [CI] 0.802–0.944) and 0.903 (95% CI 0.838–0.968) for significant fibrosis (F≥2) (Fig. 3A), 0.897 (95% CI 0.846–0.949) and 0.907 (95% CI 0.862–0.952) for advanced fibrosis (F≥3) (Fig. 3B), and 0.910 (95% CI 0.867–0.953) and 0.866 (0.815–0.918) for cirrhosis (F = 4) (Fig. 3C), respectively (Table 2). There were no significant differences between AUROC values of LS and FT (all $p>0.05$ by Hanley and McNeil test) [29].

3. Determination of the optimal cutoffs for LS and FT

The most discriminant cutoff values for LS and FT were determined from the ROC curves to maximize the sum of sensitivity and specificity [30] (Table 2). LS cutoff values of 8.8, 10.2, and 14.1 kPa generated sensitivity of 78.0%, specificity of 86.7%, NPV of 41.9%, and PPV of 97.0% for F≥2; sensitivity of 86.3%, specificity of 90.4%, NPV of 86.3%, and PPV of 90.4% for F≥3; and sensitivity of 84.0%, specificity of 84.9%, NPV of 89.4%, and PPV of 77.8% for F = 4, respectively. Similarly, FT cutoff scores of 0.32, 0.52, and 0.68 generated sensitivity of 79.3%, specificity of 93.3%, NPV of 45.2%, and PPV of 98.5% for F≥2; sensitivity of 86.0%, specificity of 90.0%, NPV of 81.8%, and PPV of 92.5% for F≥3; and sensitivity of 80.0%, specificity of 84.0%, NPV of 87.0%, and PPV of 75.9% for F = 4, respectively.

LS agreed with liver biopsy on the diagnosis of F<2 vs. F≥2 in 154 patients (79.3%), F<3 vs. F≥3 in 172 patients (88.7%), and F<4 vs. F = 4 in 164 patients (84.5%), while FT agreed on the diagnosis of F<2 vs. F≥2 in 158 patients (81.4%), F<3 vs. F≥3 in 170 patients (87.6%), and F<4 vs. F = 4 in 160 patients (82.5%) (Table 3). In addition, when using the suggested cutoffs of LS and FT to diagnose each histological fibrosis stage (F1, F2, F3, and F4), 124 (63.9%) and 123 (63.4%) patients (gray-colored area in Table 3) were correctly classified consistent with liver biopsy examination, respectively, and they could avoid liver biopsy according to the corresponding results by noninvasive methods (Table 3).

Table 3. Distribution and agreement of fibrosis stages according to histology and LS or FT (n = 194).

Fibrosis stage estimated by histology	Total	Fibrosis stage estimated by LS				Fibrosis stage estimated by FT			
		F1	F2	F3	F4	F1	F2	F3	F4
		LS<8.8 kPa	8.8≤LS<10.2 kPa	10.2≤LS<14.1 kPa	LS≥14.1 kPa	FT<0.32	0.32≤FT<0.52	0.52≤FT<0.68	FT≥0.68
F1	30	26	1	2	1	28	1	0	1
F2	50	29	13	1	7	24	19	5	2
F3	39	5	2	22	10	5	2	16	16
F4	75	2	2	8	63	5	4	6	60
Total	194	62	18	33	81	62	26	27	79

LS, liver stiffness; FT, FibroTest.

4. Agreement between LS and FT

Irrespective of matching with histological fibrosis stages, 152 patients (78.3%) showed agreement in fibrosis staging using LS and FT for noninvasive estimation of F<2 vs. F≥2, 158 patients (81.4%) for F<3 vs. F≥3, and 146 patients (75.3%) for F<4 vs. F = 4. Thus, when LS and FT agreed for noninvasive prediction of F<2 vs. F≥2, F<3 vs. F≥3, and F<4 vs. F = 4, these results agreed with those of liver biopsy examination in 88.8% (134 of 152 patients), 96.8% (153 of 158 patients), and 94.5% (138 of 146 patients), respectively.

Overall agreement between each fibrosis stage (F1, F2, F3, and F4) estimated by LS and FT was observed in 111 patients. Among them, 88 patients (79.3%) were correctly classified with reference to liver biopsy examinations, and they could avoid liver biopsy based upon concordant results between the two tests (gray-colored area in Table 4).

5. Discordance between LS and FT

Discordant results between fibrosis stages estimated by LS and FT were identified in 83 patients (42.8%). On multivariate analysis, only the presence of histological cirrhosis was identified as a single significant factor, which showed a negative association with discordance between LS and FT ($p = 0.009$; odds ratio 0.151, 95% CI 0.036–0.628). Among these patients with discordance between LS and FT, 41 and 42 patients showed higher fibrosis stage by LS and by FT, respectively. The baseline characteristics were compared between these two groups, and none was identified as a significant factor capable of explaining this difference.

6. Combined use of LS and FT

Based on a previous report by Castéra et al. [31], we examined the diagnostic performance of a combination formula adding LS to FT (LS+FT). It showed a non-significant trend toward better AUROC than LS, but was worse than FT in prediction of F≥2 (0.885, 95% CI 0.816–0.953) and F≥3 (0.905, 95% CI 0.856–0.955). With regard to prediction of cirrhosis, the combination formula showed better AUROC (0.915, 95% CI 0.874–0.956) than LS and FT alone.

Furthermore, we examined the diagnostic performance of another combination formula multiplying LS by FT (LS×FT), which showed the best AUROC for prediction of F≥2 (0.941, 95% CI 0.908–0.975), F≥3 (0.931, 95% CI 0.889–0.974), and F = 4 (0.929, 95% CI 0.894–0.965), compared to LS, FT, and LS+FT. The optimized cutoff values of combination formula, LS+FT and LS×FT, are described in detail in Table 5.

Using the above cutoffs, LS+FT agreed with liver biopsy on the diagnosis of F<2 vs. F≥2 in 164 patients (84.5%), F<3 vs. F≥3 in 176 patients (90.7%), and F<4 vs. F = 4 in 169 patients (87.1%), while LS×FT agreed on the diagnosis of F<2 vs. F≥2 in 165 patients (85.1%), F<3 vs. F≥3 in 175 patients (90.2%), and F<4 vs. F = 4 in 170 patients (87.6%). Overall, 129 (66.5%) and 130 (67.0%) patients were correctly classified consistent with each histological fibrosis stage (F1, F2, F3, and F4) using LS+FT and LS×FT, respectively.

Discussion

FT, a good surrogate marker for liver biopsy, has been widely studied regarding its usefulness for noninvasive prediction of fibrosis stage primarily in western populations with HCV infection [10]. However, only a few investigations have been conducted in populations with CHB [21,22,23,24,25]. To the best of our knowledge, we are the first to assess the diagnostic value of FT and to define new cutoff values for each fibrosis stage optimized for a

Table 4. Agreements of histological fibrosis stages among patients who showed concordant results between LS and FT (n = 111).

	Total	Fibrosis stage estimated by concordant LS and FT results			
		F1	F2	F3	F4
Fibrosis stage estimated by histology		LS<8.8 kPa	8.8 kPa≤LS<10.2 kPa	10.2 kPa≤LS<14.1 kPa	LS≥14.1 kPa
		& FT<0.32	& 0.32≤FT<0.52	& 0.52≤FT<0.68	& FT≥0.68
F1	24	24	0	0	0
F2	21	16	3	1	1
F3	11	1	0	8	2
F4	55	0	0	2	53
Total	111	41	3	11	56

LS, liver stiffness; FT, FibroTest.

homogenous Asian population with CHB. As there may be a varied spectrum in diagnostic cutoffs of such noninvasive indices based on biochemical parameters, even among studies in patients with the same etiology, a new study to generate standardized, generalized results in Asian patients with CHB is warranted.

Although the underlying mechanisms of fibrosis progression in chronic viral hepatitis are expected to be similar, several differences according to etiology may affect diagnostic accuracy [32,33]. For example, patients with CHC often have steatosis, which may influence baseline biochemical parameters, and have micronodular cirrhosis. Those with CHB more frequently experience a wide range of fluctuations in necroinflammatory activity and have macronodular cirrhosis leading to relatively lower fibrotic contents than those with CHC [33]. These clinicopathological differences have been suggested to partially explain the relatively lower cutoff LS values in patients with CHB than in those with CHC [27]. Hence, in the present study recruiting Asian patients primarily with CHB, we investigated the accuracy and applicability of FT, which is the most accurate index among patients with CHC.

This study has several strengths. First, we prospectively recruited patients who underwent the baseline blood tests and LS on the same day as liver biopsy, and the diagnostic performance of FT was compared to LS, which has already shown excellent diagnostic value in Asian populations with CHB [26,34,35,36]. Furthermore, a relatively large number of subjects from a single center were consecutively enrolled in this study, and the distribution of our population was homogeneous and representative of patients with CHB seen in clinical practice. Therefore, the optimal cutoff values of FT derived from our study are ultimately expected to be used as reference values for future studies to elaborate on the role of FT in Asian patients with CHB.

In the present study, the diagnostic performance of FT was comparable to that of LS for diagnosing fibrosis stages: 0.903 vs. 0.873 for significant fibrosis (F≥2), 0.907 vs. 0.897 for advanced fibrosis (F≥3), and 0.866 vs. 0.910 for cirrhosis (F = 4), respectively. Using the Youden method [30], we suggested FT cutoff values of 0.32, 0.52, and 0.68 for F≥2, F≥3, and F = 4, respectively. All of these values were slightly lower than the suggested cutoff values for CHB by BioPredictive (0.49, 0.59, and 0.75, respectively). Although several studies have investigated FT in patients with CHB [21,22,23,24,25], the optimal cutoffs for each fibrosis stage have not been proposed. Thus, another external validation is required for our new thresholds for Asian CHB subjects.

Among subjects where LS and FT agreed with prediction of F≥2, F≥3, and F = 4 regardless of matching with histological examinations, concordance with liver biopsy examination was observed in 88.8%, 96.8%, and 94.5%, respectively. Furthermore, overall agreement between each fibrosis stage (F1, F2, F3, and F4) estimated by LS and FT was observed in 111 patients (57.2%). Among them, 88 patients (79.3%) were correctly classified with reference to liver biopsy examinations, and they could avoid liver biopsy based on the concordant results between the two tests (Table 4). In contrast to other studies, we demonstrated the concordance between two tests for noninvasive prediction of each

Table 5. Diagnostic performances of combination formula using LS and FT and their suggested optimal cutoff values.

Method	Fibrosis stage	AUROC (95% CI)	Cutoffs	Sensitivity (%)	Specificity (%)	NPV (%)	PPV (%)
LS+FT	F≥2	0.885 (0.816–0.953)	8.2	84.8	83.3	50.0	96.5
	F≥3	0.905 (0.856–0.955)	10.7	93.0	87.5	89.7	91.4
	F = 4	0.915 (0.874–0.956)	16.8	76.0	94.1	86.2	89.1
LS×FT	F≥2	0.941 (0.908–0.975)	2.3	82.9	96.7	50.9	99.3
	F≥3	0.931 (0.889–0.974)	4.7	92.1	87.5	88.6	91.3
	F = 4	0.929 (0.894–0.965)	9.8	80.0	92.4	88.0	87.0

LS, liver stiffness; FT, FibroTest; AUROC, area under the receiver operating characteristics curve; CI, confidence interval; NPV, negative predictive value; PPV, positive predictive value.

fibrosis stage (F1, F2, F3, and F4) along with F≥2, F≥3, and F = 4. Such a high level of diagnostic accuracy consistent with previous investigations is the reason why many experts recommend that liver biopsy should be avoided for those with concordance between two noninvasive tests [20,31]. In fact, based on these advantages of LS and FT, these two markers have been used as the first-line estimates of fibrosis in France instead of liver biopsy [37]. However, for noninvasive prediction of each fibrosis stage, 83 patients (42.8%) had discordant results between LS and FT, and liver biopsy should still be strongly considered in such cases, although several investigators have recently pointed out that the liver biopsy examination has an error rate of up to 20% in disease staging even when an experienced physician performs the liver biopsy examination and an expert pathologist interprets the results [38,39]. One of the most important methods to minimize such inherent limitations of liver biopsy examination is to obtain the reliable biopsy specimens of adequate sizes [40]. From this viewpoint, we only enrolled patients with so-called reliable biopsy specimens (≥20 mm size) from the beginning of the study.

With regard to discordance between LS and FT, among various baseline factors, only the presence of histological cirrhosis was identified as a single significant factor with a negative association with such discrepancies. Consistent with a previous study [41], patients with histological cirrhosis have a higher rate of non-discordance (84.0%) between LS and histology than those without histological cirrhosis (51.3%, p<0.001). The similar result was maintained for FT in our study (non-discordance of 80.0% in patient without histological cirrhosis vs. 47.1%, in subjects with histological cirrhosis, p<0.001). This negative correlation between the presence of histological cirrhosis and discordances in the present study can be explained in part by the different level of ALT in patients with and without histological cirrhosis (mean value 43.2 vs. 68.1 IU/L, respectively; $p = 0.008$). Because the higher ALT has been known as a well-known overestimating confounder of LS [42] and the same phenomenon was observed for FT in our cohort (p = 0.018) by linear regression analysis with adjusting other variables, patients without cirrhosis were more likely to have discordance between LS (or FT) and liver biopsy. Accordingly, patients with histological cirrhosis and with relatively lower ALT level can have a greater likelihood of non-discordance between LS and FT by diminishing the influence of ALT on LS or FT. However, further validation studies are required to elucidate this issue.

Several investigators [25,31] tested the combination formula with addition of LS to FT (LS+FT), suggesting that it is likely that a combination of serum biomarkers and LS will complement each other and enhance accuracy of fibrosis detection. However, this method did not always show definitely superior results. In the present study, LS+FT had better AUROC than LS, but was poorer than FT in prediction of F≥2 and F≥3, while it had better AUROCs than LS or FT alone in prediction of F = 4. Next, we assessed the diagnostic value of LS×FT, which consistently showed better AUROCs than LS or FT alone in prediction of F≥2, F≥3, and F = 4. When compared to LS+FT, LS×FT had better outcomes for diagnosing fibrosis stage. However, further studies are required to determine which is the better option for noninvasive diagnosis of fibrosis.

This study is limited in that its design was cross-sectional. It is not clear whether repeated determination of FT score may be useful for tracking the progression of fibrosis and related clinical outcomes, such as occurrence of hepatic decompensation and HCC in individual patients. Therefore, the diagnostic value for predicting the subsequent development of cirrhosis and its various complications with sequential FT measurements during long-term follow-up must be examined further in a longitudinal study. Second, our population did not include patients with F0. As our institute is a tertiary referral hospital and one of the largest medical centers in Korea, patients with relatively more advanced disease status are likely to be referred for close follow-up. It might have resulted in a selection bias and eventually a spectrum bias, since the diagnostic performance of a given noninvasive test tends to increase in general in a cohort with the high disease prevalence and thus the diagnostic performances of LS and FT might have been overestimated in our cohort accordingly. Therefore, another independent external validation study in a population with minimal fibrotic burden should be performed to provide more generalizable results in patients with CHB-related chronic liver disease.

In summary, in a prospective study, we first assessed FT in Asian patients with CHB, demonstrating its comparable diagnostic accuracy to LS for predicting histological fibrosis stage. The optimal suggested cutoff values are expected to be useful as reference values for future studies in Asian patients with CHB. Our results suggest that combined use of LS and FT could avoid invasive liver biopsy in most patients with CHB. We hope that other researchers will evaluate the reproducibility of FT for the noninvasive diagnosis of fibrosis stage in independent populations.

Author Contributions

Conceived and designed the experiments: BKK SUK DYK. Performed the experiments: JYP SHA CYC YNP. Analyzed the data: BKK SUK. Contributed reagents/materials/analysis tools: HSK JYP SHA CYC IRC DHJ YNP KHH DYK. Wrote the paper: BKK SUK.

References

1. Lok AS, McMahon BJ (2007) Chronic hepatitis B. Hepatology 45: 507–539.
2. Degertekin B, Lok AS (2009) Indications for therapy in hepatitis B. Hepatology 49: S129–137.
3. Liaw YF, Sung JJ, Chow WC, Farrell G, Lee CZ, et al. (2004) Lamivudine for patients with chronic hepatitis B and advanced liver disease. New England Journal of Medicine 351: 1521–1531.
4. de Franchis R (2008) Non-invasive (and minimally invasive) diagnosis of oesophageal varices. J Hepatol 49: 520–527.
5. Spinzi G, Terruzzi V, Minoli G (2001) Liver biopsy. New England Journal of Medicine 344: 2030.
6. Poynard T, Halfon P, Castera L, Charlotte F, Le Bail B, et al. (2007) Variability of the area under the receiver operating characteristic curves in the diagnostic evaluation of liver fibrosis markers: impact of biopsy length and fragmentation. Alimentary Pharmacology and Therapeutics 25: 733–739.
7. Wai CT, Greenson JK, Fontana RJ, Kalbfleisch JD, Marrero JA, et al. (2003) A simple noninvasive index can predict both significant fibrosis and cirrhosis in patients with chronic hepatitis C. Hepatology 38: 518–526.
8. Sheth SG, Flamm SL, Gordon FD, Chopra S (1998) AST/ALT ratio predicts cirrhosis in patients with chronic hepatitis C virus infection. The American journal of gastroenterology 93: 44–48.
9. Forns X, Ampurdanès S, Llovet JM, Aponte J, Quintó L, et al. (2002) Identification of chronic hepatitis C patients without hepatic fibrosis by a simple predictive model. Hepatology 36: 986–992.
10. Imbert-Bismut F, Ratziu V, Pieroni L, Charlotte F, Benhamou Y, et al. (2001) Biochemical markers of liver fibrosis in patients with hepatitis C virus infection: a prospective study. Lancet 357: 1069–1075.
11. Lim SG, Oo AM, Mak B, Chua W, Chan E, et al. (2006) Non-invasive models for predicting histology in patients with chronic hepatitis B. Liver international 26: 666–672.
12. Han KH, Yoon KT (2008) New diagnostic method for liver fibrosis and cirrhosis. Intervirology 51 Suppl 1: 11–16.
13. Lackner C, Struber G, Liegl B, Leibl S, Ofner P, et al. (2005) Comparison and validation of simple noninvasive tests for prediction of fibrosis in chronic hepatitis C. Hepatology 41: 1376–1382.
14. Castera L, Vergniol J, Foucher J, Le Bail B, Chanteloup E, et al. (2005) Prospective comparison of transient elastography, Fibrotest, APRI, and liver

biopsy for the assessment of fibrosis in chronic hepatitis C. Gastroenterology 128: 343–350.
15. Friedrich-Rust M, Ong MF, Martens S, Sarrazin C, Bojunga J, et al. (2008) Performance of transient elastography for the staging of liver fibrosis: a meta-analysis. Gastroenterology 134: 960–974.
16. Ziol M, Handra-Luca A, Kettaneh A, Christidis C, Mal F, et al. (2005) Noninvasive assessment of liver fibrosis by measurement of stiffness in patients with chronic hepatitis C. Hepatology 41: 48–54.
17. Kim SU, Han KH, Ahn SH (2010) Transient elastography in chronic hepatitis B: an Asian perspective. World J Gastroenterol 16: 5173–5180.
18. Shaheen AA, Wan AF, Myers RP (2007) FibroTest and FibroScan for the prediction of hepatitis C-related fibrosis: a systematic review of diagnostic test accuracy. Am J Gastroenterol 102: 2589–2600.
19. Poynard T, Morra R, Halfon P, Castera L, Ratziu V, et al. (2007) Meta-analyses of FibroTest diagnostic value in chronic liver disease. BMC Gastroenterol 7: 40.
20. Halfon P, Munteanu M, Poynard T (2008) FibroTest-ActiTest as a non-invasive marker of liver fibrosis. Gastroenterol Clin Biol 32: 22–39.
21. Myers RP, Tainturier MH, Ratziu V, Piton A, Thibault V, et al. (2003) Prediction of liver histological lesions with biochemical markers in patients with chronic hepatitis B. J Hepatol 39: 222–230.
22. Sebastiani G, Vario A, Guido M, Alberti A (2007) Sequential algorithms combining non-invasive markers and biopsy for the assessment of liver fibrosis in chronic hepatitis B. World J Gastroenterol 13: 525–531.
23. Poynard T, Zoulim F, Ratziu V, Degos F, Imbert-Bismut F, et al. (2005) Longitudinal assessment of histology surrogate markers (FibroTest-ActiTest) during lamivudine therapy in patients with chronic hepatitis B infection. Am J Gastroenterol 100: 1970–1980.
24. Stibbe KJ, Verveer C, Francke J, Hansen BE, Zondervan PE, et al. (2011) Comparison of non-invasive assessment to diagnose liver fibrosis in chronic hepatitis B and C patients. Scand J Gastroenterol 46: 962–972.
25. Raftopoulos SC, George J, Bourliere M, Rossi E, de Boer WB, et al. (2011) Comparison of noninvasive models of fibrosis in chronic hepatitis B. Hepatol Int.
26. Kim SU, Ahn SH, Park JY, Kang W, Kim DY, et al. (2008) Liver Stiffness Measurement in Combination With Noninvasive Markers for the Improved Diagnosis of B-viral Liver Cirrhosis. J Clin Gastroenterol 43: 267–271.
27. Castera L, Forns X, Alberti A (2008) Non-invasive evaluation of liver fibrosis using transient elastography. J Hepatol 48: 835–847.
28. Batts KP, Ludwig J (1995) Chronic hepatitis. An update on terminology and reporting. American journal of surgical pathology 19: 1409–1417.
29. Hanley JA, McNeil BJ (1983) A method of comparing the areas under receiver operating characteristic curves derived from the same cases. Radiology 148: 839–843.
30. Fluss R, Faraggi D, Reiser B (2005) Estimation of the Youden Index and its associated cutoff point. Biom J 47: 458–472.
31. Castéra L, Vergniol J, Foucher J, Le Bail B, Chanteloup E, et al. (2005) Prospective comparison of transient elastography, Fibrotest, APRI, and liver biopsy for the assessment of fibrosis in chronic hepatitis C. Gastroenterology 128: 343–350.
32. Kim BK, Kim do Y, Park JY, Ahn SH, Chon CY, et al. (2010) Validation of FIB-4 and comparison with other simple noninvasive indices for predicting liver fibrosis and cirrhosis in hepatitis B virus-infected patients. Liver int 30: 546–553.
33. Chang PE, Lui HF, Chau YP, Lim KH, Yap WM, et al. (2008) Prospective evaluation of transient elastography for the diagnosis of hepatic fibrosis in Asians: comparison with liver biopsy and aspartate transaminase platelet ratio index. Alimentary pharmacology & therapeutics 28: 51–61.
34. Kim BK, Han KH, Park JY, Ahn SH, Chon CY, et al. (2010) A novel liver stiffness measurement-based prediction model for cirrhosis in hepatitis B patients. Liver int 30: 1073–1081.
35. Jung KS, Kim SU, Ahn SH, Park YN, Kim do Y, et al. (2011) Risk assessment of hepatitis B virus-related hepatocellular carcinoma development using liver stiffness measurement (FibroScan). Hepatology 53: 885–894.
36. Kim do Y, Kim SU, Ahn SH, Park JY, Lee JM, et al. (2009) Usefulness of FibroScan for detection of early compensated liver cirrhosis in chronic hepatitis B. Dig Dis Sci 54: 1758–1763.
37. Fontaine H, Petitprez K, Roudot-Thoraval F, Trinchet JC (2007) Guidelines for the diagnosis of uncomplicated cirrhosis. Gastroenterol Clin Biol 31: 504–509.
38. Afdhal NH (2003) Diagnosing fibrosis in hepatitis C: is the pendulum swinging from biopsy to blood tests? Hepatology 37: 972–974.
39. Poynard T, Munteanu M, Imbert-Bismut F, Charlotte F, Thabut D, et al. (2004) Prospective analysis of discordant results between biochemical markers and biopsy in patients with chronic hepatitis C. Clin Chem 50: 1344–1355.
40. Bedossa P, Dargere D, Paradis V (2003) Sampling variability of liver fibrosis in chronic hepatitis C. Hepatology 38: 1449–1457.
41. Kim SU, Seo YS, Cheong JY, Kim MY, Kim JK, et al. (2010) Factors that affect the diagnostic accuracy of liver fibrosis measurement by Fibroscan in patients with chronic hepatitis B. Aliment Pharmacol Ther 32: 498–505.
42. Fung J, Lai CL, Cheng C, Wu R, Wong DK, et al. (2011) Mild-to-moderate elevation of alanine aminotransferase increases liver stiffness measurement by transient elastography in patients with chronic hepatitis B. Am J Gastroenterol 106: 492–496.

17

Serum γ-glutamyl Transferase Levels, Insulin Resistance and Liver Fibrosis in Patients with Chronic Liver Diseases

Salvatore Petta[1]*, Fabio Salvatore Macaluso[1], Maria Rosa Barcellona[1], Calogero Cammà[1], Daniela Cabibi[2], Vito Di Marco[1], Antonio Craxì[1]

1 Sezione di Gastroenterologia, DiBiMIS, University of Palermo, Palermo, Italy, **2** Cattedra di Anatomia Patologica, University of Palermo, Palermo, Italy

Abstract

Background and Aims: Serum levels of γ-glutamyl-transpeptidase(γ-GT) were associated with liver disease severity and metabolic alterations, which in turn are able to affect hepatic damage. In patients with nonalcoholic fatty liver disease (NAFLD), genotype 1 chronic hepatitis C (G1CHC) and chronic hepatitis B (CHB), we assessed the link between liver fibrosis and γ-GT serum levels, and we evaluated if normal or high γ-GT serum levels affect the association between insulin resistance (IR) and severity of liver fibrosis.

Methods: 843 consecutive patients with chronic liver disease (CLD)(193 NAFLD, 481 G1CHC, 169 CHB) were evaluated by liver biopsy (Kleiner and Scheuer scores) and clinical and metabolic measurements. IR was diagnosed if HOMA>3. A serum γ-GT concentration of >36 IU/L in females and >61 IU/L in males was considered the threshold value for identifying high levels of γ-GT.

Results: By multivariate logistic regression analysis, abnormal γ-GT serum levels were independently linked to severe liver fibrosis in patients with NAFLD (OR2.711,CI1.120–6.564,p = 0.02), G1CHC (OR3.461,CI2.138–5.603,p<0.001) and CHB (OR2.778,CI1.042–7.414,p = 0.04), together with IR and liver necroinflammation, and with a negative predictive value>80%. Interestingly, among patients with high or normal γ-GT values, even if IR prevalence was significantly higher in patients with severe fibrosis compared to those without, IR remained significantly associated with severe fibrosis in patients with abnormal γ-GT values only (OR4.150,CI1.079–15.970,p = 0.03 for NAFLD; OR2.250,CI1.211–4.181,p = 0.01 for G1CHC; OR3.096,CI2.050–34.220,p = 0.01 for CHB).

Conclusions: In patients with CLD, IR is independently linked to liver fibrosis only in patients with abnormal γ-GT values, without differences according to liver disease etiology, and suggesting a role of γ-GT as a marker of metabolic-induced liver damage. These data could be useful for the clinical and pharmacologic management of patients with CLD.

Editor: Sang-Hoon Ahn, Yonsei University College of Medicine, Republic of Korea

Funding: The authors have no support or funding to report.

Competing Interests: The authors have declared that no competing interests exist.

* E-mail: petsa@inwind.it

Introduction

The prognosis of patients with chronic liver diseases (CLD), independently of the underlying etiology, is ultimately decided by the amount of liver fibrosis that will accumulate over the years as a consequence of several mechanisms of tissue injury, with the ultimate development of cirrhosis and its complicances [1,2]. Other than conventional host and viral factors known to affect liver fibrosis progression, metabolic factors, and especially insulin resistance (IR) act as major disease modifiers associated with the severity of hepatic damage. Specifically, IR is the key determinant of nonalcoholic fatty liver disease (NAFLD) and its severity [3], is common in western patients with chronic hepatitis C (CHC) [4], due to both viral and host factors [5], and associated with the severity of fibrosis and its progression independently of steatosis and visceral obesity [6,7], and finally seems also associated with the severity of liver fibrosis in patients with chronic hepatitis B (CHB) [8].

However, nevertheless these data, it is probably that the impact of IR on the severity of liver fibrosis is different according to the clinical setting. These considerations in fact arise from contrasting evidences about the association between liver fibrosis and IR observed in some studies on patients with CHC [4,9] or CHB [10], and from the evidences that insulin-sensitizer therapies obtain an improvement in histological outcomes in a proportion of NAFLD patients only [11,12].

γ-glutamyl transpeptidase (γ-GT) is a hepatic and biliary enzyme synthesized by hepatocytes as well as epithelial cells of intra-hepatic bile ducts [13,14]. Several cross-sectional and prospective studies showed that plasma γ-GT is associated with metabolic syndrome risk factors and with markers of inflammation [15–18], also representing in large population studies an independent predictor of all-cause, liver-related, diabetes-related, and cancer-related death [13]. In this line, recent studies suggest that plasma γ-GT is a significant predictor of NAFLD, independently of alcohol intake [14,15,19], and that more specifically elevated γ-GT levels are associated with a more severe histological spectrum of NAFLD, namely the presence of NASH and fibrosis [16], whereas reductions in γ-GT predict histological improvement in NAFLD following bariatric surgery [15,20]. Similarly, different cross-sectional studies also showed that higher γ-GT serum levels are predictive of the severity of liver fibrosis in patients with both CHC and CHB, being this test also included in non-invasive scores for hepatic fibrosis assessment [21,22].

All these data therefore could suggest that γ-GT is expression of an environmental and probably genetic state of inflammation and metabolic dysfunction, affecting the spectrum of the severity of liver disease.

In light of these facts, we aimed to confirm the association between severity of liver disease and γ-GT serum levels in patients with an histological diagnosis of CLD, due to NAFLD, CHC and CHB, and to evaluate, in these patients, if the presence of normal or high γ-GT serum levels affects the association between IR and severity of liver fibrosis.

Materials and Methods

Patients

Eight-hundred and forty-three consecutive patients with CLD, due to viral or metabolic etiology (193 with NAFLD, 481 with genotype 1 CHC, and 169 with CHB), recruited at the Gastrointestinal & Liver Unit at the University Hospital in Palermo and fulfilling all inclusion and exclusion criteria detailed below, were assessed. (a) histological diagnosis of NAFLD, or G1 CHC, or CHB on a liver biopsy performed less than 6 months before enrollment; (b) NAFLD diagnosed on the basis of chronically elevated ALT for at least 6 months, alcohol consumption of <20 g/day, steatosis (>5% of hepatocytes) at histology with necroinflammation and/or fibrosis, and negative anti-HCV and HBsAG; (c) G1 CHC characterized by the presence of anti-HCV and HCVRNA, with persistently abnormal alanine aminotransferase (ALT), alcohol consumption of <20 g/day in the last 12 months or more, naive to antiviral therapy, and negative HBsAg; (d) CHB characterized by the presence of HBsAg and HBVDNA >2000 IU/ml, with persistently abnormal alanine aminotransferase (ALT), alcohol consumption of <20 g/day in the last 12 months or more, naive to antiviral therapy, and negative anti-HCV. Exclusion criteria were: (1) advanced cirrhosis; (2) hepatocellular carcinoma; (3) other causes of liver disease or mixed aetiologies; (4) human immunodeficiency virus infection; (5) previous treatment with antiviral therapy, immunosuppressive drugs and/or regular use of steatosis-inducing drugs, evaluated by interview; (6) active intravenous drug addiction.

The study was carried out in accordance with the principles of the Declaration of Helsinki and its appendices, and with local and national laws. Approval was obtained from the hospital's Internal Review Board and its Ethics Committee, and written informed consent was obtained from all patients and controls.

Clinical and Laboratory Assessment

Clinical and anthropometric data were collected at the time of liver biopsy. Body mass index (BMI) was calculated on the basis of weight in kilograms and height in meters, and patients were classified as normal weight (BMI, 18.5–24.9 kg/m^2), overweight (BMI, 25–29.9), or obese (BMI ≥30). A diagnosis of arterial hypertension was based on the following criteria: systolic blood pressure ≥130 mm Hg and/or diastolic blood pressure ≥85 mm Hg (measured three times in 30 minutes, in the sitting position and using a brachial sphygmomanometer), or use of blood-pressure-lowering agents. A diagnosis of type 2 diabetes was based on the revised criteria of the American Diabetes Association, using a value of fasting blood glucose ≥126 mg/dL on at least two occasions [23]. In patients with a previous diagnosis of type 2 diabetes, current therapy with insulin or oral hypoglycemic agents was documented.

A 12-hour overnight fasting blood sample was drawn at the time of biopsy to determine serum levels of ALT, total cholesterol, triglycerides, plasma glucose concentration, insulin, and platelet count. Insulin resistance (IR) was determined by the homeostasis model assessment (HOMA) method, using the following equation [24]: insulin resistance (HOMA-IR) = fasting insulin (μU/mL) x fasting glucose (mmol/L)/22.5. HOMA-IR has been validated in comparison with the euglycemic/hyperinsulinemic clamp technique in both diabetic and non-diabetic patients [25]. HOMA-IR values >3 were considered to indicate IR [26].

Commercially available enzymatic colorimetric test was used for serum γ-GT assays. In accordance with the kit's instructions, a serum γ-GT concentration of >36 IU/L in females, and >61 IU/L in males was considered the threshold value for identifying high levels of γ-GT.

HCV-infected individuals were tested at the time of biopsy for HCV-RNA using qualitative PCR (Cobas Amplicor HCV Test version 2.0; limit of detection: 50 IU/ml). HCVRNA-positive samples were quantified by Versant HCV-RNA 3.0 bDNA (Bayer Co. Tarrytown, NY, USA) expressed in IU/ml. Genotyping was performed by INNOLiPA (HCV II, Bayer HealthCare, Berkeley, CA, USA). Hepatitis B virus-infected patients were tested at the time of biopsy for HBs, HBeAg, anti-HBe and anti-HDV IgG, using commercial enzyme immunoassays (Dia Sorin, Saluggia, Italy). HBV-DNA was quantified by bDNA (Versant HBV 3.0, Siemens Medical Solutions Diagnostics Europe, Dublin, Ireland; range 357–17 857 000 IU/ml).

Histology

Slides were coded and read by one pathologist (D.C.), who was unaware of the patient's identity and history. Steatosis was assessed as the percentage of hepatocytes containing fat droplets (minimum 5%), and evaluated as a continuous variable. Steatosis was classified according to Kleiner classification as: absent <5%; mild 5%–33%; moderate >33%–66%; and severe >66%. In the NAFLD group, the Kleiner classification [27] was used to compute the NAFLD activity score (from 0 to 8, on a scale including separate scores for steatosis, lobular inflammation, and hepatocellular ballooning) and to stage fibrosis from 0 to 4. Biopsies of CHC and CHB patients were classified for grade and stage according to Scheuer's system [28].

Statistics

Continuous variables were summarized as mean±SD, and categorical variables as frequency and percentage. The Student's t-test and chi-square test were used when appropriate. Multiple logistic regression analyses were done to identify factors independently associated with severe fibrosis in NAFLD, CHC and CHB patients considered separately, and in the sub-groups with high or normal γ-GT serum levels. As candidate risk factors, we selected age, gender, BMI, baseline ALT, normal or high γ-GT (only in the entire populations), triglycerides, total cholesterol, blood glucose, insulin, HOMA score, IR, diabetes, arterial hypertension, steatosis grade, lobular inflammation, ballooning, NAS score, and fibrosis. In these models, the dependent variable was severe fibrosis coded as 1 = present (F3–F4) versus 0 = absent (F0–F2).

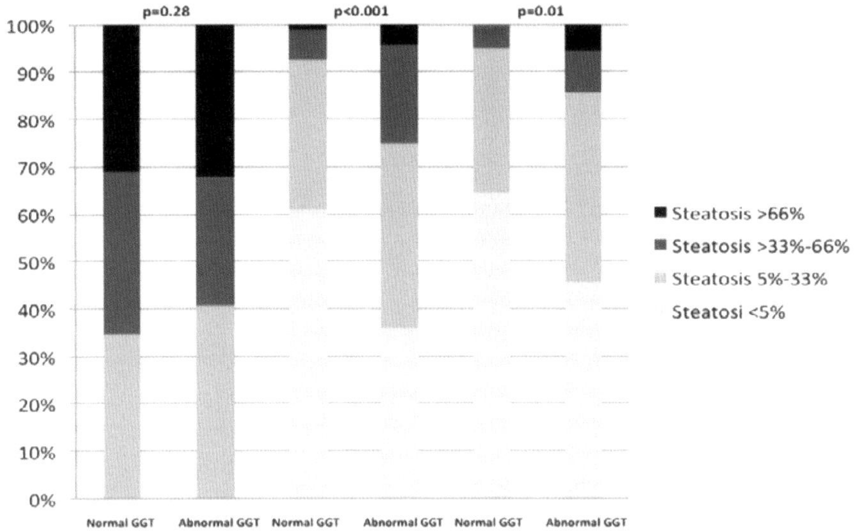

Figure 1A NAFLD CHC CHB

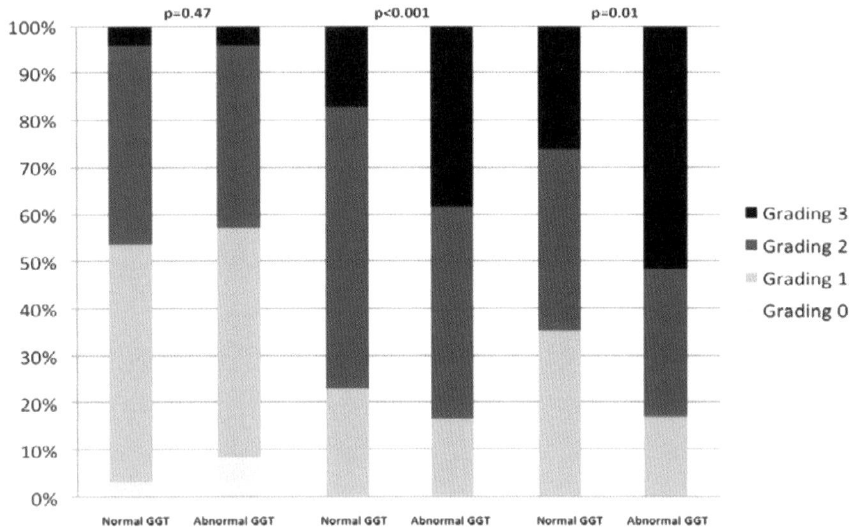

Figure 1B NAFLD CHC CHB

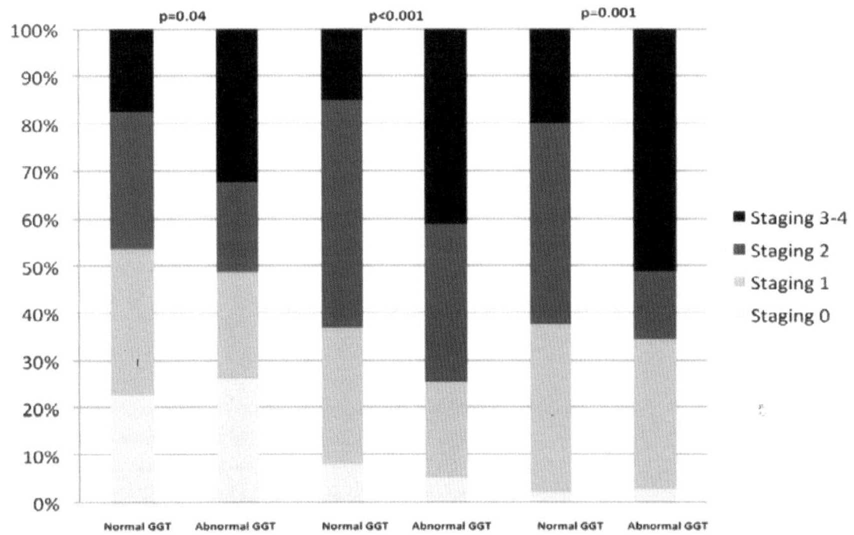

Figure 1C NAFLD CHC CHB

Figure 1. Histological characteristics of patients. (A) Steatosis grade according to liver disease etiology and normal/abnormal γ-GT values; (B) Grade of liver inflammation, according to liver disease etiology (Kleiner score for NAFLD, Scheuer score for CHC and CHB) and normal/abnormal γ-GT values; (C) Stage of liver fibrosis, according to liver disease etiology (Kleiner score for NAFLD, Scheuer score for CHC and CHB) and normal/abnormal γ-GT values.

Receiver operating characteristic (ROC) curves were applied to identify the area under ROC curve (AUC) of γ-GT and other variables to discriminate the presence of severe liver fibrosis.

Variables associated with the dependent variable on univariate analysis (probability threshold, $p \leq 0.10$) were included in the multivariate regression models. To avoid the effect of colinearity, diabetes, IR, HOMA score, blood glucose levels, and insulin levels, as well as NAS score and its components, were not included in the same multivariate model. Regression analyses were done using Proc Logistic, Proc Reg and subroutine in SAS (SAS Institute, Inc., Cary, North Carolina, U.S.A.) [29].

Results

Patient Characteristics and Histology

Abnormal values of serum γ-GT levels were observed in 49.7%, 43.2% and 20.7% of NAFLD, G1 CHC and CHB patients, respectively. The baseline characteristics of the 843 patients according to the etiology of liver disease, and to the presence of normal or high γ-GT serum levels are shown in Table 1 and in Supplemental Table S1. Overall, patients with abnormal γ-GT serum levels had higher ALT serum levels and, considering liver histological features, a more severe liver disease, in term of fibrosis in NAFLD, and of steatosis, inflammatory activity and fibrosis in both CHC and CHB (Figure 1). In addition, patients with abnormal γ-GT had more frequent metabolic alterations, namely higher cholesterol and triglycerides levels in NAFLD, higher triglycerides levels and a higher prevalence of IR and diabetes in CHC, and higher cholesterol and triglycerides and a higher prevalence of IR and hypertension in CHB.

Due to the evidence of a higher prevalence of IR in CHC and CHB patients with abnormal γ-GT values compared to their counterpart, in both CHC and CHB groups we tested if this association was maintained at multivariate analysis. We found that, after confirming older age (OR 1.025, CI 1.006–1.045, $p = 0.01$ for CHC), and higher BMI (OR 1.171, CI 1.105–1.242, $p < 0.001$ for CHC; OR 1.211, CI 1.071–1.369, $p = 0.002$ for CHB) as independent predictors of IR, abnormal γ-GT values remained independently associated with IR in CHC patients only (OR 1.861, CI 1.228–2.821, $p = 0.003$). In this group of patients the AUC of γ-GT values for IR prediction was 0.652 (C.I. 0.603–0.705), compared to 0.609 (C.I. 0.603–0.705) ($p = 0.22$) of age, and 0.689 (C.I. 0.642–0.736) ($p = 0.27$) of BMI. Finally, the positive predictive value (PPV) of abnormal γ-GT for IR prediction was 55.2%, while the negative predictive value (NPV) of normal γ-GT was 64.1%.

Factors Associated with Severe Liver Fibrosis in the Entire Cohort of Patients with CLD

Severe fibrosis (F2–F4) was independently associated with abnormal γGT values in NAFLD (OR 2.711, CI 1.120–6.564, $p = 0.02$), G1 CHC (OR 3.461, CI 2.138–5.603, $p < 0.001$), and CHB (OR 2.778, CI 1.042–7.414, $p = 0.04$) patients, together with other well known risk factors for fibrosis like older age, IR and lobular inflammation in NAFLD (Table 2 up), older age, lower cholesterol, IR and moderate-severe necroinflammatory activity in G1 CHC (Table 2 medium), and older age, virological status, IR and moderate-severe necroinflammatory activity in CHB (Table 2 bottom) patients. The AUC of the entire models were 0.830 (C.I. 0.769–0.880) for NAFLD, 0.798 (C.I. 0.759–0.833) for CHC, and 0.855 (C.I. 0.793–0.904) for CHB. The PPV and NPV of abnormal and normal γGT values, respectively, for severe fibrosis prediction, were reported in table 3.

Finally, when replacing in the model γGT as categorical variable, with γGT as continuous variable, the latter remained significantly associated with severe fibrosis in NAFLD (OR 1.003, CI 1.001–1.006, $p = 0.04$), G1 CHC (OR 1.004, CI 1.001–1.007, $p = 0.004$), and CHB patients (OR 1.022, CI 1.005–1.039, $p = 0.01$). The AUC of γGT values for severe fibrosis prediction, compared to those of the other variables, were reported in table 3.

Factors Associated with Liver Fibrosis in Patients with CLD and with Normal γGT Serum Levels

In patients with normal γGT values, severe fibrosis was independently associated with older age (OR 1.070, CI 1.013–1.129, $p = 0.01$) and lobular inflammation (OR 3.215, CI 1.150–8.987, $p = 0.02$) in NAFLD (Table 4 up), older age (OR 1.034, CI 1.001–1.070, $p = 0.04$), no male gender (OR 0.295, CI 0.129–0.673, $p = 0.004$), and lower cholesterol levels (OR 0.981, CI 0.969–0.993, $p = 0.003$) in G1 CHC (Table 4 medium), and with only moderate-severe liver necroinflammatroy activity (OR 15.985, CI 1.894–134.893, $p = 0.01$) in CHB (Table 4 bottom) patients.

Factors Associated with Liver Fibrosis in Patients with CLD and with Abnormal γGT Serum Levels

In patients with abnormal γGT values, severe fibrosis was independently associated with older age (OR 1.061, CI 1.015–1.111, $p = 0.01$), lower cholesterol levels (OR 0.982, CI 0.968–0.996, $p = 0.01$), IR (OR 4.150, CI 1.079–15.970, $p = 0.03$), and lobular inflammation (OR 6.824, CI 2.228–20.904, $p = 0.001$) in NAFLD (Table 5 up), with older age (OR 1.049, CI 1.020–1.079, $p = 0.001$), IR (OR 2.250, CI 1.211–4.181, $p = 0.01$), and moderate-severe liver necroinflammatory activity (OR 8.970, CI 2.559–31.447, $p = 0.001$) in G1 CHC (Table 5 medium), and with virological status (OR 13.757, CI 1.013–189.931, $p = 0.04$), and IR (OR 3.096, CI 2.050–34.220, $p = 0.01$) in CHB (Table 5 bottom) patients.

Discussion

In a large cohort of patients with an histological diagnosis of CLD, other than to confirm the independent association between higher γ-GT serum levels and severity of liver fibrosis, we showed that, IR is independently associated with severe fibrosis only in patients with abnormal γ-GT values, without differences according to the metabolic (NAFLD) or viral (HCV or HBV) etiology of the underlying liver disease.

In patients with CLD the severity of liver fibrosis is the strongest predictor of liver related morbidity and mortality, being, in a context of genetic predisposition, IR and liver necroinflammation two of the most important factors associated with the severity and the progression of liver disease [3–8]. Specifically, IR has been clearly associated with fibrosis severity in NAFLD and CHC patients, while contrasting data exist in CHB. In our study, we confirmed both IR and liver necroinflammation as independently

Table 1. Demographic, Clinical, Biochemical, and Histological Features of 843 Patients with Metabolic and Viral Chronic Liver Diseases, According to the Etiology and to γ-glutamiltranspherase Serum Levels.

Variable	Non-alcoholic Fatty Liver Disease N = 193			Genotype 1 Chronic Hepatitis C N = 481			Chronic Hepatitis B N = 169		
	normal γGT (n = 97)	abnormal γGT (n = 96)	P value	normal γGT n = 273	abnormal γGT n = 208	P value	normal γGT n = 134	abnormal γGT n = 35	P value
Mean age – yrs	44.7±13.6	46.7±13.2	0.31	51.9±12.1	54.2±11.8	0.03	38.6±13.7	46.7±13.1	0.002
Male Gender	78	50	<0.001	131	111	0.24	102	21	0.05
Mean body mass index – kg/m^2	30.0±4.5	29.5±4.8	0.42	26.2±4.2	26.7±4.1	0.22	25.4±3.2	26.0±3.3	0.37
Alanine aminotransferase – IU/L	70.0±56.7	89.2±52.9	0.01	61.7±38.2	128.4±128.8	<0.001	93.7±94.9	138.5±99.5	0.01
γ-glutamiltranspherase –IU/L	32.8±13.7	155.9±143.2	<0.001	27.5±13.4	135.4±155.5	<0.001	28.5±13.3	83.5±46.9	<0.001
Cholesterol – mg/Dl	192.8±42.0	217.0±49.9	<0.001	175.9±36.0	173.8±36.4	0.53	185.2±39.1	211.7±57.7	0.01
Triglycerides – mg/dL	136.4±69.8	161.9±83.1	0.02	88.2±40.0	107.2±49.1	<0.001	96.7±33.2	117.2±66.6	0.01
Blood glucose – mg/dL	97.4±23.0	101.1±37.8	0.41	92.9±25.4	103.7±42.3	0.001	88.5±16.8	98.0±28.5	0.01
Insulin – μU/mL	16.3±18.5	18.2±11.8	0.20	12.3±8.9	14.1±7.5	0.02	10.0±6.9	12.0±8.0	0.15
HOMA-score	4.05±2.95	4.73±3.93	0.18	2.97±2.23	3.56±2.64	0.001	2.21±1.60	3.02±2.37	0.01
Insulin Resistance	44	49	0.43	98	115	<0.001	29	13	0.05
Type 2 diabetes	17	16	0.84	29	40	0.008	3	3	0.07
Stage of Fibrosis*									
0	22	25		22	11		7	1	
1	30	22		79	42		46	11	
2	28	18		131	69		55	5	
3	15	20		29	48		18	8	
4	2	11	0.04	12	38	<0.001	8	10	0.001

Data are given as mean ± SD or as number of cases. Yrs, indicates years; HOMA, homeostasis model assessment. * Kleiner score for non-alcoholic fatty liver disease patients, and Scheuer score for genotype 1 chronic hepatitis C, and chronic hepatitis B patients.

Table 2. Univariate and Multivariate Analysis of Risk Factors Associated with Severe Fibrosis (F3–F4) in 843 Patients with Metabolic and Viral Chronic Liver Diseases by Logistic Regression Analysis.

Variable	No Severe Fibrosis (F0–F2)	Severe Fibrosis (F3–F4)	Univariate Analysis *p* value	Multivariate Analysis OR (95% CI) *p* value
Non-alcoholic Fatty Liver Disease				
	n = 144	**n = 49**		
Age - yrs	42.9±12.6	54.0±12.3	<0.001	1.063 (1.028–1.100) <0.001
Male Gender	104	40	0.003	1.079 (0.457–2.546) 0.86
Body Mass Index - Kg/m2	29.3±4.7	31.1±4.2	0.01	1.044 (0.948–1.150) 0.37
Abnormal γ-GT	65	31	0.02	2.711 (1.120–6.564) 0.02
Insulin Resistance	57	36	<0.001	2.749 (1.153–6.556) 0.02
Histology at Biopsy				
Lobular Inflammation 0/1/2/3	11/84/46/3	0/12/32/5	<0.001	4.531 (2.244–9.147) <0.001
Genotype 1 Chronic Hepatitis C				
	n = 354	**n = 127**		
Age - yrs	51.1±12.3	57.8±9.5	<0.001	1.044 (1.022–1.067) <0.001
Male Gender	185	54	0.06	0.639 (0.397–1.028) 0.07
Abnormal γ-GT	122	86	<0.001	3.461 (2.138–5.603) <0.001
Cholesterol - mg/Dl	178.1±34.9	166.5±38.2	<0.001	0.991 (0.984–0.998) 0.01
Insulin Resistance	133	80	<0.001	1.688 (1.043–2.731) 0.03
Histology at Biopsy				
Steatosis grade 0/1/2/3	198/118/32/6	43/50/28/6	<0.001	1.275 (0.950–1.711) 0.10
Grading 1 vs 2–3	92/262	6/121	<0.001	5.767 (2.327–14.289) <0.001
Chronic Hepatitis B				
	n = 125	**n = 44**		
Age - yrs	37.0±13.6	49.4±10.8	<0.001	1.044 (1.003–1.088) 0.03
Abnormal γ-GT	17	18	<0.001	2.778 (1.041–7.414) 0.04
Virological status				
HBe+/HBe−/HBe-Anti-HDV+	26/94/5	2/33/9	<0.001	3.303 (1.229–8.877) 0.01
Insulin Resistance	105/20	22/22	<0.001	2.405 (1.038–6.197) 0.04
Histology at Biopsy				
Steatosis grade 0/1/2/3	88/30/7/0	14/25/3/2	<0.001	1.929 (0.978–3.804) 0.07
Grading 1 vs 2–3	50/75	3/41	<0.001	7.326 (1.690–31.754) 0.008

Data are given as mean±SD or as number of cases. Yrs, indicates years; γ-GT, γ-glutamiltranspherase.

related to the severity of liver fibrosis in patients with NAFLD and CHC, adding data pros this association in CHB.

In our study, we identified in high γ-GT serum levels a risk factor for severe fibrosis. This feature is in accord not only to when highlighted by other authors in NASH [19], and to the evidences about an association between γ-GT serum levels reduction and regression of liver damage in NAFLD patients after bariatric surgery [20], but also to different studies showing an independent link between higher γ-GT serum levels and severity of fibrosis in both CHC [21] and CHB patients [22], and potentially to the role of γ-GT serum levels as predictor of all-cause deaths, including liver-related death [20]. Interestingly, in our cohort, the presence of abnormal γ-GT, had a NPV of more than 80% for rule-out severe fibrosis in all patients, independently of the aetiology of liver disease. This data is encouraging, even if, in clinical practice, we are not confident to suggest to use γ-GT as a single test to predict or rule-out fibrosis severity, but as a potential useful component of noninvasive scores.

Considering therefore the association between γ-GT and liver disease severity, the evidences about a link between γ-GT values and metabolic alterations, like visceral obesity, diabetes, etc, in both cross-sectional and prospective studies [15,16], and also observed in our population, and the sometime contrasting evidences on the role of IR in liver disease severity [4,9,10] and in NAFLD treatment [11,12], we speculated that discriminating NAFLD patients according to normal or abnormal γ-GT values, we can identify different patterns of liver disease where metabolic alterations, and in particular IR, could have a different

Table 3. Diagnostic performance of GGT in predicting severe liver fibrosis.

AUC of variables for severe liver fibrosis prediction

	AUC	C.I. 95%	p*
	Non-alcoholic fatty liver disease		
γ-GT	0.574	0.484–0.664	–
Age	0.739	0.654–0.834	0.009
HOMA	0.752	0.670–0.834	0.004
	Chronic Hepatitis C		
γ-GT	0.712	0.661–0.764	–
Age	0.659	0.606–0.712	0.16
HOMA	0.615	0.556–0.673	0.007
Total cholesterol	0.607	0.562–0.651	0.01
	Chronic Hepatitis B		
γ-GT	0.770	0.696–0.845	–
Age	0.759	0.683–0.836	0.81
HOMA	0.693	0.598–0.787	0.007

PPV and NPV of abnormal/normal γ-GT for predicting severe liver fibrosis

	PPV (%)	NPV (%)
NAFLD	**32.2**	**81.4**
CHC	**41.3**	**84.9**
CHB	**51.4**	**80.5**

HOMA, homeostasis model assessment; γ-GT, γ-glutamiltranspherase; PPV, positive predictive value; NPV, negative predictive value. * p value of corresponding AUC compared to γ-GT AUC (pairwise comparison).

impact. In this line, for the first time to our knowledge, we found that, while classical host and viral risk factors were confirmed as independently linked to the severity of liver fibrosis in NAFLD, CHC and CHB patients with high or normal γ-GT values, by contrast IR remained significantly associated with liver fibrosis only in patients with abnormal γ-GT levels nevertheless similar HOMA values were observed in those with normal or high γ-GT levels, and independently of the etiology of the underlying liver disease.

Although this study was not designed to clarify this interesting finding, a few hypotheses may be put forward according to the literature. A German cohort study found that hepatic steatosis is a significant predictor of all-cause and cardiac-related mortality in men only when it was associated with high γ-GT levels [30]. Another population Italian study also showed that, considering a non-invasive index for steatosis diagnosis (fatty liver index) composed by different metabolic traits including γ-GT, only γ-GT was predictive of all-cause mortality in a context of presence of other metabolic alterations [31]. Finally it has recently been described that serum γ-GT levels have shared genetic determinants which may include the b-2 adrenergic receptor gene [32] and loci interacting with cardiometabolic disease alterations [33]. Overall these data could suggest that γ-GT, in a context of metabolic disturbances, may reflect genetic and metabolic determinants which are associated with poorer outcomes. In this line, according to these data and to our findings on patients with CLD due to metabolic or viral ones, it should be possible to speculate that high γ-GT levels identify a group of liver patients whit a metabolic milieu probably also influenced by genetic background, and able to participate in liver damage affecting the severity of disease. Instead normal γ-GT levels probably identify another group of patients with CLD where metabolic alterations, and in particular IR, even if present, have not a dominant role in affecting disease severity. By contrast in these patients conventional risk factors, like liver inflammation, are the main determinant of disease severity, suggesting a potential dominant role of inflammatory genetic background. In this line we recently reported that IL28B polymorphisms are able to affect severity of liver inflammation in NAFLD patients independently of metabolic alterations [34].

From a clinical standpoint, the identification of these two different patterns of CLD according to γ-GT values, could be useful in the management of these patients. In fact overall our results might also suggest to evaluate if γ-GT can identify NAFLD, CHC and CHB patients at different liver disease progression risk and with different natural history, or where the correction of IR is of further help. In this line our data could help to better understand because: 1) IR is associated with fibrosis severity in a great proportion but not in all studies on CHC patients; and 2) very contrasting results exist about the association between IR and severity of fibrosis in CHB. In addition, considering NAFLD, even if is well known that lifestyle correction is the gold standard treatment for these patients [35], conflicting results exist about pharmacologic therapy. In particular literature data showed that insulin sensitizer [11] and antioxidant drugs [12] could improve liver histological damage, but only in a proportion of NAFLD patients. The discrimination of NAFLD patients according to γ-GT values could therefore help to distinguish patients more sensitive to an approach (lifestyle and/or pharmacological)

Table 4. Univariate and Multivariate Analysis of Risk Factors Associated with Severe Fibrosis (F3–F4) in 504 Patients with Metabolic and Viral Chronic Liver Disease and normal GGT values, by Logistic Regression Analysis.

Variable	No Severe Fibrosis (F0–F2)	Severe Fibrosis (F3–F4)	Univariate Analysis *p* value	Multivariate Analysis OR (95% CI) *p* value
Non-alcoholic Fatty Liver Disease				
	n = 79	**n = 18**		
Mean age – yrs	42.5±13.1	54.6±11.1	0.01	1.070 (1.013–1.129) 0.01
Male Gender	12	7	0.02	2.132 (0.538–8.458) 0.28
Mean body mass index – kg/m²	29.6±4.5	31.8±3.9	0.05	1.028 (0.881–1.199) 0.72
Insulin Resistance	32	12	0.04	2.555 (0.671–9.727) 0.16
Histology				
Lobular inflammation 0/1/2/3	3/45/28/3	0/4/13/1	0.02	3.215 (1.150–8.987) 0.02
Genotype 1 Chronic Hepatitis C				
	n = 232	**n = 41**		
Age – yrs	50.9±12.3	57.3±8.5	0.002	1.034 (1.001–1.070) 0.04
Male Gender	100	31	<0.001	0.295 (0.129–0.673) 0.004
Cholesterol – mg/Dl	179.5±35.5	155.6±31.8	<0.001	0.981 (0.969–0.993) 0.003
Insulin Resistance	76	22	0.01	1.331 (0.613–2.889) 0.46
Histology at Biopsy				
Steatosis grade 0/1/2/3	148/71/11/2	18/16/6/1	0.02	1.605 (0.910–2.830) 0.10
Grading 1 vs 2–3	60/172	3/38	0.009	3.143 (0.873–11.316) 0.08
Chronic Hepatitis B				
	n = 108	**n = 26**		
Age – yrs	36.5±13.5	47.1±11.6	<0.001	1.037 (0.992–1.085) 0.10
Virological status				
HBe+/HBe−/HBe-Anti-HDV+	22/81/5	1/20/5	0.009	2.666 (0.879–8.087) 0.08
Insulin Resistance	19	10	0.02	1.383 (0.460–4.155) 0.56
Histology at Biopsy				
Steatosis grade 0/1/2/3	76/27/5/0	10/14/2/0	0.009	1.917 (0.831–4.425) 0.12
Grading 1 vs 2–3	46/62	1/25	<0.001	15.985 (1.894–134.892) 0.01

Data are given as mean ± SD or as number of cases. Yrs, indicates years; γ-GT, γ-glutamiltranspherase.

aimed to correct metabolic dysfunctions, to patients more sensitive to drugs acting on oxidative stress and liver inflammation. Our hypotheses would seem to suggest using γ-GT as a way of stratify NAFLD patients in intervention trials, even if, clearly, further studies must be done, in diverse settings and with larger cohorts of patients, before applying this method in clinical practice.

The main limitation of this study lies in its cross-sectional nature, making it impossible to dissect the temporal relation among γ-GT values, liver fibrosis, and both metabolic and liver inflammatory findings in patients with CLD. A further methodological question is the potentially limited external validity of the results for different populations and settings. Our study included a cohort of Italian patients enrolled at a tertiary care center, who may be different from the majority of cases of CLD in the general population. In particular we enrolled patients with abnormal ALT levels and, for CHC and CHB, with a high viral load; therefore our results could be applied only to this setting of patients and not to those with a milder liver disease. An hidden alcohol abuse, and lack of data on genetic polymorphisms affecting CLD severity and γ-GT serum levels may also have affected interpretation of the results.

In conclusion, we confirmed γ-GT serum levels as a marker of fibrosis in patients with CLD useful to be included in noninvasive scores, and observed that IR is independently linked to liver fibrosis only in patients with abnormal γ-GT values, without differences according to the metabolic (NAFLD) or viral (HCV or HBV) etiology of the underlying liver disease, and suggesting a role of γ-GT as a marker of metabolic-induced liver damage. These data need further validation in independent, large scale studies, potentially representing an useful tools for the clinical and pharmacologic management of patients with CLD.

Table 5. Univariate and Multivariate Analysis of Risk Factors Associated with Severe Fibrosis (F3–F4) in 339 Patients with chronic liver disease (Chronic Hepatitis C, Non-alcoholic Fatty Liver Disease and Chronic Hepatitis B) and abnormal GGT values, by Logistic Regression Analysis.

Variable	No Severe Fibrosis (F0–F2)	Severe Fibrosis (F3–F4)	Univariate Analysis *p* value	Multivariate Analysis OR (95% CI) *p* value
Non-alcoholic Fatty Liver Disease				
	n = 65	n = 31		
Mean age - yrs	43.6±11.5	49.7±14.2	0.02	1.061 (1.015–1.111) 0.01
Mean body mass index - kg/m^2	28.9±4.9	30.7±4.3	0.08	1.046 (0.911–1.201) 0.52
Cholesterol - mg/Dl	225.6±49.3	200.4±47.6	0.02	0.982 (0.968–0.996) 0.01
Insulin Resistance	25	24	<0.001	4.150 (1.079–15.970) 0.03
Histology				
Lobular inflammation 0/1/2/3	8/39/18/0	0/8/19/4	<0.001	6.824 (2.228–20.904) 0.001
Genotype 1 Chronic Hepatitis C				
	n = 122	n = 86		
Age - yrs	51.6±12.3	58.0±10.0	<0.001	1.049 (1.020–1.079) 0.001
Insulin Resistance	65/57	28/58	0.003	2.250 (1.211–4.181) 0.01
Histology at Biopsy				
Grading 1 vs 2–3	32/90	3/83	<0.001	8.970 (2.559–31.447) 0.001
Chronic Hepatitis B				
	n = 17	n = 18		
Virological status				
HBe+/HBe−/HBe-Anti-HDV+	4/13/0	1/13/4	0.05	13.757 (1.013–189.931) 0.04
Insulin Resistance	16/1	6/12	<0.001	3.096 (2.050–34.220) 0.01
Histology at Biopsy				
Steatosis grade 0/1/2/3	12/13/2/0	4/11/1/2	0.01	1.706 (0.316–9.209) 0.53

Data are given as mean ± SD or as number of cases. Yrs, indicates years; γ-GT, γ-glutamiltranspherase.

Author Contributions

Conceived and designed the experiments: SP CC VD AC. Performed the experiments: FSM MRB DC. Analyzed the data: SP. Wrote the paper: SP.

References

1. Herzer K, Sprinzl MF, Galle PR (2007) Hepatitis viruses: Live and let die. Liver Int 27: 293–301.
2. Petta S, Muratore C, Craxì A (2009) Non-alcoholic fatty liver disease pathogenesis: the present and the future. Dig Liver Dis 41: 615–25.
3. Petta S, Craxì A (2010) Hepatocellular carcinoma and non-alcoholic fatty liver disease: from a clinical to a molecular association. Curr Pharm Des 16: 741–52.
4. Petta S, Amato M, Cabibi D, Cammà C, Di Marco V, et al (2010) Visceral adiposity index is associated with histological findings and high viral load in patients with chronic hepatitis C due to genotype 1. Hepatology 52: 1543–52.
5. Cammà C, Petta S (2009) Insulin resistance in HCV mono-infected and in HIV/HCV co-infected patients: Looking to the future. J Hepatol 50: 648–51.
6. Petta S, Cammà C, Di Marco V, Alessi N, Cabibi D, et al (2008) Insulin resistance and diabetes increase fibrosis in the liver of patients with genotype 1 HCV infection. Am J Gastroenterol 103: 1136–44.
7. Everhart JE, Lok AS, Kim HY, Morgan TR, Lindsay KL, et al (2009) HALT-C Trial Group. Weight-related effects on disease progression in the hepatitis C antiviral long-term treatment against cirrhosis trial. Gastroenterology 137: 549–57.
8. Petta S, Cammà C, Di Marco V, Macaluso FS, Maida M, et al (2011) Hepatic steatosis and insulin resistance are associated with severe fibrosis in patients with chronic hepatitis caused by HBV or HCV infection. Liver Int 31: 507–15.
9. Cammà C, Bruno S, Di Marco V, Di Bona D, Rumi M, et al (2006) Insulin resistance is associated with steatosis in nondiabetic patients with genotype 1 chronic hepatitis C. Hepatology 43: 64–71.
10. Park SH, Kim DJ, Lee HY (2009) Insulin resistance is not associated with histologic severity in nondiabetic, noncirrhotic patients with chronic hepatitis B virus infection. Am J Gastroenterol 104: 1135–9.
11. Belfort R, Harrison SA, Brown K, Darland C, Finch J, et al (2006) A Placebo-Controlled Trial of Pioglitazone in Subjects with Nonalcoholic Steatohepatitis. NEJM 355;22997–2307.
12. Sanyal AJ, Chalasani N, Kowdley KV, McCullough A, Diehl AM, et al (2010) Pioglitazone, Vitamin E, or Placebo for Nonalcoholic Steatohepatitis. NEJM 362: 1675–85.
13. Nemesanszky E, Lott JA (1985) Gamma-glutamyltransferase and its isoenzymes: progress and problems. Clin Chem 31: 797–803.

14. Whitfield JB. Gamma glutamyl transferase (2001) Crit Rev Clin Lab Sci 38: 263–355.
15. Lee DS, Evans JC, Robins SJ, Wilson PW, Albano I, et al (2007) Gamma glutamyl transferase and metabolic syndrome, cardiovascular disease, and mortality risk: the Framingham Heart Study. Arterioscler Thromb Vasc Biol 27: 127–133.
16. Lee DH, Jacobs DR Jr, Gross M, Kiefe CI, Roseman J, et al (2003) Gammaglutamyltransferase is a predictor of incident diabetes and hypertension: the Coronary Artery Risk Development in Young Adults (CARDIA) Study. Clin Chem 49: 1358–1366.
17. Kazemi-Shirazi L, Endler G, Winkler S, Schickbauer T, Wagner O, et al (2007) Gamma glutamyltransferase and long-term survival: is it just the liver? Clin Chem 53: 940–946.
18. Jo SK, Lee WY, Rhee EJ, Won JC, Jung CH, et al (2009) Serum gamma-glutamyl transferase activity predicts future development of metabolic syndrome defined by 2 different criteria. Clin Chim Acta 403: 234–40.
19. Leite NC, Villela-Nogueira CA, Pannain VL, Bottino AC, Rezende GF, et al (2011) Histopathological stages of nonalcoholic fatty liver disease in type 2 diabetes: prevalences and correlated factors. Liver Int 31: 700–6.
20. Dixon JB, Bhathal PS, O'Brien PE (2006) Weight loss and non-alcoholic fatty liver disease: falls in gamma-glutamyl transferase concentrations are associated with histologic improvement. Obes Surg 16: 1278–1286.
21. Poynard T, Imbert-Bismut F, Ratziu V, Chevret S, Jardel C, et al (2002) Biochemical markers of liver fibrosis in patients infected by hepatitis C virus: longitudinal validation in a randomized trial. J Viral Hepat 9: 128–33.
22. Seto WK, Lee CF, Lai CL, Ip PP, Fong DY, et al (2011) A new model using routinely available clinical parameters to predict significant liver fibrosis in chronic hepatitis B. PLoS One 6(8): e23077.
23. American Diabetes Association. Report of the Expert Committee on the diagnosis and classification of diabetes mellitus (2000) American Diabetes Association: Clinical Practice Recommendations 2000 Committee Report. Diabetes Care 23: S4–19.
24. Matthews DR, Hosker JP, Rudenski AS, Naylor BA, Treacher DF, et al (1985) Homeostasis model assessment: insulin resistance and beta-cell function from fasting plasma glucose and insulin concentrations in man. Diabetologia 28: 412–419.
25. Ikeda Y, Suehiro T, Nakamura T, Kumon Y, Hashimoto K (2001) Clinical significance of the insulin resistance index as assessed by homeostasis model assessment. Endocr J 48: 81–86.
26. Moucari R, Asselah T, Cazals-Hatem D, Voitot H, Boyer N, et al (2008) Insulin resistance in chronic hepatitis C: association with genotypes 1 and 4, serum HCV RNA level, and liver fibrosis. Gastroenterology 134: 416–23.
27. Kleiner DE, Brunt EM, Van Natta M, Behling C, Contos MJ, et al (2005) Design and validation of a histological scoring system for nonalcoholic fatty liver disease. Hepatology 411: 313–321.
28. Scheuer PJ (1991) Classification of chronic viral hepatitis: a need for reassessment. J Hepatol 13: 372–4.
29. SAS Technical Report (1992) SAS/STAT software: changes and enhancement, Release 6.07. Cary, NC: SAS Institute, Inc.
30. Haring R, Wallaschofski H, Nauck M, Dörr M, Baumeister SE, et al (2009) Ultrasonographic hepatic steatosis increases prediction of mortality risk from elevated serum gamma-glutamyl transpeptidase levels. HEPATOLOGY 50: 1403–1411.
31. Calori G, Lattuada G, Ragogna F, Garancini MP, Crosignani P, et al (2011) Fatty liver index (FLI) and mortality: The cremona study at the 15(th) year of follow up. HEPATOLOGY 54: 145–152.
32. Loomba R, Rao F, Zhang L, Khandrika S, Ziegler MG, et al (2010) Genetic covariance between gamma-glutamyl transpeptidase and fatty liver risk factors: role of beta2-adrenergic receptor genetic variation in twins. Gastroenterology 139: 836–845.
33. Middelberg RP, Benyamin B, de Moor MH, Warrington NM, Gordon S, et al (2011) Loci affecting gamma-glutamyl transferase in adults and adolescents show age × SNP interaction and cardiometabolic disease associations. Hum Mol Genet 21: 446–55.
34. Petta S, Grimaudo S, Cammà C, Cabibi D, Di Marco V, et al (2011) IL28B and PNPLA3 Polymorphisms Affect Histological Liver Damage in Patients with Non-alcoholic Fatty Liver Disease. J Hep 2012 56: 1356–62.
35. Promrat K, Kleiner DE, Niemeier HM, Jackvony E, Kearns M, et al (2010) Randomized controlled trial testing the effects of weight loss on nonalcoholic steatohepatitis. Hepatology 51: 121–9.

Decrypting Cryptogenic Hepatocellular Carcinoma: Clinical Manifestations, Prognostic Factors and Long-Term Survival by Propensity Score Model

Chia-Yang Hsu[1,4,7], Yun-Hsuan Lee[1,4], Po-Hong Liu[1,4], Cheng-Yuan Hsia[1,5], Yi-Hsiang Huang[2,4], Han-Chieh Lin[1,4], Yi-You Chiou[1,6], Fa-Yauh Lee[1,4], Teh-Ia Huo[3,4]*

1 Faculty of Medicine, National Yang-Ming University School of Medicine, Taipei, Taiwan, **2** Institute of Clinical Medicine, National Yang-Ming University School of Medicine, Taipei, Taiwan, **3** Institute of Pharmacology, National Yang-Ming University School of Medicine, Taipei, Taiwan, **4** Department of Medicine, Taipei Veterans General Hospital, Taipei, Taiwan, **5** Department of Surgery, Taipei Veterans General Hospital, Taipei, Taiwan, **6** Department of Radiology, Taipei Veterans General Hospital, Taipei, Taiwan, **7** Department of Biostatistics, UCLA, Los Angeles, California, United States of America

Abstract

Background and Aims: The clinical aspects of cryptogenic hepatocellular carcinoma (HCC), defined as HCC in patients without hepatitis B, C or alcoholism, are not clear. We investigated its clinical presentations, long-term survival and prognostic predictors.

Methods: A total of 2645 HCC patients were studied. One-to-one matched pairs between viral/alcoholic and cryptogenic HCC patients were generated by using the propensity model. The survival analysis was performed with the Kaplan-Meier method and log-rank test, and hazard ratios were calculated with Cox proportional hazards model.

Results: Among 366 (14%) patients with cryptogenic HCC, 34% of patients were presented with abdominal discomfort, and 31% of patients were identified incidentally. Compared to patients with viral/alcoholic HCC, cryptogenic HCC patients were significantly older ($p<0.0001$), with poorer performance status ($p=0.0031$) and less often underwent curative treatment ($p=0.0041$). They also had larger tumor burden ($p<0.0001$), poorer renal function ($p<0.0001$), lower α-fetoprotein level ($p<0.0001$), and more advanced Barcelona Clinic Liver Cancer stages ($p<0.0001$). With propensity score model, 366 pairs of similar HCC patients were selected and similar long-term survival between the two groups of patients was found ($p=0.1038$). For cryptogenic HCC patients, α-fetoprotein $\geq$49 ng/mL (hazard ratio [HR]: 1.955, $p=0.0002$), Child-Turcotte-Pugh class B/C (HR: 2.798, $p<0.0001$), performance status $\geq$1 (HR: 2.463, $p<0.0001$) and vascular invasion (HR: 1.608, $p=0.0257$) were independent predictors of poor prognosis.

Conclusions: Patients with cryptogenic HCC are usually diagnosed with poor general condition at late stages. However, cryptogenic HCC patients have similar prognostic predictors and long-term survival compared with viral/alcoholic HCC patients. Diagnosis at an early stage may improve their clinical outcomes.

Editor: Isabelle A. Chemin, CRCL-INSERM, France

Funding: This study was supported by grants from the Center of Excellence for Cancer Research at Taipei Veterans General Hospital (DOH102-TD-C-111-007), Taiwan, from Taipei Veterans General Hospital (V102C-012), Taipei, Taiwan, and from the Ministry of Education, Aim for the Top University Plan (101AC-D101), Taiwan. The funders had no role in study design, data collection and analysis, decision to publish, or preparation of the manuscript.

Competing Interests: The authors have declared that no competing interests exist.

* E-mail: tihuo@vghtpe.gov.tw

Introduction

Hepatocellular carcinoma (HCC) is one of the most common malignant neoplasms worldwide [1]. For patients diagnosed at early stages, curative treatments including surgical resection, percutaneous ablation and transplantation provide the chance of long-term remission with 5-year survival rate of up to 75% [1]. Unfortunately, for symptomatic patients, the majority of them are not suitable to undergo aggressive treatments because of poor hepatic reserve or overwhelming tumor burden. Most of them receive palliative treatments such as transarterial chemoembolization (TACE), targeted therapy and best palliative management to prolong survival or improve the quality of life [2,3].

Hepatitis B, hepatitis C and alcoholic hepatitis are common chronic liver diseases which could result in liver cirrhosis and HCC. Hepatitis B is the major risk factor of HCC in Asia and Africa, whereas hepatitis C is the predominant etiology in Japan and Western countries [4]. In the past decade, the importance of nonalcoholic steatohepatitis (NASH) related cirrhosis or HCC has increased gradually due to the obese population in developed countries [5]. However, there is still a substantial portion of HCC patients without definite history of chronic liver disease at the time of diagnosis [6,7]. In countries with high prevalence rate of hepatitis B or C, prevention programs such as hepatitis B vaccination and regular follow-up for chronic liver diseases have been carried out in order to reduce the incidence of HCC [8,9]. As for patients with non-viral and non-alcoholic HCC, there are few studies addressing the adequate surveillance strategy, clinical features or long-term prognosis, and most of them are diagnosed at advanced stages when symptoms surface.

Cryptogenic HCC, defined as non-viral, non-alcoholic HCC and no other known etiology of chronic liver disease, has been seldom systemically studied. In addition, most conclusions were obtained from small HCC cohort and the long-term survival of these patients was not fully examined [10,11]. In this study, we have investigated its clinical presentations, demographic characteristics, and predictors of long-term outcome in a prospectively collected cohort; the survival distributions of patients with cryptogenic or viral/alcoholic HCC were compared in the propensity model.

Patients and Methods

Patients

A prospective database of patients with HCC collected during an 11-year period from 2002 to 2013 at Taipei Veterans General Hospital, Taiwan, formed the basis of this study. A total of 2645 treatment-naïve HCC patients were identified. The baseline information, including patient characteristics, causes of chronic liver disease, serum biochemistry, severity of cirrhosis, performance status and cancer stages, were recorded when the diagnosis was made. Part of the study patients had been enrolled in our previous studies [12,13]. This study has been approved by the institutional review board of Taipei Veterans General Hospital, Taiwan, and complies with the standards of Declaration of Helsinki and current ethical guidelines. All medical records were de-identified prior to analysis.

Diagnosis and Definitions

The diagnosis of HCC was based on the findings of typical radiological characteristics in at least two imaging modalities including ultrasound, hepatic arterial angiography, magnetic resonance (MR) imaging and contrast-enhanced dynamic computed tomography (CT); or histologically confirmed or by a single positive imaging technique accompanied with serum α-fetoprotein (AFP) level >400 ng/mL [14,15]. Alcoholism was diagnosed in patients with daily consumption of at least 40 g of alcohol for 5 years or more [16]. Patients were considered to have hepatitis C virus (HCV) infection if they were seropositive for antibody against HCV (anti-HCV) by a second-generation enzyme immunoassay (Abbott Laboratories). Hepatitis B virus (HBV) infection was diagnosed if hepatitis B surface antigen (HBsAg) was found serologically (RIA kits, Abbott Laboratories). Ascites defined as free peritoneal fluid was discovered by abdominal sonography, CT or MR imaging [17]. Performance status was determined at entry according to the Eastern Cooperative Oncology Group (ECOG) criteria [18].

The estimated glomerular filtration rate (eGFR) was calculated by using the modification of diet in renal disease formula [19]. Vascular invasion was diagnosed by contrast-enhanced imaging modalities. Total tumor volume was calculated according to mathematical equations as described in our previous studies [20].

Treatment

Surgical resection, transplantation and percutaneous ablation (acetic or ethanol acid injection and radiofrequency ablation) were collectively classified as curative treatment in this study [21]. TACE, targeted therapy, systemic chemotherapy and best supportive care were classified as non-curative treatment [22].

Propensity Score Analysis

To compare the overall survival between patients with viral/alcoholic and cryptogenic HCC in a prospectively collected cohort, a propensity score model and greedy algorithm matching without replacement were used with an attempt to reduce potential biases in survival analysis [23,24]. Possible variables associated with long-term survival of HCC patients, including age, sex, tumor burden, severity of cirrhosis, performance status, vascular invasion, renal function, AFP, curative treatments, the Barcelona-Clinic Liver Cancer (BCLC) and Cancer of the Liver Italian Program (CLIP) staging systems were included comprehensively for propensity score generation. With these selected variables, a logistic regression was applied to generate a continuous propensity score from 0 to 1. One-to-one matches between patients with viral/alcoholic and cryptogenic HCC were introduced into the subsequent analysis.

Statistics

Categorical data were compared with chi-squared test between patients with viral/alcoholic and cryptogenic HCC. Continuous demographic characteristics were compared with Mann-Whitney ranked sum test. The comparison of survival distribution was performed by the Kaplan-Meier method with a log-rank test. For prognostic predictor analysis, continuous variables were split by the median or clinically meaningful cut-off values and treated as dichotomous covariates. Each possible prognostic predictor was tested by the Kaplan-Meier method initially; and factors which were significant in the univariate analysis were introduced into the multivariate Cox proportional hazards model to calculate the adjusted hazard ratios. A p value was considered statistically significant when it was less than 0.05. All statistical analyses were conducted with the SAS 9.0 (SAS institute, North Carolina).

Results

Patients Characteristics

Patients were classified as cryptogenic HCC if there was no evidence of hepatitis B, hepatitis C or alcoholism-related HCC. In addition, 10 patients with known etiologies of chronic liver disease such as primary biliary cirrhosis, hemochromatosis, and Wilson's disease were excluded. A total of 366 (14%) cryptogenic HCC patients were identified. As shown in Table 1, cryptogenic HCC patients were significantly older ($p<0.0001$), with poorer performance status ($p=0.0031$) and poorer renal function ($p<0.0001$). They also had significantly larger tumor size and total tumor volume (both $p<0.0001$), advanced BCLC stages ($p<0.0001$) and more often to receive non-curative therapy ($p=0.0041$).

For patients with viral/alcoholic HCC, they had more tumor nodules ($p=0.0043$), higher serum bilirubin and AFP levels (both $p<0.0001$) and longer prothrombin time ($p<0.0001$). Otherwise there were no significant differences in gender ($p=0.9619$), Child-Turcotte-Pugh (CTP) classification ($p=0.8538$), prevalence of ascites and vascular invasion ($p=0.7662$ and 0.9441), serum levels of albumin and sodium ($p=0.1617$ and 0.7036) and the CLIP score ($p=0.1225$) between viral/alcoholic and cryptogenic HCC patients.

Primary Presentations

As indicated in Table 2, one-third (34%) of cryptogenic HCC patients were presented to the hospital due to abdominal discomfort, including dull or sharp pain, and fullness sensation over upper abdomen. The second most common presentation was incidental finding (31%), which was so defined that the diagnosis of HCC was made during medical management not related to

Table 1. Comparison of demographic characteristics between patients with cryptogenic HCC and viral/alcoholic HCC.

Variables	Viral and alcoholic HCC (n = 2269)	Cryptogenic HCC (n = 366)	P
Age (years, mean ± SD)	63±13	72±13	<0.0001
Male (%)	1757 (77)	283 (77)	0.9619
Chronic liver disease			
Positive HBsAg (%)	1456 (64)	0	
Positive anti-HCV (%)	810 (36)	0	
HBV+HCV (%)	116 (5)	0	
Alcoholism (%)	447 (20)	0	
CTP class A (%)	1641 (72)	263 (72)	0.8538
Ascites (%)	554 (24)	92 (25)	0.7662
Tumor size ≥ 3 cm (%)	1496 (67)	289 (79)	<0.0001
Multiple tumors (%)	929 (41)	121 (33)	0.0043
Tumor volume (cm^3, median)	357±711 (44)	466±793 (144)	<0.0001
Performance status 0 (%)	1340 (59)	186 (51)	0.0031
Vascular invasion (%)	655 (29)	105 (29)	0.9441
Biochemistry (mean ± SD)			
Albumin (g/dL)	3.7±0.6	3.7±0.7	0.1617
Bilirubin (mg/dL)	1.6±2.8	1.3±2.2	<0.0001
Creatinine (mg/dL)	1.2±1.1	1.3±0.8	<0.0001
INR of PT	1.09±0.2	1.05±0.2	<0.0001
Sodium (mmol/L)	138±3.9	138±4.1	0.7036
Estimated GFR (mL/min/1.73 m^2)	77±32 (75)	66±28 (64)	<0.0001
AFP (ng/mL, median)	26,823±252,893 (57)	20,958±158,676 (14)	<0.0001
BCLC stage 0/A/B/C/D (%)	6/23/13/44/14	4/16/16/44/21	<0.0001
CLIP score 0/1/2/3/4/5/6 (%)	27/25/16/12/12/7/2	28/22/14/17/10/7/2	0.1225
Curative treatments (%)	1057 (47)	141 (39)	0.0041

AFP, α-fetoprotein; BCLC, Barcelona Clinic Liver Cancer; CLIP, Cancer of the Liver Italian Program; CTP, Child-Turcotte-Pugh; GFR, glomerular filtration rate; HBV, hepatitis B virus; HCV, hepatitis C virus; INR, international ratio; PT, prothrombin time; SD, standard deviation.
Curative treatments include resection, radiofrequency ablation, percutaneous alcohol/acetic acid injection, and transplantation.

liver disease, or physical check-up for asymptomatic patients without a prior history of liver disease. Systematic presentations including poor appetite (6%), general weakness (6%), body weight loss (3%) and fever (2%) were noted at the time of diagnosis. There were only 21 patients (6%) under regular follow-up programs for non-viral/alcoholic hepatitis related cirrhosis when HCC was diagnosed.

Survival Comparison Between Viral/alcoholic and Cryptogenic HCC Patients

The comparison of long-term survival between viral/alcoholic and cryptogenic HCC patients was given in Fig. 1. During a mean follow-up period of 27±26 months, cryptogenic HCC patients had a significantly shorter survival than did patients with viral/alcoholic etiologies (p = 0.0084).

Characteristics of Patients Selected in the Propensity Model

By using the propensity model, 366 pairs of matched HCC patients were selected (Table 3). Among matched patients stratified by the etiology of HCC, there were no significant differences in age, sex, severity of cirrhosis, tumor burden, performance status, prevalence of ascites and vascular invasion,

Table 2. Primary complaint or presentation at diagnosis of patients with cryptogenic HCC.

Cryptogenic HCC patients (n = 366)	Number (%)
Abdominal discomfort	125 (34)
Incidental finding	112 (31)
Poor appetite	22 (6)
Non-viral, non-alcoholic cirrhosis under regular surveillance	21 (6)
General weakness	21 (6)
Elevated liver enzymes	20 (6)
Body weight loss	10 (3)
Yellowish skin/tea-color urine	8 (2)
Fever	8 (2)
Gastrointestinal bleeding	7 (2)
Lower leg edema	5 (1)
Palpable abdominal mass	4 (1)
Nausea and/or vomiting	3 (1)

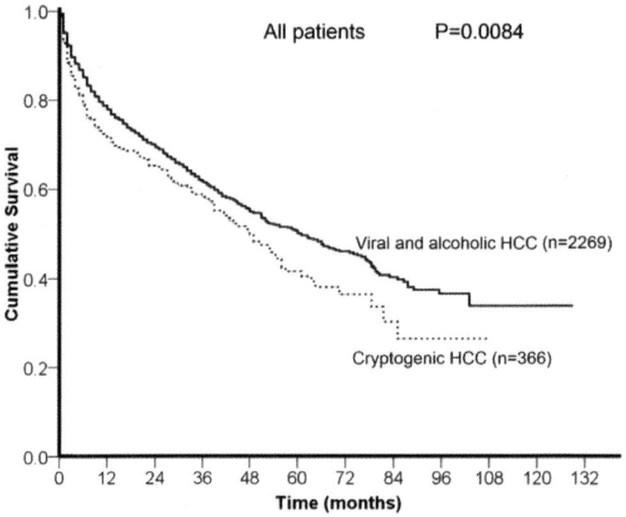

Figure 1. Comparison of the survival distribution between patients with cryptogenic HCC and viral/alcoholic HCC. Cryptogenic HCC patients had a significantly worse survival than viral/alcoholic HCC patients (p = 0.0084).

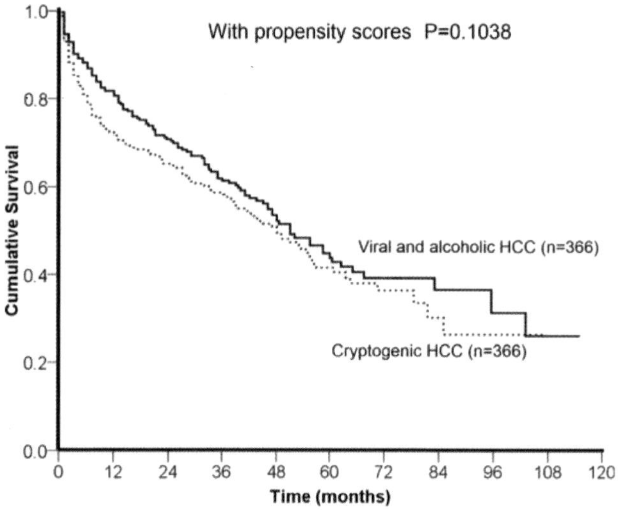

Figure 2. Comparison of the survival distribution of cryptogenic and viral/alcoholic HCC patients in the propensity model. There was no significant difference of overall survival between patients with cryptogenic and viral/alcoholic HCC (p = 0.1038).

renal function, serum AFP level, treatment modalities and the scores of BCLC and CLIP systems (all p>0.05).

Survival Analysis in the Propensity Model

During a mean follow-up period of 26±25 months, the comparison of long-term survival between patients with viral/alcoholic and cryptogenic HCC showed no significant difference in the propensity model (p = 0.1038; Fig. 2).

Predictors of Long-term Survival in Cryptogenic HCC Patients

Potential prognostic predictors including age, gender, number and size of tumor nodules, total tumor volume, CTP class, presence of ascites and vascular invasion, serum AFP level, performance status, renal function, and treatment modalities were examined by using the Kaplan-Meier analysis and log-rank test. Factors associated with decreased overall survival were older age (p = 0.0159), advanced CTP classification (p<0.0001), ascites (p<0.0001), larger tumor size (p = 0.0007), multiple tumors (p = 0.0312), larger tumor volume (p<0.0001), poorer performance status (p<0.0001), vascular invasion (p<0.0001), poorer renal function (p = 0.0005), higher AFP level (p<0.0001), and non-curative treatments (p<0.0001). When these variable were introduced into the Cox proportional hazards model to generate adjusted hazard ratios, four predictive factors, including serum AFP level ≥49 ng/mL (hazard ratio [HR]: 1.955, 95% confidence interval [CI]: 1.371–2.787, p = 0.0002), CTP class B

Table 3. Comparison of demographic characteristics between patients with cryptogenic HCC and viral/alcoholic HCC in the propensity model.

Variables	Viral and alcoholic HCC (n = 366)	Cryptogenic HCC (n = 366)	P
Age ≥ 65 years (%)	273 (75)	273 (75)	1
Male (%)	284 (78)	283 (77)	0.9295
CTP class A (%)	249 (68)	263 (72)	0.2591
Ascites (%)	92 (25)	92 (25)	1
Tumor size ≥ 3 cm (%)	273 (75)	289 (79)	0.1614
Multiple tumors (%)	118 (32)	121 (33)	0.8131
Tumor volume ≥ 50.9 cm^3	231 (63)	236 (64)	0.7006
Performance status 0 (%)	201 (55)	186 (51)	0.2667
Vascular invasion (%)	114 (31)	105 (29)	0.4676
Estimated GFR ≥ 60 mL/min/1.73 m^2	214 (58)	214 (58)	1
AFP ≥ 49 ng/mL	141 (39)	141 (39)	1
BCLC stage 0/A/B/C/D (%)	6/17/17/45/15	4/16/16/44/21	0.2185
CLIP score 0/1/2/3/4/5/6 (%)	28/25/15/12/12/7/1	28/22/14/17/10/7/2	0.5112
Curative treatments (%)	147 (40)	141 (39)	0.6499

Table 4. Independent predictors of poor prognosis in patients with cryptogenic HCC in Cox proportional hazard model.

	Hazard ratio	95% CI	P
Cryptogenic HCC (n = 366)			
AFP ≥ 49 ng/mL	1.955	1.371–2.787	0.0002
CTP class B or C	2.798	1.694–4.621	<0.0001
Performance status ≥ 1	2.463	1.64–3.697	<0.0001
Vascular invasion	1.608	1.059–2.44	0.0257

CI, confidence interval.

or C (HR: 2.798, 95% CI: 1.694–4.621, p<0.0001), performance status ≥1 (HR: 2.463, 95% CI: 1.640–3.697, p<0.0001), and vascular invasion (HR: 1.608, 95% CI: 1.059–2.44, p = 0.0257), were identified as independent predictors of poor prognosis (Table 4).

Discussion

Hepatitis B, hepatitis C and alcoholism are considered three major etiologies of chronic liver diseases that could subsequently result in cirrhosis or HCC. Genetic liver disease, autoimmune liver disease and NASH are also associated with chronic liver injury and various complications. In general, cryptogenic HCC is used to describe HCC in patients without viral/alcoholic hepatitis after other known etiologies such as autoimmune, genetic, toxin-related liver diseases, NASH, Wilson's disease and hemochromatosis are excluded. The prevalence rate, associated factors, and distribution of long-term survival of cryptogenic HCC were not fully investigated due to insufficient case number and variable definitions from different research groups [7,25]. In this study, cryptogenic HCC was diagnosed in 14% of HCC patients from a large prospective patient cohort. Cryptogenic HCC patients usually had poor general condition and larger tumor(s) at the time of diagnosis. After potential biases caused by different baseline characteristics were removed in the propensity model, we found that there was no significant difference of long-term survival between cryptogenic and viral/alcoholic HCC patients. Our results indicate that early diagnosis with effective surveillance program may enhance the survival in these patients.

Small HCC(s) seldom causes clinical symptoms, therefore it is often very difficult to diagnose small HCC(s) in patients without a prior history of liver disease. When clinical symptoms develop, HCC patients are usually presented with large tumor burden and poor general condition. Hence, most of them could only receive non-curative treatments and are associated with a less favorable prognosis [26,27]. In our study, nearly two-thirds of patients with cryptogenic HCC were diagnosed when clinical manifestations were apparent. About 17% of patients presented with systemic symptoms such as poor appetite, weakness, body weight loss and fever. For these patients, it is more challenging for physicians to reach a definite diagnosis. Only 6% of cryptogenic HCC patients were diagnosed under regular chronic liver disease follow-up program. In comparison to patients with viral/alcoholic HCC, who received regular follow-up after the diagnosis of viral hepatitis or alcoholic liver disease was made, patients with cryptogenic HCC often do not receive regular follow-up until symptomatic cirrhosis develop. Advanced cirrhosis *per se* could preclude the possibility of patients with cryptogenic HCC to receive aggressive treatments due to the status of liver decompensation. Taken together, the majority of cryptogenic HCC patients did not receive comprehensive liver studies until symptoms of HCC developed. This could result in delayed diagnosis, limited choice of treatment and poor prognosis.

Comparison of baseline characteristics between viral/alcoholic and cryptogenic HCC (Table 1) highlighted the different compositions in these two groups. Patients with cryptogenic HCC were significantly older and had poorer performance status and renal function; in addition, cryptogenic HCC patients had significantly larger tumor size and total tumor volume. Not surprisingly, cryptogenic HCC patients had more advanced BCLC stages that make curative therapy less likely to perform. Importantly, the analysis of overall survival might be confounded by these crucial baseline differences (Fig. 1). In this study, propensity score analysis with one-to-one nearest neighbor matching selected 366 pairs of similar patients (Table 3). After baseline confounders were removed, the survival analysis showed comparable long-term survival distribution. There findings not only show the evidence of confounding effects caused by larger tumor burden and poor general condition, but also suggest that cryptogenic HCC patients might have an improved prognosis if the diagnosis of HCC could be made earlier.

Patients with viral/alcoholic cirrhosis had significantly higher AFP level, which might be associated with ongoing hepatitis at the time of diagnosis [28,29]; they also had significantly higher serum bilirubin and longer prothrombin time in comparison with cryptogenic HCC patients. However, these differences were not large enough to make an impact on CTP classification. It is noteworthy that more viral/alcoholic HCC patients had multiple tumors in our study. This is possibly because that liver parenchyma in patients with viral/alcoholic HCC suffered from chronic liver injury for decades, and the whole liver may become fertile soil for the development of HCC nodule(s).

Non-alcoholic fatty liver disease (NAFLD), including NASH, has been increasingly considered an underlying cause of HCC [25,30]. However, several reasons make NAFLD-related HCC a difficult-to-diagnose clinical entity: (1) for patients with viral hepatitis and possible simultaneous NAFLD, usually they were classified as viral hepatitis-related HCC, (2) for patients with chronic liver disease, cirrhosis or HCC, most of them did not receive liver biopsy on a routine basis, and (3) with the progression of liver injury, the typical pathologic features of NAFLD/NASH may disappear when cirrhosis develops. For our HCC cohort, which enrolled every patient when the diagnosis of HCC was made, it was difficult to evaluate the presence of NAFLD/NASH even with biopsied or resected liver tissue [31]. Hence, we did not specifically exclude NAFLD-related HCC from cryptogenic HCC in this study, and further studies are required to delineate the role of NASH in cryptogenic HCC.

The prognostic predictors of patients with cryptogenic HCC had not been comprehensively studied due to very limited case number in published literatures. In this study, we have determined the predictors of long-term survival by using a large, prospectively enrolled HCC cohort. High serum AFP level and vascular invasion, which are both associated with large tumor burden, are identified as independent predictors of poor outcome. The association between advanced CTP class and poor survival further discloses the importance of hepatic reserve. In addition, consistent with published series, the multivariate Cox model shows that poor performance status was a strong predictor of decreased long-term survival [18]. These findings suggest that in spite of different underlying etiologies, cryptogenic HCC shares similar prognostic predictors with patients with viral/alcoholic HCC [32,33].

There are a few potential limitations of this study. Firstly, in this study, more than half of our patients had evidence of hepatitis B infection. This feature is distinctly different from countries where hepatitis C infection and NAFLD were the predominant etiologies of chronic liver disease [34]. Secondly, patients with hepatitis B or C might have received anti-viral treatment to suppress viral activity some time during the follow-up period, and this may alter the prognosis [35,36].

In conclusion, our results indicate that cryptogenic HCC are often diagnosed at late stages in older patients. However, cryptogenic HCC is not associated with a poor prognosis after confounding effects are abolished. For these patients, early diagnosis could substantially improve their long-term survival. Our findings also imply that a subset of HCC patients might have a chance to benefit from adequate surveillance program. The optimal surveillance guidelines for this particular patient group need further studies to establish.

Author Contributions

Conceived and designed the experiments: CY.Hsu TIH. Performed the experiments: PHL YHL CY.Hsia YHH HCL. Analyzed the data: CY.Hsu TIH. Contributed reagents/materials/analysis tools: YYC FYL. Wrote the paper: CY.Hsu.

References

1. El-Serag HB, Marrero JA, Rudolph L, Reddy KR (2008) Diagnosis and treatment of hepatocellular carcinoma. Gastroenterology134: 1752–1763.
2. Hsu CY, Hsia CY, Huang YH, Su CW, Lin HC, et al. (2010) Selecting an optimal staging system for hepatocellular carcinoma: comparison of 5 currently used prognostic models. Cancer 116: 3006–3014.
3. Tsai YJ, Hsu CY, Huang YH, Su CW, Lin HC, et al. (2011) Early identification of poor responders to transarterial chemoembolization for hepatocellular carcinoma. Hepatol Int 5: 975–984.
4. Pekow JR, Bhan AK, Zheng H, Chung RT (2007) Hepatic steatosis is associated with increased frequency of hepatocellular carcinoma in patients with hepatitis C-related cirrhosis. Cancer 109: 2490–2496.
5. Neuschwander-Tetri BA, Caldwell SH (2003) Nonalcoholic steatohepatitis: summary of an AASLD Single Topic Conference. Hepatology 37: 1202–1219.
6. Bedogni G, Miglioli L, Masutti F, Tiribelli C, Marchesini G, et al. (2005) Prevalence of and risk factors for nonalcoholic fatty liver disease: the Dionysos nutrition and liver study. Hepatology 42: 44–52.
7. Lee SS, Jeong SH, Byoun YS, Chung SM, Seong MH, et al. (2013) Clinical features and outcome of cryptogenic hepatocellular carcinoma compared to those of viral and alcoholic hepatocellular carcinoma. BMC Cancer 13: 335.
8. Chang CH, Lin JW, Wu LC, Liu CH, Lai MS (2013) National antiviral treatment program and the incidence of hepatocellular carcinoma and associated mortality in Taiwan: a preliminary report. Med Care 51: 908–913.
9. Yeh YP, Hu TH, Cho PY, Chen HH, Yen AM, et al. (2013) Evaluation of abdominal ultrasonography mass screening for hepatocellular carcinoma in Taiwan. Hepatology (in press). doi: 10.1002/hep.26703.
10. Tokushige K, Hashimoto E, Horie Y, Taniai M, Higuchi S (2011) Hepatocellular carcinoma in Japanese patients with nonalcoholic fatty liver disease, alcoholic liver disease, and chronic liver disease of unknown etiology: report of the nationwide survey. J Gastroenterol 46: 1230–1237.
11. Yokoi Y, Suzuki S, Baba S, Inaba K, Konno H, et al. (2005) Clinicopathological features of hepatocellular carcinomas (HCCs) arising in patients without chronic viral infection or alcohol abuse: a retrospective study of patients undergoing hepatic resection. J Gastroenterol 40: 274–282.
12. Lee YH, Hsu CY, Huang YH, Su CW, Lin HC, et al. (2013) Alpha-fetoprotein-to-total tumor volume ratio predicts post-operative tumor recurrence in hepatocellular carcinoma. J Gastrointest Surg 17: 730–738.
13. Lee YH, Hsu CY, Hsia CY, Huang YH, Su CW, et al. (2012) A prognostic model for patients with hepatocellular carcinoma within the Milan criteria undergoing non-transplant therapies, based on 1106 patients. Aliment Pharmacol Ther 36: 551–559.
14. Bruix J, Sherman M, Llovet JM, Beaugrand M, Lencioni R, et al. (2001) Clinical management of hepatocellular carcinoma. Conclusions of the Barcelona-2000 EASL conference. European Association for the Study of the Liver. J Hepatol 35: 421–430.
15. Bruix J, Sherman M (2005) Management of hepatocellular carcinoma. Hepatology 42: 1208–1236.
16. Lee YH, Hsu CY, Hsia CY, Huang YH, Su CW, et al. (2013) Alcoholism worsens the survival of patients with hepatitis B virus and C virus-related hepatocellular carcinoma. Hepatol Int 7: 645–654.
17. Hsu CY, Lee YH, Huang YH, Hsia CY, Su CW, et al. (2013) Ascites in patients with hepatocellular carcinoma: prevalence, associated factors, prognostic impact, and staging strategy. Hepatol Int 7: 188–198.
18. Hsu CY, Lee YH, Hsia CY, Huang YH, Su CW, et al. (2013) Performance status in patients with hepatocellular carcinoma: determinants, prognostic impact, and ability to improve the Barcelona Clinic Liver Cancer system. Hepatology 57: 112–119.
19. Lee YH, Hsu CY, Huang YH, Su CW, Lin HC et al. (2012) Selecting a prognostic renal surrogate for patients with hepatocellular carcinoma undergoing transarterial chemoembolization. J Gastroenterol Hepatol 27: 1581–1588.
20. Hsu CY, Huang YH, Hsia CY, Su CW, Lin HC, et al. (2010) A new prognostic model for hepatocellular carcinoma based on total tumor volume: the Taipei Integrated Scoring System. J Hepatol 53: 108–117.
21. Lin ZZ, Shau WY, Hsu C, Shao YY, Yeh YC, et al. (2013) Radiofrequency ablation is superior to ethanol injection in early-stage hepatocellular carcinoma irrespective of tumor size. PLoS One 8: e80276.
22. Lee S, Kim BK, Kim SU, Park Y, Chang S, et al. (2013) Efficacy of sorafenib monotherapy versus sorafenib-based loco-regional treatments in advanced hepatocellular carcinoma. PloS One 8: e77240.
23. Hsu CY, Lee YH, Hsia CY, Huang YH, Su CW, et al. (2013) Performance status enhances the selection of treatment for patients with hepatocellular carcinoma within the milan criteria. Ann Surg Oncol 20: 2035–2042.
24. Austin PC (2013) A comparison of 12 algorithms for matching on the propensity score. Stat Med (in press). doi: 10.1002/sim.6004.
25. Ertle J, Dechene A, Sowa JP, Penndorf V, Herzer K, et al. (2011) Non-alcoholic fatty liver disease progresses to hepatocellular carcinoma in the absence of apparent cirrhosis. Int J Cancer 128: 2436–2443.
26. Gellert L, Jalaludin B, Levy M (2007) Hepatocellular carcinoma in Sydney South West: late symptomatic presentation and poor outcome for most. Intern Med J 37: 516–522.
27. Lee CS, Sung JL, Hwang LY, Sheu JC, Chen DS, et al. (1986) Surgical treatment of 109 patients with symptomatic and asymptomatic hepatocellular carcinoma. Surgery 99: 481–490.
28. Akuta N, Suzuki F, Kobayashi M, Hara T, Sezaki H, et al. (2014) Correlation between hepatitis B virus surface antigen level and alpha-fetoprotein in patients free of hepatocellular carcinoma or severe hepatitis. J Med Virol 86: 131–138.
29. Gopal P, Yopp AC, Waljee AK, Chiang J, Nehra M, et al. (2013) Factors that Affect Accuracy of alpha-Fetoprotein Test in Detection of Hepatocellular Carcinoma in Patients with Cirrhosis. Clin Gastroenterol Hepatol (in press). doi: 10.1016/j.cgh.2013.09.053.
30. Reddy SK, Steel JL, Chen HW, DeMateo DJ, Cardinal J, et al. (2012) Outcomes of curative treatment for hepatocellular cancer in nonalcoholic steatohepatitis versus hepatitis C and alcoholic liver disease. Hepatology 55: 1809–1819.
31. Caldwell SH, Crespo DM (2004) The spectrum expanded: cryptogenic cirrhosis and the natural history of non-alcoholic fatty liver disease. J Hepatol 40: 578–584.
32. Bruix J, Llovet JM (2002) Prognostic prediction and treatment strategy in hepatocellular carcinoma. Hepatology 35: 519–524.
33. Kao WY, Su CW, Chau GY, Lui WY, Wu CW, et al. (2011) A comparison of prognosis between patients with hepatitis B and C virus-related hepatocellular carcinoma undergoing resection surgery. World J Surg 35: 858–867.
34. Tokushige K, Hashimoto E, Yatsuji S, Tobari M, Taniai M, et al. (2010) Prospective study of hepatocellular carcinoma in nonalcoholic steatohepatitis in comparison with hepatocellular carcinoma caused by chronic hepatitis C. J Gastroenterol 45: 960–967.
35. Kudo M (2011) Adjuvant therapy after curative treatment for hepatocellular carcinoma. Oncology 81 Suppl 1: 50–55.
36. Kubo S, Takemura S, Sakata C, Urata Y, Uenishi T (2013) Adjuvant Therapy after Curative Resection for Hepatocellular Carcinoma Associated with Hepatitis Virus. Liver Cancer 2: 40–46.

Longitudinal Change of HBsAg in HBeAg-negative Patients with Genotype B or C Infection

Tung-Hung Su[1,2,3], Chun-Jen Liu[1,2,3], Tai-Chung Tseng[2,4], Chen-Hua Liu[1,2,3], Hung-Chih Yang[1,5], Chi-Ling Chen[2], Pei-Jer Chen[1,2,3], Jia-Horng Kao[1,2,3*], Ding-Shinn Chen[1,2,3]

1 Department of Internal Medicine, National Taiwan University Hospital, Taipei, Taiwan, **2** Graduate Institute of Clinical Medicine, National Taiwan University College of Medicine, Taipei, Taiwan, **3** Hepatitis Research Center, National Taiwan University Hospital, Taipei, Taiwan, **4** Division of Gastroenterology, Department of Internal Medicine, Buddhist Tzu Chi General Hospital Taipei Branch, Taipei, Taiwan, **5** Department of Microbiology, National Taiwan University College of Medicine, Taipei, Taiwan

Abstract

Background & Aims: Quantitative HBsAg has been recognized to assist in the management of chronic hepatitis B virus (HBV) infection. However, its role in disease monitoring of HBeAg-negative patients remains unclear. We aimed to investigate the longitudinal HBsAg change in HBeAg-negative carriers with HBV genotype B or C infection.

Methods: This is a retrospective cohort study conducted in a university hospital. Treatment-naïve HBeAg-negative carriers followed for more than 3 years were recruited. Their hepatitis activities were categorized by longitudinal HBV-DNA levels into high viral-load (HVL: HBV-DNA >/= 2000 IU/mL persistently), low viral-load (LVL: HBV-DNA <2000 IU/mL persistently) and fluctuated viral-load (FVL: HBV-DNA between HVL and LVL). The baseline and end-of-follow-up (EOF) HBsAg levels were quantified for analyses.

Results: We recruited 187 patients with a median follow-up of 8 years. LVL patients had a significantly lower HBsAg at baseline and EOF and a significantly greater annualized HBsAg decline compared with the FVL and HVL. The longitudinal HBsAg change was independent of genotype B or C. The lower baseline HBsAg level predicted the HBsAg decline and HBsAg loss, whereas the higher baseline HBV-DNA predicted the hepatitis flare. A baseline HBsAg <50 IU/mL predicted subsequent HBsAg loss with a sensitivity of 82% and specificity of 67%. The annualized HBsAg decline appeared non-linear, and accelerated as the HBsAg level lowered (0.054, 0.091, 0.126 $\log_{10}$ IU/mL in patients with baseline HBsAg >1000, 100–999, <100 IU/mL, respectively, P for trend = .014).

Conclusions: In genotype B or C HBeAg-negative carriers, baseline HBsAg levels correlate with future disease activities and help to predict HBsAg decline or loss. Inactive carriers with lower baseline HBsAg levels have a greater and accelerating HBsAg decline over time, regardless of HBV genotypes.

Editor: James Fung, The University of Hong Kong, Hong Kong

Funding: This work was supported by grants from the National Taiwan University Hospital (NTUH 100-S1914), the Department of Health, and the National Science Council, Executive Yuan, Taiwan. The funders had no role in study design, data collection and analysis, decision to publish, or preparation of the manuscript.

Competing Interests: Jia-Horng Kao: Consultant for Abbott, Bristol-Myers Squibb, Gilead Sciences, GlaxoSmithKline, Merck Sharp & Dohme, Novartis, Omrix, Roche; on speaker's Cover Letter bureau for Abbott, Roche, Bayer, Bristol-Myers Squibb, GlaxoSmithKline, Novartis; Ding-Shinn Chen: Consultant for Novartis and GlaxoSmithKline; Pei-Jer Chen: Consultant for Gilead Sciences, Novartis and Roche; All other authors declare no competing interests.

* E-mail: kaojh@ntu.edu.tw

Introduction

The natural history of hepatitis B virus (HBV) carriers who acquire the virus in early life can be divided into 4 dynamic phases based on virus-host interactions, including: immune tolerance, immune clearance, inactive carrier state and reactivation phase. [1,2] After hepatitis B e antigen (HBeAg) seroconversion, patients usually enter the inactive state, with low viral load and normal alanine aminotransferase (ALT) level. However, a certain proportion of inactive carriers may experience HBV reactivation, which accelerates the disease progression to end-stage liver disease, including cirrhosis and hepatocellular carcinoma (HCC). [3] Therefore, patients in the HBeAg-negative phase should still receive regular monitoring of the hepatitis activity.

The introduction of HBsAg quantification has provided a new diagnostic tool in the management of chronic hepatitis B (CHB), such as the prediction of disease activity, HBsAg loss, and development of HCC in the natural history,[4–9] as well as the responses to treatment.[10–12] Several cross-sectional studies have shown the dynamic change of HBsAg levels during the natural course of HBV infection: higher in the immune tolerance and clearance phase, lower in the inactive phase and increases again in the reactivation phase.[13–16] In an European study with 3 years of longitudinal follow-up of 209 genotype D HBeAg-negative patients, HBsAg levels correlated with disease activity and helped to predict the inactive carrier state. [8] In another longitudinal study on 68 genotype B or C HBeAg-negative patients, HBsAg levels tended to be higher in the active carriers. [14] These lines of evidence suggest that, HBsAg quantification can be utilized for monitoring in patients with chronic hepatitis B infection because of its dynamic change and complementary role to HBV-DNA.

However, most of the previous studies looking at the clinical significance of HBsAg level were of cross-sectional design with a limited follow-up duration or case numbers. The definition of disease activities mostly relied on the short-term observation of HBV-DNA; however, the HBV-DNA tended to fluctuate overtime. Therefore, larger studies with longer observation period are still needed for validation, especially in Asian countries where most chronic HBV infections are acquired early in life. To that end, we conducted a study to investigate the longitudinal HBsAg change in HBeAg-negative patients with genotype B or C infection, and to explore the role of baseline HBsAg level in predicting disease progression in this special clinical setting.

Materials and Methods

Patient Cohort

A total of 187 HBeAg-negative carriers were recruited from the Gastroenterology Clinics in National Taiwan University Hospital between 1993 and 2006. All of them fulfilled the criteria of >20 years old, HBsAg-positive and HBeAg-negative >6 months, and had never received anti-HBV treatment. Patients should have available baseline and end-of-follow-up (EOF) sera stored at −20°C refrigerators in the Hepatitis Research Center and a follow-up duration >3 years. Patients with malignancy, autoimmune disease, hemochromatosis, Wilson's disease, alcohol intake >40 gm/day, and HIV, HCV or HDV co-infection were excluded. At first, 221 patients fulfilled the inclusion criteria, but 34 were excluded due to follow-up duration <3 years in 25 patients, HCC at baseline in 6 patients and unavailable baseline or EOF serum sample in 3 patients [Figure 1]. The study conformed to the ethical guidelines of the 1975 Declaration of Helsinki and was approved by the Institutional Review Board of the National Taiwan University Hospital. Written informed consents were obtained from all patients at enrollment.

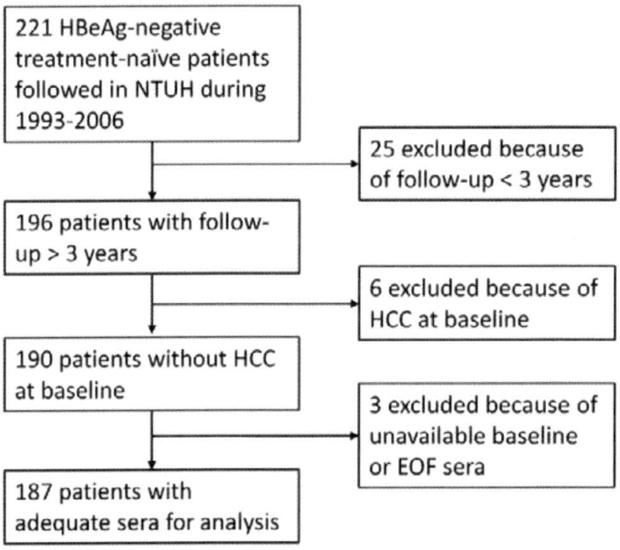

Figure 1. The flow chart of patient enrollment. EOF = end-of-follow-up, HCC = hepatocellular carcinoma.

Data Collection

Throughout the follow-up period, liver function tests and alpha-fetoprotein were assayed every 6 months if ALT levels were within normal limits (</ = 40 U/L) and at least every 3 months if ALT levels were elevated. Pertinent clinical information was collected from the patient's medical records. The EOF was defined as the date of the last visit, the start of anti-HBV therapy or December 31, 2010, whichever came first.

HBV Serological and Virological Assays

Serum HBeAg, anti-HBe, anti-HCV and anti-HDV were tested by using commercial kits. (Abbott Laboratories, Abbott Park, IL, USA). Serum HBsAg titer was quantified by Architect HBsAg QT assay (Abbott Laboratories) with a diagnostic range from 0.05 IU/mL to 250 IU/mL. Serial 1:100 to 1:1000 dilutions were performed if the HBsAg >250 IU/mL according to the manufacturer's instructions. The HBsAg levels were quantified in all cases at baseline, and at EOF. Among them, 165 patients with available first-year sera were also quantified for HBsAg.

Serum HBV-DNA was extracted from 200 μL of serum by QIAmp DNA Blood Mini Kit (QIAGEN Inc, Valencia, CA, USA) and quantified by a real-time PCR amplification assay using LightCycler (Roche Diagnostics, Basel, Switzerland) with a detection sensitivity of 20 IU/mL. [17] The HBV genotype was determined by the the melting curve analysis followed by the real-time PCR. [17].

Definition of HBV Hepatitis Activity

Because HBV-DNA levels fluctuate with time, it is inadequate to define the disease activity by a short period of observation (eg. 1 year) of HBV-DNA level. In order to know the true disease activities, we classified these HBV carriers according to their longitudinal HBV-DNA level: (1) high viral-load (HVL): HBV-DNA >/ = 2000 IU/mL persistently; (2) low viral-load (LVL) HBV-DNA level <2000 IU/mL persistently; (3) fluctuated viral-load (FVL): HBV-DNA level between HVL and LVL during follow-up.

HBsAg loss was defined as two consecutive HBsAg levels of <0.05 IU/mL at least 6 months apart. Hepatitis flare was defined as ALT >5 times of the upper normal limit (</ = 40 U/L) with a concomitant serum HBV-DNA level >2000 IU/mL, [18] at least 6 months after inclusion. Cirrhosis was defined by histological or ultrasonographic findings (two consecutive examinations 6 months apart for confirmation) along with clinical features of splenomegaly, esophageal varices, or ascites. [19] HCC was diagnosed either by histology/cytology or by typical dynamic imaging study (CT, MRI or angiography) plus a serum alpha-fetoprotein level >200 ng/mL. [20].

Statistics

Continuous variables were expressed as median (25–75th percentile) and categorical variables were expressed as number (percentage) as appropriate. The HBsAg, HBV-DNA and HBV-DNA/HBsAg levels were logarithmically transformed for analysis. For those with HBsAg or HBV-DNA level below the detection limit (0.05 IU/mL for HBsAg and 20 IU/mL for HBV-DNA), an arbitrary value of 0.025 IU/mL for HBsAg and 10 IU/mL for HBV-DNA were assigned for analysis. Differences between subgroups were analyzed using one-way ANOVA tests or Student's t test as appropriate. Categorical variables were compared by the Chi-square test as appropriate. The decline of HBsAg and HBV-DNA were calculated by the value at baseline – value at EOF. Paired t test was used to compare the decline of

HBsAg and HBV-DNA levels between the baseline and EOF. The annualized rate of HBsAg decline was computed by dividing the HBsAg decline by individual duration of follow-up. Nonparametric trend test was used for trend across ordered groups. Receiver Operating Characteristic (ROC) analysis was used for a cut-off HBsAg level to predict HBsAg loss in the LVL group. The statistical analysis was performed by STATA (version 11.0; Stata Corp, College Station, TX, USA). All tests were 2-sided and a p value <0.05 was considered significant.

Results

Baseline and End-of-follow-up HBsAg and HBV-DNA Levels Differed Significantly between Active and Inactive Carriers

The baseline and EOF data of our patients are shown in Table 1. The distribution of HBV genotypes was mostly B (126/166, 76%), followed by C (38/166, 23%), B+C (2/166, 1%) and was undetermined in 21 patients because of low viral-load. The median follow-up duration was 8 years. Two patients developed HCC during the longitudinal follow-up in the HVL and FVL groups, respectively.

The baseline characteristics were comparable in terms of gender, genotype, and percentage of liver cirrhosis among three groups [Table 1]. The baseline HBsAg and HBV-DNA levels were significantly lower in the LVL group compared with the FVL and HVL groups (HBsAg: 2.84, 3.43 and 3.37 $\log_{10}$ IU/mL, P<.001; HBV-DNA: 1.77, 3.43 and 4.78 $\log_{10}$ IU/mL, P<.001). Among them, HBsAg was quantified in 165 patients (LVL/FVL/HVL: 39/101/25) with available first-year sera. The median first-year HBsAg were 2.59, 3.29 and 3.22 in the LVL, FVL and HVL groups, respectively. Compared with the FVL and LVL groups, the HVL group had significantly higher ALT, HBsAg and HBV-DNA levels at EOF. The HBV-DNA/HBsAg ratios were significantly higher in active carriers both at baseline and EOF (all P<.001).

Long-term Events of the Individual Group

The long-term events of each group were compared in Table 2. The maximal ALT level during follow-up was significantly higher in the HVL group (median: 168 U/L). A significant HBsAg decline was observed in LVL, FVL and HVL groups when compared with the baseline level (0.99, 0.52 and 0.20 $\log_{10}$ IU/mL, respectively). The decline of HBV-DNA levels were insignificant in 3 groups (P = .248). There was no hepatitis flare in the LVL group, compared with 16% and 30% in the FVL and HVL groups, respectively (P = .001). A significant trend of increasing cirrhosis at EOF was observed in FVL and HVL groups (11% and 27%, respectively) compared with LVL group (5%, P = .017) [Table 1]. About 43% of patients in the HVL group finally received anti-viral therapy, which was significantly higher than the FVL and LVL groups (17% and 5%, respectively). Nineteen patients (10%) achieved HBsAg loss during the follow-up and 56% of them developed anti-HBs (>10 mIU/mL) spontaneously.

A significantly higher frequency of HBsAg loss was observed in the LVL (21%) and FVL (9%) groups, but none in the HVL group. Furthermore, the annualized HBsAg decline was 0.101, 0.067 and 0.040 $\log_{10}$ IU/mL in LVL, FVL and HVL groups, respectively (P for trend = .006).

Genotype C was Associated with More Cirrhosis and HBV-DNA Reduction at End-of-follow-up

HBV genotype B and C patients had comparable baseline age, gender, ALT, HBsAg and HBV-DNA levels [Table 3]. However, genotype C patients had a higher percentage of cirrhosis than

Table 1. Characteristics of HBeAg-negative HBsAg carriers according to their hepatitis activities.

Characteristics	Low viral-load	Fluctuated viral-load	High viral-load	P value
	n = 43	n = 114	n = 30	
Age at enrollment	38 (33, 48)	43 (36, 51)	47 (41, 55)	.004
Male, n(%)	25 (58)	78 (68)	16 (53)	.216
Genotype B, n(%) n = 166	19 (73)	81 (74)	26 (87)	.543
Baseline				
ALT (U/L)	22 (14, 37)	30 (20, 45)	40 (25, 66)	<.001
HBsAg ($\log_{10}$ IU/mL)	2.84 (1.54, 3.34)	3.43 (2.85, 3.77)	3.37 (3.01, 3.64)	<.001
HBV-DNA ($\log_{10}$ IU/mL)	1.77 (1.00, 2.82)	3.43 (2.48, 4.08)	4.78 (3.85, 5.85)	<.001
HBV-DNA/HBsAg	−0.51 (−1.64, 0.58)	0.09 (−0.88, 1.24)	1.60 (0.77, 2.28)	<.001
Liver cirrhosis, n(%)	2 (5)	6 (5)	4 (13)	.239
End-of-follow-up				
ALT (U/L)	22 (18, 37)	34 (22, 56)	48 (30, 121)	.002
HBsAg ($\log_{10}$ IU/mL)	1.31 (−0.74, 2.90)	2.92 (1.79, 3.49)	3.13 (2.54, 3.54)	<.001
HBV-DNA ($\log_{10}$ IU/mL)	1.00 (1.00, 2.36)	3.31 (2.53, 4.65)	5.05 (4.39, 6.10)	<.001
HBV-DNA/HBsAg	0.19 (−0.43, 2.22)	1.15 (0.29, 2.28)	1.98 (1.46, 3.01)	<.001
Liver cirrhosis, n (%)	2 (5)	13 (11)	8 (27)	.017
Number of HBV DNA exams	4 (3, 5)	6 (4, 8)	7 (3, 7)	<.001
Percentage of HBV-DNA <2000 IU/mL	100 (100, 100)	50 (33, 67)	0 (0, 0)	<.001
Duration of FU, year	9.7 (4.9, 12.2)	8.7 (4.7, 11.8)	5.2 (4.3, 7.1)	.007

Data are expressed as median (25th, 75th quartile) or number (percentage) as indicated.

Table 2. Long-term events of groups according to their hepatitis activities.

Characteristics	Low viral-load	Fluctuated viral-load	High viral-load	P value
	n = 43	n = 114	n = 30	
Maximal ALT level (U/L)	41 (29, 75)	70 (39, 162)	168 (113, 246)	.006
HBsAg decline (log_{10} IU/mL)	0.99 (0.26, 2.05)†	0.52 (0.07, 1.06)†	0.20 (−0.04, 0.53)*	.004
Annualized HBsAg decline (log_{10} IU/mL)	0.101 (0.039, 0.203)	0.067 (0.008, 0.162)	0.040 (−0.008, 0.101)	.006‡
HBV-DNA decline (log_{10} IU/mL)	0 (0, 1.22)	−0.09 (−1.69, 1.34)	−0.54 (−1.43, 1.09)	.248
Hepatitis flare, n(%)	0 (0)	18 (16)	9 (30)	.001
Received treatment, n(%)	2 (5)	19 (17)	13 (43)	<.001
HBsAg loss, n(%)	9 (21)	10 (9)	0 (0)	.010

Data are expressed as median (25th, 75th quartile) or number (percentage) as indicated.
†P<.001,
*P<.05 compared with its baseline level.
‡P for trend.

genotype B patients either at baseline (16 vs. 5%) or EOF (24 vs. 11%). Genotype C patients had a significantly lower HBV-DNA level (2.74 vs. 3.77 log_{10} IU/mL, P = .041) and HBV-DNA/HBsAg ratio (0.65 vs. 1.40, P = .044) at EOF compared with genotype B. The HBsAg decline during the follow-up was comparable between genotype B and C.

Predictors for HBsAg Decline/Loss and Hepatitis Flare

After adjustment for age, gender, genotype, ALT and HBV-DNA level at study entry, baseline HBsAg (1 log_{10} IU/mL increment) independently predicted both HBsAg decline >1 log_{10} IU/mL at EOF (OR: 0.64, 95% CI = 0.43–0.94, P = .023) and HBsAg loss at EOF (OR = 0.37, 95% CI = 0.21–0.65, P = .001) [Table 4]. On the other hand, multivariate analysis showed that male gender (OR = 3.48, 95%CI = 1.14–10.63, P = .028) and baseline HBV-DNA level (1 log_{10} IU/mL increment, OR = 1.50, 95%CI = 1.11–2.03, P = .009) could predict hepatitis flare during the follow-up period. The ROC analysis showed a baseline HBsAg level <50 IU/mL in the LVL group could predict subsequent HBsAg loss with a sensitivity of 82% and specificity of 67%.

The Dynamic Change of HBsAg According to Baseline HBsAg Level

Patients were further stratified by their baseline HBsAg levels into <100, 100–999 and >1000 IU/mL. The median HBsAg levels were 1.28, 2.65 and 3.54 log_{10} IU/mL at baseline, 1.20, 2.53

Table 3. Characteristics of patients according to HBV genotype B or C.

Characteristics	Genotype B	Genotype C	P value
	n = 126	n = 38	
Age	44 (36, 52)	42 (35, 50)	.317
Male, n(%)	78 (62)	26 (68)	.465
Baseline			
ALT (U/L)	29 (19, 44)	37 (22, 66)	.459
HBsAg (log_{10} IU/mL)	3.35 (2.80, 3.64)	3.62 (3.11, 3.97)	.280
HBV-DNA (log_{10} IU/mL)	3.45 (2.66, 4.56)	3.41 (2.27, 3.90)	.920
HBV-DNA/HBsAg	0.45 (−0.66, 1.54)	0.40 (−1.22, 0.96)	.462
Liver cirrhosis, n(%)	6 (5)	6 (16)	.022
End-of-follow-up			
ALT (U/L)	32 (22, 55)	35 (21, 75)	.132
HBsAg (log_{10} IU/mL)	2.94 (1.83, 3.42)	2.91 (1.64, 3.76)	.727
HBV-DNA (log_{10} IU/mL)	3.77 (2.69, 4.87)	2.74 (1.26, 4.47)	.041
HBV-DNA/HBsAg	1.40 (0.38, 2.51)	0.65 (−0.47, 2.22)	.044
Liver cirrhosis, n (%)	14 (11)	9 (24)	.050
HBsAg decline (log_{10} IU/mL)	0.42 (0.04, 0.99)†	0.55 (0.10, 1.22)†	.173
HBV DNA decline (log_{10} IU/mL)	−0.45 (−1.59, 0.99)	0.47 (−0.09, 1.59)	.065
Duration of FU, year	8.0 (4.7, 11.8)	6.3 (4.3, 10.0)	.105

Data are expressed as median (25th, 75th quartile) or number (percentage) as indicated.
†P<.001 compared with its baseline level.

Table 4. Predictors for HBsAg decline >1 log at end-of-follow-up, HBsAg loss and HBeAg-negative hepatitis by multivariate analysis.

Baseline parameters	HBsAg decline >1 log		HBsAg loss		HBeAg-negative hepatitis	
	OR	95% CI	OR	95% CI	OR	95% CI
Age (1 yr increment)	1.01	0.98–1.05	1.02	0.97–1.08	1.00	0.95–1.04
Male vs. female	1.62	0.73–3.60	1.86	0.44–7.86	3.48*	1.14–10.63
Genotype B vs non-B	0.63	0.27–1.44	0.49	1.12–1.98	1.23	0.41–3.63
ALT (1 U/L increment)	1.00	1.00–1.00	1.00	0.98–1.01	1.00	1.00–1.00
HBsAg (1 $\log_{10}$ IU/mL increment)	0.64*	0.43–0.94	0.37†	0.21–0.65	1.50	0.77–2.90
HBV-DNA (1 $\log_{10}$ IU/mL increment)	0.86	0.66–1.10	0.99	0.61–1.61	1.50*	1.11–2.03

†P = .001,
*P<.05.

and 3.39 $\log_{10}$ IU/mL at the first year and −0.23, 1.83 and 3.22 $\log_{10}$ IU/mL at EOF [Figure 2]. A significantly greater HBsAg decline was observed in patients with lower baseline HBsAg levels (1.22, 0.64 and 0.42 $\log_{10}$ IU/mL, respectively, P for trend = .006). The estimated annualized rate of HBsAg decline was 0.126, 0.091, 0.054 $\log_{10}$ IU/mL in those with baseline HBsAg <100, 100–999 and >1000 IU/mL, respectively (P for trend = .014).

Discussion

In this study, a large cohort of HBeAg-negative treatment-naïve patients was used to demonstrate the longitudinal changes of HBsAg titer. It is known that HBV-DNA level and hepatitis activity fluctuate during the HBeAg-negative phase of chronic HBV infection; therefore, we categorized our patients according to longitudinal HBV-DNA measurements. In agreement with previous results, [8,14] patients with inactive diseases had significantly lower HBsAg, HBV-DNA level and HBV-DNA/HBsAg ratios, not only at EOF but also at the start of the study recruitment 8 years ago. However, the baseline HBsAg levels were indistinguishable between the FVL and HVL groups, suggesting the predicting role of HBsAg in identifying inactive diseases.

The substantial reduction of HBsAg levels in inactive carriers observed in this study was consistent with the results from genotype D chronic hepatitis B patients, showing that HBsAg was stable in active carriers but declined in inactive ones. [8] The

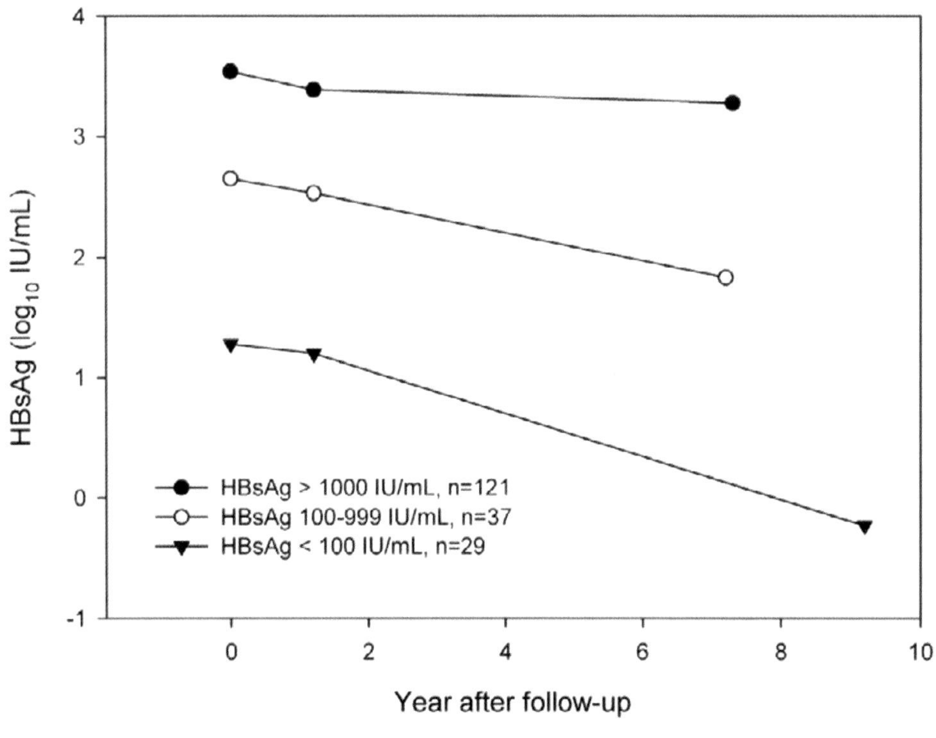

Figure 2. The dynamic change of HBsAg after stratification according to baseline HBsAg level of <100, 100–999 and >1000 IU/mL. The median follow-up duration was 9.2, 7.0 and 7.3 years, respectively. 165 patients (n = 25, 33 and 107 in baseline HBsAg level of <100, 100–999 and >1000 IU/mL) with available first-year HBsAg levels were also plotted. A greater HBsAg decline was observed in patients with lower baseline HBsAg levels (1.22, 0.64, 0.42 $\log_{10}$ IU/mL in HBsAg <100, 100–999 and >1000 IU/mL, P for trend = .006).

annualized rate of HBsAg decline was reported to be 0.012–0.041 $\log_{10}$ IU/mL in active carriers and 0.043–0.077 $\log_{10}$ IU/mL in inactive ones. [8,14] We found this trend similarly in patients with genotype B or C infection. Furthermore, after stratification according to the baseline HBsAg levels, an increasing HBsAg reduction rate was observed in patients with lower baseline HBsAg levels. Taking these lines of evidence together, the annualized rate of HBsAg decline appears non-linear, and may accelerate as the HBsAg level decreases. This information is clinically important for the management of inactive HBV carriers.

It is generally believed that HBsAg level may reflect the "transcriptionally active" cccDNA or the integrated form of HBV genome and is considered to be a surrogate marker of infected hepatocytes. [4] Therefore HBsAg decline indicates a (1) higher clearance and/or (2) a lower production of HBsAg; that is, a reduction of HBsAg mRNA being translated from cccDNA or integrated HBV genome. [21] The dynamics of both mechanisms may contribute to the non-linear and accelerating decline of HBsAg in lower levels. The low HBsAg level suggests host immune taking control over the HBV infection to achieve and sustain an inactive HBV state. [8] In the scenario of acute hepatitis B, the half-life of HBsAg shortened continually after infection: an initial slow decay or non-specific removal of HBsAg, and is followed by the more rapid immunological neutralization with anti-HBs. [22] Besides, a greater decline in HBsAg level is seen after immuno-modulatory interferon therapy, compared with direct antiviral nucleos(t)ide analogues. [10,13,23] In this study, a lower HBV-DNA/HBsAg ratio was found in LVL and FVL group at baseline and EOF; implicating HBV was less productive in patients with milder liver diseases. [8] Whether the HBsAg decline is associated with inhibition of HBsAg expression and clearance of cccDNA or the integrated form of HBV genome under immunological pressure needs to be clarified by further studies.

HBV genotype is an important viral parameter in predicting disease progression and therapeutic outcome.[24–28] In vitro studies demonstrated genotype-specific patterns of intracellular and extracellular HBV-DNA and HBsAg expressions: the HBsAg secretion was most abundant for genotype A followed by B, C and less in D. [29] A genotypic-specific HBsAg decline during pegylated-interferon treatment was also demonstrated, which was higher in genotype A, intermediate in B and D, and lower in C and E. [28,30] In our study, genotype C patients had a significantly higher percentage of cirrhosis and decline of HBV-DNA, but not HBsAg. This may partly be explained by immunologic attack against HBV-infected hepatocytes, resulting in disease progression to cirrhosis and decline in HBV-DNA but there is still insufficient immune control over HBV infection with HBsAg persistence in genotype C patients. [24,25] However, further larger studies with special focus on immune functions are needed to validate this important and interesting issue.

Recent studies indicated that a lower HBsAg level can better predict the clinical outcomes, especially HBsAg loss. [6,31,32] In this study, we confirmed that HBsAg level positively predicted both HBsAg decline >1 log and HBsAg loss over time, indicating a good immunological control and viral clearance. [14] We found a cut-off HBsAg level <50 IU/mL could predict subsequent HBsAg loss. On the other hand, the predictors for hepatitis flare included male gender and baseline HBV-DNA level, but not HBsAg level. These findings were consistent with our previous data that HBV-DNA levels >/ = 2000 IU/mL can predict HBeAg-negative hepatitis and hepatitis flare among HBeAg seroconverters. [18] Nevertheless, in patients with HBV-DNA <2000 IU/mL (n = 95), HBsAg seemed to predict HBeAg-negative hepatitis flare (OR: 4.29, 95%CI = 0.91–20.27, P = .066) though the statistic power was suboptimal. This fact again supports the complementary role of HBsAg level in low HBV-DNA patients to predict adverse outcomes. In our patients, 10% achieved HBsAg loss during the follow-up and 56% of them developed anti-HBs (>10 mIU/mL) spontaneously. For patients who lost HBsAg without seroconversion to anti-HBs, hepatitis B vaccination might be a strategy to generate anti-HBs. In a recent study, the response rate to the vaccination in prior HBsAg carriers was only 24%. [33] On the other hand, the overall response rate of hepatitis B vaccination in subjects with isolated hepatitis B core antibody was up to 72–86%, [34,35] and a prior history of HBsAg positivity was associated with a decreased response to vaccination. [36] The reduced response to hepatitis B vaccination was possibly due to the prolonged carriage of HBsAg with ineffective immunity on repeated exposure to HBsAg. Finally, in subjects who have recovered from previous HBV infection, the protection of anti-HBs after HBsAg seroconversion should be cautiously monitored whenever they receive rituximab-containing chemotherapy, because HBsAg seroreversion may occur. [37].

Our study had a few limitations. Due to the retrospective study design, our patients did not have frequent HBV-DNA tests, possibly leading to mis-classification of the disease status. However, the ALT levels were checked regularly, and HBV-DNA would be checked in case of significant abnormal liver function. Furthermore, liver biopsies were not a routine procedure in HBV patients with mild disease. This potential source of error in liver disease status could be partly compensated by serial HBV-DNA testing and regular ultrasonographic examinations.

In summary, patients with inactive HBV infection have a significantly lower HBsAg and HBV-DNA levels during the long-term follow-up than active HBV carriers. The HBsAg decline was significantly greater in inactive carriers with low baseline HBsAg levels, regardless of whether HBV genotype B or C. The HBsAg decline appears non-linear, and accelerates as the HBsAg level lowers. Lower baseline HBsAg level can predict HBsAg decline and loss over time, whereas higher baseline HBV-DNA level can predict HBeAg-negative hepatitis flare.

Acknowledgments

We thank the fourth Core Laboratory of the Department of Medical Research, National Taiwan University Hospital for technical assistance.

Author Contributions

Conceived and designed the experiments: THS JHK DSC. Performed the experiments: THS CJL TCT CHL HCY PJC JHK. Analyzed the data: THS CLC. Wrote the paper: THS.

References

1. Liaw YF, Chu CM (2009) Hepatitis B virus infection. Lancet 373: 582–592.
2. Chen DS (1993) From hepatitis to hepatoma: lessons from type B viral hepatitis. Science 262: 369–370.
3. Chu CM, Liaw YF (2009) Incidence and risk factors of progression to cirrhosis in inactive carriers of hepatitis B virus. Am J Gastroenterol 104: 1693–1699.
4. Liaw YF (2011) Clinical utility of hepatitis B surface antigen quantitation in patients with chronic hepatitis B: A review. Hepatology 53: 2121–2129.
5. Tseng TC, Liu CJ, Su TH, Wang CC, Chen CL, et al. (2011) Serum hepatitis B surface antigen levels predict surface antigen loss in hepatitis B e antigen seroconverters. Gastroenterology 141: 517–525.
6. Tseng TC, Liu CJ, Yang HC, Su TH, Wang CC, et al. (2012) Determinants of spontaneous surface antigen loss in hepatitis B e antigen-negative patients with a low viral load. Hepatology 55: 68–76.

7. Tseng TC, Liu CJ, Yang HC, Su TH, Wang CC, et al. (2012) High Levels of Hepatitis B Surface Antigen Increase Risk of Hepatocellular Carcinoma in Patients With Low HBV Load. Gastroenterology 142: 1140-1149.
8. Brunetto MR, Oliveri F, Colombatto P, Moriconi F, Ciccorossi P, et al. (2010) Hepatitis B surface antigen serum levels help to distinguish active from inactive hepatitis B virus genotype D carriers. Gastroenterology 139: 483-490.
9. Chan HL, Thompson A, Martinot-Peignoux M, Piratvisuth T, Cornberg M, et al. (2011) Hepatitis B surface antigen quantification: why and how to use it in 2011 - a core group report. J Hepatol 55: 1121-1131.
10. Brunetto MR, Moriconi F, Bonino F, Lau GK, Farci P, et al. (2009) Hepatitis B virus surface antigen levels: a guide to sustained response to peginterferon alfa-2a in HBeAg-negative chronic hepatitis B. Hepatology 49: 1141-1150.
11. Chan HL, Wong VW, Chim AM, Chan HY, Wong GL, et al. (2010) Serum HBsAg quantification to predict response to peginterferon therapy of e antigen positive chronic hepatitis B. Aliment Pharmacol Ther 32: 1323-1331.
12. Moucari R, Mackiewicz V, Lada O, Ripault MP, Castelnau C, et al. (2009) Early serum HBsAg drop: a strong predictor of sustained virological response to pegylated interferon alfa-2a in HBeAg-negative patients. Hepatology 49: 1151-1157.
13. Su TH, Hsu CS, Chen CL, Liu CH, Huang YW, et al. (2010) Serum hepatitis B surface antigen concentration correlates with HBV DNA level in patients with chronic hepatitis B. Antivir Ther 15: 1133-1139.
14. Chan HL, Wong VW, Wong GL, Tse CH, Chan HY, et al. (2010) A longitudinal study on the natural history of serum hepatitis B surface antigen changes in chronic hepatitis B. Hepatology 52: 1232-1241.
15. Nguyen T, Thompson AJ, Bowden S, Croagh C, Bell S, et al. (2010) Hepatitis B surface antigen levels during the natural history of chronic hepatitis B: a perspective on Asia. J Hepatol 52: 508-513.
16. Jaroszewicz J, Calle Serrano B, Wursthorn K, Deterding K, Schlue J, et al. (2010) Hepatitis B surface antigen (HBsAg) levels in the natural history of hepatitis B virus (HBV)-infection: a European perspective. J Hepatol 52: 514-522.
17. Yeh SH, Tsai CY, Kao JH, Liu CJ, Kuo TJ, et al. (2004) Quantification and genotyping of hepatitis B virus in a single reaction by real-time PCR and melting curve analysis. J Hepatol 41: 659-666.
18. Tseng TC, Liu CJ, Chen CL, Wang CC, Su TH, et al. (2012) Serum hepatitis B virus-DNA levels correlate with long-term adverse outcomes in spontaneous hepatitis B e antigen seroconverters. J Infect Dis 205: 54-63.
19. Feld JJ, Ayers M, El-Ashry D, Mazzulli T, Tellier R, et al. (2007) Hepatitis B virus DNA prediction rules for hepatitis B e antigen-negative chronic hepatitis B. Hepatology 46: 1057-1070.
20. Bruix J, Sherman M (2005) Management of hepatocellular carcinoma. Hepatology 42: 1208-1236.
21. Brunetto MR (2010) A new role for an old marker, HBsAg. J Hepatol 52: 475-477.
22. Chulanov VP, Shipulin GA, Schaefer S, Gerlich WH (2003) Kinetics of HBV DNA and HBsAg in acute hepatitis B patients with and without coinfection by other hepatitis viruses. J Med Virol 69: 313-323.
23. Reijnders JG, Rijckborst V, Sonneveld MJ, Scherbeijn SM, Boucher CA, et al. (2011) Kinetics of hepatitis B surface antigen differ between treatment with peginterferon and entecavir. J Hepatol 54: 449-454.
24. Kao JH, Chen PJ, Lai MY, Chen DS (2000) Hepatitis B genotypes correlate with clinical outcomes in patients with chronic hepatitis B. Gastroenterology 118: 554-559.
25. Kao JH, Chen PJ, Lai MY, Chen DS (2002) Genotypes and clinical phenotypes of hepatitis B virus in patients with chronic hepatitis B virus infection. J Clin Microbiol 40: 1207-1209.
26. Kao JH, Chen PJ, Lai MY, Chen DS (2004) Hepatitis B virus genotypes and spontaneous hepatitis B e antigen seroconversion in Taiwanese hepatitis B carriers. J Med Virol 72: 363-369.
27. Kao JH, Wu NH, Chen PJ, Lai MY, Chen DS (2000) Hepatitis B genotypes and the response to interferon therapy. J Hepatol 33: 998-1002.
28. Liu CJ, Kao JH, Chen DS (2005) Therapeutic implications of hepatitis B virus genotypes. Liver Int 25: 1097-1107.
29. Sugiyama M, Tanaka Y, Kato T, Orito E, Ito K, et al. (2006) Influence of hepatitis B virus genotypes on the intra- and extracellular expression of viral DNA and antigens. Hepatology 44: 915-924.
30. Moucari R, Martinot-Peignoux M, Mackiewicz V, Boyer N, Ripault MP, et al. (2009) Influence of genotype on hepatitis B surface antigen kinetics in hepatitis B e antigen-negative patients treated with pegylated interferon-alpha2a. Antivir Ther 14: 1183-1188.
31. Chen YC, Jeng WJ, Chu CM, Liaw YF (2012) Decreasing Levels of HBsAg Predict HBsAg Seroclearance in Patients With Inactive Chronic Hepatitis B Virus Infection. Clin Gastroenterol Hepatol 10: 297-302.
32. Chan HL, Wong GL, Tse CH, Chan HY, Wong VW (2011) Viral determinants of hepatitis B surface antigen seroclearance in hepatitis B e antigen-negative chronic hepatitis B patients. J Infect Dis 204: 408-414.
33. Taheri H, Hasanjani Roushan MR, Soleimani Amiri MJ, Pouralijan M, Bijani A (2011) Efficacy of Hepatitis B vaccine in those who lost Hepatitis B surface antigen during follow-up: Efficacy of HBV vaccine in those who lost HBsAg. Hepat Mon 11: 119-122.
34. Lok AS, Lai CL, Wu PC (1988) Prevalence of isolated antibody to hepatitis B core antigen in an area endemic for hepatitis B virus infection: implications in hepatitis B vaccination programs. Hepatology 8: 766-770.
35. Tseng KC, Lei HY, Cheng PN, Young KC, Jen CM, et al. (2003) Immune response to hepatitis B vaccine of subjects with isolated antibody to hepatitis B core antigen. Hepatogastroenterology 50: 1474-1477.
36. Kabir A, Keshvari M, Kashani AH, Alavian SM (2008) Predicting response to HBV vaccination in people with positive anti-HBc but negative HBsAg and anti-HBs. Hum Vaccin 4: 379-383.
37. Pei SN, Ma MC, Wang MC, Kuo CY, Rau KM, et al. (2012) Analysis of hepatitis B surface antibody titers in B cell lymphoma patients after rituximab therapy. Ann Hematol 91: 1007-1012.

20

Enhanced HBsAg Synthesis Correlates with Increased Severity of Fibrosis in Chronic Hepatitis B Patients

Mei-Zhu Hong[1], Wen-Qi Huang[1], Feng Min[1], Jin-Chao Xu[1], Zhen Lin[2], Kuang-Nan Fang[3]*, Jin-Shui Pan[4]*

1 Department of Infectious Diseases, Chenggong Hospital affiliated to Xiamen University (The 174th Hospital of PLA), Xiamen, China, **2** Department of Pathology, Chenggong Hospital affiliated with Xiamen University (The 174th Hospital of PLA), Xiamen, China, **3** Department of Statistics, School of Economics, Xiamen University, Xiamen, China, **4** Department of Gastroenterology, Zhongshan Hospital affiliated with Xiamen University, Xiamen, China

Abstract

Background and Aims: Little is known about whether low serum HBsAg levels result from impaired HBsAg synthesis or a reduced number of hepatocytes caused by advanced liver fibrosis. Therefore, we investigated the capacity for HBsAg synthesis in a cross-sectional cohort of treatment-naïve chronic hepatitis B patients.

Methods: Chronic hepatitis B patients (n = 362) were enrolled; liver biopsies were performed and liver histology was scored, and serum HBsAg and HBV DNA levels were investigated. In the enrolled patients, 183 out of 362 have quantitative serum HBsAg levels. Tissue HBsAg was determined by immunohistochemistry.

Results: A positive correlation between serum HBsAg and HBV DNA levels was revealed in HBeAg(+) patients ($r = 0.2613$, $p = 0.0050$). In HBeAg(+) patients, serum HBsAg and severity of fibrosis were inversely correlated ($p = 0.0094$), whereas tissue HBsAg levels correlated positively with the stage of fibrosis ($p = 0.0280$). After applying the mean aminopyrine breath test as a correction factor, adjusted serum HBsAg showed a strong positive correlation with fibrosis severity in HBeAg(+) patients ($r = 0.5655$, $p < 0.0001$). The adjusted serum HBsAg values predicted 'moderate to severe' fibrosis with nearly perfect performance in both HBeAg(+) patients (area under the curve: 0.994, 95% CI: 0.983–1.000) and HBeAg(−) patients (area under the curve: 1.000, 95% CI: 1.000–1.000).

Conclusions: Although serum HBsAg levels were negatively correlated with fibrosis severity in HBeAg(+) patients, aminopyrine breath test-adjusted serum HBsAg and tissue HBsAg, two indices that are unaffected by the number of residual hepatocytes, were positively correlated with fibrosis severity. Furthermore, adjusted serum HBsAg has an accurate prediction capability.

Editor: Wenyu Lin, Harvard Medical School, United States of America

Funding: The study was funded by National Science Foundation for Young Scholars, China (No. 81100285) http://www.nsfc.gov.cn/Portal0/default152.htm; Natural Science Foundation of Fujian Province, China (No. 2010J05086) http://www.fjkjt.gov.cn/; Science Fund for Distinguished Young Scholars of Xiamen, China (No. 3502Z20105011) http://www.xminfo.net.cn/. The funders had no role in study design, data collection and analysis, decision to publish, or preparation of the manuscript.

Competing Interests: The authors have declared that no competing interests exist.

* E-mail: ruiqwy@163.com (KNF); j.s.pan76@gmail.com (JSP)

Introduction

Chronic hepatitis B (CHB) remains one of the most common infectious diseases worldwide, and in Asia and Africa in particular. Interferon α (or pegylated-interferon) and nucleosides (or nucleotide analogues) are prescribed widely for the treatment of CHB. Following effective therapy, a marked decline in hepatitis B virus (HBV) DNA load and/or quantified serum hepatitis B surface antigen (HBsAg) can be observed. There is a positive correlation between HBV DNA level and liver cirrhosis and hepatocellular carcinoma (HCC) [1,2]. In the past several years, the role of quantified serum HBsAg in the surveillance of treatment efficacy has attracted interest. HBsAg seroclearance confers a favorable prognosis in cirrhosis and HCC [3–6]. The risk of hepatocellular tumorigenesis is lower in the patients with clearance of serum HBsAg after interferon α-based antiviral therapy [7]. High levels of HBsAg increase the risk of HCC and vice versa [8]. Moreover, a clinical association between serum HBsAg quantification and liver histology has been reported [9,10].

Recently, two studies have reported on the negative correlation between serum HBsAg level and the severity of liver fibrosis [11,12]. However, the number of viable hepatocytes and the capacity for synthesis of HBsAg critically affect serum HBsAg levels. Therefore, it is not clear whether the diminished serum HBsAg levels in patients with advanced fibrosis are due to a decrease in the number of residual hepatocytes or to impaired secretion of HBsAg, and the results of these two studies may have been misinterpreted in terms of the beneficial effect of HBsAg in the control of liver fibrosis. Furthermore, these studies are based on cross-sectional observations, yielding insufficient information on the role of serum HBsAg in liver fibrosis. Thus, clinical investigation is necessary to explore the cause of diminished serum HBsAg in the patients with advanced liver fibrosis.

HBsAg is secreted into the circulation as tubular forms or spherical particles by HBV-infected hepatocytes. Patients with CHB usually express different levels of HBsAg when assayed by immunohistochemistry. In patients with advanced fibrosis, residual hepatocytes diminish dramatically, which has a profound effect on serum HBsAg quantification, but not on intrahepatic HBsAg (tissue HBsAg) quantification. Tissue HBsAg levels are determined by the establishing the percentage of HBsAg-positive hepatocytes and the grade of staining reflected by immunohistochemistry. Therefore, the number of hepatocytes has limited effects on tissue HBsAg levels.

Research by Herold *et al.* [13] reported on the use of the aminopyrine breath test (ABT), which measures the metabolic capacity of hepatocytes, in a series of patients with different stages of fibrosis and grades of inflammatory activity. Increasing fibrosis or inflammatory activity was associated with decreasing ABT values. Thus, the ABT value may reflect the number of hepatocytes to some degree. In order to rule out the effect of the number of hepatocytes on serum HBsAg levels, the present study aims at investigating the correlation between ABT adjusted serum HBsAg and fibrosis in a large cohort of treatment-naïve CHB patients. The potential relationship between intrahepatic HBsAg and the severity of liver histology will be also discussed.

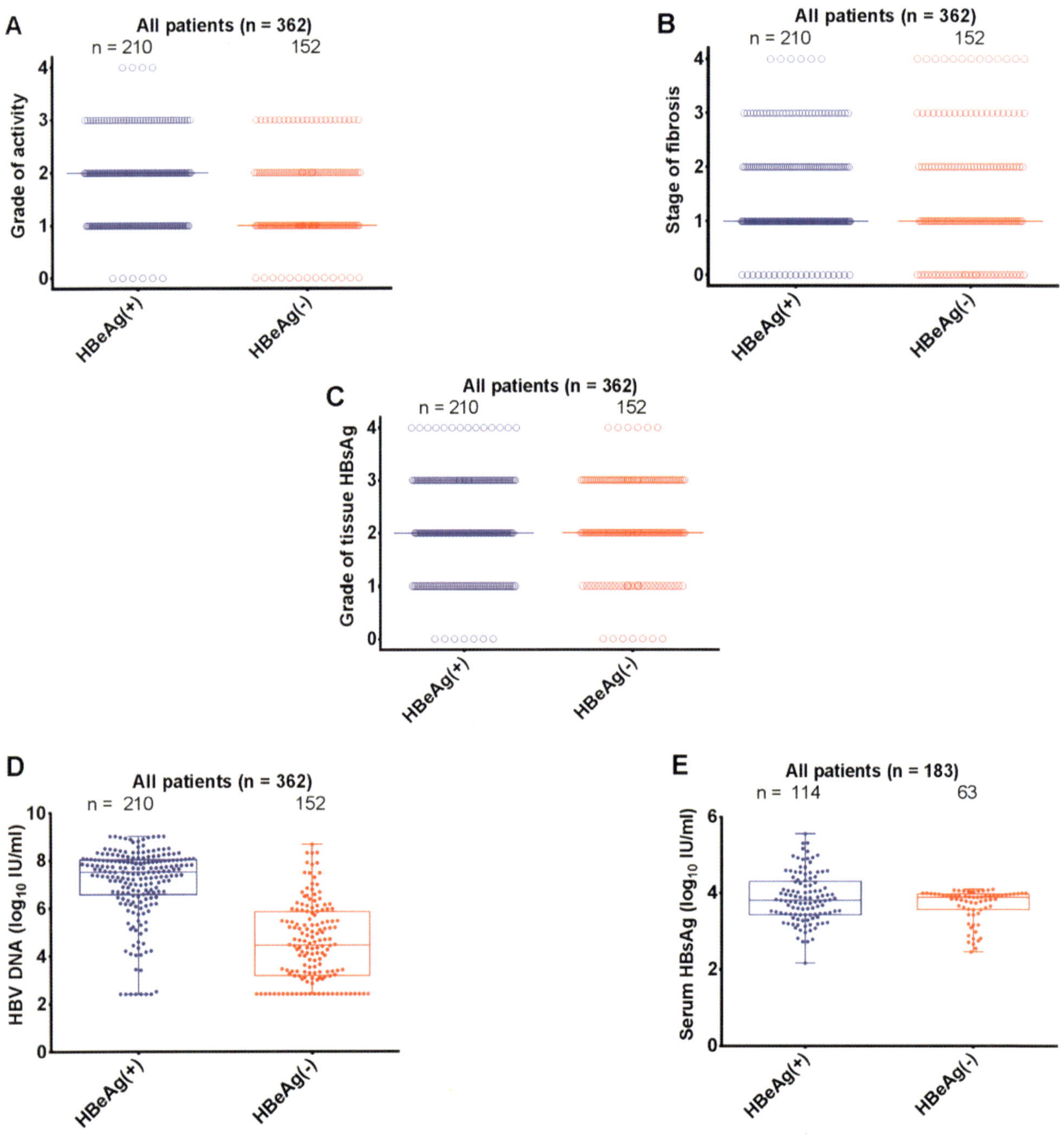

Figure 1. Patients' characteristics stratified according to HBeAg status. (A) grade of inflammatory activity; (B) stage of fibrosis; (C) immunohistochemistry grade of tissue HBsAg; (D) HBV DNA (log10 IU/ml); (E) serum HBsAg (log10 IU/ml).

Materials and Methods

Patients

Treatment-naïve CHB patients reporting to the 174th Hospital of the PLA in Fujian, China, between 2010 and 2013 were enrolled. Patients were investigated retrospectively and informed consent was obtained from all the patients. The present study was approved by the Institutional Ethics Board of Chenggong Hospital (the 174th Hospital of the PLA) and Zhongshan Hospital, Xiamen University. All patients provided written consent prior to liver biopsy and study entry. Entire study was conducted according to the principles of the Declaration of Helsinki. Inclusion criteria for patients were: HBsAg-positive, known HBeAg status, and scheduled liver biopsy. Patients were excluded in the following situations: Hepatitis C virus, Hepatitis D virus, or Human Immunodeficiency Virus co-infection, significant steatosis, alcoholic fatty liver, and decompensated cirrhosis. A total of 362 treatment-naïve CHB patients were included in the present study.

Liver biopsies were performed on the same day that serum samples were collected, or in less than 2 days thereafter.

Diagnostic Tests

HBsAg levels were assayed using the HBsAg assay kit (Wantai Biological Co., Beijing, China). HBV DNA levels were determined by quantitative fluorescence PCR on an ABI 7000 (Applied Biosystems, Carlsbad, USA), with a lower limit of detection of 500 IU/ml. HBsAg and HBV DNA were expressed as log IU/ml. Serum ALT and AST levels were expressed as IU/ml. Liver histology was assessed using the Scheuer scoring system [14]. Liver histology was evaluated by two independent pathologists who were blind to the study design. If the two pathologists could not agree on the pathological diagnosis, histological scores were made and confirmed by a panel of pathologists. Intrahepatic HBsAg was determined by immunohistochemistry. The primary antibody for HBsAg was purchased from Maixin Company (catalog no. MAB-0587; Fuzhou, China). Grade of tissue HBsAg was defined according to the percentile of anti-HBsAg staining hepatocytes, as per the following metrics: 0+, 0~1.9%; 1+, 2.0~24.9%; 2+, 25~49.9%; 3+, 50~74.9%; 4+, 75~100%.

Data Analysis

Quantitative testing of liver functions in a large sample of fibrosis patients related to chronic hepatitis have been reported by Herold *et al.* [13]. Since the investigated objects in our study were

Table 1. Patient characteristics.

Patient group	All(N = 362)	HBeAg(+) (n = 210)	HBeAg(−) (n = 152)	*p* value*
Age, yr (Mean ± SD)	35.5±9.9	32.7±8.7	40.2±9.6	<0.0001
Male, n (%)	285 (78.7)	160 (76.2)	125 (82.2)	0.1935
ALT, IU/L (Mean ± SD)	144.7±207.0	176.6±236.9	100.2±145.2	<0.0001
Normal ALT, n (%)	62 (17.1)	19 (9.0)	43 (28.3)	<0.0001
AST, IU/L (Mean ± SD)	77.0±111.9	92.6±133.2	55.5±67.6	<0.0001
Normal AST, n (%)	163 (45.0)	73 (34.8)	90 (59.2)	<0.0001
Liver histology†				
Activity, n (%)				
G0	19 (5.2)	6 (2.9)	13 (8.6)	0.0290
G1	145 (40.1)	75 (35.7)	70 (46.0)	0.0511
G2	132 (36.5)	86 (40.9)	46 (30.3)	0.0463
G3	62 (17.1)	39 (18.6)	23 (15.1)	0.4800
G4	4 (1.1)	4 (1.9)	0 (0)	0.1423
Fibrosis, n (%)				
S0	53 (14.6)	21 (10.0)	32 (21.1)	0.0041
S1	152 (42.0)	99 (47.1)	53 (34.9)	0.0234
S2	84 (23.2)	51 (24.3)	33 (21.7)	0.6148
S3	54 (15.0)	33 (15.7)	21 (13.8)	0.0083
S4	19 (5.2)	6 (2.9)	13 (8.5)	0.0290
Tissue HBsAg, n (%)				
0	14 (3.9)	7 (3.3)	7 (4.6)	0.5875
1	83 (22.9)	55 (26.2)	28 (18.4)	0.0905
2	134 (37.0)	73 (34.8)	61 (40.1)	0.3217
3	111 (30.7)	61 (29.0)	50 (32.9)	0.4886
4	20 (5.5)	14 (6.7)	6 (4.0)	0.3526
HBV DNA, $\log_{10}$ IU/ml (Mean ± SD)	6.01±1.98	7.07±1.49	4.55±1.63	<0.0001

*HBeAg(+) vs. HBeAg(−);
†According to the Scheuer scoring system.
The study cohort was analyzed both as a whole and stratified according to HBeAg status.

Table 2. Characteristics of the 183 patients with quantitative serum HBsAg levels.

Patient group	All (N = 183)	HBeAg(+) (n = 113)	HBeAg(−) (n = 69)	*p* value*
Age, yr (Mean ± SD)	34.7±10.2	31.0±8.1	40.9±10.3	<0.0001
Male, n (%)	147 (80.3)	86 (75.4)	61 (88.4)	0.0358
ALT, IU/L (Mean ± SD)	143.2±199.6	168.3±220.0	101.1±152.0	<0.0001
Normal ALT, n (%)	30 (16.4)	10 (8.8)	20 (29.0)	0.0007
AST, IU/L (Mean ± SD)	72.8±92.8	83.8±104.9	54.3±64.4	<0.0001
Normal AST, n (%)	87 (47.5)	46 (40.7)	41 (59.4)	0.0152
Liver histology[†]				
Activity, n (%)				
G0	10 (5.5)	4 (3.5)	6 (8.7)	0.1824
G1	75 (41.0)	45 (39.5)	30 (43.5)	0.6444
G2	67 (36.5)	47 (41.2)	20 (29.0)	0.1130
G3	27 (14.8)	14 (12.3)	13 (18.8)	0.2837
G4	4 (2.2)	4 (3.5)	0 (0)	0.2990
Fibrosis, n (%)				
S0	25 (13.6)	14 (12.3)	11 (15.9)	0.5127
S1	81 (44.3)	55 (48.2)	26 (37.7)	0.1681
S2	38 (20.8)	26 (22.8)	12 (17.4)	0.4531
S3	26 (14.2)	14 (12.3)	12 (17.4)	0.3864
S4	13 (7.1)	5 (4.4)	8 (11.6)	0.0807
Tissue HBsAg, n (%)				
0	6 (3.3)	3 (3.3)	3 (4.6)	0.6748
1	40 (21.9)	27 (26.2)	13 (18.4)	0.4654
2	64 (35.0)	36 (34.8)	28 (40.1)	0.2641
3	59 (32.2)	37 (29.0)	22 (32.9)	1.0000
4	14 (7.6)	11 (6.7)	3 (4.0)	0.2553
HBsAg, log_{10} IU/ml (n, Mean ± SD)	183, 3.80±0.58	114, 3.87±0.64	69, 3.68±0.44	0.2600
HBV DNA, log_{10} IU/ml (Mean ± SD)	6.05±2.08	7.17±1.45	4.20±1.58	<0.0001

[†]According to the Scheuer scoring system.
The study cohort was analyzed both as a whole and stratified according to HBeAg status.

patients with CHB, it seems reasonable that mean ABT values in our study is comparable to that of Herold *et al.* Mean values of ABT in patients with different stages of fibrosis and grades of inflammatory activity have been shown by Herold *et al.* Gm is the grade of inflammatory activity and Sn is the stage of fibrosis of a group of CHB patients. According to the Scheuer scoring system, inflammatory grade and fibrosis stage were scored as 0, 1, 2, 3, or 4. Thus, Gm represented anyone of G0, G1, G2, G3 or G4 while Sn represented anyone of S0, S1, S2, S3 or S4. If the liver histology of a group of patients was GmSn, the mean value of ABT of this group, ABT(GmSn), was calculated from the data provided by Herold *et al.* [13] by using the following expression: ABT(GmSn) = ABT(Gm) × ABT(Sn).

Statistical analyses were performed using R platform (version 3.0.1, http://www.R-project.org) or GraphPad Prism 6.01. Quantitative data conformed to Gaussian distribution were tested using ANOVA. Qualitative data or quantitative data that did not pass a Gaussian distribution test were analyzed using a nonparametric test, such as the Kruskal-Wallis test. The correlation of quantitative data was determined by the Pearson correlation test. Correlation of ordinal data was tested using the Spearman rank correlation test. All tests were two-sided and $p<0.05$ was regarded as statistically significant. HBV DNA and HBsAg levels were logarithmically transformed. For patients with HBV DNA levels lower than 500 IU/ml, a value of 250 IU/ml was assigned.

Results

Patients' Characteristics

Among the 362 enrolled patients, 210 (58.0%) were HBeAg(+) and 152 (42.0%) were HBeAg(−) (Table 1). In both HBeAg(+) and HBeAg(−) groups, there were more men (n = 285; 78.7%) than women. Patients who were HBeAg(+) tended to younger than HBeAg(−) patients ($p<0.0001$). The mean alanine aminotransferase (ALT) levels and mean aspartate aminotransferase (AST) levels were significantly higher in HBeAg(+) patients than in HBeAg(−) patients ($p<0.0001$). Proportions of patients with normal ALT or AST in the HBeAg(−) group were significantly greater than in the HBeAg(+) group ($p<0.0001$). The grade of inflammation activity observed in HBeAg(+) patients was significantly higher compared with that seen in HBeAg(−) patients (median:2.0 vs. 1.0, Mann Whitney test, $p = 0.0018$; Fig. 1A). However, there was no statistically significant difference regarding the stage of fibrosis between the two groups (median: 1.0 vs. 1.0, Mann Whitney test, $p = 0.6253$; Fig. 1B). The expression of tissue

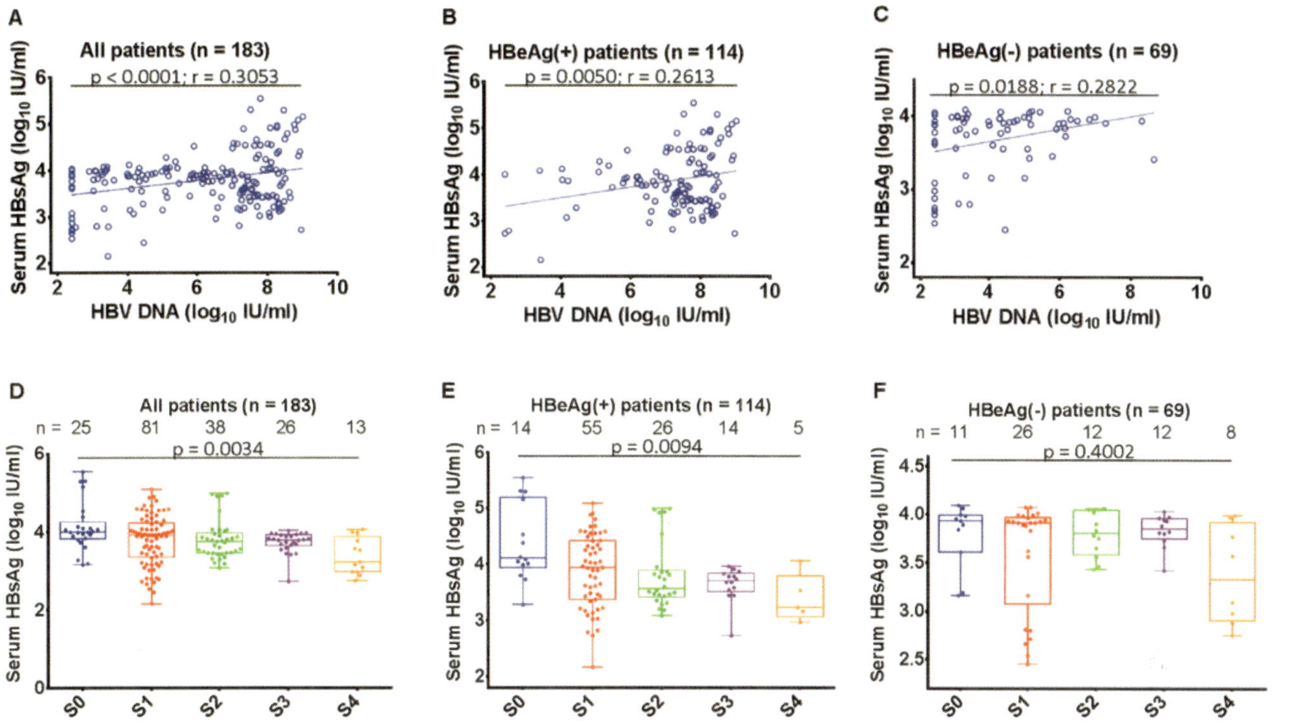

Figure 2. Correlation between serum HBsAg and HBV DNA and stage of fibrosis in treatment-naïve CHB patients. (A–C) correlation between serum HBsAg (log10 IU/ml) and HBV DNA (log10 IU/ml) in 183 patients with quantified serum HBsAg values, HBeAg(+) patients, and HBeAg(−) patients, respectively. (D–F) correlation between serum HBsAg (log10 IU/ml) and stage of fibrosis in 183 patients with quantified serum HBsAg values, HBeAg(+) patients, and HBeAg(−) patients, respectively.

HBsAg was similar in both groups (median: 2.0 vs. 2.0, Mann Whitney test, $p = 0.5703$; Fig. 1C).

All patients underwent an HBV DNA assay. However, due to cost, quantitative HBsAg measurement was performed in only 183 of the 362 enrolled patients. Detailed informations of the 183 patients were listed in Table 2. HBeAg(+) patients exhibited significantly higher serum levels of HBV DNA compared with HBeAg(−) patients ($p<0.0001$; Fig. 1D). HBeAg(+) patients tended to have higher serum HBsAg levels than did HBeAg(−) patients, although there was no statistically significant difference between the two groups (mean ± SD: 3.87±0.64 vs. 3.68±0.44, $p = 0.2600$; Fig. 1E).

Table 3. Mean value of aminopyrine breath test (ABT) in different stage of fibrosis and grade of activity.

	S0*	S1	S2	S3	S4
G0	0.55	0.40	0.42	0.24	0.21
G1	0.52	0.38	0.40	0.22	0.19
G2	0.47	0.34	0.36	0.20	0.17
G3	0.48	0.35	0.37	0.21	0.18
G4	0.43	0.31	0.33	0.19	0.16

*Herold *et al.* [13] did not provided the mean value of ABT in S0. The mean value of ABT in the control group was used as the mean value of ABT in S0.

Positive Correlation between Serum HBsAg and HBV DNA Levels

In the 183 patients in whom serum HBsAg levels were quantified, there was a positive correlation between serum HBsAg and HBV DNA levels ($r = 0.3053$, $p<0.0001$; Fig. 2A). After stratifying the patients according to HBeAg status, a correlation was found between HBsAg and HBV DNA levels in HBeAg(+) patients ($r = 0.2613$, $p = 0.0050$; Fig. 2B) as well as in HBeAg(−) patients ($r = 0.2822$, $p = 0.0188$; Fig. 2C).

Negative Correlation between Serum HBsAg Levels and Stage of Fibrosis

Severity of liver fibrosis was scored using the Scheuer system [14]. In the 183 patients with quantitative HBsAg data, increasing severity of fibrosis was associated with a decreasing serum HBsAg ($p = 0.0034$; Fig. 2D) and there was a negative correlation ($r = -0.2711$; $p = 0.0002$). In HBeAg(+) patients, this negative relationship was also significant ($p = 0.0094$; Fig. 2E) and the correlation was ($r = -0.3212$; $p = 0.0005$); however, no confirmed relationship could be seen in HBeAg(−) patients ($p = 0.4002$; Fig. 2F).

Positive Correlation between ABT-adjusted Serum HBsAg Levels and Stage of Fibrosis

Table 3 was deduced from the data reported in Herold *et al.* [13]. ABT-adjusted serum HBsAg was calculated by dividing serum HBsAg ($\log_{10}$ IU/ml) by ABT(GmSn).

In all 183 patients, or when stratifying this cohort into HBeAg(+) and HBeAg(−) patients, increasing ABT-adjusted serum HBsAg values were associated with increasing severity of fibrosis (Fig. 3A, 3B, 3C, respectively). Specifically, in the 183

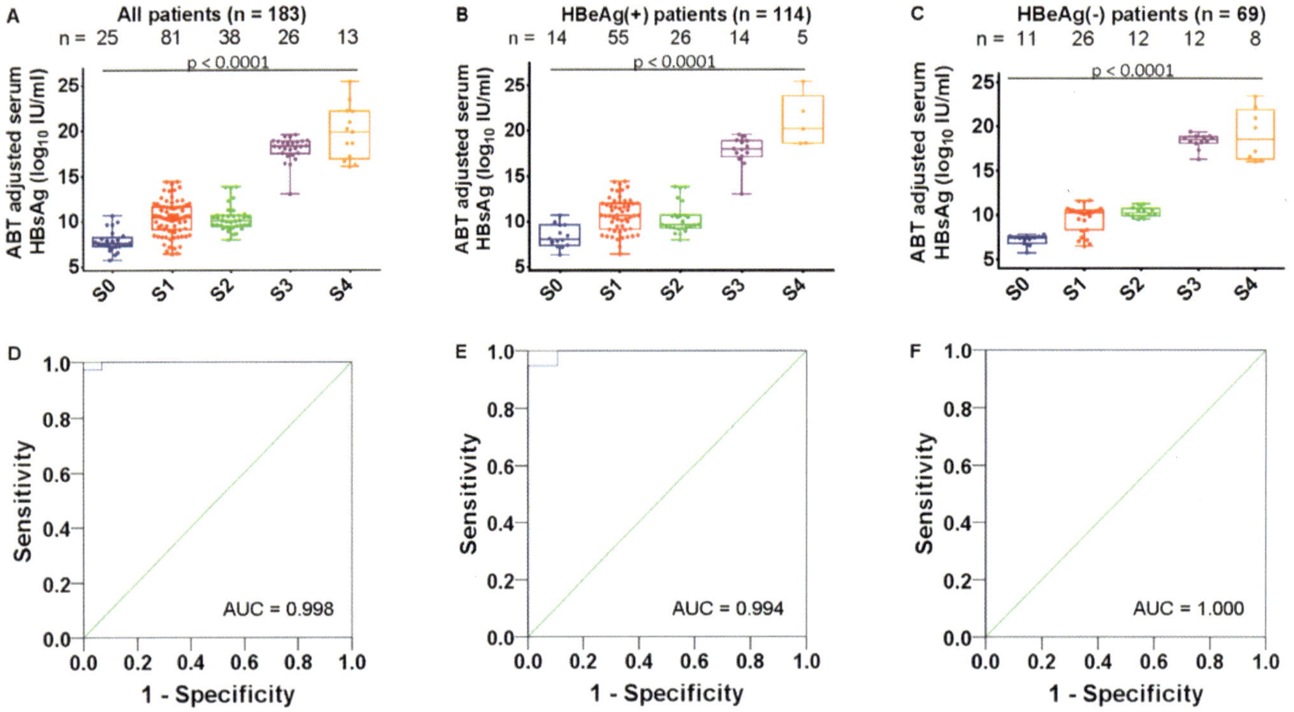

Figure 3. Correlation between aminopyrine breath test (ABT)-adjusted serum HBsAg and fibrosis severity. (A–C) correlation between ABT-adjusted serum HBsAg (log10 IU/ml) and fibrosis severity in 183 patients with quantified serum HBsAg values, HBeAg(+) patients and HBeAg(−) patients, respectively. Stage of fibrosis was determined according to the Scheuer scoring system. (D–F) diagnostic performance (AUC) of aminopyrine breath test -adjusted serum HBsAg in recognizing moderate to severe fibrosis (S3 and S4) in all of 183 patients, HBeAg(+) patients, and HBeAg(−) patients, respectively.

patients, a positive correlation was seen between severity of fibrosis and ABT-adjusted serum HBsAg values ($r = 0.6929$, $p<0.0001$); a similar phenomenon was observed in HBeAg(+) patients ($r = 0.5655$, $p<0.0001$), while in HBeAg(−) patients the correlation was even stronger ($r = 0.8289$, $p<0.0001$).

Role of ABT-adjusted Serum HBsAg Levels in Differentiating CHB Patients with no to Mild Fibrosis from those with Moderate to Severe Fibrosis

Stages S0–S1 fibrosis were defined as 'no to mild', while stages S3–S4 were defined as 'moderate to severe' fibrosis. In order to evaluate the diagnostic performance of ABT-adjusted serum HBsAg levels in differentiating patients with S0–S1 fibrosis from patients with S3–S4 fibrosis, ROC curves were generated. In the 183 patients with quantified serum HBsAg levels, the ABT-adjusted serum HBsAg values had a nearly perfect area under the curve (AUC) for differentiating stages S0–S2 from stages S3–S4 (AUC: 0.998, 95% confidence interval [CI]: 0.994–1.000; Fig. 3D). For HBeAg(+) patients, the AUC was 0.994 (95% CI: 0.983–1.000; Fig. 3E), and in HBeAg(−) patients AUC was 1.000 (95% CI: 1.000–1.000; Fig. 3F). In the 183 patients, a cut-off value for ABT-adjusted serum HBsAg (log_{10} IU/ml) of 15.0 had a sensitivity of 97.44%, a specificity of 100.00%, and a positive predictive value of 100.00%, with a negative predictive value of 99.31% for recognizing stages S3–S4 of fibrosis.

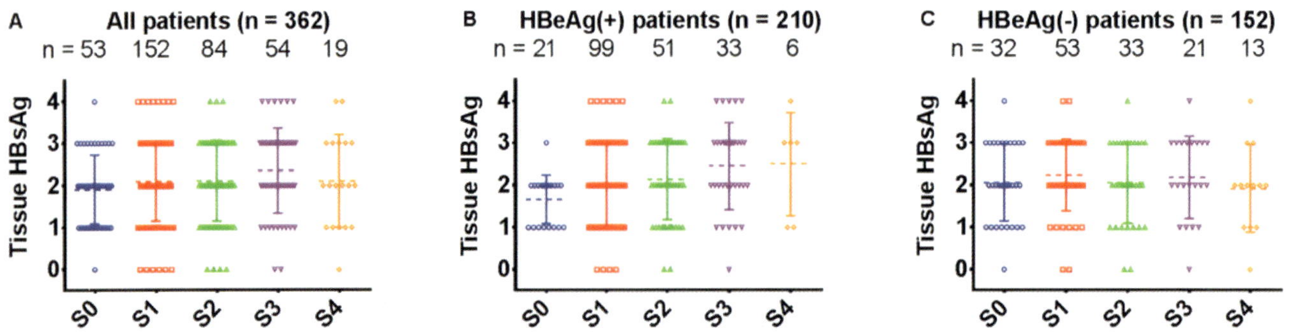

Figure 4. Expression of tissue HBsAg in patients with different stages of fibrosis. (A–C) grade of tissue HBsAg in CHB patients stratified according to the stage of fibrosis in all enrolled patients, HBeAg(+) patients, and HBeAg(−) patients, respectively. Stage of fibrosis was determined according to the Scheuer scoring system.
doi:10.1371/journal.pone.0087344.g004

Positive Correlation between Tissue HBsAg Levels and Severity of Fibrosis

When stratifying the enrolled 362 patients according to the severity of fibrosis, there was a trend toward increasing tissue HBsAg levels with increasing fibrosis severity in HBeAg(+) patients ($p = 0.0040$), as is shown in Fig. 4B. However, no confirmed relationship between tissue HBsAg and severity of fibrosis was observed in the total group of 362 patients ($p = 0.1618$; Fig. 4A), or in HBeAg(−) patients ($p = 0.7067$; Fig. 4C). A positive correlation was revealed between tissue HBsAg levels and fibrosis in the group of 362 patients (Spearman rank correlation, $r = 0.1092$, $p = 0.0378$; Fig. S1A). In HBeAg(+) group, the positive correlation was even stronger ($r = 0.2168$, $p = 0.0016$; Fig. S1B), but there was no statistically significant correlation in the HBeAg(−) group ($p = 0.7786$; Fig. S1C).

Discussion

In brief, we preformed this cross-sectional study in a group of 362 unselected CHB patients and attempted to elucidate the relationship between serum HBsAg or tissue HBsAg and severity of fibrosis. In China, due to medical insurance cover, some of the patients accepted qualitative measurement of HBsAg. Thus, quantitative HBsAg levels could be determined in only 183 patients. An investigation performed by Zeng *et al.* [15] indicated that genotype B and genotype C of HBV accounted for up to 94% of HBV infections in Chinese patients. We could not recruit sufficient patients infected with genotypes other than B and C for statistical analysis, and therefore, HBV genotyping was not performed.

We observed that HBeAg(−) patients tended to have a higher percentage of normal ALT or AST levels, lower HBV DNA load, with mild necroinflammation, as compared to HBeAg(+) patients. Loss of HBeAg may indicate that the hosts had attained a certain level of immune-control over HBV and these hosts may become 'inactive carriers' [16,17], which may partly explain the afore-mentioned phenomena. However, the severity of fibrosis in HBeAg(−) patients was similar to that in HBeAg(+) patients. Since HBeAg(−) patients tended to be older than HBeAg(+) patients, the former may have undergone repeated bouts of inflammation than the latter, although the necroinflammation was milder in HBeAg(−) patients.

In the past several years, increasing numbers of studies have been performed to establish the role of serum HBsAg quantification in the prediction of therapy response [18,19], intervention monitoring [20,21], and disease progression [22]. Quite recently, the relationship between serum HBsAg and liver histology has been discussed [9–12]. In the present study, a positive correlation between serum HBsAg and HBV DNA load was revealed in the treatment-naïve HBeAg(+) CHB patients. In HBeAg(−) CHB patients, there tended to be a similar but weaker relationship, which was in accordance with previous studies [23–25].

In treatment-naïve CHB patients, pre-core promoter mutations may lead to impaired secretion of HBeAg and HBV virions [26], which are the main source of serum HBV DNA, while pre-S region mutations would reduce serum HBsAg output [27,28]. Since these mutations do not always occur simultaneously, unbalanced production of HBsAg and HBV DNA may be observed.

Similar to previous reports [9–12], we also observed a strong inverse correlation between serum HBsAg and severity of fibrosis in HBeAg(+) CHB patients, whereas this correlation was not evident in HBeAg(−) patients (Fig. 2E, F). Interestingly, after adjusted by mean ABT (listed in Table 3), the ABT-adjusted serum HBsAg values highly positively correlated with the severity of fibrosis in both HBeAg(+) and HBeAg(−) CHB patients (Fig. 3B, C). ABT reflects the metabolic capacity of hepatocytes and essentially mirrors the quantity of viable hepatocytes. Therefore, ABT-adjusted serum HBsAg values would be unaffected by variation in the number of hepatocytes and could be regarded as a way to map the amount of HBeAg secreted by a 'single hepatocyte'.

As for the prediction of severity of fibrosis, ABT-adjusted serum HBsAg values demonstrated a nearly perfect AUC in both HBeAg(+) and HBeAg(−) CHB patients (Fig. 3E, F), which was superior to the use of serum HBsAg quantification only as a predictor of fibrosis severity [11]. Integrated application of serum HBsAg quantification data and ABT values may be necessary for precise prediction. It should be noted that the Ludwig scoring system was adopted in the study by Herold *et al.* [13], while the Scheuer scoring system was used in our investigation. However, the definitions of S1 to S4 are similar in these two systems (Table S1). Therefore, use of mean ABT values presented in the study by Herold *et al.* [13] was acceptable in our investigation.

We also found that there was a positive correlation between tissue HBsAg and the severity of fibrosis for all of the enrolled patients, and more particularly for HBeAg(+) patients. Using immunohistochemistry, tissue HBsAg was determined from the percentage and the strength of staining in hepatocytes. The number of viable hepatocytes has no effect on the expression of tissue HBsAg; thus, the positive correlation of tissue HBsAg with the severity of fibrosis further confirmed the relationship that we observed between ABT-adjusted serum HBsAg levels and the stage of fibrosis. Therefore, it seemed reasonable to deduce that the capacity for synthesis of HBsAg by individual hepatocyte is enhanced in cases with moderate to severe fibrosis.

Compared with recent studies [11,12], several key differences were exhibited in our study: (1) ABT was adopted to adjust serum HBsAg levels and more precise prediction of moderate to severe fibrosis was achieved; (2) correlation between tissue HBsAg and fibrosis severity was analyzed, which further supported the relationship between ABT-adjusted serum HBsAg and the stage of fibrosis. Thus, it was helpful to elucidate the actual value of serum HBsAg; (4) 58% of the enrolled patients were HBeAg (+), which was differed markedly from the study of Martinot-Peignoux *et al.* [11]. It is well known that there is significant heterogeneity in the genomes of HBeAg(−) HBV, which may hinder the generalization of the conclusions derived from HBeAg(−) patients. Future research with long-term follow-up in humans and laboratory animal-based research using stratification according to serum HBsAg levels are indispensable for exploring the roles of HBsAg in liver fibrosis.

Supporting Information

Figure S1 Correlation between immunohistochemistry grade of tissue HBsAg and stage of fibrosis. (A–C) grade of tissue HBsAg in CHB patients stratified according to the stage of fibrosis in all enrolled patients, HBeAg(+) patients, and HBeAg(−) patients, respectively. Stage of fibrosis was determined according to the Scheuer scoring system.

Table S1 Definition of fibrosis stage in Ludwig scoring system and Scheuer scoring system.

Acknowledgments

We are much indebted to Prof. Yu-Qing Zheng and Prof. Tian-Hai Ji for reviewing the liver histology. We thank Dr. Rong-Hua Fan, Wei-Bin Wu and Li Zhang for collecting the clinical information.

Author Contributions

Conceived and designed the experiments: MZH JSP. Performed the experiments: MZH WQH FM JCX ZL. Analyzed the data: KNF JSP. Contributed reagents/materials/analysis tools: MZH WQH FM JCX ZL. Wrote the paper: JSP.

References

1. Chen CJ, Yang HI, Su J, Jen CL, You SL, et al. (2006) Risk of hepatocellular carcinoma across a biological gradient of serum hepatitis B virus DNA level. JAMA 295: 65–73.
2. Iloeje UH, Yang HI, Su J, Jen CL, You SL, et al. (2006) Predicting cirrhosis risk based on the level of circulating hepatitis B viral load. Gastroenterology 130: 678–686.
3. Chen YC, Sheen IS, Chu CM, Liaw YF (2002) Prognosis following spontaneous HBsAg seroclearance in chronic hepatitis B patients with or without concurrent infection. Gastroenterology 123: 1084–1089.
4. Yuen MF, Wong DK, Fung J, Ip P, But D, et al. (2008) HBsAg Seroclearance in chronic hepatitis B in Asian patients: replicative level and risk of hepatocellular carcinoma. Gastroenterology 135: 1192–1199.
5. European Association For The Study Of The Liver (2012) EASL clinical practice guidelines: Management of chronic hepatitis B virus infection. J Hepatol 57: 167–185.
6. Simonetti J, Bulkow L, McMahon BJ, Homan C, Snowball M, et al. (2010) Clearance of hepatitis B surface antigen and risk of hepatocellular carcinoma in a cohort chronically infected with hepatitis B virus. Hepatology 51: 1531–1537.
7. Fattovich G, Giustina G, Sanchez-Tapias J, Quero C, Mas A, et al. (1998) Delayed clearance of serum HBsAg in compensated cirrhosis B: relation to interferon alpha therapy and disease prognosis. European Concerted Action on Viral Hepatitis (EUROHEP). Am J Gastroenterol 93: 896–900.
8. Tseng TC, Liu CJ, Yang HC, Su TH, Wang CC, et al. (2012) High levels of hepatitis B surface antigen increase risk of hepatocellular carcinoma in patients with low HBV load. Gastroenterology 142: 1140–1149 e1143; quiz e1113–1144.
9. Cheng PN, Tsai HW, Chiu YC, Ho CH, Wu IC, et al. (2013) Clinical significance of serum HBsAg levels and association with liver histology in HBeAg positive chronic hepatitis B. J Clin Virol 57: 323–330.
10. Xun YH, Zang GQ, Guo JC, Yu XL, Liu H, et al. (2013) Serum HBsAg Quantification as a useful assessment for significant fibrosis in HBeAg positive hepatitis B virus carriers. J Gastroenterol Hepatol.
11. Martinot-Peignoux M, Carvalho-Filho R, Lapalus M, Netto-Cardoso AC, Lada O, et al. (2013) Hepatitis B surface antigen serum level is associated with fibrosis severity in treatment-naive, e antigen-positive patients. J Hepatol 58: 1089–1095.
12. Seto WK, Wong DK, Fung J, Ip PP, Yuen JC, et al. (2012) High hepatitis B surface antigen levels predict insignificant fibrosis in hepatitis B e antigen positive chronic hepatitis B. PLoS One 7: e43087.
13. Herold C, Heinz R, Niedobitek G, Schneider T, Hahn EG, et al. (2001) Quantitative testing of liver function in relation to fibrosis in patients with chronic hepatitis B and C. Liver 21: 260–265.
14. Scheuer PJ (1991) Classification of chronic viral hepatitis: a need for reassessment. J Hepatol 13: 372–374.
15. Zeng G, Wang Z, Wen S, Jiang J, Wang L, et al. (2005) Geographic distribution, virologic and clinical characteristics of hepatitis B virus genotypes in China. J Viral Hepat 12: 609–617.
16. Bortolotti F, Guido M, Bartolacci S, Cadrobbi P, Crivellaro C, et al. (2006) Chronic hepatitis B in children after e antigen seroclearance: final report of a 29-year longitudinal study. Hepatology 43: 556–562.
17. Lok AS, Lai CL, Wu PC, Leung EK, Lam TS (1987) Spontaneous hepatitis B e antigen to antibody seroconversion and reversion in Chinese patients with chronic hepatitis B virus infection. Gastroenterology 92: 1839–1843.
18. Chan HL, Wong VW, Tse AM, Tse CH, Chim AM, et al. (2007) Serum hepatitis B surface antigen quantitation can reflect hepatitis B virus in the liver and predict treatment response. Clin Gastroenterol Hepatol 5: 1462–1468.
19. Moucari R, Mackiewicz V, Lada O, Ripault MP, Castelnau C, et al. (2009) Early serum HBsAg drop: a strong predictor of sustained virological response to pegylated interferon alfa-2a in HBeAg-negative patients. Hepatology 49: 1151–1157.
20. Ahmed SN, Ecochard M, Zoulim F (2010) End points of therapy in chronic hepatitis B. Expert Rev Gastroenterol Hepatol 4: 37–49.
21. Ayoub WS, Keeffe EB (2011) Review article: current antiviral therapy of chronic hepatitis B. Aliment Pharmacol Ther 34: 1145–1158.
22. Tseng TC, Liu CJ, Yang HC, Su TH, Wang CC, et al. (2013) Serum hepatitis B surface antigen levels help predict disease progression in patients with low hepatitis B virus loads. Hepatology 57: 441–450.
23. Nguyen T, Thompson AJ, Bowden S, Croagh C, Bell S, et al. (2010) Hepatitis B surface antigen levels during the natural history of chronic hepatitis B: a perspective on Asia. J Hepatol 52: 508–513.
24. Reijnders JG, Rijckborst V, Sonneveld MJ, Scherbeijn SM, Boucher CA, et al. (2011) Kinetics of hepatitis B surface antigen differ between treatment with peginterferon and entecavir. J Hepatol 54: 449–454.
25. Su TH, Hsu CS, Chen CL, Liu CH, Huang YW, et al. (2010) Serum hepatitis B surface antigen concentration correlates with HBV DNA level in patients with chronic hepatitis B. Antivir Ther 15: 1133–1139.
26. Lok ASF, McMahon BJ (2009) Chronic hepatitis B: Update 2009. Hepatology 50: 661–662.
27. Torresi J (2002) The virological and clinical significance of mutations in the overlapping envelope and polymerase genes of hepatitis B virus. J Clin Virol 25: 97–106.
28. Bock CT, Tillmann HL, Torresi J, Klempnauer J, Locarnini S, et al. (2002) Selection of hepatitis B virus polymerase mutants with enhanced replication by lamivudine treatment after liver transplantation. Gastroenterology 122: 264–273.

21

Chronic Hepatitis B Prevalence among Children and Mothers: Results from a Nationwide, Population-Based Survey in Lao People's Democratic Republic

Anonh Xeuatvongsa[1], Kenichi Komada[2], Tomomi Kitamura[2], Phengta Vongphrachanh[3], Chansay Pathammavong[1], Kongxay Phounphenghak[1], Thongchanh Sisouk[3], Darouny Phonekeo[3], Bounthanom Sengkeopaseuth[3], Vilasak Som-Oulay[3], Koji Ishii[4], Takaji Wakita[4], Masaya Sugiyama[5], Masahiko Hachiya[2]*

1 National Immunization Program, Ministry of Health, Lao PDR, Simeuang Road, Vientiane, Lao PDR, **2** Bureau of International Cooperation, National Center for Global Health and Medicine, Shinjuku, Tokyo, Japan, **3** National Center for Laboratory and Epidemiology, Ministry of Health, Lao PDR, Simeuang Road, Vientiane, Lao PDR, **4** Department of Virology II, National Institute of Infectious Diseases, Musashi-murayama, Tokyo, Japan, **5** Hepatology Research Center, National Center for Global Health and Medicine, Ichikawa, Chiba, Japan

Abstract

Background: Hepatitis B is regarded as a serious public health issue in Lao People's Democratic Republic (Lao PDR), a Southeast Asian country. However, disease epidemiology among the general population is not well known, and thus a nationwide cross-sectional survey for hepatitis B surface antigen (HBsAg) prevalence in children and their mothers was conducted.

Methods and findings: We applied three-stage cluster sampling using probability proportionate to size. After randomly selecting child (5 to 9 years old) and mother (15 to 45 years old) pairs from the selected villages, questionnaires and HBsAg rapid tests were conducted. Data from 965 child and mother pairs were analyzed. Multivariate logistic regression analyses were used to investigate the independent association of individual background characteristics for the odds of being HBsAg positive. In total, 17 children and 27 mothers were HBsAg positive. HBsAg prevalence was estimated to be 1.7% (95% confidence interval: 0.8%-2.6%) in children, and 2.9% (95% confidence interval: 1.7%–4.2%) in their mothers after taking sampling design and weight of each sample into account. Mother's infection status was positively associated with HBsAg positivity in children ($p<0.001$), whereas other potential risk factors, such as ethnicity, proximity to health centers, and history of surgery, were not. There were no significant associations between mother's HBsAg status and history of surgery, and other sociodemographic factors.

Conclusions: Despite the slow implementation of the hepatitis B vaccination program, HBsAg prevalence among children and their mothers was not high in Lao PDR compared to reports from neighboring countries. The reasons for the differences in prevalence among these countries are unclear. We recommend that prevalence surveys be conducted in populations born before and after the implementation of a hepatitis B vaccination program to better understand the epidemiology of hepatitis B.

Editor: Pierre Roques, CEA, France

Funding: This study was supported by The Grant for Nationa Center for Global Health and Medicine (25-8). The funders had no role in study design, data collection and analysis, decision to publish, or preparation of the manuscript.

Competing Interests: The authors have declared that no competing interests exist.

* E-mail: m-hachiya@it.ncgm.go.jp

Introduction

More than two billion people have been infected with hepatitis B worldwide, and among these individuals, more than 350 million suffer from chronic hepatitis B virus (HBV) infection [1,2,3]. Infection with HBV results in 600,000 to 1.2 million deaths per year due to chronic hepatitis, cirrhosis, and hepatocellular carcinoma [2,4]. HBV is responsible for 60% to 80% of the world's hepatocellular carcinoma cases, one of the major three causes of death in Africa, Asia, and the Pacific Rim, and accordingly, has been categorized as a Group 1 carcinogenic agent to humans by the International Agency for Research on Cancer [5].

The prevalence of hepatitis B differs throughout the world. Southeast Asian countries have been estimated to have a chronic HBV infection rate of more than 8% before the introduction of hepatitis B vaccination [6]. The Western Pacific region of the World Health Organization (WHO), to which most of the Southeast Asian countries belong, is assumed to have a high prevalence of hepatitis B [7]. Specifically, the prevalence is estimated to be 9% to 12% among women of childbearing age [8] and 8% to 10% among children in pre-vaccine era [9]. The WHO

estimates that the region has 28% of the global population, while it accounts for almost half of all chronic hepatitis B infections worldwide [10].

Hepatitis B vaccination, especially within 24 hours after childbirth, is considered the most effective and efficient preventive measure against hepatitis B infection [3,11]. Based on these assumptions, the WHO set goals to lower the prevalence of chronic hepatitis B among children over 5 years of age to 2% by 2012 and 1% by 2017. To achieve these goals, the WHO plans to increase immunization coverage to 65% for the birth dose and 80% for the third dose of the hepatitis B vaccine [7].

Lao People's Democratic Republic (Lao PDR) is a Southeast Asian country, located in the center of the Indochina peninsula. The country is landlocked and surrounded by China, Vietnam, Cambodia, Thailand, and Myanmar. The neighboring countries report relatively high hepatitis B prevalence compared to other parts of the world. For example, a survey from two provinces in Cambodia reported a hepatitis B surface antigen (HBsAg) prevalence of 7.7% (95% CI: 6.2%–9.3%) among healthy volunteer adults [12]. Another population-based survey in a province in rural Vietnam found that 18.8% (95% CI: 15.7%–21.9%) of adults and 12.5% (95% CI: 9.7%–15.3%) of infants were HBsAg positive at the time of the survey [13]. Thus, Lao PDR has been regarded as one of the hyperendemic countries for hepatitis B for quite some time and is ranked as a priority country by the WHO [7,9] despite a lack of data on the prevalence in a representative population. Pre-vaccine era prevalence was estimated as 11.8% [4], 8–10% [9], or 8% or more [6] for Lao PDR and Indochina countries. In response to this situation, Lao PDR has implemented the hepatitis B vaccine into the routine immunization program since 2002 (at 6, 10, and 14 weeks after birth), as well as birth dosing since 2004. The birth dosing was initiated at referral hospitals in the capital city, and then gradually expanded into rural hospitals (2006), and eventually home deliveries (2010). However, since then, no direct investigation has been conducted, and thus a nationwide survey is warranted [7,9]. The routine immunization coverage is reported as 56% for BCG, 50% for the third DPT, 50% for the third hepatitis B, 40% for measles, and 46% for oral polio vaccine in 2007, when a proportion of target children were born [14].

The primary objective of the present study was to estimate the chronic HBV infection rates by measuring the seroprevalence of HBsAg among children aged 5 to 9 years, and their mothers aged 15 to 45 years.

Methods

Ethical considerations

The survey protocol was reviewed and approved by the Ethical Committee of the Ministry of Health, Lao PDR, and the institutional review board of the National Center for Global Health and Medicine, Japan (NCGM-G-001130-00). Access to selected households was granted by the Ministry of Health, and the provincial and district government authorities.

After obtaining approval to conduct the survey from local authorities, surveyors explained the purpose of the survey to village leaders, selected participants, and their caregivers, assured them that all information would be strictly confidential and that no names would be gathered, and that there would be no benefit or penalties for agreeing or refusing to participate. Written informed consent was obtained from each mother on behalf of her child for each pair. Written informed consent was obtained from legal representatives (next of kin, caregivers, or guardians) when mothers were illiterate. The respondents' names were not recorded on the questionnaire sheets.

Study population

The target population was children aged 5 to 9 years (date of birth: January 2, 2002 to January 1, 2007) and their mothers aged 15 to 45 years (date of birth: January 2, 1966 to January 1, 1997) living in the selected cluster at the time of the survey. The reasons for this selection criteria are: 1) the national and regional hepatitis control policy target is to reduce chronic hepatitis B prevalence among children aged 5 years or older [7]; 2) Lao PDR does not have reliable HBsAg prevalence data among healthy adults, and mothers of childbearing age are considered the major source of hepatitis B infection for children; and 3) our pilot survey revealed that between 20 and 25 mother and child pairs can be practically sampled from each village.

Calculation of sample size

The equation used to calculate the required sample size is as follows [15,16]:

$$n = Z^2 \times p(1-p)DEFF \times 2/(d^2 \times RR)$$

where n = sample size
Z = significance level for 95% confidence
p = expected prevalence
$DEFF$ = design effect
d = precision
RR = response rate

The sample size (n) of 961 was calculated on the basis of an expected HBsAg seroprevalence (p) of 5%, a 5% level of significance (Z), precision (d) of ±2.0%, design effect ($DEFF$) of 2.0, two strata, and response rate (RR) of 95%. For field practicability, we requested 24 survey teams to sample 21 child and mother pairs from each cluster, with the aim of gathering 1,008 pairs in total.

Survey design and sampling

The survey applied a stratified three-stage random cluster sampling design, a type of probability sampling recommended by the WHO [15,17]. The survey was carried out by 24 survey teams (two members per team). Team members were recruited from the same districts that were under investigation to implement the survey more smoothly. The survey teams consisted of epidemiology, surveillance, or laboratory staff. The survey teams were supervised by 11 national personnel (six from the National Immunization Program and five from the National Center for Laboratory and Epidemiology, Ministry of Health) as well as 13 provincial officers.

For stratified multistage cluster sampling, immunization coverage by district and population data were obtained from the National Immunization Program, the Ministry of Health, and the Department of Statistics, Lao PDR. For post-survey weight adjustment, the survey teams obtained the latest population data from village leaders or health volunteers.

All 143 districts in Lao PDR were stratified into two strata, one having high (more than 76%) and the other having low (76% or less) immunization coverage for the third diphtheria, pertussis, tetanus, and hepatitis B (DPT-HepB)vaccines as reported in 2010. For the first stage, we selected 12 districts from each stratum using probability proportionate to size (PPS) sampling based on the population census of 2005. For the second stage, we selected two villages from each selected district by PPS sampling, and 48

villages were randomly sampled in total. In the instances in which the selected village lacked a sufficient number of children or the survey team could not approach the selected village due to safety or security reasons, the nearest village on the way back to the district center was selected. For each selected village, surveyors obtained a list of households, including age and sex, primarily from the poverty reduction program data with the assistance of the village leader, women's union, and/or healthcare volunteer. From these lists, 21 mothers aged 15 to 45 years old with children aged 5 to 9 years were randomly selected using a paper-based lottery system. When a mother had multiple children aged 5 to 9 years old, the youngest child was chosen for the survey. Special attention was paid to ensure that the child's biological mother was surveyed, as adoption is common in rural Lao PDR.

The survey was carried out from January 25th to February 4th, 2012. Each survey team successfully approached their assigned villages, with the exception of one village, which could not be visited because of road difficulties. An alternative village was chosen according to the predetermined selection criteria. In total, 1,008 children and 1,008 mothers were sampled. The overall response rate for HBsAg was 100%; however, 43 pairs were excluded from the analysis due to age ineligibility. That is, one child was over 9 years of age and 33 were less than 5 years of age. Furthermore, three mothers were over 45 years of age and six were less than 15 years of age. This happened as 43 mothers confused calendar age with traditional age. In rural areas, newborns start at one year old and a year is added to their age for each passing of a Lunar New Year. The surveyors asked participants for their age in years and their date of birth, and checked that they matched. A total of 965 pairs were included for analysis.

Questionnaires

A brief face-to-face questionnaire was administered to the sampled mother. The questionnaire consisted of 25 questions in four domains of inquiry: sociodemographic background of the family (i.e., ethnicity, family head's occupation, and mother's education level), family history of liver diseases, including mother, demographic characteristics of the child (i.e., age, sex, and place of birth), and immunization records. Additionally, questions were asked regarding exposure to potential risk factors for acquiring hepatitis B infection (e.g., history of blood transfusion, surgical operation, and sharing of toothbrush). The questionnaire was developed in English, translated into Lao, back-translated into English, and then compared and revised by bilingual staff members. A small pilot test was conducted prior to the data collection.

Testing for HBsAg

We used a simple and rapid test (Alere Determine HBsAg test card; Alere Medical Co. Ltd., Chiba, Japan) rather than the traditional ELISA test, as it was better suited to use in the field [14]. The sensitivity and specificity of the test were reported as high in two Asian countries [18,19]. In Vietnam, the Determine HBsAg test validity was measured based on comparison with HBsAg EIA. Results were 100% in both sensitivity and specificity in 328 samples [18]. In China, the Determine HBsAg performance was evaluated in comparison with HBsAg EIA for 671 samples. The sensitivity was reported to be 98.9% and specificity 100% [19]. The Determine HBsAg examination kit is one of the most reliable point-of-care HBsAg tests, and is recommended by the WHO [15]. HBsAg testing was performed according to the manufacturer's instructions. Blood was collected from a finger prick using a safety lancet (BD Safety Lancet, Becton Dickinson, NJ, USA) and glass capillary tube, and the blood was applied onto the sample pad of the rapid test kit. After applying the chase buffer, surveyors assessed the results after at least 15 minutes, but no longer than 24 hours. When no control bar appeared after 15 minutes, the test results were considered invalid, and the test was repeated. Blood spots were collected onto filter paper for further testing. A 2-day training session was organized for surveyors and supervisors on the use of the rapid test and the completion of the questionnaire. To ensure the safety of the blood collection procedure, surveyors always used a new pair of latex gloves. Surveyors were instructed to place all capillary tubes and lancets into safety boxes immediately after use.

Data entry and statistical analysis

All of the completed questionnaires were brought to a centralized location and the data were entered into a Microsoft Excel 2007 spreadsheet. Data were double-entered and cross-checked. Logistic regression tests and odds ratios were used to examine the relationship between the independent variables and HBsAg results. Multivariate logistic regression was used to investigate the independent association of different household and individual characteristics with the odds of being HBsAg positive. All estimates and standard errors were calculated by taking the multistage clustered sampling design and the weight of each sample into account to give representative, unbiased results. A p value <0.05 was considered statistically significant.

In our regression analyses, we adjusted for potential confounders by using the following variables: third DPT-HepB immunization coverage at the location of current residence, mother's age, ethnic group, mother's education level, family head's occupation, and mother's HBsAg status. For multivariate logistic regression analyses, multicollinearity was tested by calculating the variance inflation factors for each independent variable, and a value of more than 10 was considered as having multicollinearity.

All statistical analyses were carried out using STATA version 12 (Stata Corp., College Station, TX). Means and proportions were calculated using STATA's 'svy' function, with each sample weighted according to estimated population size.

Results

Socioeconomic backgrounds

The baseline characteristics of the 965 mothers and their children are summarized in Table 1. The mean age of the mothers was 29.1 years (95% CI: 26.2–33.1), and the mean age of the children was 5.8 years (95% CI: 5.4–6.3). Of the sampled children, 474 (49.4%) were male and 486 (50.6%) were female (five were unknown).

HBsAg prevalence among the general population

Of the 965 pairs included in the study, 17 children and 27 mothers were positive for HBsAg. Six child and mother pairs were HBsAg positive. The estimated prevalence was 1.7% for children (95% CI: 0.8%–2.6%) and 2.9% for mothers (95% CI: 1.7%–4.2%) after taking the sampling design and weight of each sample into account. HBsAg prevalence did not change significantly between DPT-HepB3 high and low coverage districts in both children and mothers (Table 2).

Potential risk factors

To determine whether background characteristics affect HBsAg status, we conducted multivariate logistic regression analysis in children and their mothers. In children, the mother's HBsAg status was positively associated with hepatitis B infection (Table 3),

Table 1. HBsAg prevalence among children (5 to 9 years old) and mothers (15 to 45 years old) in Lao PDR by selected background characteristics.

		n	%	Children's HBsAg (+)	%	95% CI	Mothers' HBsAg (+)	%	95% CI
Mothers' age(n = 965)	15–19	4	0.41	0	0.00		0	0.00	
	20–24	85	8.80	1	1.18	0.00–3.52	3	3.53	0.00–7.53
	25–29	294	30.47	7	2.38	0.63–4.13	8	2.72	0.85–4.59
	30–34	275	28.50	6	2.18	0.44–3.92	9	3.27	1.16–5.39
	35–39	176	18.24	3	1.70	0.00–3.64	3	1.70	0.00–3.64
	40–45	131	13.58	0	0.00		4	3.05	0.07–6.04
Ethnicity (n = 963)	Low land Lao	651	67.60	9	1.38	0.48–2.28	19	2.92	1.62–4.22
	Mid land Lao	248	25.75	6	2.42	0.49–4.34	5	2.02	0.25–3.78
	High land Lao	64	6.65	2	3.13	0.00–7.51	3	4.69	0.00–10.01
[1]Transportation (n = 939)	on foot	298	31.74	1	0.34	0.00–1.00	6	2.01	0.41–3.62
	bicycle	14	1.49	0	0.00		0	0.00	
	motor bike	364	38.76	7	1.92	0.51–3.34	10	2.75	1.06–4.43
	car	183	19.49	5	2.73	0.35–5.12	6	3.28	0.67–5.88
	hand tractor	66	7.03	3	4.55	0.00–9.71	4	6.06	0.15–11.97
	other	14	1.49	0	0.00		0	0.00	
[2]Time (n = 901)	< 5 minutes	31	3.44	0	0.00		1	3.23	0.00–9.81
	5 to 15 minutes	274	30.41	3	1.09	0.15–2.33	6	2.19	0.45–3.93
	15 to 30 minutes	231	25.64	5	2.16	0.27–4.06	11	4.76	2.00–7.53
	30 to 60 minutes	209	23.20	5	2.39	0.30–4.48	4	1.91	0.04–3.79
	> 60 minutes	156	17.31	3	1.56	0.00–4.68	4	2.56	0.06–5.07
[3]Education (n = 962)	did not finish primary school	307	31.91	7	2.28	0.60–3.96	12	3.91	1.73–6.09
	primary school	374	38.88	5	1.34	0.17–2.51	10	2.67	1.03–4.32
	junior high	185	19.23	3	1.62	0.00–3.46	2	1.08	0.00–2.59
	high school	73	7.59	0	0.00		1	1.37	0.00–4.10
	college/univ	20	2.08	1	5.00	0.00–15.47	2	10.00	0.00–24.41
	other or unknown	3	0.31	1	33.33	0.00–100.00	0	0.00	
[4]Occupation (n = 963)	farmer	683	70.92	13	1.90	0.88–2.93	19	2.78	1.55–4.02
	fisherman	5	0.52	0	0.00		0	0.00	
	laborer	92	9.55	1	1.09	0.00–3.25	5	5.43	0.71–10.16
	public officer	88	9.14	1	1.14	0.00–3.40	3	6.25	1.70–10.80
	factory employee	8	0.83	0	0.00		0	0.00	
	general employee	16	1.66	1	6.25	0.00–19.57	0	0.00	
	merchant	63	6.54	1	1.59	0.00–4.76	0	0.00	
	others	8	0.83	0	0.00		0	0.00	
Mother's surgery (n = 962)	yes	95	9.88	2	2.11	0.00–5.05	3	3.16	0.00–6.74
	no	867	90.12	15	1.73	0.86–2.60	24	2.77	1.67–3.86
Child's sex (n = 960)	male	474	49.38	9	1.89	0.67–3.13			
	female	486	50.63	7	1.44	0.38–2.50			
Place of delivery (n = 961)	province hospital	207	21.54	4	1.93	0.04–3.82	6	2.90	0.59–5.20
	district hospital	105	10.93	2	1.90	0.00–4.56	5	4.76	0.62–8.90
	health center	10	1.04	0	0.00		0	0.00	
	private clinic	11	1.14	0	0.00		1	9.09	0.00–29.35
	at home	569	59.21	8	1.41	0.44–2.38	14	2.46	1.18–3.74
	in the forest	56	5.83	3	5.36	0.00–11.44	1	1.79	0.00–5.36
	other health facility	3	0.32	0	0.00		0	0.00	
Child's surgery (n = 960)	yes	22	2.29	0	0.00				

Table 1. Cont.

	n	%	Children's HBsAg (+)	%	95% CI	Mothers' HBsAg (+)	%	95% CI
no	938	97.71	16	1.71	0.88–2.54			

[1]Transportation to the nearest health facility, [2] Time to the nearest health facility, [3] Mothers' completed education, [4] Family head's occupation.

whereas the other potential risk factors were not associated according to the adjusted odds ratio. We did not obtain information regarding the type of delivery, and we did not find significant differences in HBsAg prevalence associated with delivery settings. No independent factor was positively associated with HBsAg positivity in mothers, according to the adjusted odds ratio (Table 4).

Immunization status

Written immunization records were available for 213 out of 965 children (22.1%). One hundred ninety eight children were vaccinated with three doses of hepatitis B vaccine, and 34 children were immunized on the day of birth or the following day. Five out of 213 children with immunization records were HBsAg positive (2.35%; 95% CI: 0.30–4.40%), while 12 of 752 without immunization records were HBsAg positive (1.60%; 95% CI: 0.70–2.49%). The differences between the two groups were not significant ($p = 0.46$).

Discussion

HBsAg prevalence among the general population

The estimated HBsAg prevalence in the general population was much lower in both children and adults than that of previous reports from neighboring countries and Lao PDR. For example, HBsAg prevalence in adults in Cambodia, Thailand, and Vietnam was reported to be 7.7% (95% CI: 6.2%–9.3%) [12], 6 to 10% [15,20], and 18.8% (95% CI: 15.7%–21.9%) [13], respectively. Data on HBsAg prevalence amongst children was relatively scarce, and reported to be 3.5% (95% CI: 2.4%–4.8%) in Cambodia [21], and 18.4% (95% CI: 13.4%–23.4%) in Vietnam [13]. In Lao PDR, studies in blood donors, hospitalized patients, and Lao migrant workers tested in Thailand showed HBsAg prevalence of 8.73% (95% CI: 8.69%–8.77%) [22], 17.99% (95% CI: 17.81%–18.17%) [23], and 6.86% (95% CI: 6.80%–6.92%) [24] based on the given numerators and denominators in the articles, respectively.

Since the study objective was to estimate the nationwide HBsAg prevalence among the general population of Lao PDR, and thus the study design is a cross sectional survey, it is difficult to explain the reasons for the unexpectedly low prevalence. There are several potential explanations for this observation. The survey methodology used was very different from that used for blood donors, patients, and migrant workers. We used probability sampling and thus the results are representative of the whole population, whereas studies of blood donors, hospitalized patients, and migrant workers used non-probability sampling and therefore the results are restricted to these populations. The primary objective of our survey was to estimate HBsAg prevalence among the general population, so probability sampling was the most appropriate choice. Demographic conditions among the sampled population are determined by survey methodology, and therefore the results showed discrepancy. The WHO strongly recommends probability sampling for hepatitis B prevalence survey [7,15,17]. Although Lao PDR has the lowest population density of the Indochina peninsula countries [25], the precise effects on hepatitis B prevalence of the reduced frequency of human to human contact due to the country's relatively low population density and less developed infrastructure remain unclear.

The number of HBsAg positives varied from 0 to 4 per cluster. Since the sampling design of the survey aimed to estimate the prevalence in the whole country, it is difficult to determine whether these differences reflect the local endemic status.

Potential risk factors

Our survey revealed that no potential risk factors were significantly associated with the children's infection status, with the exception of the mothers' hepatitis B infection status. HBsAg prevalence surveys in other countries revealed that history of surgery [26,27], level of education [26], and ethnicity [28] were independently associated with hepatitis B infection. The reason why we could not find any potential risk factors positively associated with hepatitis B infection among children is not clear. However, it should be noted that the primary objective of the present study was to assess HBsAg prevalence, and not its risk factors. Additionally, some reports found that HIV positive individuals are positively associated with hepatitis B virus infection

Table 2. HBsAg prevalence among children (5 to 9 years old) and mothers (15 to 45 years old).

	Children's HBsAg (+)	%	95% CI	Standard error	Design effect	Mothers' HBsAg (+)	%	95% CI	Standard error	Design effect
High coverage districts (n = 486)	6	1.14	0.23–2.04	0.44	0.82	18	3.79	1.79–5.79	0.97	1.24
Low coverage districts (n = 479)	11	2.39	0.75–4.03	0.79	1.27	9	1.88	0.49–3.37	0.69	1.22
Total (n = 965)	17	1.72	0.81–2.63	0.44	1.10	27	2.93	1.65–4.20	0.61	1.28

Table 3. Unadjusted and adjusted odds ratio for being HBsAg positive among children from five to nine years old in Lao PDR by selected background characteristics.

		Unadjusted odds ratio	95% CI	p	Adjusted odds ratio	95% CI	p
DPT3 coverage	high	1(reference)					
	low	2.13	0.73–6.21	0.16	3.47	0.77–15.64	0.10
Mothers' age	15 to 29	1(reference)					
	30 to 45	0.70	0.28–1.78	0.44	0.87	0.31–2.47	0.79
Ethnicity	Low land Lao	1(reference)					
	others	1.90	0.67–5.40	0.22	1.41	0.26–7.72	0.68
Education	none	1(reference)					
	finished primary school or upper	1.50	0.67–3.36	0.30	1.03	0.27–3.89	0.96
Occupation	white collar	1(reference)					
	blue collar	1.15	0.37–3.64	0.80	0.60	0.18–1.96	0.38
Sex	male	1(reference)					
	female	0.75	0.21–2.62	0.63	0.65	0.21–2.08	0.46
Birth place	health facility	1(reference)					
	non-health facility	0.98	0.39–2.49	0.97	0.79	0.28–2.21	0.64
Mothers' HBsAg	negative	1(reference)					
	positive	24.02	9.45–61.07	0.00	28.13	10.21–77.53	0.00

[29,30]; however, we did not investigate HIV due to limited budget.

WHO's regional target

The interim target of the WHO is to reduce HBsAg prevalence to less than 2% in children aged at least 5 years old by 2012 [7,31]. The point prevalence is used for monitoring the control of hepatitis B. The Regional Office for the Western pacific recommended that the country conduct a national HBsAg prevalence survey to verify whether the country has reached the regional prevalence target [9]. Following these criteria, Lao PDR had already achieved its goal. However, it is unlikely that Lao PDR achieved the target through the immunization program alone because the country has the lowest immunization coverage of all countries in the region [7,9]. Considering the relatively lower HBsAg seroprevalence among the mothers compared to those reported in previous studies, it is likely that Lao PDR had a lower prevalence even before the introduction of the hepatitis B immunization program. Therefore, the final target of reducing HBsAg prevalence to less than 1% in children aged at least 5 years could be difficult to achieve if the country simply continues its current immunization policy.

A nationwide prevalence survey targeting the general population is ideally conducted before implementing the immunization

Table 4. Unadjusted and adjusted odds ratio for being HBsAg positive among mothers from 15 to 45 years old in Lao PDR by selected background characteristics.

		Unadjusted odds ratio	95% CI	p	Adjusted odds ratio	95% CI	p
DPT3 coverage	high	1(reference)					
	low	0.50	0.20–1.28	0.14	0.47	0.19–1.16	0.10
Mothers' age	15 to 29	1(reference)					
	30 to 45	1.03	0.43–2.51	0.94	0.94	0.39–2.25	0.88
Ethnicity	Low land Lao	1(reference)					
	others	0.80	0.30–2.17	0.65	0.68	0.25–1.85	0.44
Education	none	1(reference)					
	finished primary school or upper	1.68	0.70–4.01	0.23	2.04	0.89–4.68	0.09
Occupation	white collar	1(reference)					
	blue collar	1.71	0.53–5.55	0.35	1.93	0.68–5.50	0.21
History of surgery	no	1(reference)					
	yes	1.28	0.39–4.25	0.67	1.30	0.35–4.78	0.68

strategy to evaluate hepatitis B epidemiology. However, we were able to understand the epidemiology to some degree, even after implementation of immunization policy, because adults usually represent the pre-vaccination era [15,17].

Strengths of the study

The present study is the first nationwide survey on the prevalence of hepatitis B in the general population both before and after the implementation of a hepatitis B immunization policy in Lao PDR and other Southeast Asian countries. We applied multistage stratified cluster sampling to better represent the general population. The design effect of prevalence was calculated between 0.8 and 1.3, which was acceptable as we set it around 2.0 before the survey.

The background characteristics of our sampled population were similar to those of another nationwide population-based study, the Lao PDR Reproductive Health Survey (LRHS) [32] conducted in 2005. For example, the locations of current residence (north, central, and south) were 33.3%, 41.7%, and 25.0% in our survey, and 38.6%, 38.9%, and 22.5% in the LRHS. The levels of mothers' completed education (none, primary school, secondary school or more) were 31.9%, 38.9%, and 29.2% in our survey, and 28.8%, 43.7%, and 27.5% in the LRHS. The LRHS applied the multistage stratified cluster sampling method and surveyed more than 13,000 women all over the country. A direct comparison of the populations sampled by the two different surveys is difficult to perform as the primary objectives were different. Despite this, our sampled population is considered to likely represent the general population in Lao PDR.

Limitations of the study

There are several limitations in our study that should be addressed. First, the population data is based on the census conducted in 2005. After 2005, the population distribution may have changed and some of the villages could have merged, thereby creating bias in the findings. Fortunately, we did not survey any villages that disappeared or merged.

Second, floating or marginal populations are likely to be missed from the residential lists, and these populations could be a source of HIV and hepatitis B virus infections [33]. In future seroprevalence surveys, these subpopulations should be accounted for by using specific approaches, such as oversampling.

Third, population immunity levels were difficult to measure or estimate. The possession of immunization certificates was low, because many participants had already finished their scheduled vaccinations before 12 months of age, and relevant documents were lost. In the present study, we did not have enough data from health centers due to time and budget limitations. Since we did not examine immunization markers, such as HBsAb, herd immunity levels are unknown.

Lastly, adult men were not included in the survey. Serological studies in the past indicated that men have higher HBsAg rates than women [8,21,28]. In Lao PDR, male blood donors presented with 9.7% HBsAg positive prevalence, while the prevalence in females was 6.2% [22]. When considering the disease burden of hepatitis B virus infections, it is better to include both sexes [26].

To the best of our knowledge, this is the first nationwide, population-based serological survey on chronic hepatitis B virus infections both before and after implementation of hepatitis B immunization in Southeast Asia, where disease burden is high. As such, our results provide valuable information on a hepatitis B immunization program and a useful baseline against which to compare future assessments in this region.

National immunization policy should be based on the disease epidemiology [3]. However, in Southeast Asia, understanding of the epidemiology of hepatitis B remains unsatisfactory. Even when a country implements a hepatitis B immunization program for children and the prevalence of disease reaches the target (i.e., less than 2% among children aged 5 years or older), we cannot conclude that the immunization program alone contributed to reduced disease prevalence without comparing it to the disease prevalence in the pre-vaccine generation, i.e., adults. Nationwide surveys assessing disease prevalence in the generations before and after the implementation of a vaccination program will provide valuable information for understanding hepatitis B epidemiology. Therefore, we recommend surveying hepatitis B seroprevalence in both generations.

Conclusions

We determined the nationwide HBsAg prevalence among children (1.7%; 95% CI: 0.8%–2.6%) and their mothers (2.9%; 95% CI: 1.6%–4.2%) in Lao PDR. This is the first report to estimate the nationwide prevalence of chronic hepatitis B in pre- and post-hepatitis B immunization generations in Southeast Asia, where hepatitis B infections are a substantial burden. The estimated prevalence was below that of previous studies, suggesting that our understanding of this disease's epidemiology is lacking and warrants further investigation. We recommend that the prevalence among the pre- and post-vaccine eras should be investigated when conducting hepatitis B seroprevalence surveys.

Acknowledgments

We would like to express our sincere thanks to the sampled children, mothers, and caregivers for their voluntary participation in the survey. We are grateful to all of the surveyors and supervisors from the National Immunization Program, National Center for Laboratory and Epidemiology, Ministry of Health, and staff from the provincial and district Departments of Health. We would also like to thank Dr. H. Murakami for advising on the survey methodology, and Drs. S. Noda, Y. Sugiura, H. Okabayashi, A. Iwamoto, and M. Anami for their critical comments regarding the field survey, and Dr. Y. Horikoshi for geographical analysis.

Author Contributions

Conceived and designed the experiments: AX MH KI TW MS. Performed the experiments: KK TK PV CP KP DP BS VSO TS. Analyzed the data: KK TK MH. Contributed reagents/materials/analysis tools: KI TW MS. Wrote the paper: AX PV MH. Revised the manuscript: KK TK PV CP KP DP BS VSO KI TW MS. Arranged laboratory for diagnosis: PV KI TW MS.

References

1. Kane MA (1996) Global status of hepatitis B immunization. Lancet 348: 696.
2. Lee WM (1997) Hepatitis B virus infection. N Engl J Med 337: 1733–1745.
3. World Health Organization (2009) Hepatitis B vaccines. Wkly Epidemiol Rec 84: 405–419.
4. Goldstein ST, Zhou F, Hadler SC, Bell BP, Mast EE, et al. (2005) A mathematical model to estimate global hepatitis B disease burden and vaccination impact. Int J Epidemiol 34: 1329–1339.
5. IARC (2012) Agents classified by the IARC monographs. Available: http://monographs.iarc.fr/ENG/Classification/ClassificationsGroupOrder.pdf Accessed 1 June 2013.
6. Damme PV, Ward J, Shouval D, Wiersma S, Zanetti A (2012) Hepatitis B vaccines. In: Plotzkin SA, Orenstein WA, Offit PA, editors, Vaccines 6th ed. Philadelphia PA: Elsevier Saunders. pp. 205–234.
7. Rani M, Yang BP, Nesbit R (2009) Hepatitis B control by 2012 in the WHO Western Pacific Region: rationale and implications. WHO Bull 87: 707–713.

8. Lueng N (2009) Chronic hepatitis B in Asian women of childbearing age. Hepatol Int 3: S24–S31.
9. World Health Organization (2011) Progress towards meeting the 2012 hepatitis B control milestone: WHO Western Pacific Region, 2011. Wkly Epidemiol Rec 86: 180–188.
10. Clements CJ, Baoping Y, Crouch A, Hipgrave D, Mansoor O, et al. (2006) Progress in the control of hepatitis B infection in the Western pacific Region. Vaccine 24: 1975–82.
11. Murakami H, Cuong NV, Huynh L, Hipgrave DB (2008) Implementation of and costs associated with providing a birth-dose of hepatitis B vaccine in Viet Nam. Vaccine 26: 1411–1419.
12. Ol HS, Bjoerkvoll B, Sothy S, Heng YV, Hoel H, et al. (2009) Prevalence of hepatitis B and hepatitis C virus infections in potential blood donors in rural Cambodia. Southeast Asian J Trop Med Public Health 40: 963–971.
13. Hipgrave DB, Van NT, Huong VM, Long HT, Dat DT, et al (2003) Hepatitis B infection in rural Vietnam and the implications for a national program of infant immunization. Am J Trop Med Hyg 69: 288–294.
14. WHO/UNICEF (2013) Immunization coverage estimates. Available: http://apps.who.int/immunization_monitoring/globalsummary/timeseries/tswucoveragebcg.html. Accessed 25 October 2013.
15. World Health Organization (2011) Documenting the impact of hepatitis b immunization: best practices for conducting a serosurvey (WHO/IVB/11.08). Available: http://whqlibdoc.who.int/hq/2011/WHO_IVB_11.08_eng.pdf. Accessed 12 September 2012.
16. Naing L, Winn T, Rusli BN (2006) Practical issues in calculating the sample size for prevalence studies. Arch Orofac Sci 1: 9–14.
17. World Health Organization (2007) Western Pacific Regional plan for hepatitis B control through immunization ((WP)/ICP/EPI/5.2/001-E). Available: http://www.wpro.who.int/immunization/documents/docs/POA_HepB.pdf. Accessed 25 October 2013.
18. Lien TX, Tien NTK, Chanpong GF, Cuc CT, Yen VT, et al. (2000) Evaluation of rapid diagnostic tests for the detection of human immunodeficiency virus types 1 and 2, hepatitis B surface antigen, and syphilis in Ho Chi Minh City, Vietnam. Am J Trop Med Hyg 62: 301–309.
19. Lin YH, Wang Y, Loua A, Day GJ, Qiu Y, et al. (2008) Evaluation of a new hepatitis B virus surface antigen rapid test with improved sensitivity. J Clin Microbiol 46: 3319–3324.
20. Merican I, Guan R, Amarapuka D, Alexander MJ, Chutaputti A, et al. (2000) Chronic hepatitis B virus infection in Asian countries. J Gasroenterol Hepatol 15: 1356–1361.
21. Soeung SC, Rani M, Huong V, Sarath S, Kimly C, et al (2009) Results from nationwide hepatitis B serosurvey in Cambodia using simple and rapid laboratory test: implications for national immunization program. Am J Trop Med Hyg 81: 252–257.
22. Jutavijittum P, Yousukh A, Samountry B, Samountry K, Ounavong A, et al. (2007) Seroprevalence of hepatitis B and C virus infections among Lao blood donors. Southeast Asian J Trop Med Public Health 38: 674–679.
23. Syhavong B, Rasachack B, Smythe L, Rolain JM, Roque-Afonso AM, et al. (2010) The infective causes of hepatitis and jaundice amongst hospitalised patients in Vientiane, Laos. Trans R Soc Trop Med Hyg 104: 475–483.
24. Sa-nguanmoo P, Tangkijvanich P, Thawornsuk N, Vichaiwattana P, Prianantathavorn K, et al. (2010) Molecular epidemiological study of hepatitis B virus among migrant workers from Cambodia, Laos, and Myanmar to Thailand. J Med Virol 82: 1341–1349.
25. World Bank (2012) Population density per square km. Available: http://data.worldbank.org/indicator/EN.POP.DNST. Accessed 1 June 2013.
26. Duong TH, Nguyen PH, Henley K, Peters M (2009) Risk factors for hepatitis B infection in rural Vietnam. Asian Pacific J Cancer Prev 10: 97–102.
27. Ashraf H, Alam NH, Rothermundt C, Brooks A, Bardhan P, et al. (2010) Prevalence and risk factors of hepatitis B and C virus infections in an impoverished urban community in Dhaka, Bangladesh. BMC Infect Dis 10: 208.
28. Liang XF, Bi SL, Yang WZ, Wang LD, Cui G, et al (2009) Epidemiological serosurvey of hepatitis B in China-declining HBV prevalence due to hepatitis B vaccination. Vaccine 27: 6550–6557.
29. Alter MJ (2006) Epidemiology of viral hepatitis and HIV co-infection. J Hepatol 44: S6–S9.
30. Dunford L, Carr MJ, Dean J, Nguyen LT, Thi THT, et al. (2012) A multicentre molecular analysis of hepatitis B and blood-borne virus coinfections in Viet Nam. PLOS ONE 7(6): e39027. doi: 10.1371/journal.pone.0039027.
31. World Health Organization (2005) WPR/RC56.R8. Measles elimination, hepatitis B control and poliomyelitis eradication. Available: http://www2.wpro.who.int/rcm/en/archives/rc56/rc_resolutions/wpr_rc56_r08.htm. Accessed 25 May 2013.
32. United Nations Population Fund (2005) Lao Reproductive Health Survey 2005. Available: http://countryoffice.unfpa.org/lao/drive/LAOREPRODUCTIVEHEALTHSURVEY.pdf. Accessed 25 May 2013.
33. Rossi C, Shrier I, Marshall L, Cnossen S, Schwartzman K, et al. (2012) Seroprevalence of chronic hepatitis B virus infection and prior immunity in immigrants and refugees: a systematic review and meta-analysis. PLOS ONE 7(9): e44611.

Efficacy and Tolerability of Telaprevir for Chronic Hepatitis Virus C Genotype 1 Infection: A Meta-Analysis

Yuan Kong[1]¶, Xiaoping Wang[1]¶, Yushu Shang[1]¶, Paul M. Schroder[2], Wenhua Liang[1], Xiaoting Ling[1], Zhiyong Guo[1]*, Xiaoshun He[1]*

1 Organ Transplant Center, The First Affiliated Hospital, Sun Yat-sen University, Guangzhou, China, **2** Department of Medical Microbiology and Immunology, University of Toledo College of Medicine, Toledo, Ohio, United States of America

Abstract

Background: Chronic hepatitis C virus (HCV) infection is one of the leading causes of hepatic cirrhosis and hepatocellular carcinoma, and HCV genotype 1 is the most prevalent genotype and is resistant to current standard therapy. We performed this meta-analysis to evaluate the efficacy and safety of telaprevir-based therapy for chronic HCV genotype 1 infection.

Methods: We included randomized controlled trials with no year or language restriction. All data were analyzed using a random-effects model by Review Manager v5.0. The primary outcome was the proportion of patients achieving sustained virologic response (SVR), and the secondary outcomes were HCV relapse rate, incidence of severe adverse events (SAEs), and discontinuation due to adverse events.

Results: The proportion of achieving SVR was significantly higher in the telaprevir group (odds ratio [OR] = 3.40 [1.92, 6.00], $P<0.0001$; $I^2=87\%$) regardless of a patients' previous treatment status. It was also significantly higher in the 24-week and 48-week treatment groups (OR = 4.52 [2.08, 9.81], $P<0.001$; $I^2=85\%$, and OR = 4.05 [1.56, 10.56], $P=0.004$; $I^2=92\%$, respectively), while it was comparable in the 12-week treatment group (OR = 1.32 [0.63, 2.75], $P=0.46$; $I^2=35\%$). In addition, the HCV relapse rate was significantly reduced in the telaprevir group (OR = 0.28 [0.16, 0.49], $P<0.001$; $I^2=76\%$). However, the incidence of SAE (OR = 1.56 [1.15, 2.10], $P=0.004$; $I^2=0\%$) and study discontinuation due to adverse events (OR = 2.24 [1.43, 3.50], $P<0.001$; $I^2=37\%$) were significantly higher in the telaprevir group.

Conclusion: Despite its higher incidence of SAEs and discontinuation due to adverse events, telaprevir-based therapy can increase the proportion of achieving SVR in both previously treated and untreated chronic HCV-1 infected patients.

Editor: John E. Tavis, Saint Louis University, United States of America

Funding: This study was supported by the Key Clinical Project from the Ministry of Health (159), National Natural Science Foundation of China (30972951, 81102244, 81102245 and 81170448) (http://www.nsfc.gov.cn/), and special fund for science research by the Ministry of Health (201002004). The funders had no role in study design, data collection and analysis, decision to publish, or preparation of the manuscript.

Competing Interests: The authors have declared that no competing interests exist.

* E-mail: rockyucsf1981@126.com (ZG); gdtrc@126.com (XH)

¶ These authors contributed equally to this work.

Introduction

Hepatitis C virus (HCV) infection is a serious public health concern that affects 170 million people worldwide and has become the leading indication for liver transplantation [1]. Approximately 80% of infected patients fail to clear the virus and less than 10% may develop severe liver diseases such as chronic hepatitis, liver cirrhosis, or hepatocellular carcinoma, which can compromise patient survival [2]. And the number of people requiring treatment for chronic HCV infection is expected to increase over the next 10–20 years [3].

The current standard treatment of chronic hepatitis C recommended by the 2009 American Association for Study of Liver diseases Practice Guidelines [4] is the combined use of the nucleoside analog ribavirin and pegylated interferon alpha, the success of achieving sustained virologic response (SVR) under such treatment depends largely on the viral genotype [5]. Among the 6 known HCV genotypes (1–6), HCV genotype 1 (HCV-1) is the most prevalent circulating strain in Western Europe and North America and its infection is most refractory to the therapy. For patients with HCV-1 infection, less than 50% could achieve SVR with treatment of peginterferon alfa-2a and ribavirin [6], compared to the 80% SVR in genotypes 2 and 3 patients [7]. However, apart from its significant performance in achieving SVR, there is little evidence supporting the effect of such treatment on clinical outcomes. In addition, this drug combination has been associated with severe adverse effects such as fatigue, nausea and depression, thus precluding treatment for many individuals [8]. All the issues above address the need to develop novel anti-HCV drugs with greater anti-virus effect and safety.

Recent studies of new treatment strategies for chronic hepatitis C have been focused on specifically targeted antiviral therapy, novel interferon products and nucleoside analogs, among which the treatment efficacy of direct acting antiviral agents (DAAs) appears to be the most promising. The advanced DAAs for HCV

include inhibitors of the viral NS3/4A protease and the viral NS5B RNA-dependent RNA polymerase [9–11]. Telaprevir (VX 950, Vertex), as one of the linear NS3/4A protease inhibitors, has been shown in several clinical trials to substantially enhance SVR in chronic HCV-1 infected patients when used in combination with peginterferon and ribavirin, and potentially shorten the treatment period [12–16].

Herein, we performed a meta-analysis of the current reported data in clinical trials to gain a meta-analyzed profile of the efficacy and safety of telaprevir-based therapy in chronic HCV-1 infected patients. This study provides important insights capable of better informing clinical physicians regarding the updated treatment strategy for chronic HCV infection.

Methods

Patients and Methods

This meta-analysis was carried out according to the Cochrane Reviewer's Handbook recommended by The Cochrane Collaboration.

Study Objective

The primary end point was to identify the effects of telaprevir plus peginterferon and ribavirin combination therapy on the proportion of patients who achieved SVR, which was defined as the patients who had undetectable plasma HCV RNA 24 weeks after the last planned dose of the study treatment. The secondary end points were relapse rate, which was defined as a detectable HCV RNA level during the post-treatment follow up period in a patient who had undetectable levels of HCV RNA at the end of the treatment period, and safety, as assessed by the percentage of patients who discontinued therapy due to adverse events and the incidence of severe adverse events (SAE).

Literature Search

Studies were retrieved using Medline, Embase, Cochrane Database of Systematic Reviews and manual searches with no year or language restrictions. Searching strategies were described as #1: "telaprevir" OR "VX-950" OR "Vertex" OR "NS3/4A protease inhibitor"; #2: "chronic hepatitis C" OR "chronic HCV infection"; or #1 AND #2. General reviews, meta-analyses, and references from published randomized controlled trials (RCTs) and presentation to the International Association for the Study of the Liver, the European Association for the Study of the Liver, and the American Association for the Study of Liver Diseases meetings, were also searched for additional citations.

Inclusion Criteria

We selected RCTs published as full articles in journals and RCTs published as abstracts in international, European, or American meetings, evaluating telaprevir plus peginterferon and ribavirin combination therapy in chronic hepatitis C genotype 1 patients, with the current standard peginterferon and ribavirin therapy as the control group. Reported results must include the proportion of achieving SVR, relapse rate, incidence of discontinuation and severe adverse events.

Exclusion Criteria

Nonrandomized trials, trials that included patients with non-type C hepatitis or non-genotype 1 HCV infection, and trials that included patients infected by more than one type of hepatitis virus or HCV genotype but failed to provide the specific outcome data for genotype 1 HCV infected patients were excluded. Trials that did not use the peginterferon and ribavirin combination therapy for 48 weeks as control were excluded as were trials using response-guided therapy. RCTs were also excluded when they didn't use SVR as an outcome. And trials labeled as being at "high risk of bias" during assessment of bias risks should be excluded from the analyses. In the event of unpublished virologic data, a request for information was made to investigators before excluding the trials from this report.

Patient Characteristics, Diagnoses, and Treatments

The following items were recorded as potentially useful in assessing clinical heterogeneity between RCTs: study population, method of diagnosing chronic hepatitis C, time from diagnosis, previous treatment and response status to previous treatment, baseline viral load, dose and duration of telaprevir administration, dose and duration of peginterferon and ribavirin administration.

Selection and Data Extraction

Two reviewers (YK and YS) first screened titles and abstracts, yielding potentially eligible publications. All RCTs considered for inclusion were analyzed independently by the two reviewers. When disagreements regarding bias assessment arose, a third party (ZG) was brought in to resolve the disagreement. The resutls of the individual trials were blinded to the reviewers, and the decision on inclusion or exclusion was not related to the results or conclusions of each manuscript.

Quality Assessment of Trials Included

A quality assessment was carried out for all the retrieved RCTs. Quality in a systematic review essentially refers to the absence of biases. To assess the methodological validity of the RCTs included in this meta-analysis, we used the Risk of Bias table from Review Manager 5.0 (The Cochrane Collaboration, Oxford, United Kingdom). The following aspects were evaluated: adequate sequence generation, allocation concealment, blinding, incomplete outcome data addressed, free of selective reporting, free of other bias, and intention-to-treat analysis. Trials were excluded from the analyses if they were assessed as at high risk of bias. We used Begg's funnel plot analysis to test publication bias of the included RCTs. Articles were assessed by two reviewers (YK and YS) independently. Disagreements were resolved by consultation with a third reviewer (ZG).

Statistical Analysis

All analyses were performed with the intention-to-treat (ITT) method, in which case all randomized patients were included, and patients without the outcome were considered as a treatment failure. The primary outcome was the proportion of patients achieving SVR, and secondary outcomes were HCV relapse rate, incidence of SAEs, and discontinuation due to adverse events. A primary analysis including all of the patients and subgroup analyses regarding treatment duration and previous treatment status were planned. We used the odds ratio as a measurement of effect size for SVR, relapse, drug discontinuation, and SAE. The DerSimonian and Laird model for random-effects meta-analysis was adopted to obtain summary estimates across the included studies. We tested for heterogeneity using the Cochran Q test, which follows a chi-square distribution, to make inferences about the null hypothesis of homogeneity. The I^2 value was used to demonstrate the percentage of inter-study variation in all variation (including inter-study variation and system error). If $I^2>50\%$, subgroup analysis, meta-regression analysis and sensitivity analysis would be applied if possible. All statistical analyses were performed using the statistical software Review Manager 5.0 (The Cochrane

Collaboration, Oxford, United Kingdom). This report follows the PRISMA guidelines [13] and the Cochrane collaboration guideline for reporting meta-analyses.

Results

Characteristics of Included Studies

Figure 1 shows the process of study selection. 381 citations were initially found and we included 5 RCTs with 2776 patients in this meta-analysis, including 3 phase 2 clinical trials [12–14] with 1026 patients and 2 phase 3 trials [15,16] with 1750 patients. The patients in all 5 RCTs were 18 to 70 years of age and had HCV-1 infection with evidence of chronic hepatitis, as confirmed by a liver biopsy within 18 months before enrollment. The 5 RCTs were conducted in both previously untreated and treated patients. Telaprevir was given as a single dose of 1250 or 1125 mg on study day 1 and followed by a dose of 750 mg every 8 hours orally in the 3 phase 2 trials, and administered orally at a dose of 750 mg every 8 hours with food in the 2 phase 3 trials. In all 5 RCTs, peginterferon alfa-2a was administered by subcutaneous injection at a dose of 180 ug per week, and ribavirin orally at a dose of 1000 mg per day (in patients who weighed less than 75 kg) or 1200 mg per day (in patients who weighed 75 kg or more). The duration of telaprevir treatment was 12 weeks in combination with 12, 24, or 48 weeks of peginterferon and ribavirin, while the control treatment of peginterferon and ribavirin lasted 48 weeks. Table 1 summarizes the characteristics of the included studies.

Bias Risks

To address the strength of evidence in this meta-analysis, we evaluated the risk of bias of the 5 RCTs. In general, the included trials were at low risk of bias for most of the aspects evaluated. All 5 RCTs adopted blinding and intention-to-treat analysis and were free of selective reporting or other bias. Adequate sequence was generated in 3 and allocation concealed in 2 of the 5 RCTs. Whether and how the incomplete outcome data were addressed was unclear in all 5 RCTs. Figure 2 summarizes the evaluation of risk of bias. We also tested the 5 included RCTs for publication bias in each comparison of the primary and secondary outcomes. No publication bias was identified in comparisons of SVR ($P=0.835$), relapse rate ($P=0.615$), SAE incidence ($P=0.387$), or discontinuation rate ($P=0.295$) (Figure S1, S2, S3, S4).

Effects of Telaprevir Plus Peginterferon and Ribavirin Therapy on SVR

We conducted a meta-analysis regarding SVR in all included patients receiving telaprevir-based therapy compared with patients receiving standard peginterferon and ribavirin (PR) therapy (Figure 3). The pooled estimates showed that the overall proportion of achieving SVR was significantly higher in the telaprevir group than in the PR group (OR = 3.40 [1.92, 6.00], $P<0.001$; $I^2=87\%$).

Effects of Telaprevir Plus Peginterferon and Ribavirin Therapy on SVR According to Previous Treatment

Three of the 5 RCTs compared the effect of telaprevir in combination with peginterferon and ribavirin on SVR in previously untreated patients [12,14,15], and 2 in previously treated patients [13,16]. We conducted a meta-analysis regarding SVR in patients receiving telaprevir-based therapy compared with patients receiving standard peginterferon and ribavirin (PR) therapy in subgroups defined by previous treatment status (Figure 3). In the previously untreated subgroup, the proportion of achieving SVR was significantly higher in telaprevir group than PR group (OR = 2.25 [1.35, 3.77], $P=0.002$; $I^2=77\%$). In the previously treated subgroup, it was also significantly higher than the PR group (OR = 6.70 [3.35, 13.41], $P<0.001$; $I^2=71\%$).

Effects of Telaprevir Plus Peginterferon and Ribavirin Therapy on SVR According to Treatment Duration

Two of the 5 RCTs evaluated the 12-week telaprevir in combination with 12-week PR therapy (T12PR12), 4 evaluated the 12-week telaprevir in combination with 24-week PR therapy (T12PR24), and 4 evaluated the 12-week telaprevir in combination with 48-week PR therapy (T12PR48), in comparison with the standard 48-week PR therapy. We conducted a meta-analysis regarding SVR in patients receiving telaprevir-based therapy compared with patients receiving standard PR therapy in subgroups of treatment duration (Figure 4). There was no statistically significant difference in the proportion of achieving SVR between the T12PR12 subgroup and the PR groups (OR = 1.32 [0.63, 2.75], $P=0.46$; $I^2=35\%$). In the T12PR24 subgroup, the proportion of achieving SVR was significantly higher in the telaprevir group than in the PR group (OR = 4.52 [2.08, 9.81], $P<0.001$; $I^2=85\%$). In the T12PR48 subgroup, it was also significantly higher than the PR group (OR = 4.05 [1.56, 10.56], $P<0.001$; $I^2=92\%$).

Effects of Telaprevir Plus Peginterferon and Ribavirin Therapy on HCV Relapse Rate

Three of the 5 RCTs evaluated the effects of telaprevir plus peginterferon and ribavirin on relapse rate in previously untreated patients [12,14,15], and 2 in previously treated patients [13,16]. We conducted a meta-analysis regarding relapse rate in patients receiving telaprevir-based therapy versus standard PR therapy according to the previous treatment status (Figure 5). In general, relapse was defined as a detectable HCV RNA level during the post-treatment follow up period in a patient who had undetectable levels of HCV RNA at the end of the treatment period. In the previously untreated subgroup, the incidence of relapse was significantly lower in the telaprevir group than in the PR group (OR = 0.40 [0.16, 1.00], $P=0.05$; $I^2=78\%$). In the previously treated subgroup, the incidence of relapse was also significantly lower in the telaprevir group than in the PR group (OR = 0.18 [0.09, 0.36], $P<0.001$; $I^2=71\%$). The pooled estimates showed that the overall incidence of relapse in the previously untreated and treated patients was significantly reduced in the telaprevir group (OR = 0.28 [0.16, 0.49], $P<0.001$; $I^2=76\%$).

Safety of Telaprevir Plus Peginterferon and Ribavirin Therapy

Information regarding the incidence of adverse events were sought in all 5 included RCTs, including but not limited to rash, anemia, pruritus, fatigue, flu-like syndrome, headache, nausea, insomnia, diarrhea, and pyrexia, among which rash and anemia are the most common adverse events that occur when telaprevir is added, which can lead to discontinuation of treatment in serious cases. To assess the safety profile of telaprevir-based therapy, we conducted meta-analyses regarding the incidence of SAE and therapy discontinuation due to adverse events in patients receiving telaprevir-based versus standard PR therapy. The incidence of SAE was significantly higher in the telaprevir group than in the PR group (OR = 1.56 [1.15, 2.10], $P<0.001$; $I^2=0\%$) (Figure 6). The incidence of therapy discontinuation due to adverse events was significantly higher in the telaprevir group than in the PR group (OR = 2.24 [1.43, 3.50], $P<0.001$; $I^2=37\%$) (Figure 7).

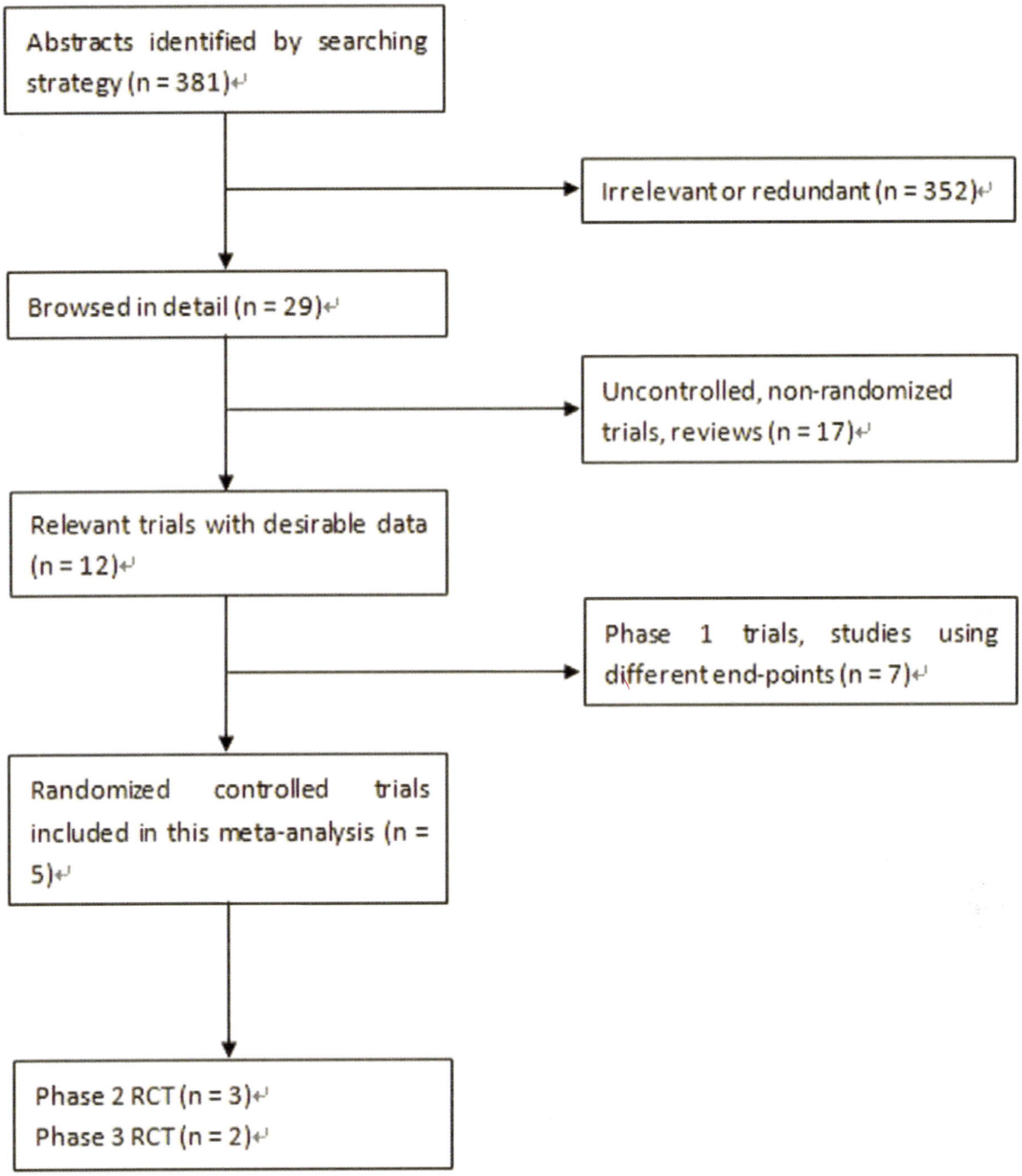

Figure 1. Flow diagram of study identification.

Additionally, meta-analyses regarding the most commonly recognized adverse events, namely rash and anemia, were carried out in patients receiving telaprevir-based versus standard PR therapy. The incidence of rash was significantly higher in the telaprevir group than in the PR group (OR = 2.11 [1.42, 3.14], P<0.001; I^2 = 68%) (Figure S5). Also, the incidence of anemia was significantly higher in the telaprevir group than in the PR group (OR = 1.88 [1.19, 2.96], P = 0.007; I^2 = 64%) (Figure S6).

Heterogeneity

Most of the heterogeneity tests for our analyses showed I^2>50%, indicating significant inter-study heterogeneity. Subgroup analyses were carried out regarding the possible factors that could cause inter-study variation, which also ended in significant heterogeneity. Ideally, a meta-regression analysis should be conducted to address this matter, but we failed to do so since the data on all the potential causes of heterogeneity were incomplete. Sensitivity analysis was carried out. Adjustment of inclusion or exclusion of individual trials or alteration of statistical models came out with the same results, suggesting that the results of these analyses were stable and reliable.

Table 1. Characteristics of included studies.

Studies	Number of Patients (Telaprevir/PR)	Gender (male/ female)	White Population	Genotype	Previous Treatment Status	Study Design	Telaprevir Dose
Hezode 2009[13]	241/82	192/131	304 (94%)	1	untreated	T12PR24/T12PR48/T12P12/ PR48	1250 mg on day 1; followed by 750 mg Q8H
McHutchison 2010[14]	339/114	306/147	402 (89%)	1	treated	T12PR24/T24PR48/T24PR24/ PR48	1125 mg on day 1; followed by 750 mg Q8H
McHutchison 2009[15]	175/75	157/93	192 (77%)	1	untreated	T12PR12/T12PR24/T12PR48/ PR48	1250 mg on day 1; followed by 750 mg Q8H
Jacobson 2011[16]	727/361	636/452	958 (88%)	1	untreated	T12PR24/T12PR48/T8PR24/ T8PR48/PR48	750 mg Q8H
Zeuzem 2011[17]	530/132	460/202	615 (93%)	1	treated	T12PR48/PR48	750 mg Q8H

T, telaprevir; P, peg-interferon; R, ribavirin; Q8H, every 8 hours.

Trial Sequential Analysis

We also conducted trial sequential analysis due to the small number of included studies and the underlying liability of type I error (Trial Sequential Analysis, Copenhagen Trial Unit, 2011). We calculated the information size required to demonstrate of reject the telaprevir-based effect of a 20% odds ratio reduction, which was 1333 patients. Information size were derived to ensure a maximum type I error of 5%. And it was heterogeneity adjusted, using the estimate of diversity D2. Information size was derived assuming and event proportion of 32% in the control group (median event proportion in this control group). The cumulative Z-curve crossed both the trial sequential monitoring boundaries and the conventional boundaries and surpassed the required information size, thereby confirming that telaprevir-based therapy is superior to PR therapy in increasing the patient proportion of achieving SVR (Figure S7).

Discussion

This meta-analysis assessed the efficacy and safety of telaprevir-based therapy and 4 major conclusions can be drawn: (1) Telaprevir-based therapy can increase the proportion of achieving SVR in HCV-1 infected patients and reduce relapse rate in comparison with PR therapy; (2) Telaprevir-based therapy can increase the proportion of achieving SVR in both previously treated and untreated patients; (3) Use of telaprevir may shorten the duration of peginterferon plus ribavirin treatment; (4) Telaprevir-based therapy is accompanied with higher incidences of SAEs and treatment discontinuation due to adverse events.

Three of the included RCTs investigated the efficacy and safety of telaprevir in previously untreated patients, and 2 in previously treated patients who were partial responders, non-responders, or relapse patients. While the difference in previous treatment status may increase the risk of heterogeneity and become a potential liability, the subgroup analysis we conducted accordingly demonstrated a boost in achieving SVR in both previously treated and untreated patient subgroup, with the OR value in previously treated subgroup higher than untreated subgroup (6.70 and 2.25, respectively). Such result indicates that HCV-1 is more susceptible to telaprevir-based therapy probably because its inhibition of NS3/4A protease is directly related to HCV replication and assembly [9]. For treatment-naïve patients, telaprevir-based therapy can be the first choice of clinical treatment since it offers a better anti-virus effect. And for previously treated patients, considering HCV-1 drug resistance is the main cause of partial response and no response, the more significant improvement in SVR presented in these patients suggests that telaprevir plus peginterferon and ribavirin therapy can somehow protect the patients from the generation of mutation in targeted genes and thus are less prone to drug-resistance. And between the options of retreatment with the same medications or telaprevir-based regimen in patients who failed the standard PR therapy, the latter may have a better chance of clearing the virus. For both previously treated and untreated patients, the use of telaprevir in combination with peginterferon and ribavirin results in a greater chance of achieving SVR. Although there hasn't been any prospective blinded study to translate SVR into clinical outcomes, several long-term follow-up studies have shown that the attainment of SVR is durable and predictive of long-term disease remission and clinical benefits in terms of histological improvement and prevention of complications [17,18]. In fact, AASLD has recently updated its guideline in 2011, recommending to use telaprevir or boceprevir in combination with peginterferon and ribavirin for the treatment of genotype-1 chronic HCV infection in both treatment-

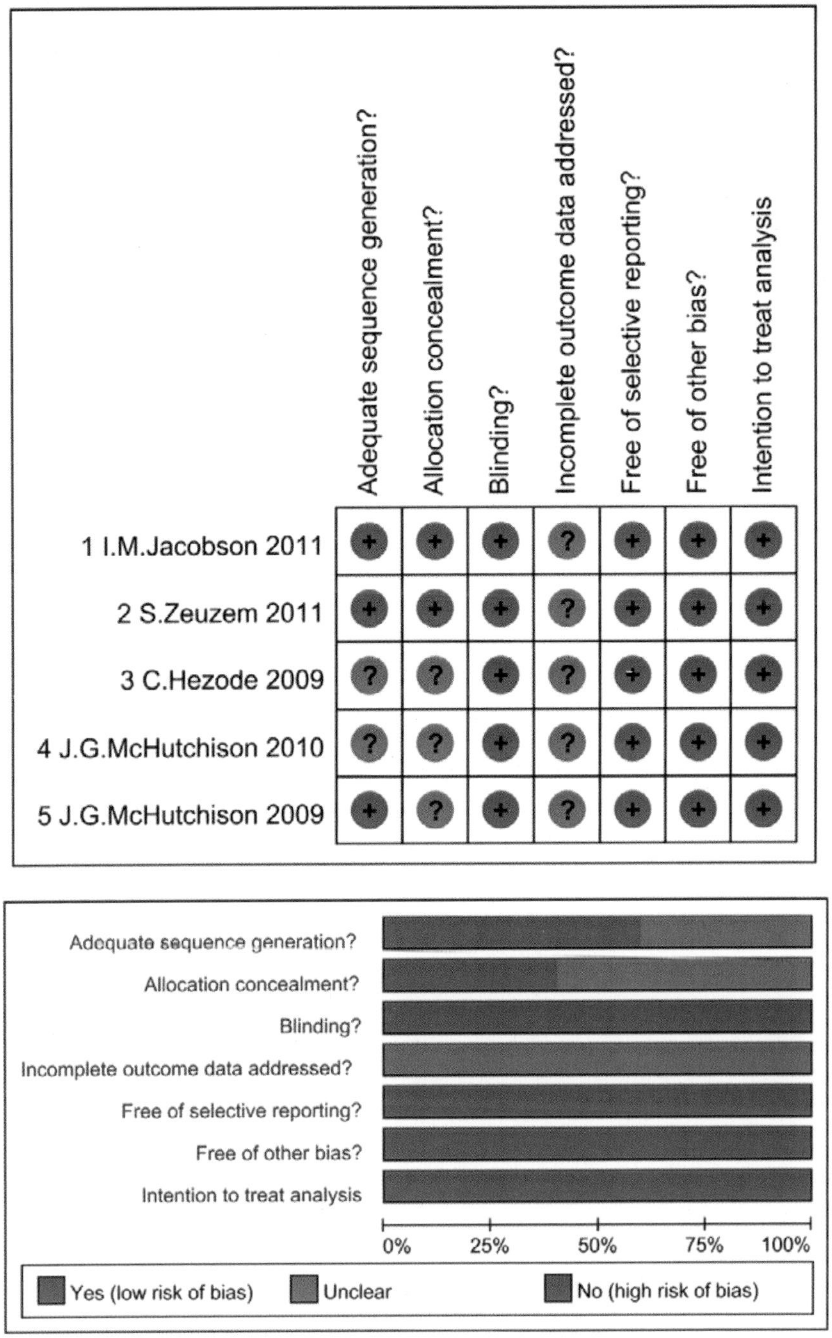

Figure 2. Risk of bias of the included studies. All 5 RCTs adopted blinding and intention-to-treat analysis and were free of selective reporting or other bias. Adequate sequence was generated in 3 and allocation concealed in 2 of the 5 RCTs. Whether and how the incomplete outcome data were addressed was unclear in all 5 RCTs. Each row represents each study and the column represents the risk of bias to be evaluated.

naïve patients and patients who have previously received therapy. The results of the current study further support this recommendation.

To address the issue of proper duration and protocol of telaprevir-based therapy, 2 of the RCTs investigated the efficacy and safety of T12PR12 treatment [12,14], 4 investigated T12PR24 [12,15] and T12PR48 treatment [13,16], respectively. Patients assigned to T12PR48 therapy demonstrated a significantly higher SVR proportion compared to the standard PR 48 therapy, which indicates that the improvement in achieving SVR and anti-virus effect can be attributed to the addition of telaprevir. Furthermore, by comparing the T12PR12 and T12PR24 protocols to the PR48 therapy, we assessed whether the addition of telaprevir could shorten the duration of therapy with peginterferon and ribavirin, which was known to cause numerous adverse events [6–8]. Patients randomly assigned to the T12PR12 protocol showed no difference in SVR proportion compared with those receiving the 48-week PR therapy in our meta-analyses, which can also be interpreted as no additional anti-virus effect gained by 12-week telaprevir therapy. On the other hand, patients assigned to

Study or Subgroup	telaprevir Events	telaprevir Total	Control Events	Control Total	Weight	Odds Ratio M-H, Random, 95% CI
1.1.1 previously untreated						
1 I.M.Jacobson 2011	521	727	158	361	22.3%	3.25 [2.50, 4.23]
3 C.Hezode 2009	133	241	38	82	19.8%	1.43 [0.86, 2.36]
5 J.G.McHutchison 2009	107	175	31	75	19.2%	2.23 [1.29, 3.87]
Subtotal (95% CI)		**1143**		**518**	**61.2%**	**2.25 [1.35, 3.77]**
Total events	761		227			
Heterogeneity: Tau² = 0.16; Chi² = 8.51, df = 2 (P = 0.01); I² = 77%						
Test for overall effect: Z = 3.09 (P = 0.002)						
1.1.2 previously treated						
2 S.Zeuzem 2011	346	530	22	132	19.9%	9.40 [5.75, 15.37]
4 J.G.McHutchison 2010	146	339	16	114	18.9%	4.63 [2.62, 8.20]
Subtotal (95% CI)		**869**		**246**	**38.8%**	**6.70 [3.35, 13.41]**
Total events	492		38			
Heterogeneity: Tau² = 0.18; Chi² = 3.40, df = 1 (P = 0.07); I² = 71%						
Test for overall effect: Z = 5.38 (P < 0.00001)						
Total (95% CI)		**2012**		**764**	**100.0%**	**3.40 [1.92, 6.00]**
Total events	1253		265			
Heterogeneity: Tau² = 0.36; Chi² = 31.54, df = 4 (P < 0.00001); I² = 87%						
Test for overall effect: Z = 4.21 (P < 0.0001)						
Test for subgroup differences: Not applicable						

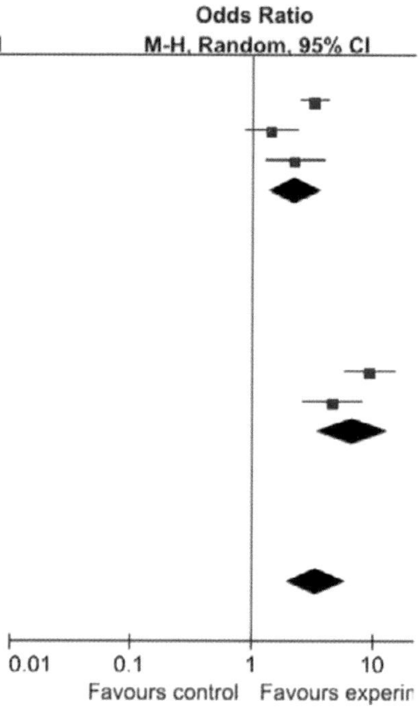

Figure 3. Meta-analysis of telaprevir plus peginterferon and ribavirin therapy on SVR according to previous treatment. The proportion of achieving SVR was significantly higher in the telaprevir group than in the PR group in the previously untreated (OR = 2.25 [1.35, 3.77], $P = 0.002$; $I^2 = 77\%$), treated (OR = 6.7 [3.35, 13.41], $P < 0.001$; $I^2 = 71\%$), and overall population (OR = 3.40 [1.92, 6.00], $P < 0.001$; $I^2 = 87\%$). OR = odds ratio, I^2 = heterogeneity index. Columns in green represent the mean difference of each study and column size represents the study weight in the analysis. Lanes represent the 95% CI of each study. Diamonds in black represent the overall effect size, and diamond width represents the overall 95% CI.

the T12PR24 protocol demonstrated clear improvement in achieving SVR compared to the 48-week PR therapy. These results support that the addition of telaprevir to the standard PR therapy has a better anti-virus effect, and the equal or even higher SVR proportion achieved by adopting the T12PR12 or T12PR24 therapy can spare the use of peginterferon and ribavirin for 24 or 36 weeks and shorten the total treatment duration.

Another issue that has been brought into sight concerning treatment duration is the application of response-guided therapy in telaprevir protocols. In another open-label study designed to investigate the effects of response-guided therapy, 150 patients with extended rapid viral response (eRVR) to telaprevir and ribavirin treatment were randomized to 24 or 48 weeks of ribavirin to evaluate whether 48-week therapy can gain further benefits [19]. The results showed no further benefit for the 12-week telaprevir plus 48-week ribavirin treatment in patients with eRVR. Collectively, the T12PR24 protocol could be more effective and shorten the therapy duration compared with the conventional PR48 protocol, thus possibly serving as the treatment of choice for chronic HCV-1 infection. However, so far there is no study that has properly addressed this issue. Therefore, whether the T12PR12 therapy has equal or greater benefits compared to the T12PR24 therapy in patients with RVR is remained to be tested.

Patients with hepatitis C are particularly prone to development of drug-resistance upon exposure to protease inhibitors and other HCV antivirals such as ribavirin [20,21]. The occurrence of drug-resistance to telaprevir is highly related to the patient's previous treatment status, indicating that HCV genetic changes are more likely to happen in previously treated patients, while in treatment-naïve patients telaprevir resistance due to the presence of HCV variants is uncommon [22]. Nevertheless, this meta-analysis suggested otherwise by showing that telaprevir-based therapy resulted in a higher proportion of achieving SVR and a lower relapse rate in both previously untreated and treated patients, with a higher OR value in the previously treated group in SVR proportion (6.70 versus 2.25) and a lower OR value in relapse rate (0.18 versus 0.40), indicating that the advantage of telaprevir-based therapy over conventional PR therapy is more significant in previously treated patients than in untreated patients and the better virologic response may result from a smaller chance of drug-resistance. However, this is not conclusive since we could not compare the previously untreated group with the treated group directly and the relation between SVR and drug-resistance could not be built in this meta-analysis. Other factors associated with resistance profiles of telaprevir are HCV-1 subtype [23,24], drug regimen [25,26] and dosing [27]. Collectively, careful evaluation of the risks of drug resistance, use of telaprevir thrice daily in combination with peginterferon and ribavirin, may prevent patients from resistance to telaprevir.

Safety is the biggest concern when telaprevir is used. Despite its encouraging efficacy in terms of enhanced SVR and decreased relapse rate, telaprevir combination treatment is coupled with an increased incidence of adverse events, including but not limited to rash, anemia, pruritus, anemia, fatigue, flu-like syndrome, headache, nausea, insomnia, diarrhea, and pyrexia, among which rash and anemia are the most common adverse events. These adverse events can lead to discontinuation of treatment in severe cases. The incidences of both SAE and discontinuation of treatment are increased with telaprevir combination treatment, as shown in this meta-analysis. Therefore, the use of telaprevir is limited to interferon-intolerant patients, and caution should be

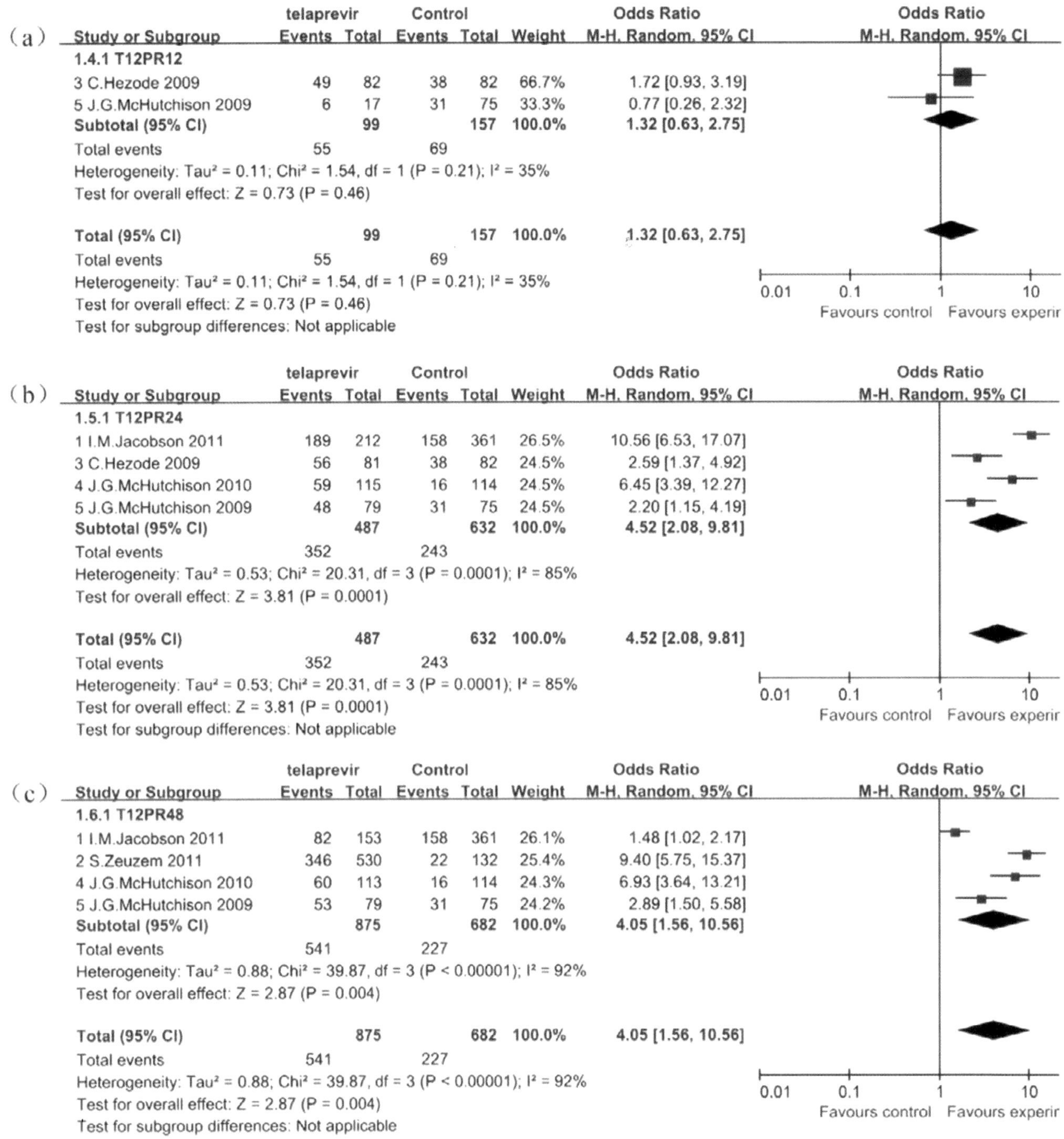

Figure 4. Meta-analysis of telaprevir plus peginterferon and ribavirin therapy on SVR according to treatment duration. There was no statistically significant difference in the proportion of patients who achieved SVR between the T12PR12 subgroup and the PR group (OR = 1.32 [0.63, 2.75], $P = 0.46$; $I^2 = 35\%$), while it was significantly higher in the T12PR24 subgroup (OR = 4.52 [2.08, 9.81], $P < 0.001$; $I^2 = 85\%$) and in the T12PR48 subgroup (OR = 4.05 [1.56, 10.56], $P = 0.004$; $I^2 = 92\%$). OR = odds ratio, I^2 = heterogeneity index. Columns in green represent the mean difference of each study and column size represents the study weight in the analysis. Lanes represent the 95% CI of each study. Diamonds in black represent the overall effect size and diamond width represents the overall 95% CI.

taken when telaprevir is used over a long period of time. Since the currently used PR therapy has already been recognized to have numerous adverse effects, we tried to discover whether the potentially shortened treatment duration by adding telaprevir can reduce the drug toxicity of peginterferon and ribavirin. However, since we failed to compare the incidence of adverse events separately in different PR duration subgroups due to lack of information, we cannot provide solid evidence on this matter and further studies focusing on how to minimize the adverse effects of telaprevir-based therapy should be done. Poor patient compliance should be noted since adherence to medications administrated thrice daily is only 59%, which requires strong and repeated

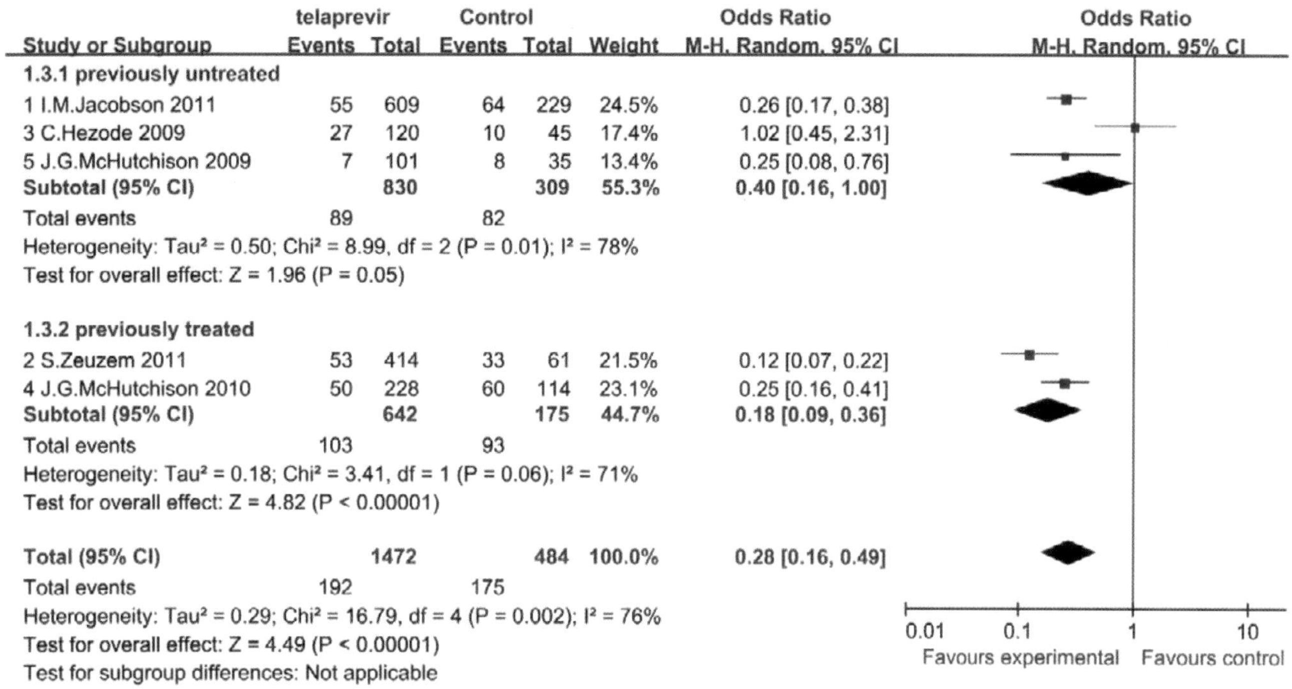

Figure 5. Meta-analysis of telaprevir plus peginterferon and ribavirin therapy on HCV relapse rate according to previous treatment. The incidence of relapse was significantly reduced in previously untreated (OR = 0.40 [0.16, 1.00], $P = 0.05$; $I^2 = 78\%$), treated (OR = 0.18 [0.09, 0.36], $P < 0.001$; $I^2 = 71\%$), and overall population (OR = 0.28 [0.16, 0.49], $P < 0.001$; $I^2 = 76\%$). OR = odds ratio, I^2 = heterogeneity index. Columns in green represent the mean difference of each study and column size represents the study weight in the analysis. Lanes represent the 95% CI of each study. Diamonds in black represent the overall effect size and diamond width represents the overall 95% CI.

encouragement from all health care providers, and a pillbox should be provided to improve patient compliance [28].

In general, this meta-analysis included all relevant RCTs from various countries and centers, probably providing the best evidence concerning telaprevir treatment for Hepatitis C. However, undoubtedly, there are several limitations in this meta-analysis. First, the primary outcome assessed here is SVR, which is a valid outcome for anti-virus effect and is associated with long-term clinical benefit [17,18,29–31]. However, with no actual clinical outcomes such as liver enzyme levels, survival, and complications being assessed, whether the achievement of SVR can be directly interpreted as clinical beneficial is still controversial. Second, there are only 5 RCTs included in this meta-analysis and all 5 studies were supported by pharmaceutical industry, which may weaken the strength of evidence demonstrated in this article, although the number of patients included in these 5 RCTs was fairly large and the risk of bias was relatively low. Third, the heterogeneity in most of these analyses is relatively high, probably due to the small number of included RCTs, different study populations and treatment durations, which indicates inter-study variation and may compromise the reliability of these results, although sensitivity analysis showed that the results were stable and reliable. Finally, most of the population studied here are whites, thus the conclusion may not be true in other races and

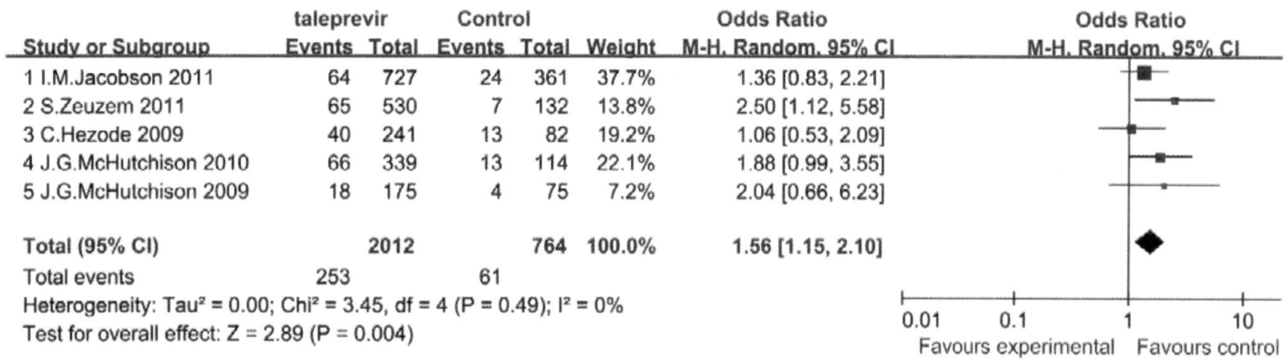

Figure 6. Meta-analysis of telaprevir plus peginterferon and ribavirin therapy on SAE incidence. The incidence of SAE was significantly higher in the telaprevir group than in the PR group (OR = 1.56 [1.15, 2.10], $P = 0.004$; $I^2 = 0\%$). OR = odds ratio, I^2 = heterogeneity index. Columns in green represent the mean difference of each study and column size represents the study weight in the analysis. Lanes represent the 95% CI of each study. Diamonds in black represent the overall effect size and diamond width represents the overall 95% CI.

Study or Subgroup	taleprevir Events	taleprevir Total	Control Events	Control Total	Weight	Odds Ratio M-H, Random, 95% CI
1 I.M.Jacobson 2011	72	727	25	361	33.9%	1.48 [0.92, 2.37]
2 S.Zeuzem 2011	68	530	4	132	14.1%	4.71 [1.69, 13.16]
3 C.Hezode 2009	28	241	6	82	16.6%	1.67 [0.66, 4.18]
4 J.G.McHutchison 2010	50	339	5	114	15.9%	3.77 [1.47, 9.71]
5 J.G.McHutchison 2009	37	175	8	75	19.4%	2.25 [0.99, 5.09]
Total (95% CI)		**2012**		**764**	**100.0%**	**2.24 [1.43, 3.50]**
Total events	255		48			

Heterogeneity: Tau² = 0.10; Chi² = 6.36, df = 4 (P = 0.17); I² = 37%

Test for overall effect: Z = 3.52 (P = 0.0004)

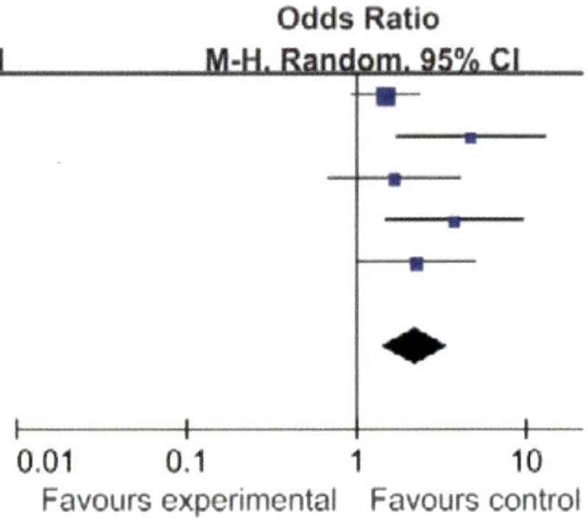

Figure 7. Meta-analysis of telaprevir plus peginterferon and ribavirin therapy on discontinuation incidence. The incidence of therapy discontinuation due to adverse events was significantly higher in the telaprevir group than in the PR group (OR = 2.24 [1.43, 3.50], $P<0.001$; $I^2 = 37\%$). OR = odds ratio, I^2 = heterogeneity index. Columns in green represent the mean difference of each study and column size represents the study weight in the analysis. Lanes represent the 95% CI of each study. Diamonds in black represent the overall effect size and diamond width represents the overall 95% CI.

areas. All these limitations point out the direction for future studies.

In conclusion, it is convincing that telaprevir is a highly potent novel drug for chronic HCV-1 hepatitis. However, cautions should be taken with telaprevir combination therapy due to increased risk of adverse events. Future studies should focus on long-term clinical outcomes of telaprevir-based therapy, applying response-guided therapy in telaprevir regimens, minimizing the adverse effects of telaprevir-based therapy, and developing second generation NS3/N4A inhibitors with less adverse effects.

Supporting Information

Figure S1 Begg's funnel plot of publication bias for the SVR comparison with pseudo 95% confidence limits. Horizontal line represents the overall effect size of the 5 RCTs. Spots represent each RCT. $P = 0.835$. No publication bias was identified.

Figure S2 Begg's funnel plot of publication bias for the relapse rate comparison with pseudo 95% confidence limits. Horizontal line represents the overall OR of the 5 RCTs. Spots represent each RCT. $P = 0.615$. No publication bias was identified.

Figure S3 Begg's funnel plot of publication bias for the comparison of SAE incidence with pseudo 95% confidence limits. Horizontal line represents the overall OR of the 5 RCTs. Spots represent each RCT. $P = 0.387$. No publication bias was identified.

Figure S4 Begg's funnel plot of publication bias for the discontinuation rate comparison with pseudo 95% confidence limits. Horizontal line represents the overall OR of the 5 RCTs. Spots represent each RCT. $P = 0.295$. No publication bias was identified.

Figure S5 Meta-analysis of telaprevir plus peginterferon and ribavirin therapy on rash incidence. The incidence of rash was significantly higher in telaprevir group than in the PR group (OR = 2.11 [1.42, 3.14], $P<0.001$; $I^2 = 68\%$). Columns in green represent the mean difference of each study and column size represents the study weight in the analysis. Lanes represent the 95% CI of each study. Diamonds in black represent the overall effect size, and diamond width represents the overall 95% CI.

Figure S6 Meta-analysis of telaprevir plus peginterferon and ribavirin therapy on anemia incidence. The incidence of anemia was significantly higher in the telaprevir group than in the PR group (OR = 1.88 [1.19, 2.96], $P = 0.007$; $I^2 = 64\%$). Columns in green represent the mean difference of each study and column size represents the study weight in the analysis. Lanes represent the 95% CI of each study. Diamonds in black represent the overall effect size, and diamond width represents the overall 95% CI.

Figure S7 The heterogeneity-adjusted required information size to demonstrate or reject a 20% odds ratio reduction of telaprevir-based therapy (with a control group proportion of 32%, an alpha of 5%) is 1333 patients (vertical red line). The rede inward-sloping line to the left make up the trial sequential monitoring boundaries and the blue line is the cumulative Z-curve.

Table S1 PRISMA checklist.

Author Contributions

Conceived and designed the experiments: YK XW YS ZG XH. Performed the experiments: YK XW YS. Analyzed the data: YK XW YS WL XL ZG XH. Contributed reagents/materials/analysis tools: YK XW YS. Wrote the paper: YK XW YS PS ZG XH.

References

1. Shepard CW, Finelli L, Alter MJ (2005) Global epidemiology of hepatitis C virus infection. Lancet Infectious Diseases 5: 9(558–567).
2. Seeff LB, Hollinger FB, Alter HJ, Wright EC, Cain CMB, et al. (2001) Long-term mortality and morbidity of transfusion-associated non-A, non-B, and type C hepatitis: a national heart, lung, and blood institute collaborative study. Hepatology 33: 2(455–463).

3. Deuffic-Burban S, Poynard T, Sulkowski MS, Wong JB (2007) Estimating the future health burden of chronic hepatitis C and human immunodeficiency virus infections in the United States. Journal of Viral Hepatitis 14: 2(107–115).
4. Ghany MG, Strader DB, Thomas DL, Seeff LB (2009) Diagnosis, management, and treatment of hepatitis C: an update. Hepatology (Baltimore) 49: 1335–1374.
5. Russo MW, Zacks SL, Fried MW (2003) Managemet of newly diagnosed hepatitis C virus infection. Cleveland Clinic Journal of Medicine 70: SUPPL. 4(S14–S20).
6. Zeuzem S, Feinman SV, Rasenack J, Heathcote EJ, Lai MY, et al. (2000) Peginterferon alfa-2a in patients with chronic hepatitis c. New England Journal of Medicine 343: 23(1666–1672).
7. Manns MP, McHutchison JG, Gordon SC (2001) Peginterferon alfa-2b plus ribavirin compared with interferon alfa-2b plus ribavirin for initial treatment of chronic hepatitis C: a randomized trial. Lancet 358: 958–65.
8. Russo MW, Fried MW (2003) Side effects of therapy for chronic hepatitis C. Gastroenterology 124: 6(1711–1719).
9. Jacobson I (2010) Emeging and novel therapies for hepatitis C. Gastroenterol Hepatol 6: 623–627.
10. Joyce MA, Tyrrell DL (2010) The cell biology of hepatitis C virus. Microbes Infect 12: 263–71.
11. Gale M, Foy E (2005) Evasion of intracellular host defence by hepatitis C virus. Nature 436(18).
12. Hezode C, Forestier N, Dusheiko G, Ferenci P, Pol S, et al. (2009) Telaprevir and peginterferon with or without ribavirin for chronic HCV infection. N Engl J Med 360: 1839–50.
13. McHutchison JG, Manns MP, Muir AJ, Terrault NA, Jacobson IM, et al. (2010) Telaprevir for previously treated chronic HCV infection. N Engl J Med 362: 1292–303.
14. McHutchison JG, Everson GT, Gordon SC, Jacobson IM, Sulkowski M, et al. (2009) Telaprevir with peginterferon and ribavirin for chronic HCV genotype 1 infection. N Engl J Med 360: 1827–38.
15. Jacobson IM, McHutchison JG, Dusheiko G, Bisceglie AM, Reddy KR, et al. (2011) Telaprevir for previously untreated chronic hepatitis C virus infection. N Engl J Med 364: 2405–16.
16. Zeuzem S, Andreone P, Pol S, Lawitz E, Diago M, et al. (2011) Telaprevir for retreatment of HCV infection. N Engl J Med 364: 2417–28.
17. Lau DT, Kleiner DE, Ghany MG, Park Y, Schmid P, et al. (1998) 10-Year follow up after interferon-alpha therapy for chronic hepatitis C. Hepatology 28: 1121–1127.
18. Fontaine H, Chaix ML, Lagneau JL, Brechot C, Pol S, et al. (2000) Recovery from chronic hepatitis C in long-term responders to ribavirin plus interferon alfa. Lancet 356: 41.
19. Sarrazin C, Zeuzem S (2010) Resistance to direct antiviral agents in patients with hepatitis C virus infection. Gastroenterology 138: 447–62.
20. McCown MF, Rajyaguru S, Le Pogam S (2008) The hepatitis C virus replicon presents a higher barrier to resistance to nucleoside analogs than to nonnucleoside polymerase or protease inhibitors. Antimicrob Agents Chemother 52: 1604–12.
21. Bartels DJ, Zhou Y, Zhang EZ (2008) Natural prevalence of hepatitis C virus variants with decreased sensitivity to NS3–4A protease inhibitors in treatment-naive subjects. J Infect Dis 198: 800–7.
22. McCown MF, Rajyaguru S, Kular S, Cammack N, Najera I, et al. (2009) GT-1a or GT-1b subtype-specific resistance profiles for hepatitis C virus inhibitors telaprevir and HCV-796. Antimicrob Agents Chemother 53: 2129–32.
23. Kuntzen T, Timm J, Berical A (2008) Naturally occurring dominant resistance mutations to hepatitis C virus protease and polymerase inhibitors in treatment-naive patients. Hepatology (Baltimore) 48: 1769–78.
24. Gentile I, Carleo MA, Borgia F, Castaldo G, Borgia G, et al. (2010) The efficacy and safety of telaprevir – a new protease inhibitor – against hepatitis C virus. Expert Opin Investig Drugs 19: 151–9.
25. Kieffer TL, Sarrazin C, Miller JS (2007) Telaprevir and pegylated interferon-alpha-2a inhibit wild-type and resistant genotype 1 hepatitis C virus replication in patients. Hepatology (Baltimore) 46: 631–9.
26. Sarrazin C, Kieffer TL, Bartels D (2007) Dynamic hepatitis C virus genotypic and phenotypic changes in patients treated with the protease inhibitor telaprevir. Gastroenterology 132: 1767–77.
27. Schmidt S, Sheikzadeh S, Beil B, Patten M, Stettin J, et al. (2008) Acceptance of telemonitoring to enhance medication compliance in patients with chronic heart failure. Telemed J E Health 14: 426–33.
28. McHutchison JG, Ware JE Jr, Bayliss MS (2001) The effects of interferon alpha-2b in combination with ribavirin on health related quality of life and work productivity. Hepatology 34: 140–7.
29. Bruno S, Stroffolini T, Colombo M (2007) Sustained virological response to interferon-alpha is associated with improved outcome in HCV-related cirrhosis: a retrospective study. Hepatology 45: 579–87.
30. Veldt BJ, Heathcote EJ, Wedemeyer H (2007) Sustained virologic response and clinical outcomes in patients with chronic hepatitis C and advanced fibrosis. Ann Intern Med 147: 677–84.
31. Manesis EK, Papaioannou C, Gioustozi A, Kafiri G, Koskinas J, et al. (1997) Biochemical and virological outcome of patients with chronic hepatitis C treated with interferon alfa-2b for 6 or 12 months: a 4-year follow-up of 211 patients. Hepatology 26: 734–739.

PEG-IFN Alpha but Not Ribavirin Alters NK Cell Phenotype and Function in Patients with Chronic Hepatitis C

Antoaneta A. Markova[1], Ulrike Mihm[2], Verena Schlaphoff[1], Sebastian Lunemann[1], Natalie Filmann[3], Birgit Bremer[1], Thomas Berg[4], Christoph Sarrazin[2], Stefan Zeuzem[2], Michael P. Manns[1], Markus Cornberg[1], Eva Herrmann[3], Heiner Wedemeyer[1]*

1 Department of Gastroenterology, Hepatology and Endocrinology, Hannover Medical School, Hannover, Germany, **2** Department of Medicine 1, JW Goethe-University Hospital, Frankfurt am Main, Germany, **3** Institute of Biostatistics and Mathematical Modelling, Faculty of Medicine, JW Goethe-University, Frankfurt am Main, Germany, **4** Department of Internal Medicine, Division of Gastroenterology and Rheumatology, University of Leipzig, Leipzig, Germany

Abstract

Background: Ribavirin (RBV) remains part of several interferon-free treatment strategies even though its mechanisms of action are still not fully understood. One hypothesis is that RBV increases responsiveness to type I interferons. Pegylated Interferon alpha (PEG-IFNa) has recently been shown to alter natural killer (NK) cell function possibly contributing to control of hepatitis C virus (HCV) infection. However, the effects of ribavirin alone or in combination with IFNa on NK cells are unknown.

Methods: Extensive ex vivo phenotyping and functional analysis of NK cells from hepatitis C patients was performed during antiviral therapy. Patients were treated for 6 weeks with RBV monotherapy (n = 11), placebo (n = 13) or PEG-IFNa-2a alone (n = 6) followed by PEG-IFNa/RBV combination therapy. The effects of RBV and PEG-IFNa-2a on NK cells were also studied in vitro after co-culture with K562 or Huh7.5 cells.

Results: Ribavirin monotherapy had no obvious effects on NK cell phenotype or function, neither ex vivo in patients nor in vitro. In contrast, PEG-IFNa-2a therapy was associated with an increase of $CD56^{bright}$ cells and distinct changes in expression profiles leading to an activated NK cell phenotype, increased functionality and decline of terminally differentiated NK cells. Ribavirin combination therapy reduced some of the IFN effects. An activated NK cell phenotype during therapy was inversely correlated with HCV viral load.

Conclusions: PEG-IFNa activates NK cells possibly contributing to virological responses independently of RBV. The role of NK cells during future IFN-free combination therapies including RBV remains to be determined.

Editor: Stephen J. Polyak, University of Washington, United States of America

Funding: This work was supported by a grant from Roche Germany, the Federal Ministry of Education and Research (BMBF; grant 01KI0788 to HW and MC) and the International Research Training Group 1273 supported by the German Research Foundation (DFG). The funders had no role in study design, data collection and analysis, decision to publish, or preparation of the manuscript.

Competing Interests: AM, UM, VS, SL, NF, BB, CS, EH and TB have declared that no competing interests exist. SZ: Consultancies for AbbVie, BMS, Boehringer, Gilead, Idenix, Janssen, Merck, Novartis, Roche, Santaris, Verte. MC: Lecture fees from Roche, Merck (MSD), Gilead, Boehringer, BMS, Falk Consultant fees from Roche, Merck (MSD), Gilead, Novartis, Boehringer Reseach support from Roche, Merck (MSD), Gilead. MPM: Consultant/Lecture fees from Abbott, Abbie, BMS, Boehringer, Falk, Gilead, JJ/Janssen-Cilag, MSD, Norgine, Novartis, Roche, Roche Diagnostics, Siemens. HW: Consultant/Lecture fees from Abbott, Abbie, Biolex, BMS, Boehringer, Falk, Gilead, ITS, JJ/Janssen-Cilag, Medgenetics, MSD, Norgine, Novartis, Roche, Roche Diagnostics, Siemens, Transgene, ViiV. Reseach support from Abbott, BMS, Gilead, Merck, Novartis, Roche, Roche Diagnostics, Siemens. The authors confirm that co-author Heiner Wedemeyer is a PLOS ONE Editorial Board member.

* E-mail: Wedemeyer.Heiner@mh-hannover.de

Introduction

Persistent hepatitis C virus (HCV) infection affects about 160–180 million individuals worldwide [1]. Hepatitis C is one of the main causes of end stage liver disease and hepatocellular carcinoma (HCC). The disease burden caused by HCV is expected to increase during the next years despite significant progress in antiviral therapy options [2].

The immunopathogenesis of chronic hepatitis C is still not completely understood - almost 25 years after the discovery of HCV. An important role of T cell responses to control early acute HCV infection is well established. Various mechanisms how the virus evades the adaptive immune system have been suggested, including viral evolution leading to T cell escape, functional exhaustion of T cells, increased frequencies of regulatory T cells, impaired CD4 T cell help and direct interference of HCV with antigen presenting cells [3,4]. Beyond T cell responses, the role of natural killer cells (NK cells) in hepatitis C virus infection has received increasing attention in recent years. NK cells are able to control viral infections by either inhibiting replication through cytokine synthesis or through direct elimination of infected cells. The activity of NK cells is regulated by a fine tuned balance between activatory and inhibitory receptors on their cell surface. Distinct combinations of specific killing inhibitory receptors (KIR), specific HLA class I molecules and their respective ligands were associated with either spontaneous clearance or chronicity of acute HCV infection [5,6]. Moreover, NK cell phenotype and function have been shown to be altered both in acute and chronic hepatitis C [7,8] and linked with either outcome of acute infection [9–11] or response to antiviral therapy [12–14].

The current standard treatment of chronic hepatitis C still includes administration of pegylated interferon alfa (PEG-IFNa) and ribavirin (RBV) [15]. In addition, HCV protease inhibitors (PIs) have been approved for HCV genotype 1 infection by FDA and EMA in 2011 [16]. HCV PIs are currently used in combination with PEG-IFNa and RBV and between 60 to 90% of patients can be successfully treated with this triple therapy. However, many patients still do not clear HCV. Response rates are in particular poor in patients with advanced liver disease [17]. Additionally, a significant proportion of HCV-infected individuals cannot be treated at all with PEG-IFNa and/or new PIs due to contraindications and co-morbidities [18]. IFN free combination therapies with different direct acting antivirals will likely become available during the next few years. Of note, RBV is still part of many new treatment regimes in clinical development (www.clinicaltrials.gov).

The detailed mode of action how IFNa and RBV provoke their antiviral effects against HCV are not completely understood. IFNa induces distinct expression of interferon stimulated genes (ISGs) which in the end leads to suppression of viral replication [19]. In addition, IFNa is believed to cause immunomodulatory effects by acting on various cells of the innate and adaptive immune system. We recently showed that IFNa induces expression of tumor necrosis factor related apoptosis inducing ligand (TRAIL) on NK cells which may contribute to control of viral replication [20]. TRAIL expression on NK cells correlated with the phase 2 decline during antiviral combination therapy [20]. However, the effects of RBV in the context of antiviral therapy of HCV infection are rather unclear. Among various suggested possible modes of action [21] ribavirin is believed to alter immune responses. For example shifts in the TH1/2 cytokine profiles have been reported both in animal models [22] as well as during ribavirin treatment of hepatitis C in humans [23]. Ribavirin is believed to increase the susceptibility of hepatocytes to IFNa stimulation [24]. Nevertheless, it is unknown if RBV may also have distinct effects on NK cells, either alone or in combination with IFNa.

We had the unique chance to study peripheral blood mononuclear cell (PBMC) samples obtained from patients during a clinical trial investigating the effects of a six-week lead-in therapy with either RBV alone, PEG-IFNa alone or placebo on the early HCV RNA kinetics [25]. We therefore aimed to address the question if RBV alters the phenotype and function of human NK cells in vivo, alone or in combination with PEG-IFNa.

Materials and Methods

Patients and Treatment

Samples were obtained as part of a prospective, randomised, partially placebo controlled clinical trial which has been described in detail previously [25]. In brief, patients with chronic HCV genotype 1 infection were treated for six weeks with either RBV monotherapy (group A, RBV 1000–1200 mg/d), placebo (group B) or PEG-IFNa alone (group C, Peginterferon alpha-2a 180 µg/week), followed by twelve weeks of PEG-IFNa-RBV combination. Subsequent antiviral treatment after the 12 weeks of therapy within this trial was administered for a total treatment duration of up to 48 weeks according to the German guidelines and under the responsibility of the investigators [25]. The initial aim of the study was to investigate early kinetics of HCV RNA in the different study arms. Blood samples were taken frequently during the first days of therapy, peripheral blood mononuclear cells (PBMC) were isolated before therapy and after 2, 14, 28, 42, 44, 56, 70, 84 and 126 days of therapy. Standard of care (SOC) was continued after week 12 according to the national treatment guidelines [26]. Patients gave written informed consent for the investigation of immunological parameters as part of the study protocol that has been approved by the ethics committee of the participating university hospitals (principal ethics committee of the medical association of Saarland and the ethics committees of the university hospitals in Berlin, Frankfurt and Hannover).

Blood samples were drawn in CDTA (citrate dextrose) tubes, peripheral blood mononuclear cells (PBMC) were separated using standard Ficoll Density Centrifugation method, washed 3 times with phosphate-buffered saline (PBS) and cryopreserved. After thawing, cells were tested for viability with trypan blue and considered for further experiments if viability was more than 90%. Altogether, vital cells were available from 30 patients: 11 in group A, 13 in group B and 6 in group C. Summary of patient characteristics are shown in Table 1 and characteristics of each individual in Table S1.

Analysis of NK Cell Phenotype and Function in Patients

NK cell phenotype and function was determined as previous described [20,27]. Detailed protocols and antibodies used in this study are provided in the Supporting Information.

Effects of Ribavirin on NK Cells in vitro

To investigate the effects of ribavirin on NK cells in vitro, NK cells from healthy blood donors were studied. Freshly isolated PBMC were cultured at 2.5×10^6 cells/ml at 37°C in complete RPMI medium alone and/or stimulated with K562 or Huh7.5 target cells. Additionally, cells were stimulated with RBV in a concentration of 0.5 µg/mL, 5 µg/ml and 50 µg/ml alone or in combination with PEG-IFN-alfa-2a in a concentration of 100 ng/mL or in combination with IL-12/IL-15.

Statistical Analyses

To evaluate the dynamics of the different immunological markers, we applied a mixed effects model with piecewise log-linear regression function for the respective treatment phases. In this way it is possible to differentiate between PEG-IFN-alfa-2a and RBV effects and the corresponding tests are more powerful than paired sample tests ignoring intermediate measurements. Nevertheless, some results for paired t-tests are also given additionally. An additional mixed effect regression model including HCV RNA was used to evaluate the effect of viral load on the different markers. Spearman rank correlations were calculated to evaluate the associations between the immunological markers and viral kinetic parameters as interferon efficacy which were previously calculated [25]. In short, the underlying mathematical model uses a standard biphasic nonlinear ordinary differential equation system accounting for varying drug levels of PEG-IFN-alfa-2a in treatment phases including PEG-IFN-alfa-2a. Estimates for mean and maximal efficacy of PEG-IFN-alfa-2a in blocking

Table 1. Patient epidemiological and clinical characteristics at baseline (day 0).

Group	Therapyd0–d42	Therapy d42–d126	Mean age, years	Mean HCV RNA, log10	Media ALT, IU/ml	Median AST, IU/ml	Gender, male/female	Mean BMI, kg/m^2
Group A (n = 11)	RBV	PEG-IFN RBV	48±10	6.1±0.9	53 (31–179)	46 (26–241)	4/7	27±5.2
Group B (n = 13)	Placebo	PEG-IFN RBV	51±15	6.1±0.9	65 (32–206)	63 (30–163)	4/9	26±4.1
Group C (n = 6)	PEG-IFN	PEG-IFN RBV	50±15	6.9±0.4	96 (57–176)	65 (38–203)	4/2	25±3.3

*ALT - alanin aminotransferase, AST - aspartate aminotransferase, BMI - body mass index.

viral production and efficacy of RBV in rendering part of the newly produced virus as non-infectious are provided as well as estimates of the infected cell loss rate. All statistical tests were two-sided with a significance level of a = 5% and account appropriately for dependencies between samples from the same patients. We used R software (R Foundation of Statistical Computing, Vienna, Austria) and the nlme package. Figures were generated using Graph Pad Prism 5 Software, Version 5.01.

Results

NK Cell Frequencies during Monotherapy with PEG-IFNa or Ribavirin and Combination Antiviral Therapy

In order to study the effects of RBV or PEG-IFNa monotherapy and the combination of both on NK cells, we first assessed frequency and phenotype of NK cells directly ex vivo in peripheral blood at several timepoints during antiviral therapy. NK cells were identified as CD3-negative, CD56 and/or CD16 positive cells after gating on lymphocytes (Fig. 1A). Gating strategies to distinguish NK cells with low and high expression levels of CD56 (CD56^{dim} vs. CD56^{bright} cells) are also shown in Figure 1A.

The frequency of NK cells was not affected by therapy in any of the three treatment groups (data not shown). However, administration of PEG-IFNa but not of ribavirin led to a shift in the frequency of NK cell subtypes (Fig. 1B). While the relative proportion of CD56^{dim} and CD56^{bright} cells did not change during ribavirin monotherapy ($p>0.05$), a marked increase in CD56^{bright} ($p<0.0001$) and a decline of CD56^{dim} ($p<0.0001$) cells was seen after the addition of PEG-IFNa until day 126 of therapy in group A patients (e.g., CD56^{bright} day 42:15±2.4% vs. day 126:39±3.7%, $p<0.0001$). A comparable change in the CD56^{dim}/CD56^{bright} ratio occurred after day 42 in patients receiving first placebo (group B) (Fig. 1B, $p<0.0001$). PEG-IFNa monotherapy also induced an increase of the CD56^{bright} population ($p<0.0001$ in the regression model; e.g., 9.8%±2.6 at baseline vs. 20%±3.5 at day 42 but not significant for paired comparison because of missing paired samples) which further augmented during subsequent combination therapy (day 126:34%±5.7, $p<0.004$ for a paired comparison with day 0).

Thus, PEG-IFNa therapy was associated with a 2–3 fold increase of CD56^{bright} cells within 12 weeks of therapy. Ribavirin had no influence on the relative CD56^{dim} vs. CD56^{bright} ratio and ribavirin pre-treatment did not alter the PEG-IFNa effect on NK cell subsets.

PEG-IFNa but not Ribavirin Induces an Activated Phenotype of NK Cells

We next aimed to investigate to what extent different treatment regimens may alter NK cell phenotypes as suggested by other studies [12,14]. Of note, ribavirin monotherapy had no effect on expression levels of NKp30 on total NK cells with stable frequencies of NKp30-positive cells until day 42 in group A (Fig. 2A) which held true for both CD56^{dim} and CD56^{bright} NK cells (Fig. S1). After adding PEG-IFNa, the percentage of NKp30-positive cells increased in all patients with mean values of 72±2.1% at day 42 and 82±2.6% at day 126 ($p = 0.006$, paired sample test). Almost similar values of NKp30 expression were observed in patients during combination therapy in group B (placebo until day 42) with a mean increase from 68±2.9% to 80±1.9% ($p = 0.005$ for the increase in group A and B in the regression model and no significant differences between both groups). PEG-IFNa monotherapy also induced a significant increase in NKp30-positive cells until day 42 ($p<0.001$) with further enhancement of NKp30 expression during subsequent

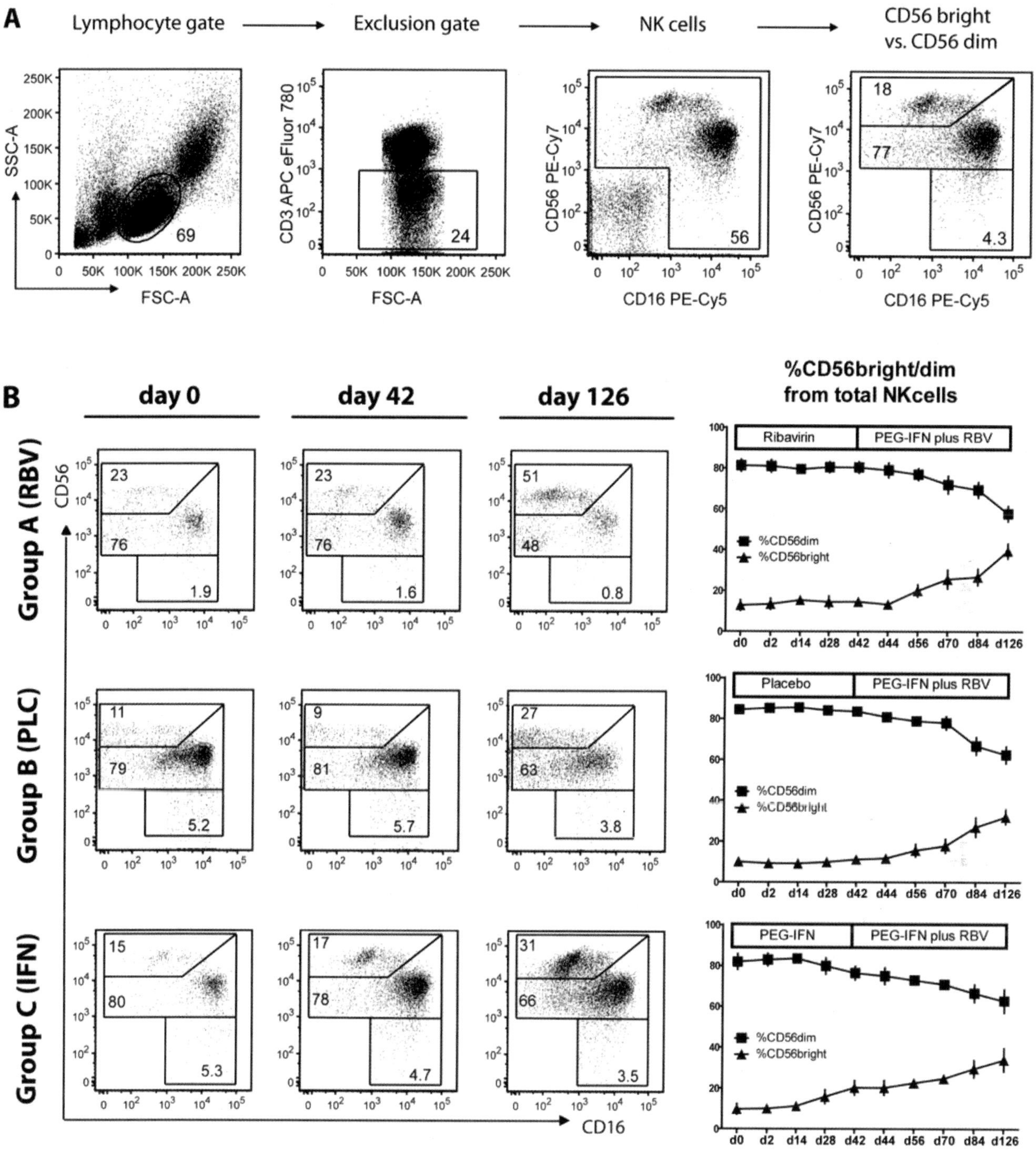

Figure 1. Frequency of NK cell subsets during therapy. (A) Gating strategy to distinguish NK cells and subgroups CD56^{dim} and CD56^{bright} cells. (B) Representative FACS plots for d0, d42 and d126 stainings and mean values for all patients are shown. d, day; RBV, Ribavirin; PLC, Placebo; PEG-IFN, pegylated Interferon.

combination treatment (Fig. 2A and Table 2). Changes of NKp30 expression during therapies were comparable for both CD56^{dim} and CD56^{bright} cells (Fig. S1).

Further, also NKp46 expression was analysed. Expression intensity measured by mean fluorescence index (MFI) increased during PEG-IFNa therapy while ribavirin did not alter NKp46 levels (Table 2 and Fig. S2A).

TRAIL expression was analysed in all the three study arms. In accordance to previous data published by our group [20], changes in TRAIL expression correlated with interferon therapy, alone or in combination with ribavirin. Ribavirin monotherapy had no significant effect on TRAIL regulation (Fig. S2C).

This data confirms previous results [12,14] that PEG-IFNa activates NK cells in vivo while we here demonstrate in addition that ribavirin does not cause any changes of NKp30 or NKp46

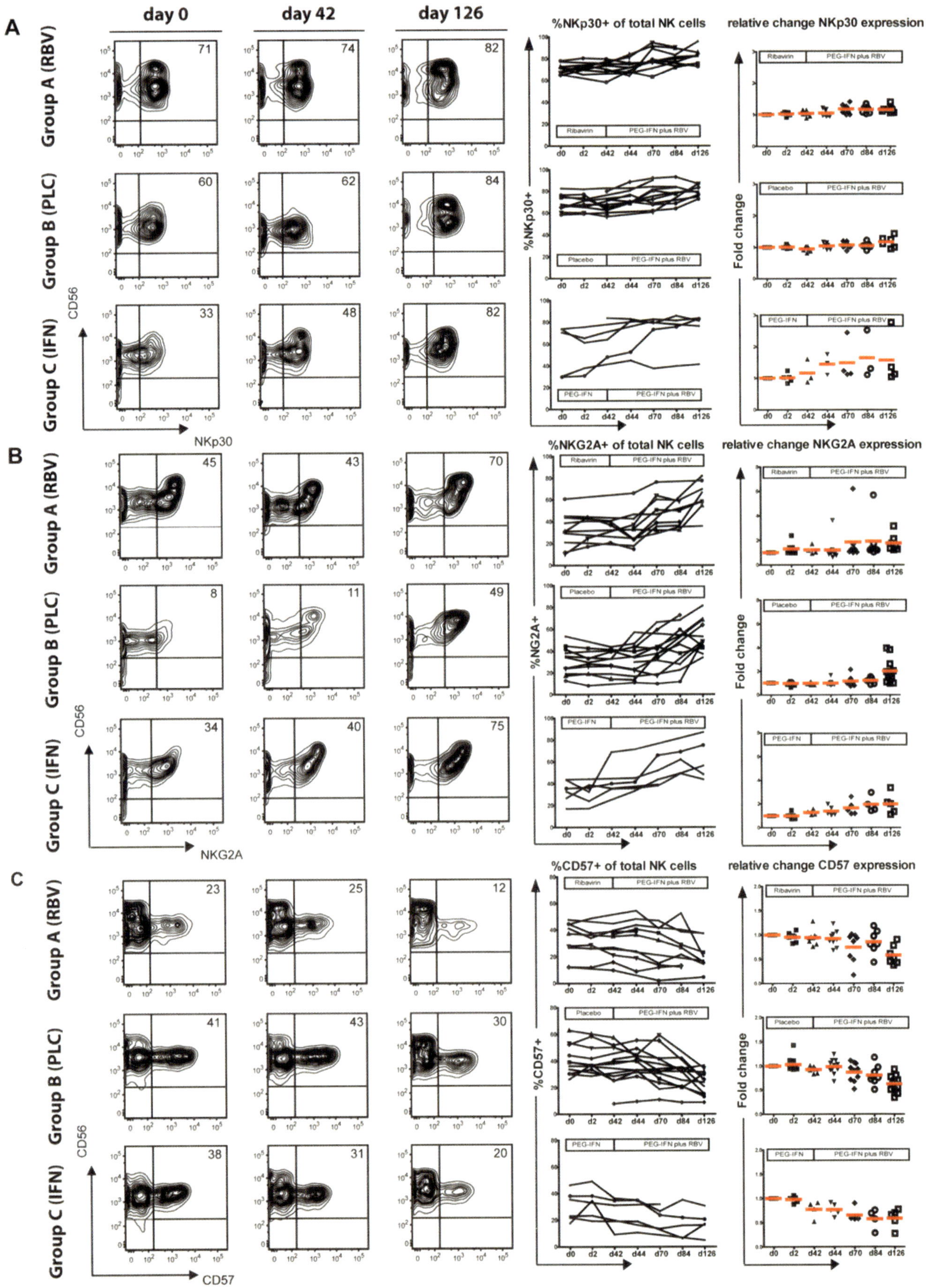
A
B
C
day 0
day 42
day 126
Group A (RBV)
Group B (PLC)
Group C (IFN)
CD56
NKp30
NKG2A
CD57
%NKp30+ of total NK cells
relative change NKp30 expression
%NKG2A+ of total NK cells
relative change NKG2A expression
%CD57+ of total NK cells
relative change CD57 expression
%NKp30+
%NG2A+
%CD57+
Fold change
Ribavirin
Placebo
PEG-IFN
PEG-IFN plus RBV
d0
d2
d42
d44
d70
d84
d126

Figure 2. Phenotypical changes during treatment with RBV, PEG-IFNa and combination therapy. PBMC from HCV patients were stained directly ex vivo. Representative FACS plots for d0, d42 and d42 and single patient courses for (A) NKp30 (B) NKG2A and (C) CD57 expression on total NK cells are shown. Percentage of positive cells as well as fold change compared to baseline expression are represented.

expression neither during monotherapy nor during combination therapy.

Decline of Terminally Differentiated NK cells during PEG-IFNa Therapy

Various infections have been linked with alterations in frequencies of immature and differentiated NK cells [28]. Interferon alpha therapy may contribute to these changes. As we had observed alterations in NK cell subsets and NK cell activation during antiviral therapy of hepatitis C, we were next interested if percentages of NKG2A-positive and CD57-positive NK cells are influenced by treatment. Indeed, PEG-IFNa therapy was associated with a 1.5–2-fold increase of NKG2A-positive NK cells (35±4.7% day 42; 63±5.1% day 126 group A; 32±3.1% day 42; 53±4.2% day 126 group B; $p<0.0001$ in the regression model with no significant differences between both groups) (Fig. 2B and Table 2), paralleled by a decline of terminally differentiated CD57-positive NK cells (29±3.6% day 42; 21±4.1% day 126 group A; 37±4.8% day 42; 24±2.5% day 126 group B; $p<0.0001$) (Fig. 2C and Table 2). These changes were most obvious after 12 weeks of therapy but even the shorter course of 6 weeks of PEG-IFNa monotherapy (group C) led already to significant changes in expression of the two markers (Figure 2B and Table 2, $p<0.0001$ for both comparisons). Changes of NKG2A+/CD57− (immature) and NGK2A−/CD57+ (terminally differentiated) cells are shown in Figure S3 and Table 2. These effects could be related to PEG-IFNa exposure alone as ribavirin monotherapy had no apparent effects on NKG2A and CD57 expression.

We also examined the CD94 expression, known as a transmembrane protein which forms heterodimers on the NK cell surface either with NKG2A or NKG2C. Increase in the expression during interferon therapy and no significant effect during ribavirin monotherapy was noted (Fig. S2B).

Hence, a reshaping of the NK cell maturation status occurs during PEG-IFNa therapy of chronic hepatitis C with a loss of

Table 2. Change of NK cell frequency, phenotype and function during monotherapy (PEG-IFNa or RBV) and combination therapy.

Parameter	PEG-IFNa alone (Group C d0–d42)	RBV alone (Group A d0–d42)	PEG-IFNa-RBV after placebo (Group B d42–d126)
% NK cells	↔	↔	↔
%CD56^{bright} cells	↑↑↑	↔	↑↑↑
%CD56^{dim} cells	↓↓↓	↔	↓↓↓
%NKp30+ NK cells	↑↑↑	↔	↑
%NKp30+ CD56^{bright} cells	↑↑↑	↔	↑
%NKp30+ CD56^{dim} cells	↑↑↑	↔	↔
MFI NKp46 NK cells	↑↑↑	↔	↔
MFI NKp46 CD56^{bright}	↑↑↑	↔	↔
MFI NKp46 CD56^{dim}	↑↑↑	↔	↔
%CD57+ NK cells	↓↓↓	↔	↓↓↓
%CD57+ CD56^{dim} cells	↓↓↓	↔	↓↓
%NKG2A+ NK cells	↑↑↑	↔	↑↑↑
%NKG2A+ CD56^{bright} cells	↑↑↑	↔	↑
%NKG2A+ CD56^{dim} cells	↑	↔	↑↑
%CD94+ NK cells	↑↑↑	↔	↑↑
%CD94+ CD56^{bright} cells	↔	↔	↔
%CD94+ CD56^{dim} cells	↑↑↑	↔	↔
%CD107+ NK-medium	↔	↔	↔
%CD107+ NK cells-K562	↑↑	↔	↔
%CD107+ NK cells-Huh7.5	↔	↔	↔
%IFNg+ NK cells-medium	↔	↑	↔
%IFNg+ NK cells-K562	↑↑↑	↑	↔
%IFNg+ NK cells-Huh7.5	↔	↔	↔
%TNF+ NK cells- medium	↔	↑↑	↔
%TNF+ NK cells-K562	↑	↔	↔
%TNF+ NK cells-Huh7.5	↔	↑	↔

*↑/↓ - $p<0.05$ in the regression model.
↑↑/↓↓ - $p<0.005$ in the regression model.
↑↑↑/↓↓↓ - $p<0.0001$ in the regression model.

terminally differentiated NK cells and a relative increase of immature cells which is not influenced by ribavirin.

Cytokine Production and Degranulation of NK Cells is Enhanced during PEG-IFNa Therapy

As NK cells were activated by PEG-IFNa therapy, we next wondered if this would translate into altered effector function. Thus, we cultured PBMC obtained before and during therapy with different target cells including hepatoma cells. Of note and in contrast to several previous studies, PBMC were not further stimulated with additional cytokines in order to reflect the in vivo situation as close as possible. NK cell degranulation was determined by CD107a expression and cytokine production was tested by interferon-gamma (IFNg) and tumor necrosis factor (TNF) expression (Fig. 3A). As shown in Figure 3B, these effector functions were significantly enhanced by PEG-IFNa therapy within few days of therapy, in particular when assessed by co-culture with the NK-target cell line K562 (here $p = 0.004$ for CD107a; $p < 0.0001$ for IFNg; $p = 0.026$ for TNF). Statistically, ribavirin monotherapy had also some effect on IFNg production and TNF expression until day 42 (Table 2) but this effect was only minor in magnitude (Fig. 3B). Interestingly, adding ribavirin after day 42 in patients which were first treated with PEG-IFNa alone (group C) did not enhance but rather shrinked degranulation and to some extent but not significantly also reduced cytokine production of NK cells (Fig. 3B).

Overall, these data clearly show that NK cell effector functions are enhanced by PEG-IFNa in vivo without any major additional effects of ribavirin.

Ribavirin does not Alter NK Cell Effector Function in vitro

Applying the above mentioned techniques, it is still possible that potential effects of ribavirin would have been overseen by ex vivo examination of cryopresevered PBMC. Thus, we aimed to investigate if ribavirin alters cytotoxicity or cytokine production of NK cells in vitro. Co-cultering NK cells with both K562 and Huh7.5 cells in presence of a wide range of ribavirin concentrations had no effect at all on the respective effector functions (Fig. 4). Similarly, ribavirin did not enhance CD107 expression, IFNg or TNF production induced by PEG-IFNa. In contrast, higher concentrations of ribavirin even reduced NK cell degranulation but not IFNg production. Adding IL-12/IL-15 to culture conditions yielded similar results as RBV exposure did not have any obvious effect on NK function even in the presence of IL-12 and IL-15 (Fig. S4). Thus, there was no evidence that potentially suboptimal assay conditions was hiding effects of ribavirin on NK cells.

Thus, these in vitro data support the observations from the clinical trial that ribavirin does not enhance NK cell effector function induced by PEG-IFNa but may even reduce NK cell degranulation.

NK Cell Phenotype and Function are Associated with HCV RNA viral Load before and during Therapy

Having shown that PEG-IFNa treatment is associated with major changes in NK cell phenotype and function, we were interested to investigate whether the IFNa effect on NK cells translates in alterations of HCV viral loads and treatment response.

Overall, NK cell subsets distribution correlated with HCV RNA levels at baseline and during the 126 days of the study as higher frequencies of $CD56^{bright}$ cells were associated with lower HCV RNA values ($p = 0.0078$). Similarly, negative associations were observed between HCV RNA levels and CD107 expression after co-culture with K562 ($p = 0.03$) and Huh7.5 cells ($p = 0.04$) as well as with IFNg expression (co-culture with K562, $p = 0.0002$).

Besides, we analysed the association between NK cell phenotype and function and the viral kinetic parameters which were fitted in by a mathematical model in [25]. Here, stronger responses to PEG-IFNa treatment which is characterized by the estimated efficacy parameter ε could be observed in patients with high baseline frequencies of CD57 positive cells in $CD56^{dim}$ cells ($p = 0.0451$) and low frequencies of CD94 positive cells on $CD56^{bright}$ cells ($p = 0.0044$).

Discussion

We here show that interferon alpha-based antiviral therapy of chronic hepatitis C is associated with major changes in the NK cell pool including an increase of $CD56^{bright}$ cells, loss of terminally differentiated cells and an overall activation of the NK cell phenotype. Moreover, NK cell function both in terms of cytotoxicity and cytokine production was significantly enhanced during therapy. Importantly, we had the unique chance to distinguish potential effects of PEG-IFNa and ribavirin on NK cell phenotype and function in this trial. Of note, ribavirin did not contribute to the stimulatory effects of PEG-IFNa and may even suppress some effector functions of NK cells. Thus, the increased efficacy of combination therapy cannot be explained by additive or even synergistic effects of both drugs on NK cells.

It is well established that type I interferons activate NK cells [29]. Since hepatitis C virus infection is treated with high doses of interferon alpha, the in vivo effect of prolonged exposure to type I interferons can be studied prospectively in patients with chronic hepatitis C. Thus, findings in patients treated for HCV infection may also have implications for other chronic inflammatory conditions where type I interferon levels are elevated. Few studies published in recent years demonstrated already some evidence that treatment with pegylated interferon alpha and ribavirin induces a shift in the NK cell subset distribution with increases of $CD56^{bright}$ cells within the first 12 weeks of therapy [12,30]. We here provide a more detailed analysis of NK cell subset kinetics and show a constant decline of $CD56^{dim}$ cells starting already about 2 weeks after initiating therapy. This effect could be attributed specifically to PEG-IFNa as 6 weeks of ribavirin monotherapy had no effect on the frequency of $CD56^{bright}$ or $CD56^{dim}$ cells. Of note, altered frequencies of $CD56^{bright}$ cells are a hallmark of various inflammatory conditions in humans including patients with HIV infection [31].

As expected, PEG-IFNa treatment induced an activatory phenotype of NK cells. NKp30 and NKp46 levels increased during therapy which is in line with previous reports showing marked changes in NK cell phenotype as early as 6–48 hours after the first dose of PEG-IFNa [12]. We here demonstrate that both markers gradually increased with continued PEG-IFNa therapy for up to 18 weeks. This activation was also associated with a loss of terminally differentiated NK cells. The relative increase in immature cells is likely to be caused by apoptosis of differentiated cells since NK cell maturation is considered irreversible [32] on the other hand migration of these cells to other organs including the liver could be an alternative explanation. On the other hand, immature cells may preferentially proliferate in response to PEG-IFNa exposure as it has been shown for other cytokines including IL-2, IL-12 or IL-15 [33–35]. Even though ribavirin has been suggested to shift cytokine responses towards a Th1-type profile [22], ribavirin did not alter IFNa-induced reshaping of the NK cell pool and had also no effects on its own during monotherapy. Thus,

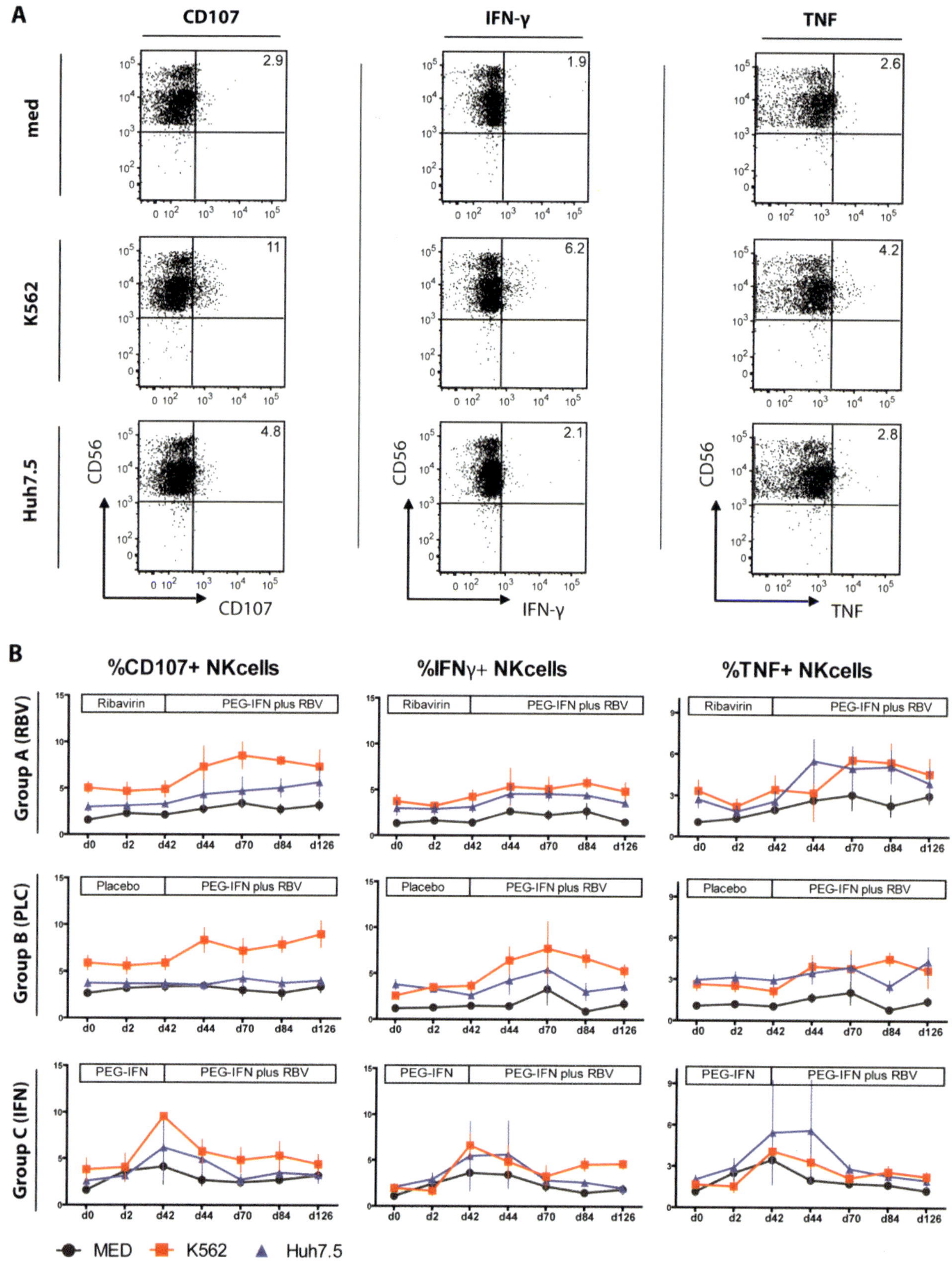

Figure 3. NK cell function during treatment. PBMC from HCV patients were cultured in medium alone or in co-culture with K562 or Huh7.5 target cells without any further cytokine stimulation. (A) Representative FACS plots for CD107a, IFNg and TNF expression on total NK cells without stimulation (MED) and after stimulation with target cells are shown. (B) Mean values of CD107a, IFNg and TNF expression on total NK cells without stimulation (MED- grey line) or upon stimulation with target cells - K562 (red line) or Huh7.5 (blue line) are shown.

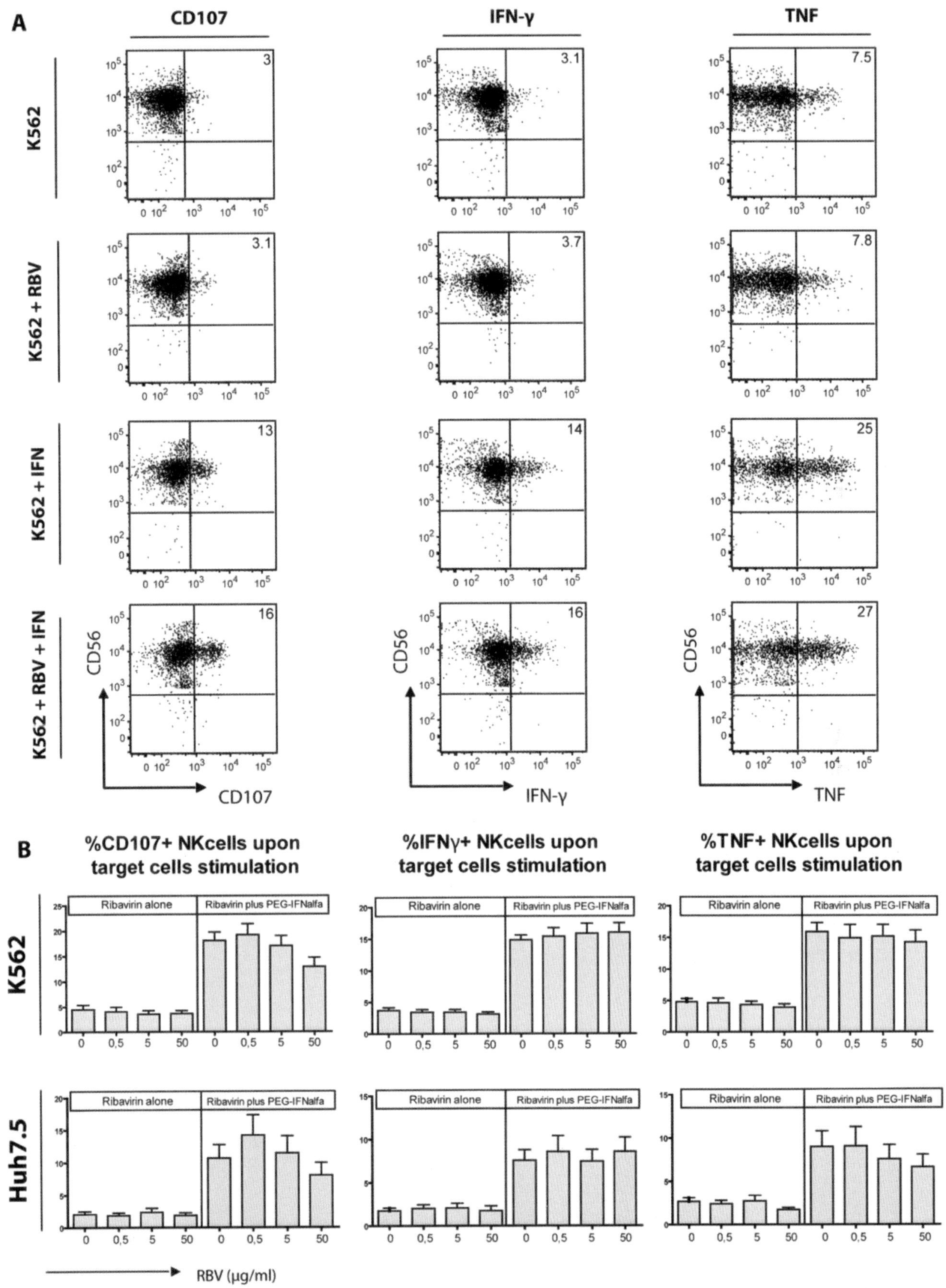

Figure 4. In vitro functionality of peripheral blood NK cells. NK cells from healthy individuals (n=11) were stimulated for 6 hours with different concentration of RBV, PEG-IFNa and combination of both. (A) Representative FACS plots for NK cells stimulated with K562 target cells alone,

with K562 target cells and RBV, with K562 target cells and PEG-IFNa, or with K562 target cells and combination of both are depicted. (B) Mean values of CD107a, IFNg and TNF expression on total NK cells upon stimulation with K562 target cells (B) and Huh7.5 hepatoma cells (C) from all healthy individuals.

this mechanism of potential immunomodulation by ribavirin does not seem to be of major importance, at least concerning NK cell maturation and proliferation.

We recently showed that in vitro stimulation of NK cells with interferon alfa increased degranulation and cytokine production after co-culture of NK cells with K562 cells and hepatoma cells [27]. Following this in vitro study, we here addressed the question if NK cells studied directly ex vivo after treatment with PEG-IFNa without any further in vitro exposure to interferon alfa would also show enhanced effector function. Previous studies investigating NK cells during antiviral therapy further stimulated the cells in vitro with different cytokines [12,36]. Thus, we here demonstrate for the first time that unmanipulated NK cells exposed only in vivo to interferon alpha display indeed stronger effector functions which was detectable as early as 2 days after first PEG-IFNa injection. Importantly, CD107a expression as a marker of degranulation and also IFNg production of NK cells were inversely correlated with HCV RNA levels during therapy suggesting a direct role of activated NK cells in the control of HCV replication during PEG-IFNa therapy.

Potential mechanisms how interferon alpha and ribavirin may influence effector functions of NK cells may involve regulation of STAT (Signal Transducers and Activators of Transcription) molecule expression and phosphorylation. Interferon alpha has been shown to alter the ratio of different STATs in NK cells with increases in STAT1 levels vs. reduction of STAT4 expression [37]. STAT1 expression and induction of STAT1-phosphorylation has been shown to be enhanced in NK cells of patients with hepatitis C which is then further increased by IFNa therapy, potentially leading to a more cytotoxic phenotype [38]. Other researchers suggested that ribavirin may further enhance IFNa-induced STAT1 and STAT3 phosphorylation in hepatocytes [39] but considering the lack of synergistic effects in this study it is unlikely that ribavirin and IFNa act in this way on NK cells. In contrast, ribavirin may even reduce phosphorylation of various signalling molecules including STAT1 in human hepatoma cells [40]. Similar mechanisms could explain the minor counterregulatory effects of ribavirin which was evident in direct ex vivo determination of NK cell degranulation of treated patients but also in the in vitro studies stimulating PBMC from healthy donors with ribavirin and PEG-IFNa.

Even though it is well established that ribavirin increases virological response to IFNa-based therapy of chronic hepatitis, the detailed modes of action are still a matter of debate [21,41]. Collectively, the data presented in this study clearly argue against a major immunomodulatory role or ribavirin involving NK cells which is based on both in vitro observations but also on ex vivo examination of treated patients. Ribavirin monotherapy was associated with declines in HCV RNA and alanin aminotransferase (ALT) levels [25] but these responses did not correlate with NK cell markers and NK cells function (data not shown). However, numbers were small and we therefore cannot exclude completely potential association. The lack of ribavirin effects on NK cells in vitro was also unlikely to be due to suboptimal cell culture conditions as even adding IL-12 and IL-15 did not reveal any different results. Overall, these findings are of potential importance for future interferon-free therapies of hepatitis C still containing ribavirin. Immune control is likely to play an important role to prevent relapse after treatment with distinct all-oral antiviral therapies. E.g., more than 30% of patients treated with sofosbuvir and ribavirin without interferon alpha experienced an HCV RNA relapse in recently published phase III trials [42]. Very preliminary data from a pilot study performed at the NIH suggested that impaired T cells but also NK cell function may be restored in part during sofosbuvir therapy which was associated with a lower likelihood of HCV relapse [43]. Based on the data from our study, we do not think that ribavirin did directly contribute to the changes in immune cell function observed in the NIH trial but this certainly warrants further investigation in future studies.

In conclusion, antiviral activities of RBV cannot be linked to apparent phenotypical or functional changes of NK cells. PEG-IFNa activates NK cells possibly contributing to virological responses independently of RBV. The role of NK cells during future IFN-free combination therapies including RBV remains to be determined.

Supporting Information

Figure S1 Phenotypical changes of NK cells during treatment with RBV, PEG-IFNa and combination therapy. PBMC were stained directly ex vivo. Single patient courses for expression of (A) NKp30 (B) NKG2A and (C) CD57 on $CD56^{bright}$ and $CD56^{dim}$ cells are shown. Percentage of positive cells as well as fold change as compared to baseline expression are represented.

Figure S2 Phenotypical changes during treatment with RBV, PEG-IFNa and combination therapy. PBMC were stained directly ex vivo. Single patient courses for expression of (A) NKp46 (B) CD94 and (C) TRAIL on NK cells are shown. MFI or percentage of positive cells as well as fold change as compared to baseline expression are represented.

Figure S3 Phenotypical changes over time during treatment with RBV, PEG-IFNa and combination therapy. PBMC were stained with the respective markers directly ex vivo. Mean values for the frequencies of (A) immature NKG2A+ CD57- and (B) mature NKG2A-CD57+ NK cells are shown.

Figure S4 In vitro functionality of peripheral blood NK cells. NK cells from healthy individuals (n = 10) were stimulated for 6 hours with different concentrations of RBV alone or in combination with IL-12/IL-15 and interferon alpha as indicated. Cells were co-cultured with K562 target cells. IFNg production on total NK cells was analysed as indicated in materials and methods. There were no statistical differences between cells stimulated with IL-12/IL-15 and IL-12/IL-15 plus ribavirin.

Table S1 Individual patient characteristics.

Methods S1

Acknowledgments

The authors thank the investigators, study coordinators, technical staff and patients involved in this study.

Author Contributions

Conceived and designed the experiments: AM VS HW. Performed the experiments: AM VS BB. Analyzed the data: AM VS SL CS NF EH HW. Contributed reagents/materials/analysis tools: UM TB CS SZ MPM. Wrote the paper: AM VS SL MC MPM EH HW.

References

1. Mohd Hanafiah K, Groeger J, Flaxman AD, Wiersma ST (2013) Global epidemiology of hepatitis C virus infection: New estimates of age-specific antibody to HCV seroprevalence Hepatology 57: 1333–1342.
2. Deuffic-Burban S, Deltenre P, Buti M, Stroffolini T, Parkes J, et al. (2012) Predicted effects of treatment for HCV infection vary among european countries Gastroenterology 143: 974–985.e14.
3. Rehermann B (2013) Pathogenesis of chronic viral hepatitis: Differential roles of T cells and NK cells Nat Med 19: 859–868.
4. Klenerman P, Thimme R. (2012) T cell responses in hepatitis C: The good, the bad and the unconventional Gut 61: 1226–1234.
5. Khakoo SI, Thio CL, Martin MP, Brooks CR, Gao X, et al. (2004) HLA and NK cell inhibitory receptor genes in resolving hepatitis C virus infection Science 305: 872–874.
6. Dring MM, Morrison MH, McSharry BP, Guinan KJ, Hagan R, et al. (2011) Innate immune genes synergize to predict increased risk of chronic disease in hepatitis C virus infection Proc Natl Acad Sci U S A 108: 5736–5741.
7. Cheent K, Khakoo SI (2011) Natural killer cells and hepatitis C: Action and reaction Gut 60: 268–278.
8. Lunemann S, Schlaphoff V, Cornberg M, Wedemeyer H (2012) NK cells in hepatitis C: Role in disease susceptibility and therapy Dig Dis 30 Suppl 1: 48–54.
9. Alter G, Jost S, Rihn S, Reyor LL, Nolan BE, et al. (2011) Reduced frequencies of NKp30+NKp46+, CD161+, and NKG2D+ NK cells in acute HCV infection may predict viral clearance J Hepatol 55: 278–288.
10. Golden-Mason L, Castelblanco N, O'Farrelly C, Rosen HR (2007) Phenotypic and functional changes of cytotoxic CD56pos natural T cells determine outcome of acute hepatitis C virus infection J Virol 81: 9292–9298.
11. Pelletier S, Drouin C, Bedard N, Khakoo SI, Bruneau J, et al. (2010) Increased degranulation of natural killer cells during acute HCV correlates with the magnitude of virus-specific T cell responses J Hepatol 53: 805–816.
12. Ahlenstiel G, Edlich B, Hogdal LJ, Rotman Y, Noureddin M, et al. (2011) Early changes in natural killer cell function indicate virologic response to interferon therapy for hepatitis C Gastroenterology 141: 1231–9, 1239.e1–2.
13. Bozzano F, Picciotto A, Costa P, Marras F, Fazio V, et al. (2011) Activating NK cell receptor expression/function (NKp30, NKp46, DNAM-1) during chronic viraemic HCV infection is associated with the outcome of combined treatment Eur J Immunol 41: 2905–2914.
14. Oliviero B, Mele D, Degasperi E, Aghemo A, Cremonesi E, et al. (2013) Natural killer cell dynamic profile is associated with treatment outcome in patients with chronic HCV infection J Hepatol.
15. European Association for the Study of the Liver (2011) EASL clinical practice guidelines: Management of hepatitis C virus infection J Hepatol 55: 245–264.
16. Sarrazin C, Hezode C, Zeuzem S, Pawlotsky JM (2012) Antiviral strategies in hepatitis C virus infection J Hepatol 56 Suppl 1: S88–100.
17. Dusheiko G, Wedemeyer H (2012) New protease inhibitors and direct-acting antivirals for hepatitis C: Interferon's long goodbye Gut 61: 1647–1652.
18. Maasoumy B, Port K, Markova AA, Serrano BC, Rogalska-Taranta M, et al. (2013) Eligibility and safety of triple therapy for hepatitis C: Lessons learned from the first experience in a real world setting PLoS One 8: e55285.
19. Schoggins JW, Wilson SJ, Panis M, Murphy MY, Jones CT, et al. (2011) A diverse range of gene products are effectors of the type I interferon antiviral response Nature 472: 481–485.
20. Stegmann KA, Bjorkstrom NK, Veber H, Ciesek S, Riese P, et al. (2010) Interferon-alpha-induced TRAIL on natural killer cells is associated with control of hepatitis C virus infection Gastroenterology 138: 1885–1897.
21. Thomas E, Ghany MG, Liang TJ (2012) The application and mechanism of action of ribavirin in therapy of hepatitis C Antivir Chem Chemother 23: 1–12.
22. Ning Q, Brown D, Parodo J, Cattral M, Gorczynski R, et al. (1998) Ribavirin inhibits viral-induced macrophage production of TNF, IL-1, the procoagulant fgl2 prothrombinase and preserves Th1 cytokine production but inhibits Th2 cytokine response J Immunol 160: 3487–3493.
23. Cramp ME, Rossol S, Chokshi S, Carucci P, Williams R, et al. (2000) Hepatitis C virus-specific T-cell reactivity during interferon and ribavirin treatment in chronic hepatitis C Gastroenterology 118: 346–355.
24. Thomas E, Feld JJ, Li Q, Hu Z, Fried MW, et al. (2011) Ribavirin potentiates interferon action by augmenting interferon-stimulated gene induction in hepatitis C virus cell culture models Hepatology 53: 32–41.
25. Mihm U, Welker M, Teuber G, Wedemeyer H, Berg T, et al. (2013; 2013) Impact of ribavirin priming on viral kinetics and treatment response in chronic hepatitis C genotype 1 infection J Viral Hepat.
26. Sarrazin C, Berg T, Ross RS, Schirmacher P, Wedemeyer H, et al. (2010) Prophylaxis, diagnosis and therapy of hepatitis C virus (HCV) infection: The german guidelines on the management of HCV infection Z Gastroenterol 48: 289–351.
27. Stegmann KA, Bjorkstrom NK, Ciesek S, Lunemann S, Jaroszewicz J, et al. (2012) Interferon alpha-stimulated natural killer cells from patients with acute hepatitis C virus (HCV) infection recognize HCV-infected and uninfected hepatoma cells via DNAX accessory molecule-1 J Infect Dis 205: 1351–1362.
28. Bjorkstrom NK, Svensson A, Malmberg KJ, Eriksson K, Ljunggren HG (2011) Characterization of natural killer cell phenotype and function during recurrent human HSV-2 infection PLoS One 6: e27664.
29. Garcia-Sastre A, Biron CA (2006) Type 1 interferons and the virus-host relationship: A lesson in detente Science 312: 879–882.
30. Lee S, Watson MW, Flexman JP, Cheng W, Hammond T, et al. (2010) Increased proportion of the CD56(bright) NK cell subset in patients chronically infected with hepatitis C virus (HCV) receiving interferon-alpha and ribavirin therapy J Med Virol 82: 568–574.
31. Meier UC, Owen RE, Taylor E, Worth A, Naoumov N, et al. (2005) Shared alterations in NK cell frequency, phenotype, and function in chronic human immunodeficiency virus and hepatitis C virus infections J Virol 79: 12365–12374.
32. Bjorkstrom NK, Riese P, Heuts F, Andersson S, Fauriat C, et al. (2010) Expression patterns of NKG2A, KIR, and CD57 define a process of CD56dim NK-cell differentiation uncoupled from NK-cell education Blood 116: 3853–3864.
33. Cooper MA, Bush JE, Fehniger TA, VanDeusen JB, Waite RE, et al. (2002) In vivo evidence for a dependence on interleukin 15 for survival of natural killer cells Blood 100: 3633–3638.
34. Guimond M, Freud AG, Mao HC, Yu J, Blaser BW, et al. (2010) In vivo role of Flt3 ligand and dendritic cells in NK cell homeostasis J Immunol 184: 2769–2775.
35. Juelke K, Killig M, Luetke-Eversloh M, Parente E, Gruen J, et al. (2010) CD62L expression identifies a unique subset of polyfunctional CD56dim NK cells Blood 116: 1299–1307.
36. Hotho DM, Kreefft K, Groothuismink ZM, Janssen HL, de Knegt RJ, et al. (2013) Natural killer cell activity and function in chronic HCV-infected patients during peg interferon and ribavirin: Early effects of active substance use Antiviral Res 97: 347–355.
37. Miyagi T, Gil MP, Wang X, Louten J, Chu WM, et al. (2007) High basal STAT4 balanced by STAT1 induction to control type 1 interferon effects in natural killer cells J Exp Med 204: 2383–2396.
38. Edlich B, Ahlenstiel G, Zabaleta Azpiroz A, Stoltzfus J, Noureddin M, et al. (2012) Early changes in interferon signaling define natural killer cell response and refractoriness to interferon-based therapy of hepatitis C patients Hepatology 55: 39–48.
39. Stevenson NJ, Murphy AG, Bourke NM, Keogh CA, Hegarty JE, et al. (2011) Ribavirin enhances IFN-alpha signalling and MxA expression: A novel immune modulation mechanism during treatment of HCV PLoS One 6: e27866.
40. Zhao LJ, Wang W, Liu Y, Ren H, Qi ZT (2012) Interference with ERK and STAT signaling pathways and inhibition of hepatitis C virus replication by ribavirin Antiviral Res 96: 260–268.
41. Hofmann WP, Herrmann E, Sarrazin C, Zeuzem S (2008) Ribavirin mode of action in chronic hepatitis C: From clinical use back to molecular mechanisms Liver Int 28: 1332–1343.
42. Jacobson IM, Gordon SC, Kowdley KV, Yoshida EM, Rodriguez-Torres M, et al. (2013) Sofosbuvir for hepatitis C genotype 2 or 3 in patients without treatment options N Engl J Med 368: 1867–1877.
43. Barrett L, Shivasabesan G, Wang C, Osinusi A, Kohli A, et al. (2013) Altered HCV specific T cell immunity very early in interferon free HCV DAA therapy. J Hepatol; 58: 1–24 2013.

TCRγδ^{+}CD4^{-}CD8^{-} T Cells Suppress the CD8^{+} T-Cell Response to Hepatitis B Virus Peptides, and Are Associated with Viral Control in Chronic Hepatitis B

Qintao Lai[1], Shiwu Ma[1,2], Jun Ge[1], Zuxiong Huang[1], Xuan Huang[1], Xiaotao Jiang[1,3], Yongyin Li[1], Mingxia Zhang[1], Xiaoyong Zhang[1], Jian Sun[1], William G. H. Abbott[1,4], Jinlin Hou[1]*

1 Hepatology Unit and Key Lab for Organ Failure Research, Department of Infectious Diseases, Nanfang Hospital, Southern Medical University, No. 1838, North Guangzhou Avenue, Guangzhou, China, **2** Department of Infectious Diseases, Kunming General Hospital of PLA, Kunming, China, **3** Department of immunology, Basic Medicine School, Southern Medical University, Auckland City Hospital, Auckland, New Zealand, **4** The New Zealand Liver Transplant Unit, Auckland City Hospital, Auckland, New Zealand

Abstract

The immune mechanisms underlying failure to achieve hepatitis B e antigen (HBeAg) seroconversion associated with viral control in chronic hepatitis B (CHB) remain unclear. Here we investigated the role of CD4^{-}CD8^{-} T (double-negative T; DNT) cells including TCRαβ^{+} DNT (αβ DNT) and TCRγδ^{+} DNT (γδ DNT) cells. Frequencies of circulating DNT cell subsets were measured by flow cytometry in a retrospective cohort of 51 telbivudine-treated HBeAg-positive CHB patients, 25 immune tolerant carriers (IT), 33 inactive carriers (IC), and 37 healthy controls (HC). We found that γδ DNT cell frequencies did not significantly change during treatment, being lower at baseline ($P = 0.019$) in patients with HBeAg seroconversion after 52 weeks of antiviral therapy ($n = 20$) than in those without ($n = 31$), and higher in the total CHB and IT than IC and HC groups ($P < 0.001$). αβ DNT cell frequencies were similar for all groups. In vitro, γδ DNT cells suppressed HBV core peptide-stimulated interferon-γ and tumor necrosis factor-α production in TCRαβ^{+}CD8^{+} T cells, which may require cell–cell contact, and could be partially reversed by anti-NKG2A. These findings suggest that γδ DNT cells limit CD8^{+} T cell response to HBV, and may impede HBeAg seroconversion in CHB.

Editor: Dimitrios Paraskevis, University of Athens, Medical School, Greece

Funding: This study was supported by grants from the National Natural Science Foundation of China (No. 30730082 and No. 81270025), Major Science and Technology Special Project of China (2012ZX10002-003). The funders had no role in study design, data collection and analysis, decision to publish, or preparation of the manuscript.

Competing Interests: The authors have declared that no competing interests exist.

* E-mail: jlhousmu@163.com

Introduction

Worldwide, more than 350 million people have chronic hepatitis B virus (HBV) infection. The serious sequelae of this disease include liver cirrhosis, liver failure, and hepatocellular carcinoma [1]. Hepatitis B e antigen (HBeAg) seroconversion, defined as the loss of serum HBeAg with development of anti-HBe, is a stage in the evolution of chronic HBV infection, which can occur either spontaneously or as a result of antiviral therapy. For HBeAg-positive patients with chronic hepatitis B (CHB), HBeAg seroconversion is one of the primary goals of antiviral treatment, as it is associated with control of viral load, cessation of liver inflammation, decreased risk for serious sequelae, and increased survival [2]. Unfortunately, most patients do not achieve HBeAg seroconversion on treatment, for reasons that are poorly understood.

Evidence that HBeAg seroconversion is the result of a host immune response to HBV has recently been summarized [3]. Genetic polymorphisms in IL-10 and IL-12 loci [4], and differences in serum IL-12 [5] and serum IL-21 [6] concentrations may predict HBeAg seroconversion. However, there is little information on the cellular immune mechanisms that might be responsible for these associations. These mechanisms need to be identified to allow optimizing treatment strategies in individual patients and developing novel immunotherapies to increase seroconversion rates. We focused on the CD4^{-}CD8^{-} subset of regulatory T cells, also known as double-negative T (DNT) cells.

DNT cells are classified into αβ DNT and γδ DNT subsets, depending on whether their TCR is comprised of αβ or γδ chains. αβ DNT cells can regulate antigen-specific T-cell responses in both mice [7] and humans [8,9], and HBeAg-activated αβDNT cells can inhibit the murine HBeAg-specific effector T-cell response [10]. γδ T cells, which are usually CD4- and CD8-negative, have a role in immunoregulation, including maintenance of oral tolerance [11], ocular tolerance [12], and hyporesponsiveness to tumors [13] in mice. Human γδ T cells also possess immune-suppressive capabilities [14,15,16,17,18]. Thus, DNT cells may involve in suppression of any cellular immune response that promotes HBeAg seroconversion. To investigate this possibility, we conducted a longitudinal study comparing DNT cell frequencies in patients with CHB who either did or did not undergo HBeAg seroconversion with antiviral therapy, and a cross-sectional comparison of DNT cell frequencies in subjects who were either HBeAg-positive or HBeAg-negative.

Materials and Methods

Human Subjects

This study was conducted according to the ethical guidelines of the 1975 Declaration of Helsinki, and was approved by the ethics committee of Nanfang Hospital. All subjects provided written informed consent.

HBeAg-positive patients with CHB for the longitudinal study (n = 51) were participating in either a phase IV, multi-center, open-label clinical trial of telbivudine (LdT 600 mg/d, n = 21, trial number CLDT600ACN07T) or the Efficacy Optimization Research of Telbivudine Therapy trial (EFFORT, n = 30, trial number NCT00962533). From each patient, 20 mL of heparinized blood was taken at baseline and at 12, 24, and 52 weeks of LdT treatment. Patients were classified as responders (n = 20) if they achieved HBeAg seroconversion by treatment week 52, and as non-responders (n = 31) if they did not. Baseline characteristics of the patients in these two groups are compared in Table 1. Sixteen responders who received LdT consolidation therapy and maintained a durable response (HBeAg-negative, anti-HBe-positive, HBV DNA <300 copies/mL, and normal alanine aminotransferase (ALT)) for 48 weeks were followed up for another 52 weeks off treatment. Virologic relapse was defined as an increase of DNA level to >10,000 copies/mL [19]. The subjects for cross-sectional study included IT (n = 25), CHB (n = 51 from the above CHB), IC (n = 33) and HC (n = 37), who were recruited according to definition in AASLD criteria (see Methods S1) [2]. Their characteristics are summarized in Table 2.

Synthetic Peptides

A panel of 26 18-mer peptides overlapping by 8 or 10 residues and covering the full HBV core open reading frame (Table S1 and S2) and HBV core18 27 (FLPSDFFPSV) were obtained (Sigma-Aldrich; St. Louis, MO, USA). 18-mer Peptides were dissolved in dimethyl sulfoxide (DMSO), pooled, and named the core peptides pool. An 18-mer HIV gag peptide (VDRFYKTLRAEQASQEVK) dissolved in DMSO was used as the negative control, while medium only as the blank control.

Cell Isolation and Flow-cytometry Analysis

Isolation of peripheral blood mononuclear cells (PBMC) [6] and liver-infiltrating lymphocytes (LIL) [20,21] was performed (see Methods S2). For analysis of the DNT cell subset frequency, cells were stained with anti-CD3-APC (UCTH1), anti-TCRγδ-FITC (11F2), anti-CD4-PE, anti-CD8-PE (all BD Biosciences, Pharmingen, San Jose, CA, USA) and anti-TCRαβ-PE-Cy7 (IP26; BioLegend, San Diego, CA, USA). Flow-cytometry analysis was performed using a FACS CanTo II flow cytometer and BD FACSDiva software (BD Biosciences).

Intracellular cytokine staining (ICS) was performed as previously described [6,22,23]. Briefly, 4×10^5 PBMC were incubated with either the core peptide pool (each peptide at a final concentration of 1 μg/mL) plus anti-CD49d (1 μg/mL) and anti-CD28 (1 μg/mL), or with anti-CD3 (OKT, 5 μg/mL) plus anti-CD28 (1 μg/mL, BD Biosciences), or with phorbol-12-myristate-13-acetate (PMA, 50 ng/mL) plus calcium ionomycin (1 nmol/mL; Sigma-Aldrich) for 1 hour in 200 μL R10 (RPMI 1640 containing 2 nmol/mL glutamine, 10% FBS, 100 U/mL penicillin, and 100 μg/mL streptomycin) in a round-bottomed 96-well plate, followed by 1 μg/mL brefeldin A (BD Biosciences) for an additional 5 hours. The cells were harvested, stained with cell surface markers, fixed, permeabilized, and stained with either anti-interferon (IFN)-γ-PerCP Cy5.5, anti-tumor necrosis factor (TNF)-α-PE or isotype controls (BD Biosciences) for flow-cytometry analysis.

The frequency of a positive $CD8^+$ T-cell response to core peptides in patients with CHB is usually <30% [23,24,25]. In this study, positive response was defined as greater production of either IFN-γ or TNF-α by core peptide-stimulated $CD8^+$ T cells compared with either culture medium-stimulated or HIV gag peptide-stimulated $CD8^+$ T cells. Patients with a positive $CD8^+$ T-cell response were chosen for the T-cell suppression assays, transwell assays, and blocking assays.

Table 1. Clinical characteristics at baseline of subjects in the cohort receiving telbivudine therapy.

Groups	Responders	Non-responders	*P* values
Cases	20	31	
Gender, M/F	14/6	26/5	0.408[b)]
Age, years[a)]	28 (25–35)	27 (24–29)	0.250[c)]
ALT, IU/L[a)]	166 (98–252)	116 (82–244)	0.370[c)]
AST, IU/L[a)]	104 (53–129)	88 (57–146)	0.946[c)]
HBV DNA, log10 copies/mL[a)]	8.16 (7.32–8.72)	8.73 (8.59–9.03)	0.002[c)]
Genotype B/C	16/4	16/15	0.080[b)]

ALT, alanine aminotransferase; AST, Aspartate aminotransferase; HBV, hepatitis B virus; M/F: Male/female.
[a)]Data are median (interquartile range).
[b)]Compared by χ^2 test (continuity correction).
[c)]Compared by Mann-Whitney *U*-test.

T-cell Suppression Assays

Because the proportion of $CD4^+$ γδ T cells in the γδ T-cell pool is extremely low (<1%), the isolation of γδ DNT was carried out using magnetic beads (Miltenyi Biotech, Bergisch Gladbach, Germany) to remove $CD8^+$ cells from PBMC, followed by positive selection of γδ T cells. γδ T(−) PBMC were obtained by direct removal of γδ T cells. The γδ DNT : γδ T(−) PBMC co-cultures were set up at a ratio of 1:2 with a total of 4.5×10^5 cells/well. After overnight incubation, both the γδ DNT : γδ T(−) PBMC and γδ T(−) PBMC were cultured with the core peptide pool, and the production of IFN-γ in $TCR\alpha\beta^+CD8^+$ T ($CD8^+$ αβ T) cells was detected by ICS. Negative or blank controls were 4.5×10^5 γδ T(−) PBMC cultured with or without the HIV gag peptide, respectively.

Transwell Assays

Transwell assays were performed using cell-culture inserts with a 1 μm polycarbonate membrane to avoid direct cell contact between the top and bottom chambers in 96-well plates (Transwell; Corning Inc., Corning, NY, USA). The γδ T(−) PBMC (4.5×10^5) were added to the bottom chamber, while γδ DNT cells (1.5×10^5) were added to either the top or the bottom chamber. Production of IFN-γ and TNF-α in core peptide-stimulated $CD8^+$αβ T cells in the bottom chamber was detected by ICS.

Blocking Assays

For more sensitive detection, blocking assays were performed as previously described [24,26,27], with minor modifications. Briefly, 1×10^5 γδ DNT cells were respectively incubated with anti-NKG2A (Z199, 10 μg/mL; Beckman Coulter Inc., Brea, CA, USA), anti-HLA-E(3D12, 10 μg/mL), or mouse IgG1 isotype

Table 2. Clinical characteristics of subjects in cross-sectional study.

Groups	IT	CHB	IC	HC
Cases	25	51	33	37
Gender, M/F	11/14	40/11	10/23	15/22
Age, years[a]	26 (23–30)	27 (24–33)	29 (24–38)	24 (23–26)
ALT, IU/L[a]	27 (17–32)	127 (88–244)	19 (16.5–25)	13(8–22)
AST, IU/L[a]	25 (22–27)	99 (57–137)	24 (21–28)	20 (16.5–24)
HBV DNA, log10 copies/mL[a]	7.80 (7.49–8.30)	8.62 (8.00–8.90)	<3.00(<3.00)	NA
HBeAg/anti-HBe	25/0	51/0	0/33	0/0

ALT, alanine aminotransferase; AST, Aspartate aminotransferase; HBeAg, HBV e antigen; HC, healthy controls; IC, inactive carriers; IT, immune tolerant carriers; M/F: Male/female; NA, not applicable.
[a]Data are median (interquartile range).

(10 μg/mL) (both Biolegend) for 45 min at 37°C, and then co-cultured with 3×10^5 γδ T(−)PBMC in the presence of the core peptides pool, anti-CD49d, and anti-CD28 (1 μg/mL). The gag peptide was the negative control. IL-2 (25 U/mL) was added on day 4. After 10 days, cells were resuspended, and stimulated again with peptides for 1 h, then Brefeldin A was added for a further 5 h. Production of IFN-γ and TNF-α in $CD8^+$αβT cells was measured by flow-cytometry analysis.

PBMC from some patients were stained with anti-HLA-A2-PE (BD). The HLA-A2 positive patients were chose for the detection using PE-labeled pentamer complexed with HBV core 18–27 (Proimmune, Oxford, UK). With the method of blocking assays, cells were expanded and re-stimulated with HBV core18–27 (5 μg/mL), and stained with anti-CD3-FITC, anti-CD8-APC-Cy7, pentamer-PE, anti-IFN-γ-PerCP-Cy5.5 and anti-TNF-α-PE-Cy7.

Statistical Analysis

Serum HBV DNA levels were normalized by log transformation. Box and whisker plots were used to show the median, interquartile range (IQR), and range. For independent group comparisons, we used the Kruskal-Wallis *H*-test to compare all groups and the Mann-Whitney *U*-test to compare groups by pairs. For related group comparisons, the Friedman test was used to compare all groups and the Wilcoxon test to compare groups by pairs. Spearman rank order correlation was used for correlation analyses. The χ^2 test, logistic regression, and receiver-operating characteristic curves (ROC) analysis were used as appropriate, using either SPSS (version 13.0; SPSS Inc., Chicago, IL, USA), GraphPad Prism (version 5; GraphPad, San Diego, CA, USA) or SAS (SAS Inc., Cary, NC, USA). For ROC analysis, an area under the curve (AUC) of 1.0 is characteristic of an ideal test, whereas AUC <0.5 indicates a test of no diagnostic value. A (two-tailed) *P*-value of <0.05 was deemed statistically significant.

Results

Association between Frequencies of γδ DNT Cells and HBeAg Seroconversion in Antiviral Therapy

In longitudinal study, HBeAg-postive patients treated with telbivudine (LdT) were classified as responders (n = 20) if they achieved HBeAg seroconversion by treatment week 52, and as non-responders (n = 31) if they did not. Circulating frequencies of αβ DNT cells and γδ DNT cells were examined (Figure 1A) at baseline, 12, 24, and 52 weeks. There were no significant changes in frequencies of the two DNT cell subsets during 52 weeks of treatment, and no significant differences in frequencies of αβ DNT cells between the two groups (Figure 1B; Figure S1A). Frequencies of γδ DNT cells were higher in non-responders than in responders at baseline (median [IQR]: 10.3% [6.1–14.7%] vs 5.1% [3.6–11.2%], respectively; $P = 0.019$) and at 12 weeks (10.5% [7.0–16.5%] vs 5.8% [3.7–12.1%]; $P = 0.041$).

Univariate logistic regression showed that HBeAg seroconversion was associated with low baseline frequencies of both γδ DNT cells ($P = 0.04$) and HBV DNA ($P = 0.005$). Multivariate analysis identified a significant effect of HBV DNA ($P = 0.008$), and a trend towards an independent effect of γδ DNT cell frequency ($P = 0.08$). No significant interaction was found between these variables ($P = 0.77$). There were no significant correlations between frequencies of γδ DNT cells and either the serum HBV DNA levels, ALT, or aspartate aminotransferase (AST), or age of the CHB patients at baseline (Table S3).

In this cohort, ROC analysis showed that either baseline γδ DNT cell frequency or baseline serum HBV DNA level predicted the non-responders after 52 weeks of LdT therapy (Figure 1C). The optimal cut-off value for prediction was baseline γδ DNT cell frequency of 7.65% of CD3-positive PBMC, which had a sensitivity of 70.0% and specificity of 71.0%. In light of that quite a few patients who achieve HBeAg seroconversion induced by nucleotide analogues have virologic relapse off treatment [19], we observed the association between baseline γδ DNT cell frequency and viral control after 52 weeks off therapy. Sixteen patients received an average of 112 Weeks (rang 104–163 weeks) of LdT therapy before off-therapy. In the cohort of patients with baseline γδ DNT cell frequency >7.65%, five of seven patients had a virologic relapse after 52 weeks off treatment, whereas only one of nine patients with baseline γδ DNT cell frequency <7.65% had a virologic relapse ($P = 0.035$, Figure 1D). All patients (n = 4) who had recurrence of HBeAg had a high frequency of γδ DNT cells, with rates for the four patients being 10.4%, 11.3%, 14.2%, and 17.8%, respectively.

Collectively, these data indicate that a high frequency of γδ DNT cells is associated with failure to achieve durable HBeAg seroconversion induced by LdT therapy.

Association between Frequencies of γδ DNT Cells and Serum HBeAg Status in Cross-sectional Comparison

To investigate whether frequency of γδ DNT cells is associated with spontaneous HBeAg seroconversion, we compared CHB with inactive carriers (IC), immune tolerant carriers (IT), and healthy controls (HC) at baseline. Frequencies of γδ DNT cells in the two HBeAg-positive groups (IT 6.4% [4.8–9.0%] and CHB 8.4%

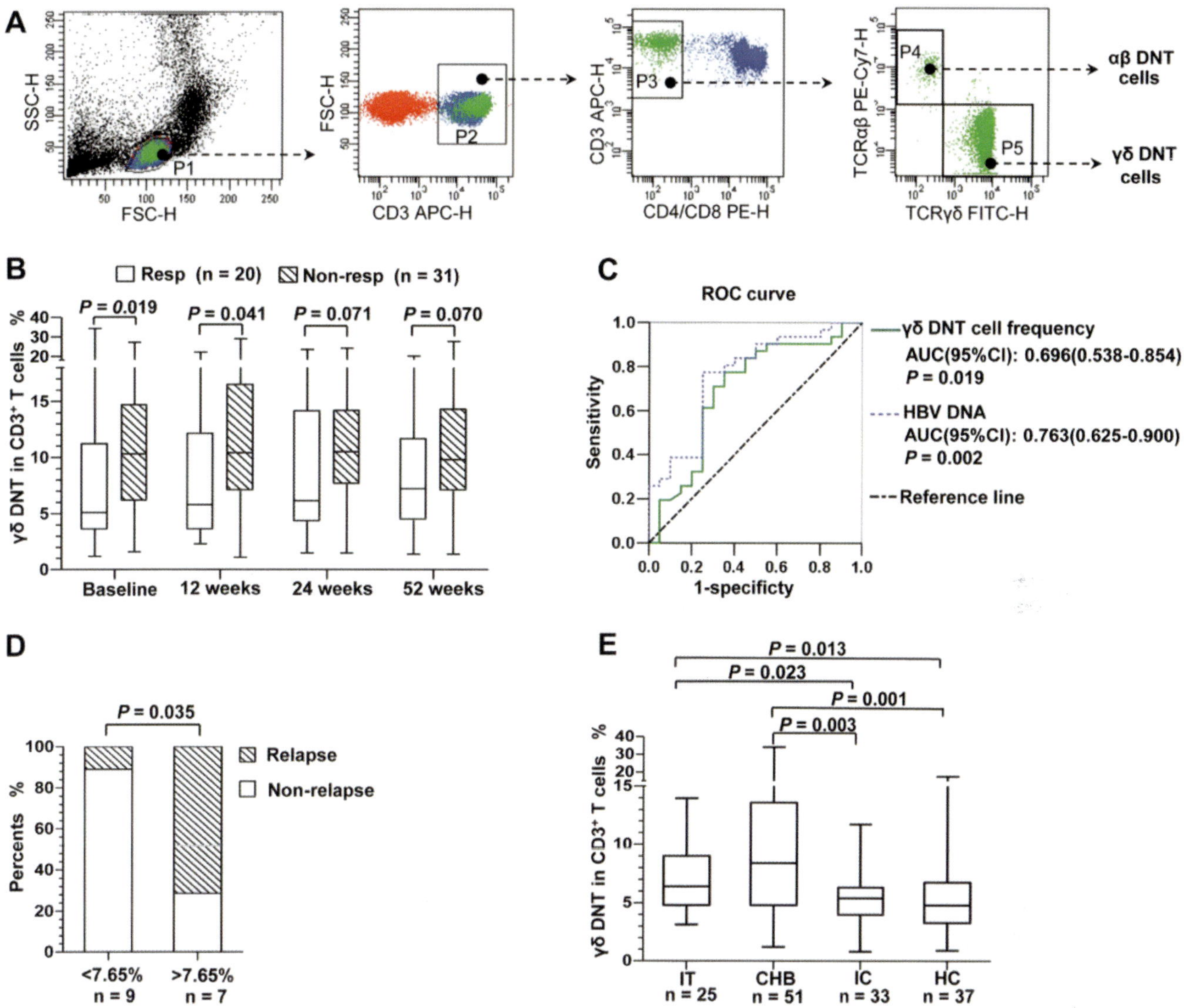

Figure 1. Comparison of the frequencies of DNT cell subsets in longitudinal and cross-sectional studies. (A) Flow-cytometry dot plots show the strategy for identifying the αβ DNT cells and γδ DNT cells. (B) The frequencies of γδ DNT cells in peripheral blood $CD3^+$ T cells were compared for responders (Resp, n = 20) and non-responders (Non-resp, n = 31) at different time points during 52 weeks of telbivudine therapy using the Mann-Whitney U test by pairs. (C) Receiver-operating characteristic curve analysis shows that either baseline γδ DNT cell frequencies or HBV DNA levels predicts the non-responders after 52 weeks of telbivudine therapy. (D) The virologic relapse rates after 52 weeks off treatment were compared between the patients with baseline γδ DNT cell frequency of >7.65% (n = 7) and <7.65% (n = 9) using χ^2 test (Fisher's exact test). (E) The frequencies of γδ DNT cells were compared in the IT, CHB, IC and HC groups using the Mann-Whitney *U* compared groups by pairs. (B, D) Data plots show the median, interquartile range (IQR), and range. αβ DNT cells, $TCR\alpha\beta^+CD4^-$ $CD8^-$ T cells; γδ DNT cells, $TCR\gamma\delta^+CD4^-CD8^-$ T cells; AUC, area under the curve; CI, confidence interval; CHB, chronic hepatitis B; DNT cells, double-negative T cells; HC, healthy controls; IC, inactive carriers; IT, immune tolerant carriers.

[4.8–13.6%]) were significantly higher than in either the IC (5.4% [4.0–6.3%]) or HC (4.8% [3.3–6.8%]) groups (Figure 1E). There were no significant differences in γδ DNT cell frequency between the CHB and IT groups, or between the IC and HC groups. These data indicate that a low γδ DNT cell frequency is associated with a state that is more likely to lead to spontaneous HBeAg seroconversion.

Suppression of Anti-HBV $CD8^+$ T cell Response by γδ DNT Cells

Together, the results of the clinical studies imply that a high frequency of γδ DNT cells is not good for viral control in CHB. Thus, we investigated whether γδ DNT cells suppress the HBV-specific $CD8^+$ T-cell responses that are known to inhibit HBV replication [28].

In the T-cell suppression assay, the median purity of isolated γδ DNT cells within the γδ T cell compartment (Figure 2A) was 89.7% (range 86.1–96.3%, n = 10). Addition of γδ DNT cells to the core peptide-stimulated cultures reduced the frequency of IFN-γ-secreting $CD8^+\alpha\beta$ T cells (P = 0.005) (Figure 2B and C). In addition, from four patients with CHB, co-cultures of γδ T cells with a γδ DNT/γδ T frequency of >80% and γδ T(−) PBMC at ratios of 0:16, 1:16, 1:4, 1:2, and 1:1 showed that a decreasing frequency of non-antigen specific, IFN-γ-producing cells in the $CD8^+$ lymphocytes cultures (P = 0.007), and decreasing prolifera-

tion of $CD8^+$ lymphocytes were accompanied by an increasing proportion of γδ T cells, which was dose-dependent ($P = 0.003$) (Figure S2A–F). However, there were no similar observations from three healthy donors (Figure S2G and H). It indicated that the suppressive function of γδ T cells was associated with the condition of chronic HBV infection.

Mechanisms Associated with the Suppression by γδ DNT Cells

In the transwell assays, production of both TNF-α and IFN-γ by core peptide-stimulated γδT(−)PBMC increased when they were separated from γδ DNT cells by inserting a membrane (Figure 3A), indicating that suppression by γδ DNT cells may require cell–cell contact. In the CHB group, few γδ DNT cells expressed cell-surface CTLA-4, FasL, PD-L1, or LAG-3, and PMA-stimulated γδ DNT cells produced almost no TGF-β or IL-10 (data not shown), implying that these molecules may not directly mediate the suppression by γδ DNT cells. More than half of γδ DNT cells expressed NKG2A, and the frequency of NKG2A expression was higher on γδ DNT cells than on αβ DNT cells, $CD4^+$ αβ T cells, NK cells, or $CD8^+$ γδ T cells. There was no significant difference between CHB and HC in the frequency of γδ DNT cells expressing NKG2A (Figure S3). Interestingly, HLA-E, the ligand of NKG2A, was expressed by all of these T-cell subsets, and the frequency of HLA-E expression on γδ DNT cells was higher than on both αβ DNT cells and $CD8^+$ αβ T cells. Moreover, frequency of HLA-E in $CD8^+$ αβ T cells was higher in CHB and IT groups compared with HC (Figure S4). To investigate whether this NKG2A-HLA-E pathway is involved in the suppression by γδ DNT cells, we used an antibody to block NKG2A or HLA-E expressed on γδ DNT cells. Figure 3B (data derived from Figure S5) shows that suppression of both core peptide pool-induced TNF-α-secreting and IFN-γ-secreting $CD8^+$ αβ T cells by γδ DNT cells was partly reversed in three patients after pre-incubation of γδ DNT cells with anti-NKG2A but not anti-HLA-E or IgG1 isotype. Furthermore, we investigated the influence of γδ DNT cells on the HBV-specific pentamer-positive $CD8^+$ T cells. As shown in Figure 4, the frequency of HBV-specific pentamer-positive $CD8^+$ T cells and the production of IFN-γ or TNF-α in these T cells decreased when γδ DNT cells were added. And such decreases can be partially reversed when γδ DNT cells were pre-incubated with anti-NKG2A in some patients.

Association between Intrahepatic γδ DNT Cells and HBeAg Seroconversion

Because the HBV-specific $CD8^+$ T-cell response mainly occurs in the liver, which is the site of HBV replication, we investigated whether the frequency of circulating γδ DNT cells reflects the frequency in the intrahepatic compartment. LIL and PBMC were obtained from 26 patients with CHB after 104 weeks of LdT treatment (10 responders and 16 non-responders). The characteristics of these patients at 104 weeks are compared between responders and non-responders in Table S4. There was no significant difference of Knodell necroinflammatory scores or Ishak fibrosis scores between these two groups. The γδ DNT cells were identified using a modified strategy (Figure S6). There was a significant correlation between frequencies of γδ DNT cells in LIL and PBMC ($r = 0.231$, $P = 0.020$, Figure 5A), both of which appeared similar ($P = 0.107$, Figure 5B). The frequency of γδ DNT cells was higher in LIL from non-responders relative to responders

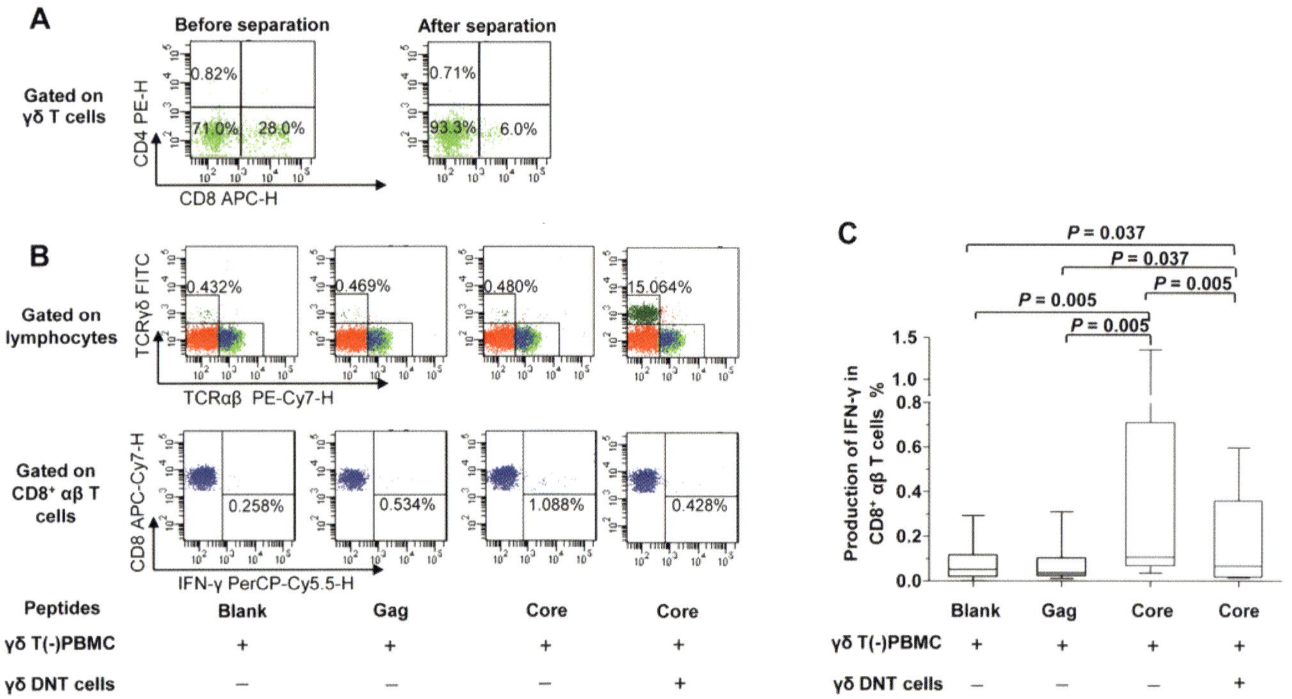

Figure 2. γδ DNT cells suppress HBV antigen-specific $CD8^+$ αβ T-cell responses. (A) One representative example shows the purity of γδ DNT cells in a γδ T-cell pool before and after separation. (B) One representative result shows that addition of γδ DNT cells reduced HBV core peptide-induced production of IFN-γ in $CD8^+$ αβ T cells. A gag peptide was used as the negative control, while medium only as the blank control. (C) The pooled results from ten patients with CHB were compared using Wilcoxon test by pairs. (blank, medium only; core, HBV core peptides pool; gag, HIV gag peptide). γδ T(−)PBMC, γδ T cell-deleted-PBMC; γδ DNT cells, CD8-deleted-γδT cells; $CD8^+$ αβ T cells, $TCR\alpha\beta^+CD8^+$ T cells; CHB, chronic hepatitis B; DNT cells, double-negative T cells; IFN, interferon; PBMC, peripheral blood mononuclear cells.

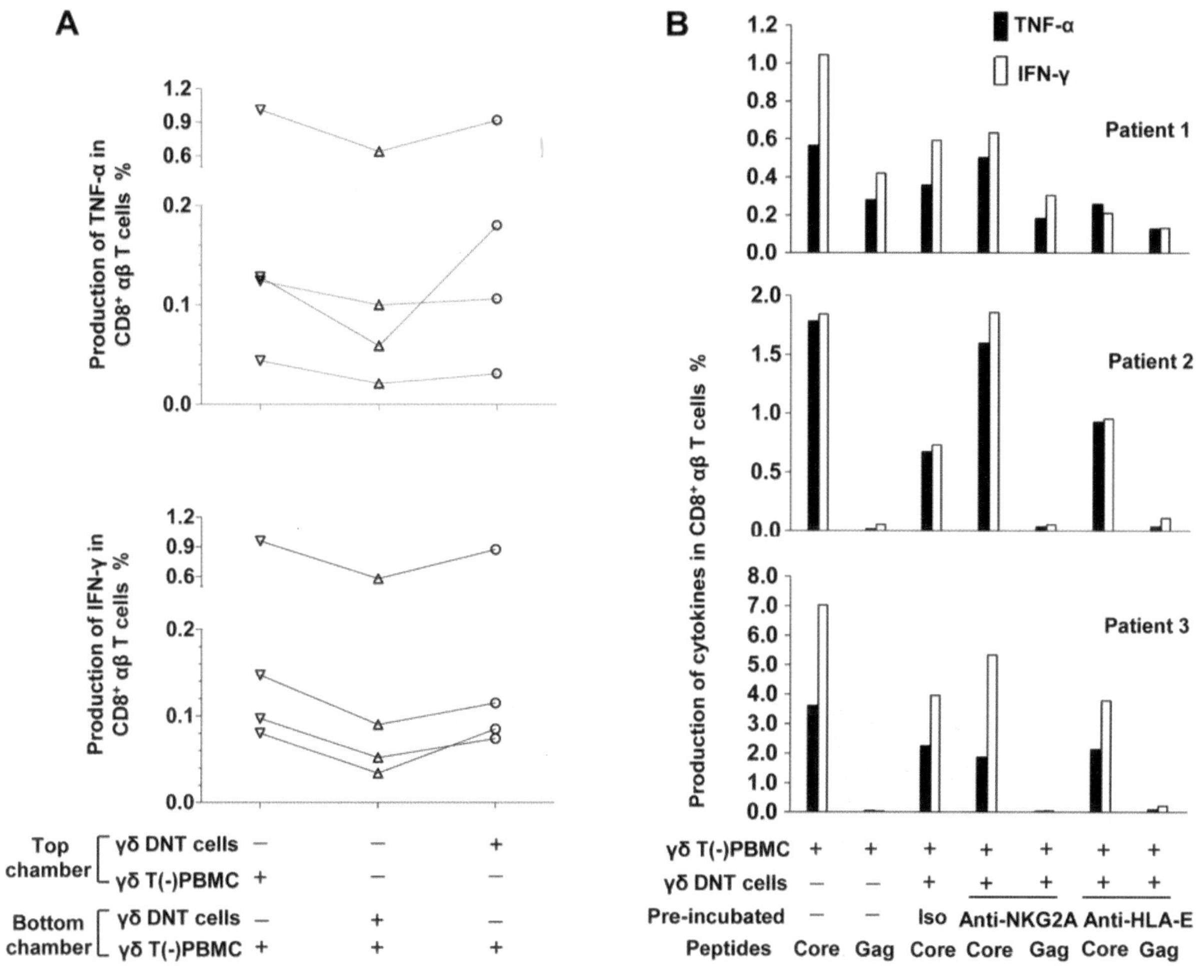

Figure 3. Mechanisms associated with the suppression by γδ DNT cells. (A) The suppression of HBV core peptide-induced production of TNF-α or IFN-γ in $CD8^+$αβ T cells could be partly abrogated by inserting a membrane between the $CD8^+$ αβ T cells and the γδ DNT cells in a transwell assay of cells from four patients with CHB. Lines link the data from the same patients. (B) γδ DNT cells were isolated and pre-incubated with either anti-NKG2A, anti-HLA-E, or mouse IgG1 isotype before being co-cultured with γδ T(−)PBMC. After 10 days of stimulation with peptides, production of TNF-α (black bars) and IFN-γ (blank bars) in $CD8^+$αβ T cells was detected. Data from three patients are shown (core, HBV core peptides pool; gag, HIV gag peptide). DNT cells, double-negative T cells; IFN, interferon; PBMC, peripheral blood mononuclear cells; TNF, tumor necrosis factor.

(8.5%, [7.1–14.0%] vs 5.2%, [4.6–8.5%]; $P = 0.035$). The higher frequency of γδ DNT cells in PBMC from non-responders relative to responders approached statistical significance (6.3%, [5.2–12.7%] vs 4.8% [2.5–8.2%]; $P = 0.051$).

Discussion

In this study, we tested the hypothesis that DNT cells are involved in failure to achieve HBeAg seroconversion associated with viral control, which is supported by several clinical observations. Firstly, the baseline frequency of γδ DNT cells in PBMC from the patients who seroconverted after antiviral therapy was half that of patients who did not seroconvert. Secondly, when antiviral therapy was discontinued, virologic relapse and recurrence of HBeAg tended to occur in those patients who had a high baseline frequency of γδ DNT cells. Thirdly, the frequency of intrahepatic γδ DNT cells was higher in patients who didn't achieve HBeAg seroconversion after 104 weeks of antiviral treatment. Finally, the frequency of γδ DNT cells was higher in the HBeAg-positive patients relative to IC, who are known to have a durable spontaneous HBeAg seroconversion. In the multivariate analysis of longitudinal data, the influence of baseline γδ DNT cell frequency on HBeAg seroconversion was not statistically independent of the influence of baseline HBV DNA level, but there was no correlation between γδ DNT cell frequency and HBV DNA level. It is difficult to determine whether these two parameters are reflections of the same underlying mechanism for HBeAg seroconversion.

Although no published evidence has shown that HBeAg seroconversion is caused by the activation of $CD8^+$ T-cell responses to HBV antigens, there is a strong association between these two events [28,29,30]. Our in vitro data showed that γδ DNT cells have the ability to suppress anti-HBV-specific $CD8^+$ T-cell responses. This raises the possibility that suppression of antiviral $CD8^+$ T-cell responses by a high level of γδ DNT cells contributes to failure to control HBV replication and achieve HBeAg seroconversion. This in vitro data also adds to the list of known mechanisms that contribute to $CD8^+$ T cell hyporesponsiveness in patients with CHB, including impaired function of dendritic cells [31], increased numbers of $CD4^+CD25^+$ regulatory T cells [32], high antigen loads [33], high levels of expression of

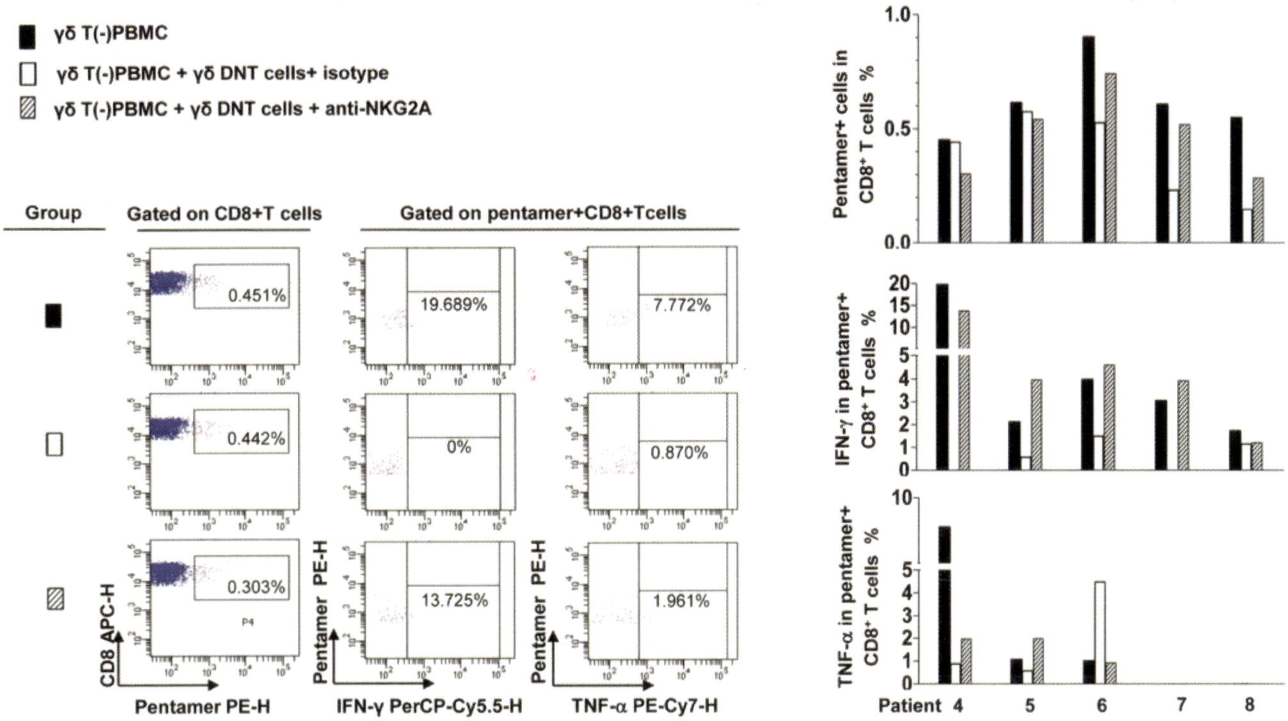

Figure 4. Influence of $\gamma\delta$ DNT cells on HBV-specific pentamer-positive CD8$^+$ T cells. $\gamma\delta$ DNT cells were isolated from HLA-A2 positive patients with CHB and pre-incubated with either anti-NKG2A (diagonal stripes bars) or mouse IgG1 isotype (blank bars) before being co-cultured with $\gamma\delta$ T(−)PBMC. The group with $\gamma\delta$ T(−)PBMC only (black bars) was also compared. Dot plots from one representative patient show the strategy for identifying the frequency of HBV pentamer-positve CD8$^+$ T cells, and the production of IFN-γ and TNF-α in pentamer-positive CD8$^+$ T cells after 10 days of stimulation with HBV core18–27. Data from five patients are shown.

PD-1 by exhausted HBV-specific CD8$^+$ T cells [26], and deletion of HBV-specific CD8$^+$ T cells by NK cells [34].

$\gamma\delta$ T cells are known to have a wide range of functions, including immune protection against pathogens in the early $\gamma\delta$ T-cell response and immunoregulation in some late $\gamma\delta$ T-cell responses [35,36]. The impaired IFN-γ production and cytotoxicity of $\gamma\delta$ T cells in persistent HBV infection have been reported previously [37]. Our study provides new insight into the immunoregulation of $\gamma\delta$ T cells in CHB. The in vitro data indicates that suppression of HBV peptide-specific CD8$^+$ T-cell responses by $\gamma\delta$ DNT cells requires cell-cell contact, and is partially mediated by the NKG2A signaling pathway. These results are in contrast to a study of human $\gamma\delta$ T cells expanded from breast tumors [15], but are consistent with a study of

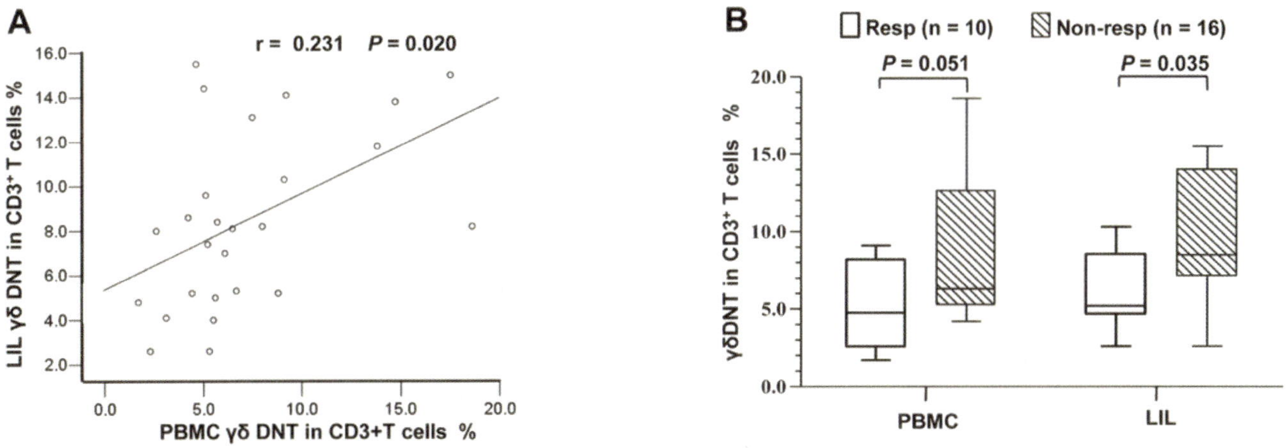

Figure 5. Frequencies of $\gamma\delta$ DNT cell subsets in LIL and PBMC. LIL and PBMC were obtained from 26 patients with CHB at the same time after 104 weeks of telbivudine treatment. (A) Spearman's correlation analysis between $\gamma\delta$ DNT cell frequencies in LIL and PBMC. (B) Comparison of the frequencies of $\gamma\delta$ DNT cells between LIL and PBMC using A Wilcoxon test, and between responders (Resp, n = 10) and non-responders (Non-resp, n = 16) using Mann-Whitney *U* test. CHB, chronic hepatitis B; DNT cells, double-negative T cells; LIL, liver-infiltrating lymphocytes; PBMC, peripheral blood mononuclear cells.

intraepithelial γδ T cells in patients with celiac disease [16]. As reviewed, NKG2A, an inhibitory receptor expressed by NK cells and $CD8^+$ T cells, plays an important role in HIV, HCV [38,39], and HBV [40] infections. NKG2A also mediates suppressive signaling in human γδ T cells [16,41]. In the current study, we found that most γδ DNT cells expressed NKG2A, and the frequency of HLA-E in $CD8^+$ αβ T cells was higher in patients with CHB. These findings suggest that two mechanisms may enhance γδ DNT cell-mediated suppression of anti-HBV $CD8^+$ T-cell responses. The first is an increase in the number rather than the activity of γδ DNT cells. The second is an increase in the expression of HLA-E on $CD8^+$ αβ T cells from HBeAg-positive subjects, which may be similar to the findings of up-regulation of HLA-E in HCV infections [42].

Pro-inflammatory cytokine or TCRγδ activation can augment γδ T-cell frequency in peripheral blood [35]. However, it seems unlikely that hepatic inflammation or viral factors are responsible for the increase in γδ DNT cell frequency seen in our study, as there were no significant changes in γδ DNT cell frequency with the decrease of ALT or serum viral components including HBV DNA, HBeAg, and hepatitis B surface antigen (HBsAg) during treatment, and there was no significant correlation between these variables at baseline. Thus, the mechanisms that regulate the circulating frequency of γδ DNT cells in CHB deserve further investigation.

We also analyzed frequencies of $CD4^+/CD8^+$ γδ T cells both in longitudinal and cross-sectional study. There was no significant difference in $CD4^+/CD8^+$ γδ T-cell frequencies between the different groups (Figure S1B and data not shown). $CD4^+$ γδ T cells make up a small proportion of γδ T cells and most of $CD4^+/CD8^+$ γδ T cells were $CD8^+$ γδ T cells. Little is known about the different properties between human $CD8^+$ γδ T cells and γδ DNT cells [16]. A recent report showed that the absolute number of $CD8^+$ γδ T cells did not change with age, whereas γδ DNT cells decreased in healthy aged people [43], Interestingly, in contrast, the cumulative lifetime incidence of HBeAg seroclearance increases with age [44]. Although we found higher frequencies of CD127, NKG2A, and HLA-DR, and lower frequencies of CD45 RA on γδ DNT cells compared with $CD8^+$ γδ T cells (unpublished data), the different functions of these two subsets in CHB require further investigation.

In conclusion, a high frequency of γδ DNT cells is associated with failure to control HBV. A low baseline frequency of γδ DNT cells in PBMC predicts HBeAg seroconversion during LdT therapy for CHB. In vitro data showing that γδ DNT cells suppress $CD8^+$ T cell responses to HBV antigens raise the possibility that the NKG2A-HLA-E signaling pathway may be a target for immunotherapy.

Supporting Information

Figure S1 Comparison of the frequencies of αβ DNT cells and $CD4^+/CD8^+$ γδ T cells in the longitudinal study.

Figure S2 Influence of different frequencies of γδ T cells on the non-specific $CD8^+$ T-cell response. CHB patients with a γδ DNT/γδ T-cell frequency of >80% were recruited into this study. γδ T cells were isolated from PBMC, and γδ T : γδ T(−)PBMC overnight co-cultures were set up at ratios of 0:16, 1:16, 1:4,1:2, and 1:1 with a total of 4.5×10^5 cells/well, and incubated in the presence of anti-CD3 and anti-CD28 antibodies to test the production of IFN-γ by ICS. (A,B) An individual experiment shows the influence of an increasing frequency of (A) γδ T cells (labeled "P1", γδ DNT/γδ T = 82.9%) on (B) the production of IFN-γ ("P2") in $CD8^+$ lymphocytes stimulated with anti-CD3 and anti-CD28. In the proliferation test, γδ T(−)PBMC labeled with 1.5 μmol/L CFSE were co-cultured with γδ T cells in the presence of anti-CD3 and anti-CD28 antibodies for 3 days, and then stained with anti-CD8-PE for analysis of the proliferation of $CD8^+$ lymphocytes by flow cytometry. (C,D) An individual experiment shows the influence of an increasing frequency of (C) γδ T cells (γδ DNT/γδ T cells = 90.3%) on (D) the proliferation of $CD8^+$ lymphocytes stimulated with anti-CD3 and anti-CD28. "P3" indicates the unlabeled γδ T cells, "P4" the γδ T(−)PBMC labeled with CFSE, and "P5" the proliferating $CD8^+$ lymphocytes. (E,F) Data from four patients with CHB were analyzed by the Friedman test. (G,H) Data from three healthy donors were also shown. CHB, chronic hepatitis B; DNT cells, double-negative T cells; ICS, intracellular cytokine staining.

Figure S3 Expression of NKG2A on γδ DNT cells. PBMC from CHB patients and HC were stained with anti-CD3-APC-Cy7, anti-TCR-γδ-FITC, anti-CD4-PE-Cy7, anti-CD8-PerCP, anti-CD56-APC and anti-NKG2A-PE. (A) Expression of NKG2A on γδ DNT, $CD8^+$γδ T, αβ DNT, $CD4^+$αβ T cells, and NK cells were measured and compared between (B) different lymphocyte subsets or (C) between the CHB and HC groups. CHB, chronic hepatitis B; DNT cells, double-negative T cells; HC, healthy controls.

Figure S4 Expression of HLA-E on γδ DNT cells. PBMC were stained with anti-CD3-APC-Cy7, anti-TCRγδ-FITC, anti-CD4-PE-Cy7, anti-CD8-PerCP, and anti-HLA-APC. Expression of HLA-E on γδ DNT, $CD8^+$ γδ T cells, αβ DNT cells, and $CD8^+$ αβ T cells was (A) measured in HC and CHB relative to the isotype control and (B) compared in the different T-cell subsets. (C,D) Expression of HLA-E on either (C) γδ DNT or (D) $CD8^+$ αβ T cells was compared in the IT, CHB, and HC groups. CHB, chronic hepatitis B; DNT cells, double-negative T cells; HC, healthy controls; IT, immune tolerant carriers.

Figure S5 γδ DNT cell-mediated suppression of cytokine production by core peptide-stimulated $CD8^+$αβ T cells is partially mediated by NKG2A. The plots were gated on $CD8^+$αβ T cells. DNT cells, double-negative T cells.

Figure S6 Strategy for gating the αβ DNT cells and γδ DNT cells from LIL. DNT cells, double-negative T cells; LIL, liver-infiltrating lymphocytes.

Table S1 The GenBank accession numbers of the sequences used to identify a panel of 26 18-mer peptides overlapping by 8 or 10 residues and covering the full HBV core open reading frame.

Table S2 The amino acid sequence of core peptides.

Table S3 Spearman's correlation analyses showing associations between the frequencies of γδ DNT cells and the clinical characteristics of the CHB patients at baseline n = 51).

Table S4 Clinical characteristics of subjects in the cohort receiving telbivudine therapy at 104 Weeks.

Methods S1 Entry criteria for study subjects.

Method S2 Isolation of peripheral blood mononuclear cells and liver-infiltrating lymphocytes.

Acknowledgments

We are grateful to all the subjects and clinicians involved in this study.

Author Contributions

Conceived and designed the experiments: QL SM JH. Performed the experiments: QL JG ZH XH XJ YL. Analyzed the data: QL MZ JS XZ WA. Contributed reagents/materials/analysis tools: QL JG ZH XH XJ YL WA. Wrote the paper: QL WA JH.

References

1. Lavanchy D (2004) Hepatitis B virus epidemiology, disease burden, treatment, and current and emerging prevention and control measures. J Viral Hepat 11: 97–107.
2. Lok AS, McMahon BJ (2009) Chronic hepatitis B: update 2009. Hepatology 50: 661–662.
3. Lau GK, Wang FS (2012) Uncover the immune biomarkers underlying hepatitis B e antigen (HBeAg) seroconversion: a need for more translational study. J Hepatol 56: 753–755.
4. Wu JF, Wu TC, Chen CH, Ni YH, Chen HL, et al. (2010) Serum levels of interleukin-10 and interleukin-12 predict early, spontaneous hepatitis B virus e antigen seroconversion. Gastroenterology 138: 165–172 e161–163.
5. Rossol S, Marinos G, Carucci P, Singer MV, Williams R, et al. (1997) Interleukin-12 induction of Th1 cytokines is important for viral clearance in chronic hepatitis B. J Clin Invest 99: 3025–3033.
6. Ma SW, Huang X, Li YY, Tang LB, Sun XF, et al. (2012) High serum IL-21 levels after 12 weeks of antiviral therapy predict HBeAg seroconversion in chronic hepatitis B. J Hepatol 56: 775–781.
7. Zhang ZX, Yang L, Young KJ, DuTemple B, Zhang L (2000) Identification of a previously unknown antigen-specific regulatory T cell and its mechanism of suppression. Nat Med 6: 782–789.
8. Fischer K, Voelkl S, Heymann J, Przybylski GK, Mondal K, et al. (2005) Isolation and characterization of human antigen-specific TCR αβ+ CD4(−)CD8- double-negative regulatory T cells. Blood 105: 2828–2835.
9. Voelkl S, Gary R, Mackensen A (2011) Characterization of the immunoregulatory function of human TCR-αβ+ CD4- CD8- double-negative T cells. Eur J Immunol 41: 739–748.
10. Lee BO, Jones JE, Peters CJ, Whitacre D, Frelin L, et al. (2011) Identification of a unique double-negative regulatory T-cell population. Immunology 134: 434–447.
11. Locke NR, Stankovic S, Funda DP, Harrison LC (2006) TCR γδ intraepithelial lymphocytes are required for self-tolerance. J Immunol 176: 6553–6559.
12. Ashour HM, Niederkorn JY (2006) γδ T cells promote anterior chamber-associated immune deviation and immune privilege through their production of IL-10. J Immunol 177: 8331–8337.
13. Seo N, Tokura Y, Takigawa M, Egawa K (1999) Depletion of IL-10- and TGF-β-producing regulatory γδT cells by administering a daunomycin-conjugated specific monoclonal antibody in early tumor lesions augments the activity of CTLs and NK cells. J Immunol 163: 242–249.
14. Kuhl AA, Pawlowski NN, Grollich K, Blessenohl M, Westermann J, et al. (2009) Human peripheral γδ T cells possess regulatory potential. Immunology 128: 580–588.
15. Peng G, Wang HY, Peng W, Kiniwa Y, Seo KH, et al. (2007) Tumor-infiltrating γδ T cells suppress T and dendritic cell function via mechanisms controlled by a unique toll-like receptor signaling pathway. Immunity 27: 334–348.
16. Bhagat G, Naiyer AJ, Shah JG, Harper J, Jabri B, et al. (2008) Small intestinal CD8+TCRγδ+NKG2A+ intraepithelial lymphocytes have attributes of regulatory cells in patients with celiac disease. J Clin Invest 118: 281–293.
17. Li X, Kang N, Zhang X, Dong X, Wei W, et al. (2011) Generation of human regulatory γδ T cells by TCRgammadelta stimulation in the presence of TGF-beta and their involvement in the pathogenesis of systemic lupus erythematosus. J Immunol 186: 6693–6700.
18. Ye J, Ma C, Hsueh EC, Eickhoff CS, Zhang Y, et al. (2013) Tumor-derived γδ regulatory T cells suppress innate and adaptive immunity through the induction of immunosenescence. J Immunol 190: 2403–2414.
19. Reijnders JG, Perquin MJ, Zhang N, Hansen BE, Janssen HL (2010) Nucleos(t)ide analogues only induce temporary hepatitis B e antigen seroconversion in most patients with chronic hepatitis B. Gastroenterology 139: 491–498.
20. Morsy MA, Norman PJ, Mitry R, Rela M, Heaton ND, et al. (2005) Isolation, purification and flow cytometric analysis of human intrahepatic lymphocytes using an improved technique. Lab Invest 85: 285–296.
21. Heydtmann M, Hardie D, Shields PL, Faint J, Buckley CD, et al. (2006) Detailed analysis of intrahepatic CD8 T cells in the normal and hepatitis C-infected liver reveals differences in specific populations of memory cells with distinct homing phenotypes. J Immunol 177: 729–738.
22. Liang M, Ma S, Hu X, Zhou B, Zhang J, et al. (2011) Cellular immune responses in patients with hepatitis B surface antigen seroclearance induced by antiviral therapy. Virol J 8: 69.
23. Chang JJ, Thompson AJ, Visvanathan K, Kent SJ, Cameron PU, et al. (2007) The phenotype of hepatitis B virus-specific T cells differ in the liver and blood in chronic hepatitis B virus infection. Hepatology 46: 1332–1340.
24. Boni C, Fisicaro P, Valdatta C, Amadei B, Di Vincenzo P, et al. (2007) Characterization of hepatitis B virus (HBV)-specific T-cell dysfunction in chronic HBV infection. J Virol 81: 4215–4225.
25. Chang JJ, Wightman F, Bartholomeusz A, Ayres A, Kent SJ, et al. (2005) Reduced hepatitis B virus (HBV)-specific CD4+ T-cell responses in human immunodeficiency virus type 1-HBV-coinfected individuals receiving HBV-active antiretroviral therapy. J Virol 79: 3038–3051.
26. Fisicaro P, Valdatta C, Massari M, Loggi E, Biasini E, et al. (2010) Antiviral intrahepatic T-cell responses can be restored by blocking programmed death-1 pathway in chronic hepatitis B. Gastroenterology 138: 682–693, 693 e681–684.
27. Ren G, Esser S, Jochum C, Schlaak JF, Gerken G, et al. (2012) Interleukin 21 augments the hepatitis B virus-specific CD8+ T-cell response in vitro in patients coinfected with HIV-1. AIDS 26: 2145–2153.
28. Phillips S, Chokshi S, Riva A, Evans A, Williams R, et al. (2010) CD8(+) T cell control of hepatitis B virus replication: direct comparison between cytolytic and noncytolytic functions. J Immunol 184: 287–295.
29. Maini MK, Boni C, Lee CK, Larrubia JR, Reignat S, et al. (2000) The role of virus-specific CD8(+) cells in liver damage and viral control during persistent hepatitis B virus infection. J Exp Med 191: 1269–1280.
30. Rehermann B, Lau D, Hoofnagle JH, Chisari FV (1996) Cytotoxic T lymphocyte responsiveness after resolution of chronic hepatitis B virus infection. J Clin Invest 97: 1655–1665.
31. van der Molen RG, Sprengers D, Binda RS, de Jong EC, Niesters HG, et al. (2004) Functional impairment of myeloid and plasmacytoid dendritic cells of patients with chronic hepatitis B. Hepatology 40: 738–746.
32. Stoop JN, van der Molen RG, Baan CC, van der Laan LJ, Kuipers EJ, et al. (2005) Regulatory T cells contribute to the impaired immune response in patients with chronic hepatitis B virus infection. Hepatology 41: 771–778.
33. Reignat S, Webster GJ, Brown D, Ogg GS, King A, et al. (2002) Escaping high viral load exhaustion: CD8 cells with altered tetramer binding in chronic hepatitis B virus infection. J Exp Med 195: 1089–1101.
34. Peppa D, Gill US, Reynolds G, Easom NJ, Pallett LJ, et al. (2013) Up-regulation of a death receptor renders antiviral T cells susceptible to NK cell-mediated deletion. J Exp Med 210: 99–114.
35. Bonneville M, O'Brien RL, Born WK (2010) γδ T cell effector functions: a blend of innate programming and acquired plasticity. Nat Rev Immunol 10: 467–478.
36. Hayday A, Tigelaar R (2003) Immunoregulation in the tissues by γδ T cells. Nat Rev Immunol 3: 233–242.
37. Chen M, Zhang D, Zhen W, Shi Q, Liu Y, et al. (2008) Characteristics of circulating T cell receptor γδ T cells from individuals chronically infected with hepatitis B virus (HBV): an association between V(δ)2 subtype and chronic HBV infection. J Infect Dis 198: 1643–1650.
38. Iwaszko M, Bogunia-Kubik K (2011) Clinical significance of the HLA-E and CD94/NKG2 interaction. Arch Immunol Ther Exp (Warsz) 59: 353–367.
39. Golden-Mason L, Bambha KM, Cheng L, Howell CD, Taylor MW, et al. (2011) Natural killer inhibitory receptor expression associated with treatment failure and interleukin-28B genotype in patients with chronic hepatitis C. Hepatology 54: 1559–1569.
40. Li F, Wei H, Gao Y, Xu L, Yin W, et al. (2013) Blocking the Natural Killer Cell Inhibitory Receptor NKG2A Increases Activity of Human Natural Killer Cells and Clears Hepatitis B Virus Infection in Mice. Gastroenterology 144: 392–401.
41. Angelini DF, Zambello R, Galandrini R, Diamantini A, Placido R, et al. (2011) NKG2A inhibits NKG2C effector functions of gammadelta T cells: implications in health and disease. J Leukoc Biol 89: 75–84.
42. Nattermann J, Nischalke HD, Hofmeister V, Ahlenstiel G, Zimmermann H, et al. (2005) The HLA-A2 restricted T cell epitope HCV core 35–44 stabilizes HLA-E expression and inhibits cytolysis mediated by natural killer cells. Am J Pathol 166: 443–453.
43. Andreu-Ballester JC, Garcia-Ballesteros C, Benet-Campos C, Amigo V, Almela-Quilis A, et al. (2012) Values for alphabeta and γδ T-lymphocytes and CD4+, CD8+, and CD56+ subsets in healthy adult subjects: assessment by age and gender. Cytometry B Clin Cytom 82: 238–244.
44. Yang HI, Hung HL, Lee MH, Liu J, Jen CL, et al. (2012) Incidence and determinants of spontaneous seroclearance of hepatitis B e antigen and DNA in patients with chronic hepatitis B. Clin Gastroenterol Hepatol 10: 527–534 e521–522.

Endoplasmic Reticulum Stress Activates the Hepatic Activator Protein 1 Complex via Mitogen Activated Protein Kinase-Dependent Signaling Pathways

Shantel Olivares, Richard M. Green, Anne S. Henkel*

Division of Gastroenterology and Hepatology, Northwestern University Feinberg School of Medicine, Chicago, Illinois, United States of America

Abstract

Background and Aims: Endoplasmic reticulum (ER) stress is induced in many forms of chronic liver disease and may promote the development of hepatocellular carcinoma. The activator protein 1 (AP-1) complex is a transcription factor that promotes hepatic carcinogenesis in response to cellular stress. The aim of this study was to determine the role of ER stress in the regulation of the hepatic AP-1 complex.

Methods: Human hepatocellular carcinoma (HepG2) cells and C57BL/6J mice were subjected to pharmacologic ER stress and the expression of AP-1-associated genes and proteins was assessed. To determine the role of MAPK signaling in ER stress-induced AP-1 activation, ER stress was induced in JNK- and ERK-inhibited HepG2 cells.

Results: Induction of ER stress promoted the activation of both Jun- and Fos-related genes and proteins of the AP-1 complex in HepG2 cells and murine liver. Inhibition of ERK phosphorylation in HepG2 cells completely prevented ER stress-induced activation of the fos-related components of AP-1 whereas activation of Jun-related components was only partially attenuated. Conversely, inhibition of JNK phosphorylation in HepG2 cells reduced ER stress-induced activation of Jun-related components but did not prevent activation of fos-related components.

Conclusions: ER stress activates the hepatic AP-1 complex via MAPK-dependent signaling pathways. ER stress-induced activation of Fos-related components is dependent primarily on ERK activation whereas ER stress-induced activation of Jun-related components is dependent primarily on JNK activation, although there is interplay between these regulatory pathways. These data implicate a novel signaling pathway by which sustained ER stress, as observed in many chronic liver diseases, may promote hepatic carcinogenesis.

Editor: Rajesh Mohanraj, UAE University, Faculty of Medicine & Health Sciences, United Arab Emirates

Funding: This work was supported by NIH/NIDDK grants R01DK080810 and K08DK095992 and an AGA Research Scholar Award. The funders had no role in study design, data collection and analysis, decision to publish, or preparation of the manuscript.

Competing Interests: The authors have declared that no competing interests exist.

* Email: a-henkel2@northwestern.edu

Introduction

The incidence of hepatocellular carcinoma (HCC) has more than doubled over the past 20 years attributable in large part to the high rate of new hepatitis C virus infection 30 to 40 years ago [1,2]. Cirrhosis is the primary risk factor for HCC, however, the underlying cause of cirrhosis impacts the risk of progressing to HCC. It is becoming increasingly evident that patients with cirrhosis secondary to nonalcoholic fatty liver disease (NAFLD) are at particularly high risk for developing HCC. In fact, recent observations suggest that NAFLD is a risk factor for HCC even in the absence of cirrhosis [3,4]. Although significant progress is being made toward curing chronic hepatitis C, the prevalence of NAFLD is rapidly escalating in the United States. As such, the burden of HCC is unlikely to decline in the foreseeable future [5,6].

Endoplasmic reticulum (ER) stress and the ensuing unfolded protein response are strongly implicated in the pathogenesis of many forms of chronic liver disease, including hepatitis C infection, alcoholic liver disease, and NAFLD [7–14]. The ER functions to maintain protein homeostasis by regulating protein synthesis, folding and processing. Under conditions of ER stress, such as glucose deprivation, aberrant calcium signaling, viral infection, lipotoxicity, and disruption of redox regulation, normal ER function becomes compromised leading to the accumulation of unfolded or misfolded proteins [15]. The accumulation of unfolded proteins triggers an evolutionarily conserved intracellular signal transduction pathway known as the unfolded protein response (UPR) [16]. The UPR initially aims to restore homeostasis and allow the cell to adapt to the stressor [17]. If homeostasis is not adequately restored, however, pathways leading to apoptosis are initiated [18,19]. Mitogen activated protein kinases (MAPKs) are activated in response to ER stress and may mediate, in part, the critical switch from restoration of homeostasis to initiation of apoptosis. In particular, cJun N-terminal kinase (JNK), a well-established downstream target of the IRE1α branch of the UPR, is thought to promote ER stress-induced apoptosis [20,21]. The role of extracellular signal-regulated protein kinase

(ERK) activation in mediating the ER stress response is less well-characterized but may function to enhance cell survival [22,23]. The mechanism by which ER stress induces ERK is incompletely understood but is thought to be at least partially mediated by PI3K and adaptor protein Nck [22,23].

Recent data suggest that ER stress and the UPR may be important in the development of hepatocellular carcinoma [24–31]. Grp78/BiP, a molecular chaperone and master regulator of the UPR, has been posited to promote malignant transformation in numerous tissues including the liver [32–34]. ER stress has also been implicated in the pathogenesis of liver cancer resulting from chronic alcohol use [35]. Sorafenib, the only approved chemotherapeutic agent to treat HCC, has been shown to modulate the UPR [26,27]. Yet, it remains unknown whether induction of ER stress contributes to the development of HCC in chronic liver diseases.

Activation of the activator protein 1 (AP-1) complex has been shown to be a critical event in the development of HCC [36]. The AP-1 complex is a dimer composed of protooncogenes from the Jun family (*cJun*, *JunD*, and *JunB*) and the Fos family (*cFos*, *FosB*, *Fra-1*, and *Fra-2*) [37,38]. In response to various types of cellular stress, the AP-1 complex is activated to function as a transcription factor targeting genes involved in cellular differentiation, proliferation, and apoptosis [37,38]. MAPKs are key regulators of numerous protooncogenes, including elements of the AP-1 complex [39,40].

In the present study we aim to determine the impact of ER stress on the regulation of the hepatic AP-1 complex. Specifically we will test our hypothesis that ER stress activates the hepatic AP-1 complex via activation of MAPK-dependent signaling pathways.

Materials and Methods

Cell culture

Human hepatocellular carcinoma (HepG2) cells (ATCC, Mannasas, VA) were cultured in DMEM with 10% fetal bovine serum and maintained at 37°C in 5% CO_2. Cells were grown to 80% confluence in 6-well plates and treated with 12 μM tunicamycin, 100 nM thapsigargin (Sigma-Aldrich, St. Louis, MO), 5 mM DL-homocysteine (Sigma-Aldrich) or vehicle (DMSO/saline) in serum-free DMEM for 6 hours. RNA isolation was performed using TRIzol Reagent (Invitrogen, Carlsbad, CA) per protocol. To determine whether the effects of tunicamycin are dependent on ERK1/2 signaling, HepG2 cells were treated with the MEK inhibitor, PD184352 (Santa Cruz Biotechnology) at a concentration of 1 μM or vehicle (DMSO/saline). To determine whether the effects of tunicamycin are dependent on cJun-N-terminal kinase (JNK) signaling, HepG2 cells were treated with the JNK inhibitor, SP600125 (Sigma-Aldrich) at a concentration of 25 μM. After one hour of exposure to PD184352 or SP600125, cells were treated with tunicamycin (10 μg/mL) (Sigma-Aldrich) in serum-free DMEM and incubated for an additional 6 hours. Cytotoxicity was assessed by measuring LDH release in cell culture media using a Cytotox 96 Nonradioactive Cytotoxicity Assay (Promega, Madison, WI). Cellular proliferation was assessed using a BrdU Cell Proliferation ELISA kit (Abcam, Cambridge, MA). In a separate experiment, cells were treated with siRNA targeting *JNK1* or control siRNA (Santa Cruz Biotechnology). HepG2 cells grown to 80% confluence were treated with *JNK1* siRNA or control siRNA per protocol. Briefly, for each transfection, 6 μL of control or *JNK1* siRNA were diluted in 100 μL of siRNA Transfection Medium (Solution A) and 6 μL of siRNA Transfection Reagent was diluted in 100 μL of siRNA Transfection Medium (Solution B). Fifty microliters of Solutions A was added to 100 μL of Solution B and allowed to incubate at room temperature for 30 minutes. After washing the cells once with Transfection Medium, 0.8 mL of the siRNA in Transfection Reagent was added to each well. Cells were incubated for 6 hours at 37°C. The transfection medium was then removed, the cells were washed and incubated in normal growth medium (DMEM with 10% FBS) for 18 hours. The cells were then treated with tunicamycin (10 μg/mL) (Sigma-Aldrich) in serum-free DMEM for 6 hours. The doses of the inhibitors/siRNA were experimentally determined to achieve near complete inhibition of ERK- and JNK-phosphorylation with PD184352 and SP600125, respectively, and an approximately 50% inhibition of JNK1 using JNK1 siRNA as confirmed by western blot (Figure S1).

Animals and Treatments

Male C57BL/6J mice (8 weeks of age) were purchased from Jackson Laboratories (Bar Harbor, ME). Mice underwent 14/10-hour light/dark cycling and were given free access to standard laboratory chow and water. Mice were treated with a single intraperitoneal injection of tunicamycin (2 mg/kg) or vehicle (20% DMSO/PBS) and sacrificed 6 or 72 hours post-injection. To examine the effects of prolonged, sublethal exposure to ER stress, an additional cohort of mice was treated with a daily injection of low-dose tunicamycin (0.1 mg/kg I.P.) for 5 days to achieve a cumulative dose of 0.5 mg/kg. At the end of the treatment protocols, mice were sacrificed by CO2 inhalation followed by cardiac puncture. The collected blood was immediately centrifuged to collect the plasma. The livers were rapidly excised, flushed with ice-cold saline and sectioned. An aliquot of liver was fixed in formalin and the remaining liver was snap-frozen in liquid nitrogen. H&E staining, TUNEL staining, and immunohistochemical staining for Ki67 were performed on liver tissue by the Northwestern University Pathology Core. Plasma ALT was measured using a colorimetric assay per manufacturer's protocol (Teco Diagnostics, Anaheim, CA). All animal protocols were approved by the Northwestern University Animal Care and Use Committee (ACUC).

Analysis of Gene Expression and Protein expression

Total RNA from frozen liver samples or HepG2 cells was isolated using TRIzol reagent and real-time quantitative PCR was performed as previously described [11,41]. Primer sequences for qPCR are shown in Table S1. Total protein was isolated from frozen liver samples and HepG2 cells and Western blotting was performed as previously described [11,41]. Protein detection was performed using polyclonal rabbit antibodies to total and phosphorylated cFos, cJun, ERK, and JNK (Cell Signaling Technology, Danvers, MA). Bound antibody was detected using goat anti-rabbit polyclonal HRP antibody (Cell Signaling Technology) and developed using ECL Western Blotting Substrate (Cell Signaling Technology). Representative Western blots of pooled samples are shown.

Statistical Analysis

Data are presented as mean ± standard deviation (SD). Comparisons between groups were performed using Student's *t*-test analysis.

Results

Endoplasmic reticulum stress activates AP-1-associated genes in human hepatocellular carcinoma cells

To determine the effect of ER stress on activation of the AP-1 complex, human hepatocellular carcinoma cells (HepG2) were treated with three well-established ER stress inducing agents, tunicamycin, thapsigargin, and homocysteine. As expected, all treatments resulted in robust activation of the unfolded protein response as evidenced by elevations in *GRP78/BIP* and *CHOP* (Figure 1 A,B). We then examined the effect of ER stress on the expression of the fos-related genes (*CFOS* and fos-related antigen 1 (*FRA1*)), and jun-related genes (*CJUN* and *JUND*) of the AP-1 complex. As shown in Figure 1, induction of ER stress by any of the three pharmacologic methods stimulated transcription of both Jun- and Fos-related genes of the AP-1 complex.

Endoplasmic reticulum stress activates AP-1 in murine liver

We next sought to determine whether ER stress activates the AP-1 complex *in vivo*. Mice were treated with a standard dose of tunicamycin (2 mg/kg I.P.) and sacrificed 6 or 72 hours later. Tunicamycin treatment resulted in significant induction of the unfolded protein response in murine liver at both time points (Figure 2 A,B). There was significant induction of hepatic *cFos*, *Fra-1*, *cJun*, and *JunD* mRNA 6 hours after exposure to tunicamycin (Figure 2A). The AP-1-associated genes were induced to an even greater degree 72 hours after tunicamycin administration (Figure 2B).

A standard experimental dose of tunicamycin (2 mg/kg) induces overwhelming ER stress from which mice are unable to restore homeostasis and do not typically survive beyond 4 days. Chronic liver diseases, however, induce low-grade ER stress over prolonged periods. Therefore, to examine the effects of prolonged, sublethal exposure to ER stress, mice were treated with daily low-dose injections of tunicamycin over 5 days to achieve a cumulative dose of 0.5 mg/kg. Robust UPR activation was achieved with this dosing strategy (Figure 2C). Mice subjected to prolonged, low-dose tunicamycin showed induction of both fos- and jun-related genes of the AP-1 complex (Figure 2C).

The AP-1 complex is also subject to regulation at the translational and post-translational levels. As shown in Figure 2, hepatic CJUN was consistently increased at the translational and post-translational level in response to 6 hours, 72 hours, or 5 days of ER stress. Total and phosphorylated CFOS were only faintly detectable at 6 hours but did demonstrate modestly enhanced expression with exposure to tunicamycin (Figure 2D). At the 72-hour and 5-day time points we observed greatly increased levels of both total and phosphorylated CFOS in response to ER stress (Figure 2 E,F).

ER stress and AP-1 activation have been shown to promote both apoptosis and cellular proliferation. We found that mice exposed to low-dose tunicamycin for 5 days developed hepatocyte ballooning and increased apoptosis in the liver but no significant increase in cellular proliferation (Figure 3A). Plasma ALT, a common marker of hepatic injury, was modestly increased in mice treated with tunicamycin (Figure 3B).

Induction of Fos-related components of AP-1 by ER stress is dependent on ERK activation

We next sought to determine the mechanism by which ER stress activates the AP-1 complex in human hepatocellular carcinoma cells. ER stress has been shown to activate MAPK signaling pathways [20,21,23]. Furthermore, ERK activation is known to promote the transcription of fos-related genes [42,43]. We therefore explored whether ER stress activates AP-1-associated genes via an ERK-dependent signaling pathway. HepG2 cells were pretreated with the potent MEK inhibitor, PD184352, which prevents ERK1/2 phosphorylation (activation), followed by treatment with tunicamycin to induce ER stress. As shown in Figure 4, treatment with tunicamycin induced ERK phosphorylation, which was completely abolished by pre-treatment with PD184352. Inhibition of ERK phosphorylation did not prevent tunicamycin-induced upregulation of ER stress markers, *GRP78/BIP* and *CHOP*, however, there was a trend toward a reduction in the degree of upregulation of these markers (Figure 4 B,C). PD184352 completely abolished the activation of *CFOS* and *FRA-1* by tunicamycin at the transcriptional level (Figure 4 D,E). Tunicamycin-induced transcription of *CJUN* and *JUND* was attenuated by ERK inhibition (Figure 4 F,G).

We found that ERK signaling also regulates AP-1 at the translational and post-translational levels (Figure 4A). Tunicamycin increased total and phosphorylated CFOS protein levels, which was completely abolished by ERK-inhibition, thus correlating with CFOS gene expression. Conversely, inhibition of ERK phosphorylation accentuated tunicamycin-induced CJUN phosphorylation. We also found that inhibition of ERK-phosphorylation increased levels of phosphorylated JNK, a key activator of CJUN.

As expected, treatment of HepG2 cells with tunicamycin increased cytotoxicity as measured by LDH release (Figure 5A). We found that ERK-inhibition did not attenuate tunicamycin-induced cell death. Induction of ER stress inhibited cellular proliferation which was also unaffected by ERK-inhibition (Figure 5B).

Induction of Jun-related components of AP-1 by ER stress is dependent on JNK activation

JNK, a MAP kinase that mediates multiple stress signaling pathways in the liver, is a well-established downstream target of the ER stress response [20,21]. Furthermore, JNK is a critical mediator of hepatic injury in fatty liver diseases and has been implicated in the development of HCC [44–46]. Given our observation that ER stress-induced activation of Jun-related genes is not completely abolished by inhibition of ERK phosphorylation, we next explored whether ER stress activates Jun-related genes via JNK activation. HepG2 cells were treated with the JNK inhibitor, SP600125, followed by treatment with tunicamycin. As expected, treatment of HepG2 cells with tunicamycin markedly induced JNK phosphorylation, which was attenuated by pretreatment with SP600125 (Figure 6A). Inhibition of JNK phosphorylation did not significantly impact tunicamycin-induced *GRP78/BIP* or *CHOP* activation however there was a trend toward reduced *GRP78/BIP* transcription in JNK-inhibited cells (Figure 6 B,C). Inhibition of JNK phosphorylation reduced tunicamycin-induced *CJUN* transcription and completely abolished upregulation of *JUND* transcription (Figure 6 D,E). *CFOS* and *FRA-1* expression was induced by tunicamycin in JNK–inhibited cells (Figure 6 C,D); however, the degree of *CFOS* induction was attenuated by JNK-inhibition, indicating that ER stress-induced *CFOS* elevation is at least partially mediated by JNK signaling.

As shown in Figure 6A, inhibition of JNK phosphorylation attenuated the induction of total and phosphorylated CJUN protein by tunicamycin. Conversely, ER stress-induced CFOS activation was not attenuated by JNK-inhibition. ER stress-induced ERK phosphorylation was enhanced in JNK-inhibited cells.

Similar to inhibition of ERK phosphorylation, inhibition of JNK phosphorylation did not attenuate tunicamycin-induced cytotoxicity (Figure 5C). Inhibition of JNK activation did, however, enhance the effects of tunicamycin on inhibition of cellular proliferation (Figure 5D).

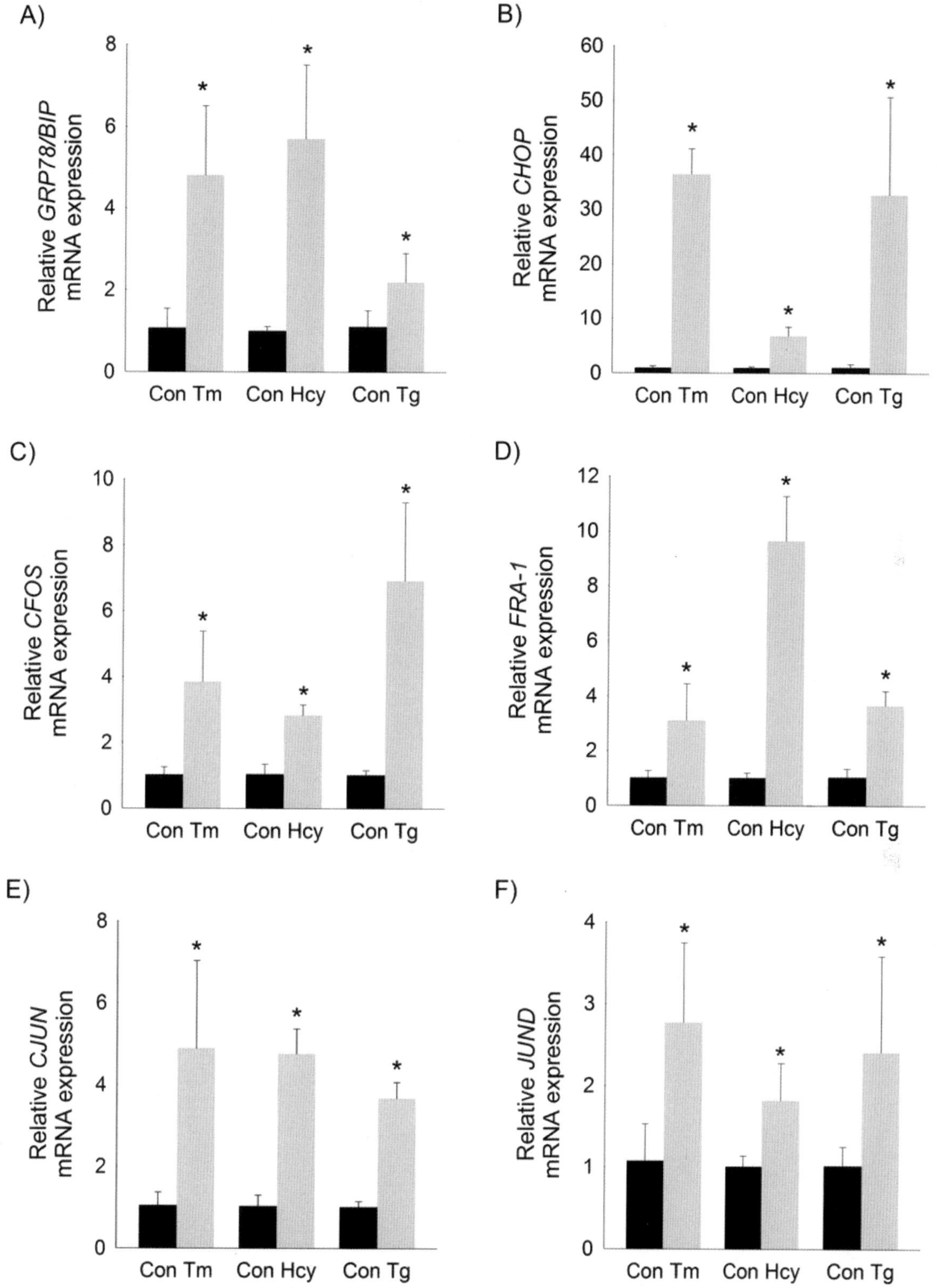

Figure 1. Induction of ER stress transcriptionally activates genes of the AP-1 complex in HepG2 cells. Relative mRNA expression of A) *GRP78/BIP*, B) *CHOP*, C) *CFOS*, D) *FRA-1*, E) *CJUN*, and F) *JUND* in HepG2 cells treated with tunicamycin (Tm), homocysteine (Hcy) or thapsigargin (Tg) for 6 hours. Mean (n = 6) ± SD. * $p<0.05$ vs vehicle-treated control cells.

Given that sustained activation of the JNK1 isoform, in particular, has been associated with steatohepatitis and the development of HCC [44–46] we confirmed the findings observed in JNK-inhibited cells using JNK1-silenced cells. Silencing of JNK1 did not effect tunicamycin-induced *GRP78/BiP* transcription but accentuated *CHOP* expression (Figure 7 A,B). Silencing

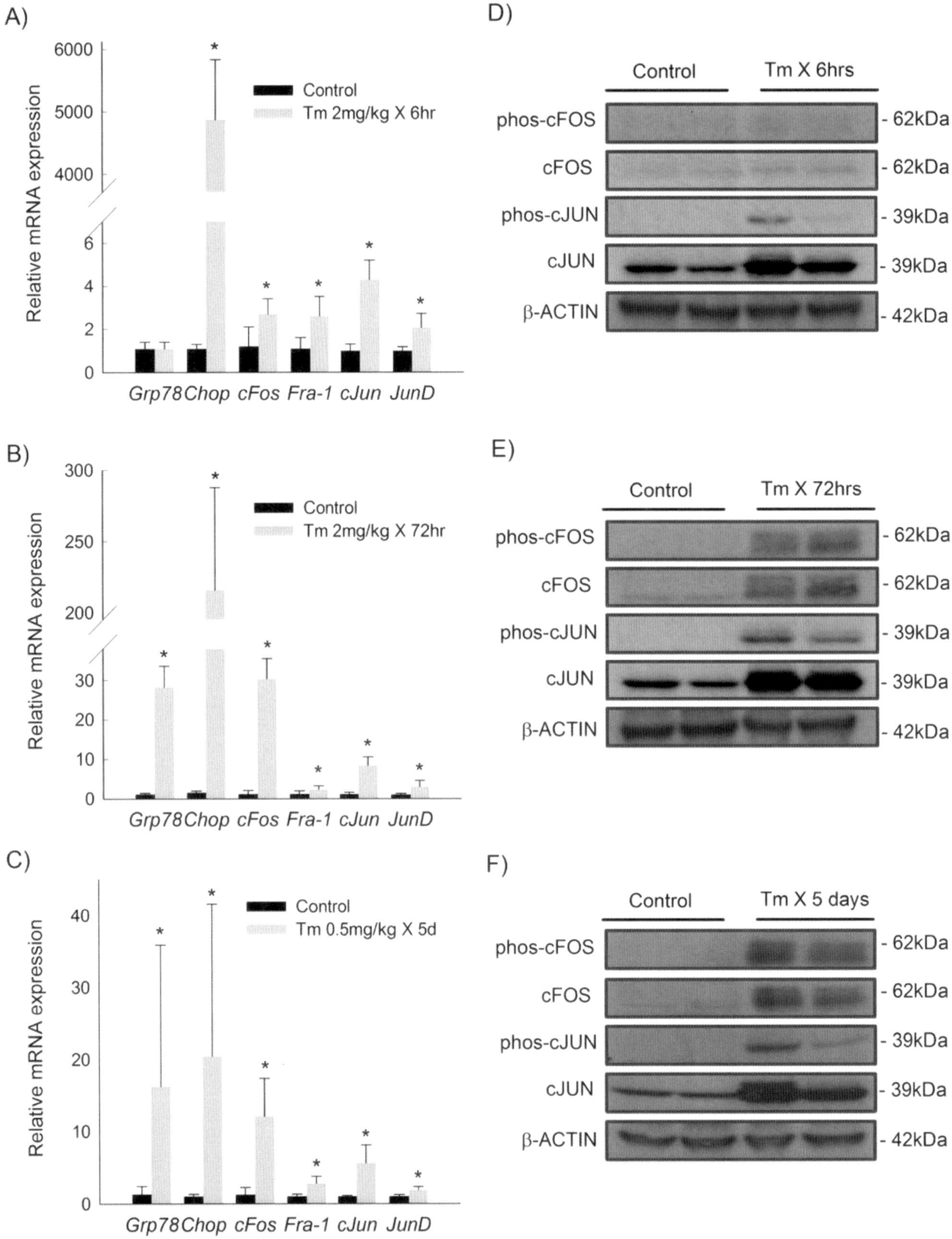

Figure 2. Induction of ER stress in mice activates the hepatic AP-1 complex. Relative hepatic mRNA expression of *Grp78/Bip*, *Chop*, *cFos*, *Fra-1*, *cJun*, and *JunD* in mice treated with tunicamycin (Tm) at doses of A) 2 mg/kg for 6 hours, B) 2 mg/kg for 72 hours, or C) 0.5 mg/kg over 5 days. Hepatic protein expression of total and phosphorylated CFOS and CJUN in mice treated with Tm at doses of D) 2 mg/kg for 6 hours, E) 2 mg/kg for 72 hours, or F) 0.5 mg/kg over 5 days. Quantitative PCR shown as mean (n = 6) ± SD. * $p<0.05$ vs vehicle-treated. Representative Western blot of pooled samples, n = 2–3.

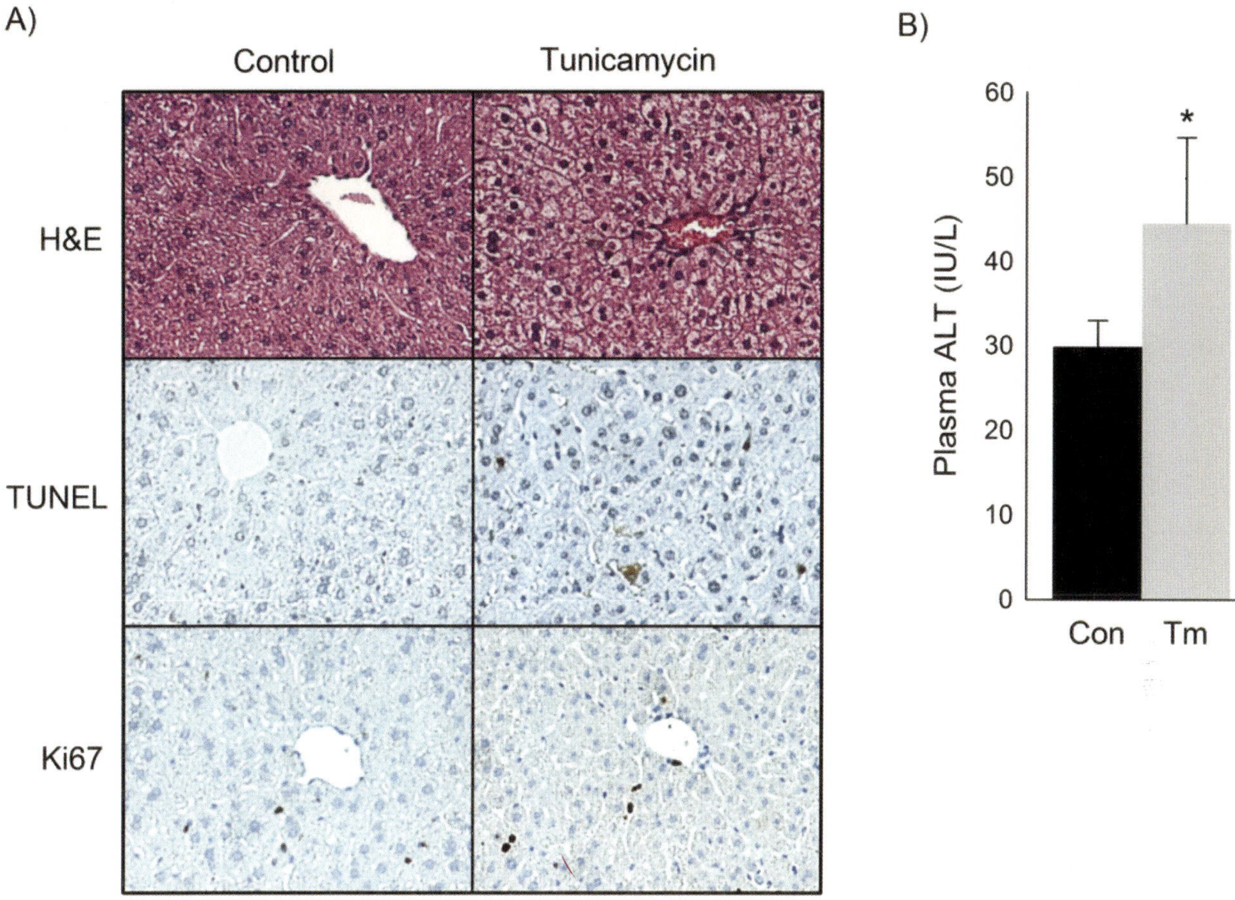

Figure 3. Prolonged low-grade ER stress promotes hepatocyte injury and apoptosis. Markers of liver injury, apoptosis, and cellular proliferation in mice treated with a cumulative dose of 0.5 mg/kg tunicamycin over 5 days. A) Representative H&E, TUNEL, and Ki67 staining of liver sections. B) Plasma ALT level (IU/L). Mean (n = 6) ± SD, *$p<0.05$.

JNK1 prevented tunicamycin-induced transcription of *CJUN* and *JUND* but not *CFOS* or *FRA-1* (Figure 7 C–F).

Discussion

Endoplasmic reticulum stress and the ensuing UPR are now recognized as mediators of numerous pathologic processes in the liver. The UPR is activated in several chronic liver diseases that ultimately promote the development of HCC including NAFLD, alcohol-induced liver disease and hepatitis C [7–13]. However, it is unknown whether activation of the UPR in these chronic liver diseases contributes to the increased risk of HCC.

The AP-1 complex is a critical regulator of hepatic carcinogenesis [36]. Here we demonstrate that induction of ER stress in human hepatocellular carcinoma cells and murine liver activates the AP-1 complex at the transcriptional, translational, and post-translational levels. We show that ER stress regulates fos-related components of the AP-1 complex primarily via activation of ERK signaling whereas the activation of jun-related components is primarily mediated by JNK. There is, however, an element of cross-talk between these pathways as evidenced by attenuated induction of *fos*-related genes in JNK-inhibited cells and attenuated induction of *jun*-related genes in ERK-inhibited cells in response to ER stress. Given the established role of AP-1 in promoting hepatic carcinogenesis, we speculate that ER stress induced AP-1 activation may be a mechanism by which chronic liver diseases promote malignant transformation.

The effect of JNK1-silencing on the expression of AP-1-associated genes paralleled that of HepG2 cells treated with SP600125 indicating that specifically the JNK1 isoform is critical for AP-1 activation. Of note, the degree of tunicamycin-induced UPR activation and resultant AP-1 gene transcription was modestly attenuated in HepG2 cells pre-treated with control (scrambled) siRNA relative to non-transfected control cells (e.g. Figures 1, 4, and 6). Although we cannot exclude the possibility that the blunted UPR was an effect of scrambled siRNA, these differences could also be due to differing cell culture conditions required for transfection (e.g. duration of serum starvation prior to tunicamycin exposure).

Mice exhibit robust activation of the unfolded protein response within 6 hours of exposure to a standard experimental dose of tunicamycin (2 mg/kg). However, beyond 72 hours this dose of tunicamycin is typically fatal. This raised the possibility that ER stress-induced AP-1 activation may occur only in the setting of overwhelming cellular stress. As such, the physiologic relevance of our observations with respect to chronic liver disease was initially uncertain. Therefore, we also subjected mice to sustained, sublethal ER stress and demonstrate robust activation of hepatic AP-1-associated genes and proteins.

AP-1 has numerous critical functions in the liver with respect to cellular differentiation, proliferation, and apoptosis. The function

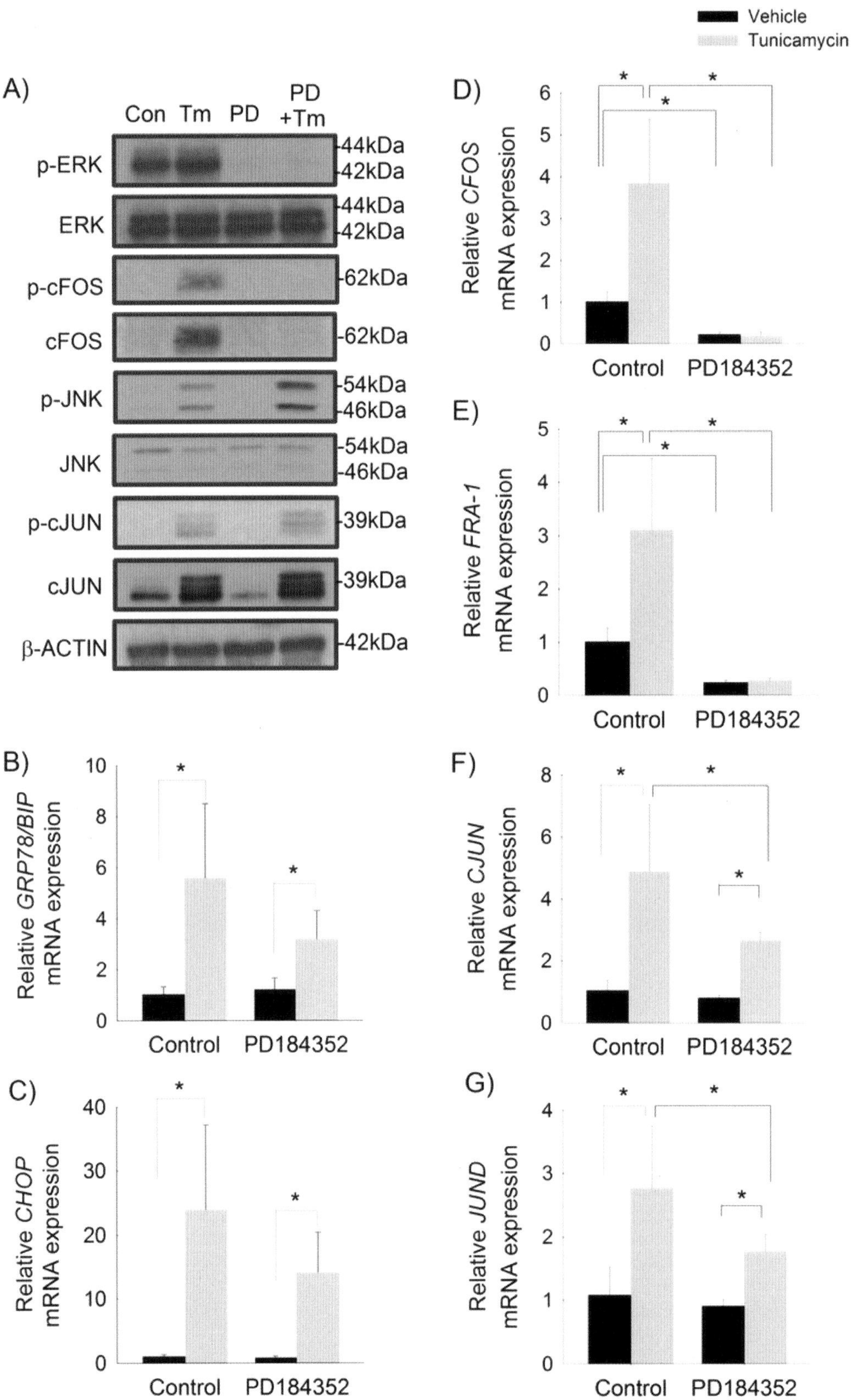

Figure 4. ER stress-induced activation of *CFOS* and *FRA-1* is mediated by ERK1/2 signaling. HepG2 cells pretreated with MEK1 inhibitor (PD) or vehicle followed by treatment with tunicamycin (Tm) or vehicle (control) for 6 hours. A) Representative Western blot of total and phosphorylated ERK, JNK, CFOS, and CJUN. Relative mRNA expression of B) *GRP78/BIP*, C) *CHOP*, D) *CFOS*, E) *FRA-1*, F) *CJUN*, and G) *JUND*. Mean (n = 6) ± SD. * $p<0.05$.

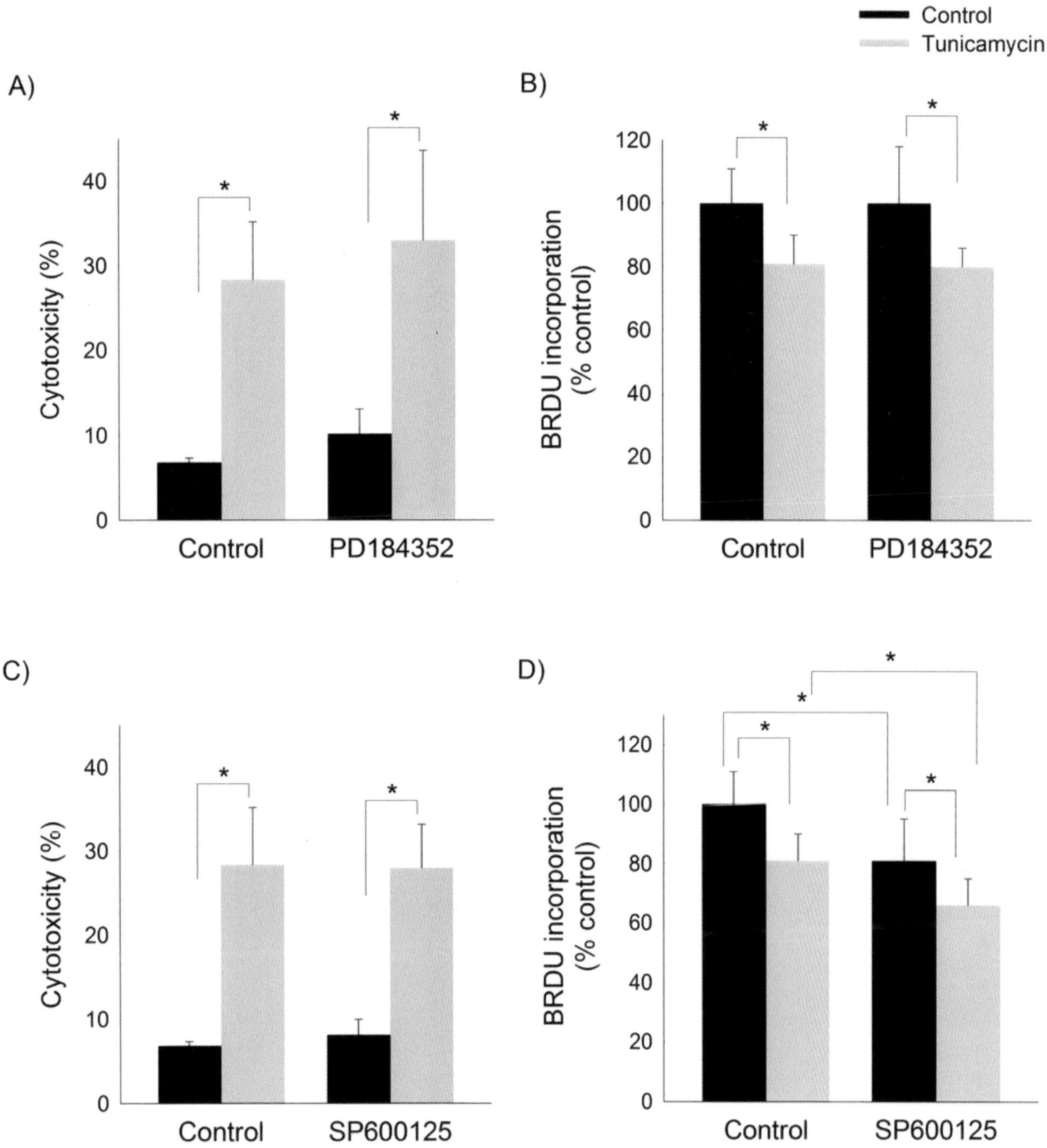

Figure 5. Effects of ERK- and JNK-inhibition on tunicamycin-induced cytotoxicity and cellular proliferation. Cytoxicity as measured by LDH release (A,C) and cellular proliferation as measured by BrdU incorporation (B,D) in HepG2 cells pretreated with MEK1 inhibitor (PD184352) or JNK inhibitor (SP600125) followed by treatment with tunicamycin or vehicle (control) for 6 hours. Mean (n = 6) ± SD. *p<0.05.

of AP-1 is determined in part by the relative activation of the various components of this heterodimeric complex. The UPR is a highly dynamic signal transduction pathway in which the various branches are preferentially activated depending on the degree and duration of ER stress. We show that the degree of induction of AP-1-associated genes in murine liver varies depending on the duration and severity of ER stress. As such, the degree and duration of ER stress may impact the transcriptional activity of the AP-1 complex by shifting the relative induction of ERK and JNK and the resultant induction of jun- and fos-related genes. Although we hypothesize that ER stress and the resultant AP-1 activation may promote hepatic carcinogenesis, it is also conceivable that under conditions of chronic low-grade ER stress, activation of the UPR may confer protection against carcinogenesis (e.g. via promoting apoptosis.) The duration of this experiment was insufficient to observe tumor formation in mice, however, future studies are warranted to determine whether inhibition of ER stress may protect against the development of HCC in mice.

At the chosen dose and time points we demonstrate that tunicamycin promotes hepatocyte injury, apoptosis, and cell death

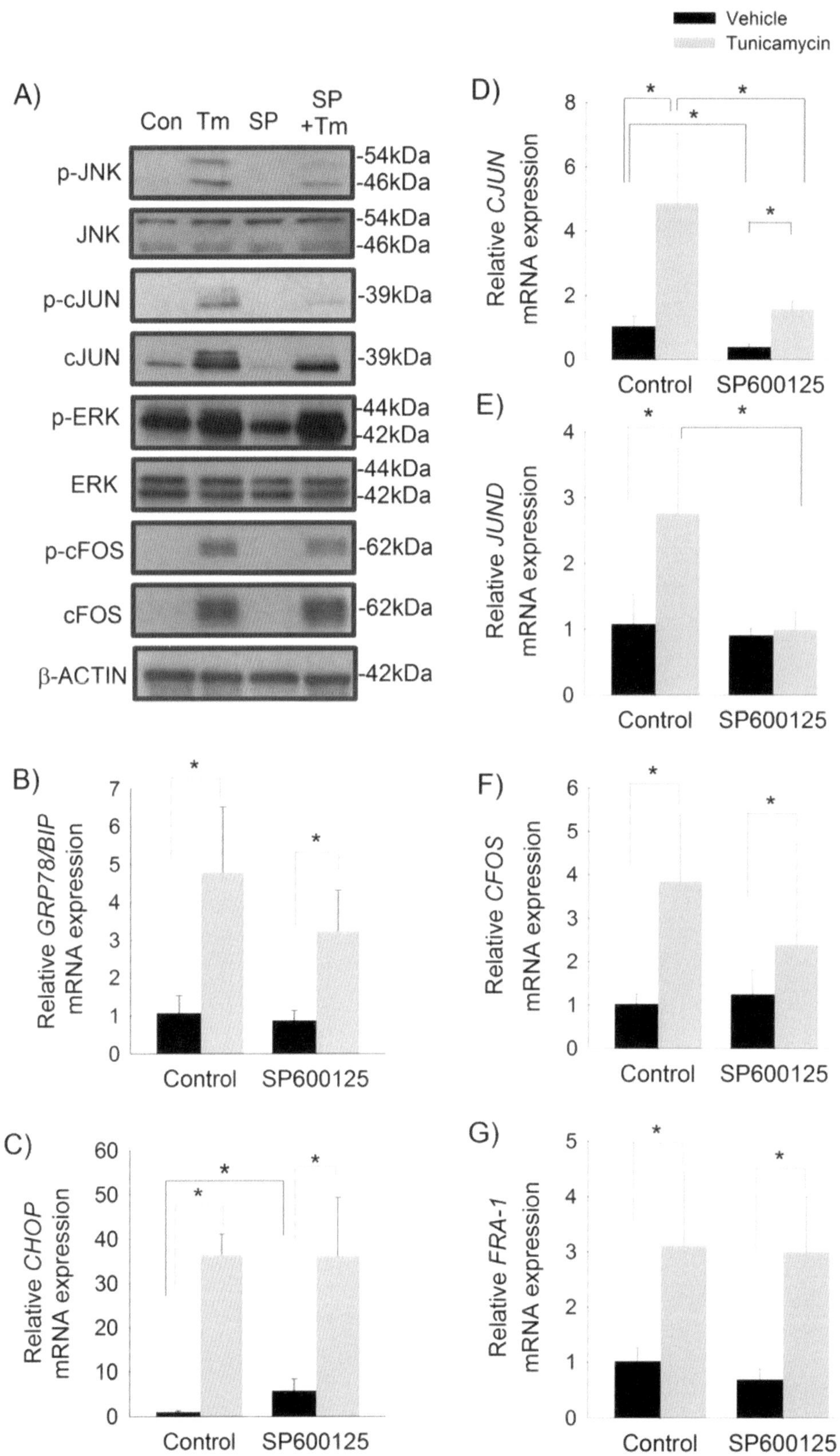

Figure 6. ER stress-induced activation of *CJUN* and *JUND* is mediated by JNK signaling. HepG2 cells pretreated with JNK inhibitor (SP600125) or vehicle followed by treatment with tunicamycin or vehicle (control) for 6 hours. A) Representative Western blot of total and phosphorylated JNK, ERK, CJUN, and CFOS. Relative mRNA expression of B) *GRP78/BIP*, C) *CHOP*, D) *CJUN*, E) *JUND*, F) *CFOS*, and G) *FRA-1*. Mean (n = 6) ± SD. * $p<0.05$.

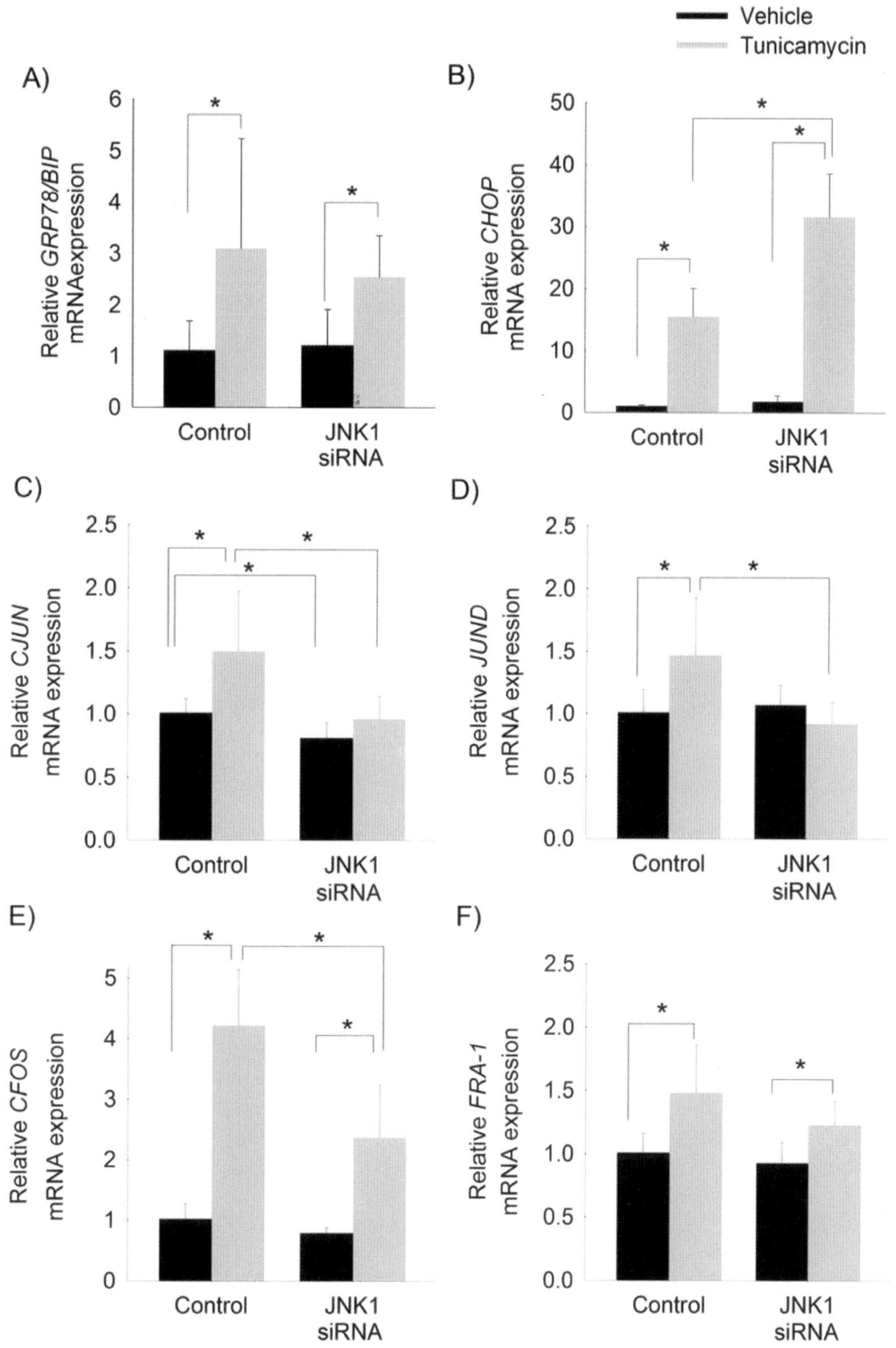

Figure 7. ER stress-induced transcriptional activation of *CJUN* and *JUND* is mediated by JNK1 signaling. Relative mRNA expression of A) *GRP78/BIP*, B) *CHOP*, C) *CJUN*, D) *JUND*, E) *CFOS*, and F) *FRA-1* in HepG2 cells pretreated with *JNK1* siRNA or control siRNA followed by treatment with tunicamycin or vehicle (control) for 6 hours. Mean (n = 6) ± SD. * $p<0.05$.

and inhibits cellular proliferation. Importantly we found that inhibition of MAPK signaling pathways did not prevent tunicamycin-induced activation of ER stress markers and did not attenuate ER stress-induced cytotoxicity. These findings indicate that the observed reduction in AP-1 activation in ERK- and JNK-inhibited cells is not a consequence of reduced cellular injury.

We propose that coordinated activation of ERK1/2 and JNK1 signaling pathways by ER stress promotes activation of the hepatic AP-1 complex. These data identify a novel pathway by which ER stress, a common feature of many chronic liver diseases, may promote hepatic carcinogenesis. Currently there are limited pharmacotherapeutic options to treat HCC. This work raises the possibility that targeting the unfolded protein response may have therapeutic benefit in the treatment or prevention of HCC in patients with chronic liver disease.

Supporting Information

Figure S1 Successful silencing of JNK1 in HepG2 cells treated with siRNA targeting JNK1. Representative Western blot of pooled samples (n = 6).

Table S1 Primer sequences for quantitative PCR.

Author Contributions

Conceived and designed the experiments: AH RG SO. Performed the experiments: AH SO. Analyzed the data: AH RG SO. Contributed reagents/materials/analysis tools: AH RG. Wrote the paper: AH.

References

1. El-Serag HB, Mason AC (1999) Rising incidence of hepatocellular carcinoma in the United States. N Engl J Med 340: 745–750.
2. Gomaa AI, Khan SA, Toledano MB, Waked I, Taylor-Robinson SD (2008) Hepatocellular carcinoma: epidemiology, risk factors and pathogenesis. World J Gastroenterol 14: 4300–4308.
3. Kawada N, Imanaka K, Kawaguchi T, Tamai C, Ishihara R, et al. (2009) Hepatocellular carcinoma arising from non-cirrhotic nonalcoholic steatohepatitis. J Gastroenterol 44: 1190–1194.
4. Ertle J, Dechene A, Sowa JP, Penndorf V, Herzer K, et al. (2011) Non-alcoholic fatty liver disease progresses to hepatocellular carcinoma in the absence of apparent cirrhosis. Int J Cancer 128: 2436–2443.
5. El-Serag HB, Rudolph KL (2007) Hepatocellular carcinoma: epidemiology and molecular carcinogenesis. Gastroenterology 132: 2557–2576.
6. Baffy G, Brunt EM, Caldwell SH (2012) Hepatocellular carcinoma in non-alcoholic fatty liver disease: an emerging menace. J Hepatol 56: 1384–1391.
7. Tardif KD, Mori K, Siddiqui A (2002) Hepatitis C virus subgenomic replicons induce endoplasmic reticulum stress activating an intracellular signaling pathway. J Virol 76: 7453–7459.
8. Li S, Ye L, Yu X, Xu B, Li K, et al. (2009) Hepatitis C virus NS4B induces unfolded protein response and endoplasmic reticulum overload response-dependent NF-kappaB activation. Virology 391: 257–264.
9. Puri P, Mirshahi F, Cheung O, Natarajan R, Maher JW, et al. (2008) Activation and dysregulation of the unfolded protein response in nonalcoholic fatty liver disease. Gastroenterology 134: 568–576.
10. Wei Y, Wang D, Topczewski F, Pagliassotti MJ (2006) Saturated fatty acids induce endoplasmic reticulum stress and apoptosis independently of ceramide in liver cells. Am J Physiol Endocrinol Metab 291: E275–281.
11. Henkel AS, Elias MS, Green RM (2009) Homocysteine supplementation attenuates the unfolded protein response in a murine nutritional model of steatohepatitis. J Biol Chem 284: 31807–31816.
12. Werstuck GH, Lentz SR, Dayal S, Hossain GS, Sood SK, et al. (2001) Homocysteine-induced endoplasmic reticulum stress causes dysregulation of the cholesterol and triglyceride biosynthetic pathways. J Clin Invest 107: 1263–1273.
13. Ji C, Kaplowitz N (2003) Betaine decreases hyperhomocysteinemia, endoplasmic reticulum stress, and liver injury in alcohol-fed mice. Gastroenterology 124: 1488–1499.
14. Wang D, Wei Y, Pagliassotti MJ (2006) Saturated fatty acids promote endoplasmic reticulum stress and liver injury in rats with hepatic steatosis. Endocrinology 147: 943–951.
15. Xu C, Bailly-Maitre B, Reed JC (2005) Endoplasmic reticulum stress: cell life and death decisions. J Clin Invest 115: 2656–2664.
16. Zhang K, Kaufman RJ (2004) Signaling the unfolded protein response from the endoplasmic reticulum. J Biol Chem 279: 25935–25938.
17. Wek RC, Cavener DR (2007) Translational control and the unfolded protein response. Antioxid Redox Signal 9: 2357–2371.
18. Marciniak SJ, Ron D (2006) Endoplasmic reticulum stress signaling in disease. Physiol Rev 86: 1133–1149.
19. Walter P, Ron D (2011) The unfolded protein response: from stress pathway to homeostatic regulation. Science 334: 1081–1086.
20. Urano F, Wang X, Bertolotti A, Zhang Y, Chung P, et al. (2000) Coupling of stress in the ER to activation of JNK protein kinases by transmembrane protein kinase IRE1. Science 287: 664–666.
21. Hu P, Han Z, Couvillon AD, Kaufman RJ, Exton JH (2006) Autocrine tumor necrosis factor alpha links endoplasmic reticulum stress to the membrane death receptor pathway through IRE1alpha-mediated NF-kappaB activation and down-regulation of TRAF2 expression. Mol Cell Biol 26: 3071–3084.
22. Nguyen DT, Kebache S, Fazel A, Wong HN, Jenna S, et al. (2004) Nck-dependent activation of extracellular signal-regulated kinase-1 and regulation of cell survival during endoplasmic reticulum stress. Molecular Biology of the Cell 15: 4248–4260.
23. Hu P, Han Z, Couvillon AD, Exton JH (2004) Critical role of endogenous Akt/IAPs and MEK1/ERK pathways in counteracting endoplasmic reticulum stress-induced cell death. J Biol Chem 279: 49420–49429.
24. Dai R, Chen R, Li H (2009) Cross-talk between PI3K/Akt and MEK/ERK pathways mediates endoplasmic reticulum stress-induced cell cycle progression and cell death in human hepatocellular carcinoma cells. Int J Oncol 34: 1749–1757.
25. Tang J, Guo YS, Zhang Y, Yu XL, Li L, et al. (2012) CD147 induces UPR to inhibit apoptosis and chemosensitivity by increasing the transcription of Bip in hepatocellular carcinoma. Cell Death Differ 19: 1779–1790.
26. Honma Y, Harada M (2013) Sorafenib enhances proteasome inhibitor-mediated cytotoxicity via inhibition of unfolded protein response and keratin phosphorylation. Exp Cell Res.
27. Yi P, Higa A, Taouji S, Bexiga MG, Marza E, et al. (2012) Sorafenib-mediated targeting of the AAA(+) ATPase p97/VCP leads to disruption of the secretory pathway, endoplasmic reticulum stress, and hepatocellular cancer cell death. Mol Cancer Ther 11: 2610–2620.
28. Xu M, Lu N, Zhang H, Dai Q, Wei L, et al. (2012) Wogonin induced cytotoxicity in human hepatocellular carcinoma cells by activation of unfolded protein response and inactivation of AKT. Hepatol Res.
29. Duan Q, Wang X, Gong W, Ni L, Chen C, et al. (2012) ER stress negatively modulates the expression of the miR-199a/214 cluster to regulates tumor survival and progression in human hepatocellular cancer. PLoS One 7: e31518.
30. Yang F, Zhang L, Wang F, Wang Y, Huo XS, et al. (2011) Modulation of the unfolded protein response is the core of microRNA-122-involved sensitivity to chemotherapy in hepatocellular carcinoma. Neoplasia 13: 590–600.
31. Chen R, Dai RY, Duan CY, Liu YP, Chen SK, et al. (2011) Unfolded protein response suppresses cisplatin-induced apoptosis via autophagy regulation in human hepatocellular carcinoma cells. Folia Biol (Praha) 57: 87–95.
32. Belfi CA, Chatterjee S, Gosky DM, Berger SJ, Berger NA (1999) Increased sensitivity of human colon cancer cells to DNA cross-linking agents after GRP78 up-regulation. Biochem Biophys Res Commun 257: 361–368.
33. Fernandez PM, Tabbara SO, Jacobs LK, Manning FC, Tsangaris TN, et al. (2000) Overexpression of the glucose-regulated stress gene GRP78 in malignant but not benign human breast lesions. Breast Cancer Res Treat 59: 15–26.
34. Shuda M, Kondoh N, Imazeki N, Tanaka K, Okada T, et al. (2003) Activation of the ATF6, XBP1 and grp78 genes in human hepatocellular carcinoma: a possible involvement of the ER stress pathway in hepatocarcinogenesis. J Hepatol 38: 605–614.
35. Han H, Hu J, Lau MY, Feng M, Petrovic LM, et al. (2013) Altered methylation and expression of ER-associated degradation factors in long-term alcohol and constitutive ER stress-induced murine hepatic tumors. Front Genet 4: 224.
36. Liu P, Kimmoun E, Legrand A, Sauvanet A, Degott C, et al. (2002) Activation of NF-kappa B, AP-1 and STAT transcription factors is a frequent and early event in human hepatocellular carcinomas. J Hepatol 37: 63–71.
37. Hess J, Angel P, Schorpp-Kistner M (2004) AP-1 subunits: quarrel and harmony among siblings. J Cell Sci 117: 5965–5973.
38. Shaulian E, Karin M (2002) AP-1 as a regulator of cell life and death. Nat Cell Biol 4: E131–136.
39. Karin M (1995) The regulation of AP-1 activity by mitogen-activated protein kinases. J Biol Chem 270: 16483–16486.
40. Johnson GL, Lapadat R (2002) Mitogen-activated protein kinase pathways mediated by ERK, JNK, and p38 protein kinases. Science 298: 1911–1912.
41. Henkel AS, Anderson KA, Dewey AM, Kavesh MH, Green RM (2011) A chronic high-cholesterol diet paradoxically suppresses hepatic CYP7A1 expression in FVB/NJ mice. J Lipid Res 52: 289–298.
42. Gille H, Kortenjann M, Thomae O, Moomaw C, Slaughter C, et al. (1995) ERK phosphorylation potentiates Elk-1-mediated ternary complex formation and transactivation. EMBO J 14: 951–962.
43. Whitmarsh AJ, Davis RJ (1996) Transcription factor AP-1 regulation by mitogen-activated protein kinase signal transduction pathways. J Mol Med (Berl) 74: 589–607.

44. Chang Q, Zhang Y, Beezhold KJ, Bhatia D, Zhao H, et al. (2009) Sustained JNK1 activation is associated with altered histone H3 methylations in human liver cancer. J Hepatol 50: 323–333.
45. Hui L, Zatloukal K, Scheuch H, Stepniak E, Wagner EF (2008) Proliferation of human HCC cells and chemically induced mouse liver cancers requires JNK1-dependent p21 downregulation. J Clin Invest 118: 3943–3953.
46. Schattenberg JM, Singh R, Wang Y, Lefkowitch JH, Rigoli RM, et al. (2006) JNK1 but not JNK2 promotes the development of steatohepatitis in mice. Hepatology 43: 163–172.

IL28B Polymorphism Correlates with Active Hepatitis in Patients with HBeAg-Negative Chronic Hepatitis B

I-Cheng Lee[1,3,6], Chen-Hao Lin[1,3], Yi-Hsiang Huang[1,3]*, Teh-Ia Huo[1,4], Chien-Wei Su[1,3], Ming-Chih Hou[1,2], Hui-Chun Huang[1], Kuei-Chuan Lee[1,3], Che-Chang Chan[1,3], Ming-Wei Lin[5], Han-Chieh Lin[1], Shou-Dong Lee[7]

1 Division of Gastroenterology, Department of Medicine, Taipei Veterans General Hospital, Taipei, Taiwan, **2** Endoscopy Center for Diagnosis and Treatment, Taipei Veterans General Hospital, Taipei, Taiwan, **3** Institute of Clinical Medicine, National Yang-Ming University School of Medicine, Taipei, Taiwan, **4** Institute of Pharmacology, National Yang-Ming University School of Medicine, Taipei, Taiwan, **5** Institute of Public Health, National Yang-Ming University School of Medicine, Taipei, Taiwan, **6** Department of Medicine, National Yang-Ming University Hospital, I-Lan, Taiwan, **7** Cheng Hsin General Hospital, Taipei, Taiwan

Abstract

Background & Aims: The clinical relevance of single nucleotide polymorphisms (SNPs) near the *IL28B* gene is controversial in patients with hepatitis B virus (HBV) infection. This study aimed to investigate the role of viral and host factors, including *IL28B* genotypes, in the natural course of chronic hepatitis B (CHB).

Methods: The study enrolled consecutive 115 treatment-naive CHB patients. HBV viral loads, genotypes, precore and basal core promotor mutations, serum hepatitis B surface antigen (HBsAg) and interferon-gamma inducible protein 10 (IP-10) levels as well as four SNPs of *IL28B* were determined. Serial alanine transaminase (ALT) levels in the previous one year before enrollment at an interval of three months were recorded. Factors associated with active hepatitis, defined as persistent ALT $>2\times$ upper limit of normal (ULN) or a peak ALT level $>5\times$ ULN, were evaluated.

Results: The prevalence of rs8105790 TT, rs12979860 CC, rs8099917 TT, and rs10853728 CC genotypes were 88.3%, 87.4%, 88.4% and 70.9%, respectively. In HBeAg-positive patients ($n = 48$), HBV viral load correlated with active hepatitis, while in HBeAg-negative patients ($n = 67$), rs10853728 CC genotype ($p = 0.032$) and a trend of higher IP-10 levels ($p = 0.092$) were associated with active hepatitis. In multivariate analysis, high viral load (HBV DNA $>10^8$ IU/mL, $p = 0.042$, odds ratio = 3.946) was significantly associated with HBeAg-positive hepatitis, whereas rs10853728 CC genotype ($p = 0.019$, odds ratio = 3.927) was the only independent factor associated with active hepatitis in HBeAg-negative population.

Conclusions: HBV viral load and IL28B rs10853728 CC genotype correlated with hepatitis activity in HBeAg-positive and HBeAg-negative CHB, respectively. Both viral and host factors play roles in disease activity during different phases of CHB.

Editor: Ming-Lung Yu, Kaohsiung Medical University Hospital, Kaohsiung Medical University, Taiwan

Funding: The study was supported by grants from the National Science Council (NSC100-2314-B-010-024) and Taipei Veterans General Hospital (V99C1-075, V100C-104 and V101C-417). The funders had no role in study design, data collection and analysis, decision to publish, or preparation of the manuscript.

Competing Interests: The authors have declared that no competing interests exist.

* E-mail: yhhuang@vghtpe.gov.tw

Introduction

Hepatitis B virus (HBV) infection is an important cause of chronic liver disease globally, with an estimated 350 million carriers worldwide [1]. Patients with chronic hepatitis B (CHB) are at increased risks of developing cirrhosis, hepatic decompensation, and hepatocellular carcinoma (HCC), either of which can lead to a liver-related death [2]. Chronic HBV infection is a dynamic state of the interactions between virus and host immune response, and the natural course varies greatly among different individuals, while some patients had frequent hepatitis flares with more rapid progression of liver disease, others were at inactive carrier state with a relative benign prognosis [3].

Several host and viral factors have been reported to be associated with the natural course of CHB [4]. Genotypes, basal core promoter (BCP) mutations and viral loads of HBV may influence the progression of HBV-related liver disease [4,5,6]. Similarly, age, sex, host immune status and metabolic factors of the host also correlate with disease progression in CHB [4,7]. Patients with higher baseline alanine transaminase (ALT) levels had a better response to interferon (IFN) therapy [8], indicating that host immune response plays an important role in eliminating HBV. Currently, the genetic determinants of host immune responses to HBV infection remain unclear.

Genome-wide association studies have shown that single-nucleotide polymorphisms (SNPs) at or near the *interleukin 28B* gene (*IL28B*) region on chromosome 19, which encodes interferon-lamda 3 (IFN-λ3), are associated with spontaneous hepatitis C virus (HCV) clearance and sustained virological response (SVR) in patients with chronic hepatitis C (CHC) treated with pegylated-interferon (PEG-IFN) and ribavirin [9,10,11,12,13]. Furthermore, a recent study showed that patients with lower serum levels of interferon gamma-inducible protein 10 (IP-10) in combination with favorable *IL28B* genotypes had higher chance of spontaneous HCV clearance [14]. Whether *IL28B* polymorphisms have influence on host immune response to HBV infection is unknown. It is possible that genetic variations at *IL28B* region determine the host susceptibility to HBV infection and influence the progression of liver disease.

Currently, whether IL28B genotypes are associated with the natural course of HBV infection and hepatitis activity in CHB is not fully understood. This study aimed to investigate the role of viral and host factors, including *IL28B* genotypes, in the natural course of chronic hepatitis B (CHB).

Materials and Methods

Patients

From April 2009 to July 2011, consecutive 115 treatment-naïve CHB patients who were willing to participate in this study at the Taipei Veterans General Hospital were enrolled. All patients were positive for serum HBsAg for more than 6 months and had documented elevation of serum ALT levels [>40 U/L, 1× upper limit of normal (ULN)] with HBV DNA >2,000 IU/mL [15,16,17]. All patients had been regularly followed with three-month interval for at least one year. Patients were negative for any of the following points: (1) coinfection with HCV, hepatitis D virus, or human immunodeficiency virus, (2) alcoholic liver disease, (3) suspected autoimmune disease with antinuclear antibody (ANA) titer ≥1:160, positive test for anti-smooth muscle antibody or anti-mitochondrial antibody, (4) use of hepatotoxic drug or Chinese herb, and (5) radiological evidence of cirrhosis or HCC (i.e., abdominal sonogram, computed tomography scan, or magnetic resonance imaging scans). This study was approved by the Institutional Review Board, Taipei Veterans General Hospital, which complied with standards of the Declaration of Helsinki and current ethical guidelines. All patients provided written informed consents for participation of the study and for use of genetic material for this study.

Peripheral blood samples were obtained from all patients for serological, virological tests and *IL28B* genotypes analyses. Serial ALT levels in the previous one year before enrollment at an interval of three months were recorded. Active hepatitis was defined as persistent ALT >2× ULN or a peak ALT level >5× ULN. Patients who did not fulfill the criteria were defined as mild hepatitis.

Liver biochemistry and viral serology tests

Serum biochemical studies were performed using a systemic multi-autoanalyzer (Technicon SMAC, Technicon Instruments Corp., Tarrytown, NY). The serum samples were tested for the presence of HBeAg and anti-HBe antibody using radio-immuno-assay (Abott Laboratories, North Chicago, IL), while a Cobas Amplicor HBV monitor determined HBV DNA (detection limit of 12 IU/mL).

IL28B genotyping

Four SNPs of *IL28B* including rs8105790, rs12979860, rs8099917 and rs10853728 were chosen according to previous reports [9,10,11,12,18,19,20]. The genotype of rs12979860 was tested using TaqMan custom-designed rs12979860 probes (Applied Biosystems, Foster City, CA; forward primer GCCTGTCGTGTACTGAACCA, reverse primer GCGCGGAGTGCAATTCAAC, and the probes TGGTTCGCGCCTTC [VIC] and CTGGTTCACGCCTTC [FAM], respectively) [21]. The genotypes of the rs8105790, rs8099917 and rs10853728 were determined with the ABI TaqMan SNP genotyping assays (Applied Biosystems) and with predesigned commercial genotyping assays (ABI assay C__43813808_10, C__11710096_10, C__11710090_10). Briefly, PCR primers and two allelic-specific probes was designed to detect a specific SNP target. The PCR reactions were performed in 96-well microplates with ABI 7900 real-time PCR (Applied Biosystems).

Detection, genotyping and sequencing of HBV DNA

Genotyping of HBV was performed by PCR restriction fragment length polymorphism (PCR-RFLP) of the surface gene of HBV [6,22]. Briefly, DNA was extracted from serum, and the fragment of the HBV genome between nucleotide position 120 and 604 was amplified by semi-nested PCR. The PCR products were subsequently treated with restriction enzymes. After incubation, the samples were run on a 4% agarose gel and stained by ethidium bromide. To confirm the correct genotyping, direct sequencing from the PCR products was done.

To detect precore G1896A and basal core promoter (BCP) A1762T/G1764A mutations, sequencing of the core region of HBV DNA was performed in all patients. Semi-nested PCR was performed by using a pair of primers: internal primers 1653F (5′-CATAAGAGGACTCTTGGACT-3′, position 1653-1672) and 1974R (5′-GGAAAGAAGTCAGAAGGC-3′, position 1974–1957); external primers: 1623F (5′-TCGCATGGAGACCACCGTCT-3′, position 1623–1640) and 2076R (5′-ATAGCTTGCCTGAGTGC-3′, position 2076–2060) as previously described [6,22].

The PCR products were then subjected to the dye-terminator cycle sequencing reaction using specific primers according to the standard protocol provided by the manufacturer (Dye terminator cycle sequencing core kit no. 402117, Perkin Elmer Cetus Corp., Norwalk, CT). To avoid false positive results, instructions to prevent cross contaminations were strictly followed.

Serum HBsAg quantification

HBsAg levels were quantified using the Elecsys HBsAg II assay (Roche Diagnostics GmbH, Mannheim, Germany) according to the manufacturer's instructions [23]. The detection limit of the Elecsys HBsAg II assay was 0.05 IU/mL.

Enzyme-linked sorbent assay (ELISA) for IP-10 detection

The concentrations of interferon gamma-inducible protein 10 (IP-10) in serum were tested by commercialized human IP-10 ELISA development kit (PeproTech, Rocky Hill, NJ) in this study. The procedure followed the instruction provided by manufactures. The lower detection limit was 8 pg/mL for IP-10.

Statistical analyses

Linkage disequilibrium (LD) between the four candidate SNP loci was assessed and haplotype blocks were constructed using Haploview 4.2 [24]. All statistical analyses were performed using the Statistical Package for Social Sciences (SPSS 17.0 for Windows, SPSS Inc, Chicago, IL). Values were expressed as median (ranges) or as mean ± standard deviation when appropriate. Pearson chi-square analysis or Fisher exact test was used to compare categorical variables, while the Student t test or Mann-Whitney U test was used to compare continuous variables. Variables with $p<0.1$ were analyzed by multivariate logistic regression analysis to identify independent variables for predicting active hepatitis. A 2-tailed p value <0.05 was considered statistically significant.

Results

Patient characteristics

The baseline characteristics of the 115 CHB patients are summarized in Table 1. Patients were predominantly male (73%) and HBeAg-negative (58.3%). Sixty-seven patients (58.3%) had active hepatitis. HBV genotypes were determined in all patients, with 3.5% genotype A, 64.3% genotypes B and 32.2% genotype C. Compared with HBeAg-positive patients, HBeAg-negative patients were older, had significantly lower HBV DNA, HBsAg and IP-10 levels (Table 1). About three-fourth of HBeAg-negative patients were infected with genotype B HBV, whereas 45% of HBeAg-positive patients were infected with genotype C HBV (p = 0.006).

Thirty-nine patients (34.2%) had BCP mutations and 55 (47.8%) had precore mutations. The prevalence of BCP mutations was comparable between HBeAg-positive and HBeAg-negative patients, whereas the prevalence of precore mutations was significantly higher in HBeAg-negative patients (Table 1). Genotype C HBV had a significantly higher prevalence of BCP mutations (26% in genotype B vs. 51.4% in genotype C, p = 0.015), whereas genotype B HBV was precore mutations predominant (54.1% in genotype B vs. 32.4% in genotype C, p = 0.051). In HBeAg-positive patients, the prevalence of BCP mutations were 16% (4/25) in genotype B and 50% (11/22) in genotype C (p = 0.029), and the prevalence of precore mutations were 38.5% (10/26) in genotype B and 22.7% (5/22) in genotype C (p = 0.390). In HBeAg-negative patients, the prevalence of BCP mutations were 25% (1/4) in genotype A, 31.3% (15/48) in genotype B and 53.3% (8/15) in genotype C (p = 0.277), and the prevalence of precore mutations were 75% (3/4) in genotype A, 62.5% (30/48) in genotype B and 46.7% (7/15) in genotype C (p = 0.448).

Distribution of *IL28B* Genotypes

Among the 115 CHB patients, 112 (97.4%) had determined rs8099917 genotype, 111 (96.5%) had determined rs8105790 and rs12979860 genotypes, and 110 (95.7%) had determined rs10853728 genotype. The distributions of the four SNPs of *IL28B* in overall patients and in patients infected with HBV genotypes A, B and C are shown in Figure 1. The prevalence of the major genotypes rs8105790 TT, rs12979860 CC, rs8099917 TT, and rs10853728 CC were 88.3%, 87.4%, 88.4% and 70.9%, respectively. The distributions of the four SNPs were not significantly different among patients infected with HBV genotypes A, B or C (p = 0.749, 0.787, 0.581 and 0.383 for rs8105790, rs12979860, rs8099917 and rs10853728, respectively). Among the four SNPs, rs8105790 and rs12979860 were highly linked, with only 1 (0.9%) patient classified discordantly ($r^2 = 0.78$, Figure 2). The rs10853728 was not so closely linked with the other 3 SNPs (Figure 2). There were no significant correlations between the HBeAg status and the four SNPs of *IL28B* (Table 1).

Factors associated with active hepatitis in CHB patients

In overall patients, serum IP-10 levels were significantly higher in patients with active hepatitis (p = 0.021, Table 2), whereas age, sex, HBeAg status, HBV genotypes, BCP or precore mutations, viral loads, HBsAg levels, or the four SNPs of *IL28B* were not correlated with active hepatitis.

We further stratified the CHB patients by HBeAg status. Factors associated with active hepatitis in HBeAg-positive and HBeAg-negative patients were shown in Table 2. In HBeAg-positive CHB patients, those with active hepatitis had significantly higher serum HBV viral load, ALT and AST levels. In contrast, serum levels of HBsAg, IP-10, HBV genotypes, precore/BCP mutations and the four SNPs of *IL28B* were not associated with hepatitis activity.

In HBeAg-negative patients, those with active hepatitis had significantly higher serum ALT and AST levels, a trend of higher

Table 1. Baseline characteristics of the 115 chronic hepatitis B patients.

	All patients n = 115	HbeAg-positive n = 48 (41.7%)	HbeAg-negative n = 67 (58.3%)	p value
Age (years)	45±13	38±11	50±12	<0.01
Male sex, n (%)	84 (73)	31 (64.6)	53 (79.1)	0.13
Active hepatitis, n (%)*	67 (58.3)	31 (64.6)	36 (53.7)	0.33
Genotype A/B/C, n (%)	4/74/37 (3.5/64.3/32.2)	0/26/22 (0/54.2/45.8)	4/48/15 (6/71.6/22.4)	<0.01
Basal core promoter mutation, n (%)	39 (34.2)	15 (31.9)	24 (35.8)	0.82
Precore mutation, n (%)	55 (47.8)	15 (31.3)	40 (59.7)	<0.01
HBV DNA (Log_{10} IU/mL)	6.52±1.36	7.39±0.98	5.90±1.26	<0.01
HBsAg (Log_{10} IU/mL)	3.49 (1.39–5.46)	4.00 (2.05–5.46)	3.14 (1.39–4.87)	<0.01
IP-10 (pg/mL)	78.6 (13.9–2078)	97.3 (19.1–2078)	65.4 (13.9–1301.7)	<0.01
ALT (U/L)	211±169	235±161	194±174	0.06
AST (U/L)	120±117	130±121	112±114	0.24
IL28B polymorphisms				
rs8105790 TT/CT + CC, n (%)	98/13 (88.3/11.7)	39/7 (84.8/15.2)	59/6 (90.8/9.2)	0.51
rs12979860 CC/CT + TT, n (%)	97/14 (87.4/12.6)	39/7 (84.8/15.2)	58/7 (89.2/10.8)	0.69
rs8099917 TT/GT + GG, n (%)	99/13 (88.4/11.6)	39/7 (84.8/15.2)	60/6 (90.9/9.1)	0.49
rs10853728 CC/CG + GG, n (%)	78/32 (70.9/29.1)	33/13 (71.7/28.3)	45/19 (70.3/29.7)	1.00

Abbreviations: HBeAg, hepatitis B e antigen; HBsAg, hepatitis B surface antigen; IP-10, interferon-gamma inducible protein 10; ALT, alanine transaminase; AST, aspartate transaminase.
*Active hepatitis was defined as persistent ALT >2× upper limit of normal (ULN) or a peak ALT level >5× ULN.

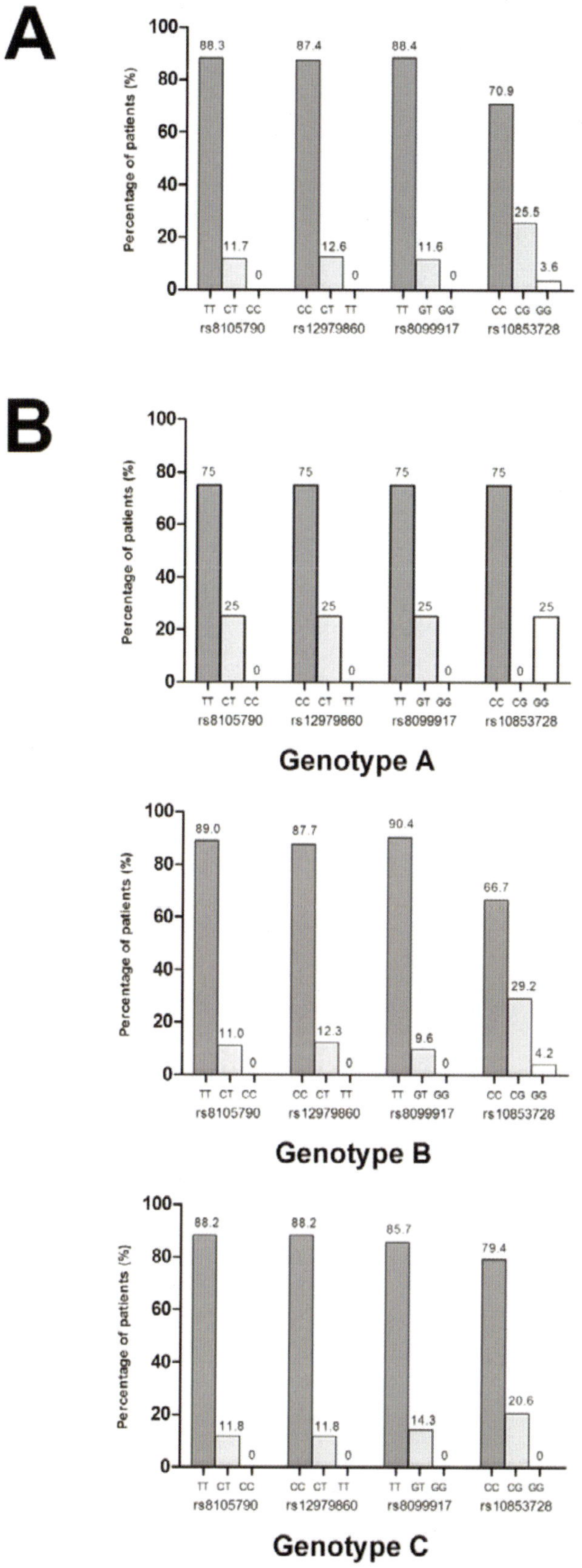

Figure 1. Distributions of *IL28B* polymorphisms. (A) Distributions of rs8105790, rs12979860, rs8099917 and rs10853728 genotypes in overall patients. (B) Distributions of rs8105790, rs12979860, rs8099917 and rs10853728 genotypes in patients infected with HBV genotypes A, B and C.

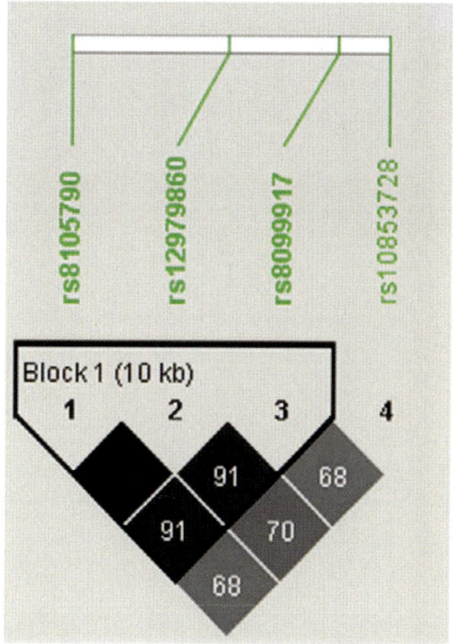

Figure 2. Pairwise linkage disequilibrium (LD) patterns of the four single nucleotide polymorphisms through *IL28B* regions. Pairwise r^2 was used for analyzing the correlation.

IP-10 levels (p = 0.092), and patients with rs10853728 CC genotype were more susceptible to active hepatitis (p = 0.032, Figure 3). In contrast, rs8105790, rs12979860, rs8099917 polymorphisms were not associated with active hepatitis. The HBV genotypes, precore/BCP mutations and HBV viral load were not associated with active hepatitis in HBeAg-negative patients.

In multivariate analysis, high viral load (HBV DNA $>10^8$ IU/mL, p = 0.042, odds ratio = 3.946) was the significant factor associated with active hepatitis in HBeAg-positive patients, while rs10853728 CC genotype (p = 0.019, odds ratio = 3.927) was the only independent factor associated with active hepatitis in HBeAg-negative population (Table 3). Among patients with lower viral loads (HBV DNA $<5\times10^7$ IU/mL), not only rs10853728 CC genotype (p = 0.041, odds ratio = 2.991) but also IP-10>75 pg/mL (p = 0.022, odds ratio = 3.062) were independently associated with active hepatitis.

Discussion

Consistent with previous reports, serum HBV viral load and HBsAg levels were lower in HBeAg-negative patients as compared with HBeAg-positive cases [25,26,27]. We also observed that serum IP-10 levels were higher in HBeAg-positive patients. There was a significant correlation between IP-10 and active hepatitis, especially in patients with lower viral loads, but IP-10 was not associated with active hepatitis in HBeAg-positive patients with high viral load. Although the role of IP-10 in the natural history of CHB is unclear, recent studies showed that IP-10 plays a major role in the immune activation during hepatic failure in CHB, and a higher IP-10 level might be associated with HBsAg seroclearance during antiviral therapy [28,29]. Both findings support that higher serum IP-10 levels in patients with active hepatitis represents stronger immune response to clear the virus. The impact of IP-10 on active hepatitis in HBeAg-positive population might be masked by viral factors.

Table 2. Characteristics of the chronic hepatitis B patients stratified by hepatitis activity*.

	All patients (n = 115)			HBeAg-positive (n = 48)			HBeAg-negative (n = 67)		
	Mild hepatitis n = 48 (41.7%)	**Active hepatitis n = 67 (58.3%)**	**p value**	**Mild hepatitis n = 17 (35.4%)**	**Active hepatitis n = 31 (64.6%)**	**p value**	**Mild hepatitis n = 31 (46.3%)**	**Active hepatitis n = 36 (53.7%)**	**p value**
Age (years)	46±13	44±14	0.38	40±13	36±11	0.39	50±11	51±12	0.72
Male sex, n (%)	34 (70.8)	50 (74.6)	0.81	8 (41.7)	23 (74.2)	0.12	26 (83.9)	27 (75)	0.56
Genotype A/B/C, n (%)	1/31/16 (2.1/64.6/33.3)	3/43/21 (4.5/64.2/31.3)	0.77	0/10/7 (0/58.8/41.2)	0/16/15 (0/51.6/48.4)	0.86	1/21/9 (3.2/67.7/29.0)	3/27/6 (8.3/75/16.7)	0.36
HBV DNA (Log_{10} IU/mL)	6.38±1.29	6.62±1.42	0.16	6.99±1.15	7.61±0.80	0.02	6.04±1.25	5.78±1.28	0.49
HBsAg (Log_{10} IU/mL)	3.46 (1.86–5.27)	3.50 (1.39–5.46)	0.63	3.59 (2.05–5.27)	4.11 (2.12–5.46)	0.58	3.30 (1.86–4.82)	3.05 (1.39–4.87)	0.55
Basal core promoter mutation, n (%)	17 (35.4)	22 (33.3)	0.98	7 (41.2)	8 (26.7)	0.48	10 (32.3)	14 (38.9)	0.76
Precore mutation, n (%)	20 (41.7)	35 (52.2)	0.35	4 (23.5)	11 (35.5)	0.60	16 (51.6)	24 (66.7)	0.32
IP-10 (pg/mL)	67.6 (19–832.9)	87.5 (13.9–2078)	0.02	93.2 (19.1–198.3)	97.3 (37.1–2078)	0.27	59.8 (19–832.9)	78.6 (13.9–1301.7)	0.09
ALT (U/L)	108±40	284±188	<0.01	111±46	303±161	<0.01	109±38	267±209	<0.01
AST (U/L)	65±25	158±139	<0.01	74±33	161±140	<0.01	61±17	156±141	<0.01
IL28B polymorphisms									
rs8105790			1.00			1.00			1.00
TT	40 (40.8%)	58 (59.2%)		14 (35.9%)	25 (64.1%)		26 (44.1%)	33 (55.9%)	
CT + CC	5 (38.5%)	8 (61.5%)		2 (28.6%)	5 (71.4%)		3 (50%)	3 (50%)	
rs12979860			1.00			1.00			0.69
CC	39 (40.2%)	58 (59.2%)		14 (35.9%)	25 (64.1%)		25 (43.1%)	33 (56.9%)	
CT + TT	6 (42.9%)	8 (57.1%)		2 (28.6%)	5 (71.4%)		4 (57.1%)	33 (56.9%)	
rs8099917			0.62			0.39			1.00
TT	42 (42.4%)	57 (57.6%)		15 (38.5%)	24 (61.5%)		27 (45%)	33 (55%)	
GT + GG	4 (30.8%)	9 (69.2%)		1 (14.3%)	6 (85.7%)		3 (50%)	3 (50%)	
rs10853728			0.15			1.00			0.03
CC	28 (35.9%)	50 (64.1%)		12 (36.4%)	21 (63.6%)		16 (35.6%)	29 (64.4%)	
CG + GG	17 (53.1%)	15 (46.9%)		4 (30.8%)	9 (69.2%)		13 (68.4%)	6 (31.6%)	

*Active hepatitis was defined as persistent ALT >2× ULN or a peak ALT level >5× ULN, while patients who did not fulfill the criteria were defined as mild hepatitis.

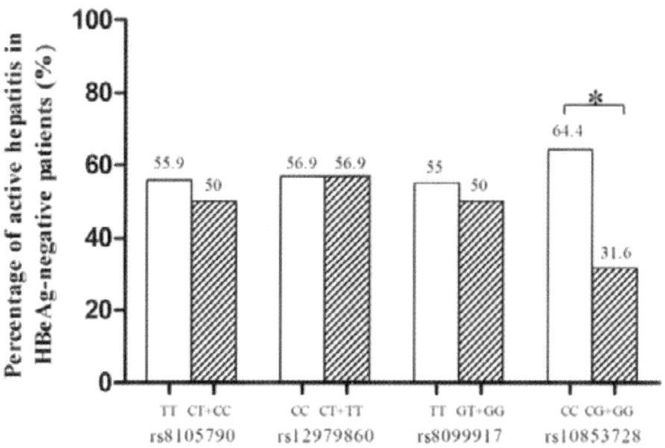

Figure 3. Association of rs8105790, rs12979860, rs8099917 and rs10853728 genotypes with hepatitis activity. *p = 0.032.

HBV genotypes also play an important role in the natural history of CHB. Consistent with previous observations that patients with genotypes B HBV have earlier HBeAg seroconversion than genotype C infection [30,31], our data showed genotype B HBV was predominant in HBeAg-negative patients whose age were older. A similar distribution of the four *IL28B* SNPs in patients infected with different HBV genotypes suggests that *IL28B* polymorphisms may not influence the susceptibility of infection to varied genotypes of HBV.

It has been recognized that BCP mutation is associated with genotype C HBV and precore mutation is associated with genotype B HBV [6,32]. In the current study, we also observed this association. BCP mutation has been shown to correlate with progression of liver fibrosis and development of HCC, whereas precore mutation was associated with reduced risk of HCC [5,33]. It is interesting that whether these mutations contribute to active hepatic necroinflammation. However, our results showed neither BCP nor precore mutations were related to active hepatitis in both HBeAg-positive and HBeAg-negative patients. The impact of the mutations on hepatic necroinflammation may not be revealed by this one-year observational study.

In our patients, the prevalence of IL28B SNPs rs8105790 TT, rs12979860 CC and rs8099917 TT genotypes were approximately 88%, while 70.9% of patients had rs10853728 CC genotype. The distributions of these four SNPs in our study were similar to that reported in CHC patients in Taiwan [18,19]. Based on linkage disequilibrium finding, rs8105790 TT, rs12979860 CC and rs8099917 TT alleles are closely linked. Therefore, either one of the three SNPs genotype can represent the other two for Taiwanese.

In this study, we demonstrated that HBV viral load correlated with active hepatitis in HBeAg-positive patients, while *IL28B* rs10853728 CC genotype was associated with active hepatitis in HBeAg-negative patients (Figure 3). The result indicates that viral factor is the major determinant of hepatic inflammation in HBeAg-positive patients, while host factor, the *IL28B* polymorphisms, may contribute to hepatic inflammation in HBeAg-negative cases, as a consequence of host immune response to HBV. Our enrolled HBeAg-positive patients with elevated liver enzymes and HBV viral load >2,000 IU/ml represents immune clearance phase in the natural history of HBV infection [3]. These patients tend to have higher HBV viral loads and therefore host factor might be overwhelmed by viral factor being responsible for disease activity. Indeed, in patients with lower viral loads, i.e. HBV DNA $<5\times10^7$ IU/mL, the role of rs10853728 CC genotype in hepatitis activity become predominant. On the contrary, in HBeAg-negative patients with a relatively lower viral load, the significance of rs10853728 CC genotype will not be masked by viral load and is the only factor associated with active hepatitis. Although rs10853728 genotype was not emphasized in studies of hepatitis C, a recent study showed that rs10853728 CC was significantly associated spontaneous HCV clearance in Chinese population [20]. Our findings suggest that certain *IL28B* genotype might relate to host immune response against viral infection. We defined "active hepatitis" as those cases might have stronger host immune response against HBV infection. A favorable *IL28B* genotype in HCV infection is associated with spontaneous and IFN-induced viral clearance, indicating that *IL28B* genes might be responsible for triggering immune response against HCV during IFN treatment. A recent study by Sonneveld MJ, et al also discovers that *IL28B* polymorphism is associated with HBeAg seroconversion in HBeAg-positive CHB under IFN treatment [34]. Although the evidence is not clear enough, this *IL28B* polymorphism might associate with a higher ALT at baseline in those patients, which is a well-known predictor of HBeAg seroconversion for HBeAg-positive patients [4,15,16,17]. In our current study, rs10853728 CC genotype correlates with a higher hepatitis activity, suggesting that the *IL28B* genotypes may also trigger intrinsic host antiviral immune response against HBV infection in HBeAg-negative patients. Although active hepatitis may induce liver disease progression, a higher ALT levels may also represent a stronger host immune response to HBV. Therefore, our finding is not descrepant with previous findings in patients with hepatitis C. The long-term outcome of IL28B related active hepatitis is still unclear and needs further extended observation.

Table 3. Factors associated with active hepatitis in HBeAg-positive and HBeAg -negative patients, by multivariate analysis.

Variables	p value	Odds ratio	95% confidence interval
HBeAg-positive patients			
HBV DNA $>10^8$ IU/mL	0.042	3.946	1.049–14.851
HBeAg-negative patients			
rs10853728 CC genotype	0.019	3.927	1.251–12.326

Currently, the association between *IL28B* polymorphisms and the outcomes of CHB remains controversial. Some studies showed that *IL28B* genotypes were not associated with recovery from HBV infection, clearance of HBeAg and HBsAg, hepatitis activity and liver cirrhosis [35,36], while other studies showed significant correlations between *IL28B* genotypes and HBV viral load, hepatic inflammation and risk of HCC [37,38]. The discrepancies between these studies may result from racial difference, and the enrolled patients were in different phases of CHB.

Two recent studies showed that *IL28B* SNP may predict response to PEG-IFN in HBeAg-positive CHB patients, indicating that host factor is important for the induction of an immune response during antiviral therapy in CHB [34,39]. Recently, Lampertico et al. also showed that *IL28B* polymorphism was associated with interferon-related HBsAg seroclearance in genotype D HBeAg-negative patients [40]. Although these studies provide promising role of *IL28B* polymorphisms in CHB, rs10853728 genotype was not tested in previous HBV studies. *IL28B* rs10853728 genotype might also have clinical implication in the treatment of HBeAg-negative CHB in the future.

There is evidence that the gene product of *IL28B*, IFN- λ3, up-regulates interferon-stimulated genes, which may regulate many of the innate cellular defenses against viral infection [41]. In addition, *IL28B* is also a regulator of the adaptive immune response by regulating the number and function of $CD8^+$ T cells [42]. The association of rs10853728 CC genotype with active hepatitis in HBeAg-negative patients implies that *IL28B* gene polymorphism may dominate host immune activity in the course of CHB.

The correlation between *IL28B* SNPs and IP-10 secretion during viral infection are not yet established. Previous studies in CHC showed that patients with rs12979860 CC genotype had lower IP-10 levels [14,43]. Our data showed that there was no correlation between *IL28B* SNPs and IP-10 levels, but in patients with low viral load (HBV DNA $<5\times10^7$ IU/mL), rs12979860 CC genotype was associated with higher IP-10 levels (mean 148.6 pg/mL in CC type vs. 128.9 pg/mL in non-CC type, $p=0.021$,). In contrast, rs10853728 CC genotype was not associated with IP-10 level. The scenario of IP-10 in response to viral infection might be different between HBV and HCV infection. Our data suggests that certain IL28B gene may relate to the susceptibility of IP-10 secretion during chronic HBV infection.

This study has some limitations. Our studied population was not large enough, which may lead to potential type I error caused by multiple comparisons. A multicenter study to include more patients to confirm the role of IL28B in the natural history of CHB is necessary in the future. Our studied population did not include inactive HBV carriers. Therefore, whether genetic variations in *IL28B* contribute to disease remission in inactive HBV carriers with persistently normal ALT could not be elucidated in this study. Our enrolled patients did not receive liver biopsy, which is currently the gold standard to evaluate hepatic necroinflammation. However, current guidelines do not suggest routine liver biopsy before antiviral therapy in CHB patients, especially those with obviously active CHB, i.e. ALT above 2 times ULN and HBV DNA >2000 IU/mL [15,16]. Furthermore, regarding the fluctuating nature of CHB, serial ALT levels may also reflect the long term course of hepatic necroinflammation.

In conclusion, HBV viral load is related to active hepatitis in HBeAg-positive CHB, while *IL28B* rs10853728 CC genotype is associated with active hepatitis in HBeAg-negative CHB. Both viral and host factors play roles in disease activity during different phases of CHB. The role of rs10853728 genotype in predicting long-term outcome and antiviral response for HBeAg-negative CHB warrants future study.

Acknowledgments

The authors thank Clinical Research Core Laboratory, Taipei Veterans General Hospital for providing their facilities to help conduct this study.

Author Contributions

Conceived and designed the experiments: I-CL Y-HH. Performed the experiments: I-CL C-HL. Analyzed the data: I-CL Y-HH M-WL. Contributed reagents/materials/analysis tools: T-IH C-WS M-CH H-CH K-CL C-CC H-CL S-DL. Wrote the paper: I-CL Y-HH.

References

1. Lavanchy D (2004) Hepatitis B virus epidemiology, disease burden, treatment, and current and emerging prevention and control measures. J Viral Hepat 11: 97–107.
2. Ganem D, Prince AM (2004) Hepatitis B virus infection – natural history and clinical consequences. N Engl J Med 350: 1118–1129.
3. Liaw YF, Chu CM (2009) Hepatitis B virus infection. Lancet 373: 582–592.
4. Liaw YF (2009) Natural history of chronic hepatitis B virus infection and long-term outcome under treatment. Liver Int 29 Suppl 1: 100–107.
5. Yang HI, Yeh SH, Chen PJ, Iloeje UH, Jen CL, et al. (2008) Associations between hepatitis B virus genotype and mutants and the risk of hepatocellular carcinoma. J Natl Cancer Inst 100: 1134–1143.
6. Huang YH, Wu JC, Chang TT, Sheen IJ, Huo TI, et al. (2006) Association of core promoter/precore mutations and viral load in e antigen-negative chronic hepatitis B patients. J Viral Hepat 13: 336–342.
7. Lee IC, Huang YH, Chan CC, Huo TI, Chu CJ, et al. (2011) Impact of body mass index and viral load on liver histology in hepatitis B e antigen-negative chronic hepatitis B. Clin Nutr 30: 647–652.
8. Perrillo R (2009) Benefits and risks of interferon therapy for hepatitis B. Hepatology 49: S103–111.
9. Thomas DL, Thio CL, Martin MP, Qi Y, Ge D, et al. (2009) Genetic variation in IL28B and spontaneous clearance of hepatitis C virus. Nature 461: 798–801.
10. Ge D, Fellay J, Thompson AJ, Simon JS, Shianna KV, et al. (2009) Genetic variation in IL28B predicts hepatitis C treatment-induced viral clearance. Nature 461: 399–401.
11. Suppiah V, Moldovan M, Ahlenstiel G, Berg T, Weltman M, et al. (2009) IL28B is associated with response to chronic hepatitis C interferon-alpha and ribavirin therapy. Nat Genet 41: 1100–1104.
12. Tanaka Y, Nishida N, Sugiyama M, Kurosaki M, Matsuura K, et al. (2009) Genome-wide association of IL28B with response to pegylated interferon-alpha and ribavirin therapy for chronic hepatitis C. Nat Genet 41: 1105–1109.
13. Balagopal A, Thomas DL, Thio CL (2010) IL28B and the control of hepatitis C virus infection. Gastroenterology 139: 1865–1876.
14. Beinhardt S, Aberle JH, Strasser M, Dulic-Lakovic E, Maieron A, et al. (2012) Serum Level of IP-10 Increases Predictive Value of IL28B Polymorphisms for Spontaneous Clearance of Acute HCV Infection. Gastroenterology 142: 78–85 e72
15. Lok AS, McMahon BJ (2009) Chronic hepatitis B: update 2009. Hepatology 50: 661–662.
16. European Association For The Study Of The L (2012) EASL Clinical Practice Guidelines: Management of chronic hepatitis B virus infection. J Hepatol 57: 167–85.
17. Liaw YF, Leung N, Kao JH, Piratvisuth T, Gane E, et al. (2008) Asian-Pacific consensus statement on the management of chronic hepatitis B: a 2008 update. Hepatol Int 2: 263–283.
18. Yu ML, Huang CF, Huang JF, Chang NC, Yang JF, et al. (2011) Role of interleukin-28B polymorphisms in the treatment of hepatitis C virus genotype 2 infection in Asian patients. Hepatology 53: 7–13.
19. Lin CY, Chen JY, Lin TN, Jeng WJ, Huang CH, et al. (2011) IL28B SNP rs12979860 is a critical predictor for on-treatment and sustained virologic response in patients with hepatitis C virus genotype-1 infection. PLoS One 6: e18322.
20. Rao HY, Sun DG, Jiang D, Yang RF, Guo F, et al. (2012) IL28B genetic variants and gender are associated with spontaneous clearance of hepatitis C virus infection. J Viral Hepat 19: 173–181.
21. Tillmann HL, Thompson AJ, Patel K, Wiese M, Tenckhoff H, et al. (2010) A polymorphism near IL28B is associated with spontaneous clearance of acute hepatitis C virus and jaundice. Gastroenterology 139: 1586–1592, 1592 e1581.
22. Huang YH, Wu JC, Chang TT, Sheen IJ, Lee PC, et al. (2003) Analysis of clinical, biochemical and viral factors associated with early relapse after lamivudine treatment for hepatitis B e antigen-negative chronic hepatitis B patients in Taiwan. J Viral Hepat 10: 277–284.
23. Wursthorn K, Jaroszewicz J, Zacher BJ, Darnedde M, Raupach R, et al. (2011) Correlation between the Elecsys HBsAg II assay and the Architect assay for the quantification of hepatitis B surface antigen (HBsAg) in the serum. J Clin Virol 50: 292–296.
24. Barrett JC, Fry B, Maller J, Daly MJ (2005) Haploview: analysis and visualization of LD and haplotype maps. Bioinformatics 21: 263–265.
25. Chan HL, Wong VW, Wong GL, Tse CH, Chan HY, et al. (2010) A longitudinal study on the natural history of serum hepatitis B surface antigen changes in chronic hepatitis B. Hepatology 52: 1232–1241.
26. Liaw YF (2011) Clinical utility of hepatitis B surface antigen quantitation in patients with chronic hepatitis B: a review. Hepatology 53: 2121–2129.
27. Nguyen T, Thompson AJ, Bowden S, Croagh C, Bell S, et al. (2010) Hepatitis B surface antigen levels during the natural history of chronic hepatitis B: a perspective on Asia. J Hepatol 52: 508–513.
28. Tan AT, Koh S, Goh W, Zhe HY, Gehring AJ, et al. (2010) A longitudinal analysis of innate and adaptive immune profile during hepatic flares in chronic hepatitis B. J Hepatol 52: 330–339.
29. Jaroszewicz J, Ho H, Markova A, Deterding K, Wursthorn K, et al. (2011) Hepatitis B surface antigen (HBsAg) decrease and serum interferon-inducible protein-10 levels as predictive markers for HBsAg loss during treatment with nucleoside/nucleotide analogues. Antivir Ther 16: 915–924.
30. Chu CJ, Hussain M, Lok AS (2002) Hepatitis B virus genotype B is associated with earlier HBeAg seroconversion compared with hepatitis B virus genotype C. Gastroenterology 122: 1756–1762.
31. Lin CL, Kao JH (2011) The clinical implications of hepatitis B virus genotype: Recent advances. J Gastroenterol Hepatol 26 Suppl 1: 123–130.

32. Chu CJ, Keeffe EB, Han SH, Perrillo RP, Min AD, et al. (2003) Prevalence of HBV precore/core promoter variants in the United States. Hepatology 38: 619–628.
33. Yotsuyanagi H, Hino K, Tomita E, Toyoda J, Yasuda K, et al. (2002) Precore and core promoter mutations, hepatitis B virus DNA levels and progressive liver injury in chronic hepatitis B. J Hepatol 37: 355–363.
34. Sonneveld MJ, Wong VW, Woltman AM, Wong GL, Cakaloglu Y, et al. (2012) Polymorphisms Near IL28B and Serologic Response to Peginterferon in HBeAg-Positive Patients With Chronic Hepatitis B. Gastroenterology 142: 513–520 e511.
35. Martin MP, Qi Y, Goedert JJ, Hussain SK, Kirk GD, et al. (2010) IL28B polymorphism does not determine outcomes of hepatitis B virus or HIV infection. The Journal of infectious diseases 202: 1749–1753.
36. Peng LJ, Guo JS, Zhang Z, Shi H, Wang J, et al. (2012) IL28B rs12979860 polymorphism does not influence outcomes of hepatitis B virus infection. Tissue Antigens 79: 302–305.
37. Li W, Jiang Y, Jin Q, Shi X, Jin J, et al. (2011) Expression and gene polymorphisms of interleukin 28B and hepatitis B virus infection in a Chinese Han population. Liver Int 31: 1118–1126.
38. Ren S, Lu J, Du X, Huang Y, Ma L, et al. (2012) Genetic variation in IL28B is associated with the development of hepatitis B-related hepatocellular carcinoma. Cancer immunology, immunotherapy 61: 1433–1439.
39. Wu X, Xin Z, Zhu X, Pan L, Li Z, et al. (2012) Evaluation of susceptibility locus for response to interferon-alpha based therapy in chronic hepatitis B patients in Chinese. Antiviral research 93: 297–300.
40. Lampertico P, Vigano M, Cheroni C, Facchetti F, Invernizzi F, et al. (2012) IL28B polymorphisms predict interferon-related HBsAg seroclearance in genotype D HBeAg-negative patients with chronic hepatitis B. Hepatology doi: 10.1002/hep.25749. [Epub ahead of print].
41. Pharm DT, Charlton M, Goldstein DB (2012) Introduction to the genetics and biology of IL28B. Hepatology 56: 361–6.
42. Morrow MP, Pankhong P, Laddy DJ, Schoenly KA, Yan J, et al. (2009) Comparative ability of IL-12 and IL-28B to regulate Treg populations and enhance adaptive cellular immunity. Blood 113: 5868–5877.
43. Lagging M, Askarieh G, Negro F, Bibert S, Soderholm J, et al. (2011) Response prediction in chronic hepatitis C by assessment of IP-10 and IL28B-related single nucleotide polymorphisms. PLoS One 6: e17232.

Biopsy-Controlled Liver Fibrosis Staging Using the Enhanced Liver Fibrosis (ELF) Score Compared to Transient Elastography

Kristin Wahl[1], William Rosenberg[2], Bernhard Vaske[3], Michael P. Manns[1], Klaus Schulze-Osthoff[4], Matthias J. Bahr[5], Heike Bantel[1]*

1 Department of Gastroenterology, Hepatology and Endocrinology, Hannover Medical School, Hannover, Germany, **2** Centre for Hepatology, University College London Institute of Liver and Digestive Health, Division of Medicine, University College London, London, United Kingdom, **3** Institute of Biometry, Hannover Medical School, Hannover, Germany, **4** Interfaculty Institute of Biochemistry, University of Tübingen, Tübingen, Germany, **5** Sana Kliniken, Lübeck, Germany

Abstract

Background and Aims: Chronic liver diseases are characterized by inflammatory and fibrotic liver injuries that often result in liver cirrhosis with its associated complications such as portal hypertension and hepatocellular carcinoma. Liver biopsy still represents the reference standard for fibrosis staging, although transient elastography is increasingly used for non-invasive monitoring of fibrosis progression. However, this method is not generally available and is associated with technical limitations emphasizing the need for serological biomarkers staging of liver fibrosis. The enhanced liver fibrosis (ELF) score was shown to accurately predict significant liver fibrosis in different liver diseases, although extracellular matrix components detected by this score may not only mirror the extent of liver fibrosis but also inflammatory processes.

Methods: In this prospective biopsy-controlled study we evaluated the utility of the ELF score in comparison to transient elastography to predict different stages of fibrosis in 102 patients with chronic liver diseases.

Results: Both techniques revealed similar area under receiver operating characteristic curve values for prediction of advanced fibrosis stages. Compared to transient elastography, the ELF score showed a broader overlap between low and moderate fibrosis stages and a stronger correlation with inflammatory liver injury.

Conclusions: Both the ELF score as well as transient elastography allowed for high quality fibrosis staging. However, the ELF score was less discriminative in low and moderate fibrosis stages and appeared more strongly influenced by inflammatory liver injury. This should be considered when making clinical interpretations on the basis of ELF score values.

Editor: Matias A. Avila, University of Navarra School of Medicine and Center for Applied Medical Research (CIMA), Spain

Funding: This study was supported by the Deutsche Forschungsgemeinschaft (SFB Transregio 77, SFB 685, BA 2092/9-1). The funders had no role in study design, data collection and analysis, decision to publish, or preparation of the manuscript.

Competing Interests: WR is an inventor of the ELF test and has received support for research studies and speaking events from Siemens Healthcare Diagnostics Inc. The proprietary assays developed for the ELF test by Siemens Healthcare Diagnostics Inc. (Tarrytown, New York, United States of America) were used and analyses were performed on an Immuno-1 auto-analyser (Siemens Healthcare Diagnostics Inc., Tarrytown, New York, United States of America). There are no further patents, products in development or marketed products to declare.

* E-mail: Bantel.Heike@mh-hannover.de

Introduction

Liver fibrosis is the consequence of a variety of chronic liver diseases and can result in liver cirrhosis. Early detection of fibrosis progression and development of cirrhosis are crucial for management of patients with chronic liver diseases since advanced fibrosis is associated with clinical complications and formation of hepatocellular carcinoma. Although liver biopsy remains the reference standard for evaluating liver fibrosis, it is limited by sampling errors and risk of complications [1,2]. In addition to sampling errors, intra- and interobserver variability may lead to misinterpretation of the fibrosis stage [3–6]. One reason for the difficulties in correctly assessing the fibrosis stages might base on biopsy specimen that only represents 1/50.000 of the total liver mass [1].

The liver volume explored by transient elastography is estimated to be 100 times larger compared to liver biopsy and might thus be more representative of the entire organ [7]. Fibrosis is a dynamic process and monitoring of fibrosis is desirable to obtain information not only about disease progression but also about treatment efficacy. Much attention has therefore been focused on the development of non-invasive methods to detect liver fibrosis. Measurement of liver stiffness by transient elastography is a widely accepted method for non-invasive liver disease staging. However, this technique is cost-intensive and its availability is largely limited to liver centers. Moreover, liver stiffness measurements can be difficult or impossible in obese patients, in those with narrow intercostal space or in patients with ascites [8] and a failure rate up to 18.9% has been reported following a review of 13,369 examinations over a 5-year period [9]. Substantial effort has been devoted to develop routine laboratory tests for fibrosis assessment, including the FibroTest®, Hepascore® and markers of extracellular matrix components or enzymes involved in their degradation or synthesis [10–15]. The combination of some of those parameters, such as hyaluronic acid (HA), tissue inhibitor of metalloproteinases-1 (TIMP-1) and aminoterminal propeptide of procollagen type III (PIIINP), has been recently proposed for fibrosis detection [16,17]. A simplified version of this panel – called enhanced liver fibrosis (ELF) score-was shown to accurately predict significant liver fibrosis in different liver diseases [11,18–21].

Extracellular matrix components may not only mirror the extent of liver fibrosis but are also involved in inflammatory processes. For instance, direct immunological impact of HA by regulating inflammatory cell recruitment and release of inflammatory cytokines has been described [22]. Vice versa, a variety of cytokines play a role in activating hepatic stellate cells for extracellular matrix production [23–25]. Moreover, hepatocyte apoptosis, which plays a role in inflammatory liver injury, has been mechanistically linked to stellate cell activation and increased fibrogenesis [26]. Activated hepatic stellate cells not only regulate fibrosis by secretion of extracellular matrix components but also induce an inflammatory response by expression of pro-inflammatory cytokines and receptors [27,28]. Thus, multiple pathways of interaction between extracellular matrix production and inflammatory responses exist.

In the present study we have evaluated the performance of the ELF test against transient elastography for non-invasive assessment of fibrosis in a prospective biopsy-controlled manner. In this context we have analyzed the influence of possible confounders, such as liver inflammation or steatosis, on fibrosis detection by ELF score and transient elastography.

Methods

Patient Characteristics and Analysis of Liver Fibrosis

We investigated sera from 102 patients (52% male, age 18–75 years, mean 46.6±1.3 years) with chronic liver diseases (viral hepatitis, n = 55; autoimmune hepatitis, n = 7; Wilson's diseases, n = 4; non-alcoholic fatty liver disease, n = 22; unknown origin, n = 14). Serum samples were analyzed for markers of the ELF score, including tissue inhibitor of matrix metalloproteinase 1 (TIMP-1), hyaluronic acid (HA), and amino-terminal propeptide of type III collagen (PIIINP). The proprietary assays developed for the ELF test by Siemens Healthcare Diagnostics Inc. (Tarrytown, New York, USA) were used and analyses were performed on an Immuno-1 auto-analyser (Siemens Healthcare Diagnostics Inc., Tarrytown, New York, USA). Results were entered into the established algorithm and expressed as score as described.[16] In addition to the ELF score alanine and aspartate aminotransferase (ALT, AST) levels were determined. At the time of blood withdrawal, all patients obtained liver biopsy and liver stiffness measurement using the Fibroscan (Echosens, Paris, France). The fibrosis stage (F1–F6) was determined according to Ishak *et al.* [29]. The percentage of liver steatosis was assessed by the same pathologist. Patients were divided in low (F0-1; n = 68), moderate (F2-4; n = 23) and severe fibrosis (F5-6; n = 11). Demographic and clinical features of the patients are shown in **Table 1**. No significant differences in ALT levels, percentage of steatosis and body mass index (BMI) were observed between the different fibrosis groups. All liver stiffness (LS) measurements were performed by a single experienced investigator (M.D.) as described [8]. The result of liver stiffness determination was expressed in kPa and was the median of at least 10 individual measurements with a success rate of >60%. Valid LS values were obtained for all patients included in this study. Written consent was obtained from the patients participating in this study, and the consent procedure and study were approved by the Ethics Committee of Hannover Medical School.

Statistical Analyses

Statistical analyses were performed by using Graphpad Prism 5.0 and SPSS 19.0 software and confirmed by a professional statistician. Data are presented as box plot and whiskers analysis as well as mean ± standard error of the mean (SEM). The results obtained with the different serum markers or liver stiffness measurements were compared using the Mann-Whitney's U test. Regression analyses were performed to calculate the Spearman rank correlation coefficient. Receiver operating characteristics (ROC) analysis was calculated. A P value <0.05 was considered significant. A multivariate logistic regression analysis was performed in order to adjust for variables found to be associated with fibrosis.

Results

Non-Invasive Assessment of Fibrosis Stages in Chronic Liver Diseases by ELF Test and Transient Elastography

The ELF test was compared with transient elastography for detection of different fibrosis stages in patients with chronic liver diseases (n = 102). Transient elastography allowed a better discrimination between low (F0-1; mean liver stiffness (LS) 6.9±0.4 kPa) and moderate (F2-4; mean LS 11.7±1.6 kPa) and between moderate and high fibrosis stages (F5-6; mean LS 27.3±4.8; **Figure 1A**) compared to the ELF score (F0-1: mean 8.6±0.1; F2-4: mean 9.3±0.3 and F5-6.11.0±0.3, **Figure 1B**). Although both noninvasive methods could significantly discriminate between the different fibrosis stages, transient elastography revealed a higher significance (p<0.001) to distinguish between low and moderate fibrosis stages compared to the ELF score (p<0.05). Accordingly, the ELF score showed a broad overlapping range of F0-1 (6.3–11.2) and F2-4 (7.6–12.9) which was not observed for transient elastography (F0-1:3.2–16.3 kPa and F2-4:4.0–43 kPa). In line with this observation, regression analyses showed a significant correlation between transient elastography or ELF score and ISHAK fibrosis stages as well as between transient elastography and ELF score (**Table 2**).

Table 1. Demographic and clinical features of patients with different stages of fibrosis.

ISHAK	F0-1	F2-4	F5-6
Patient No.	68	23	11
Mean age ± SEM	45.6±1.8	48.2±2.0	49.1±3.3
Sex (% male)	51.5	52.2	54.5
Steatosis (%)	17.9±3.1	23.7±4.6	14.3±5.3
ALT (U/L)	67.9±5.8	80.7±8.7	92.7±19.5
BMI (kg/m^2)	24.8±0.4	27.0±0.9	24.2±1.0
Biopsy Length (mm)	23.3±1.5	18.9±2.1	22.1±2.2

BMI, body mass index; SEM, standard error of the mean.

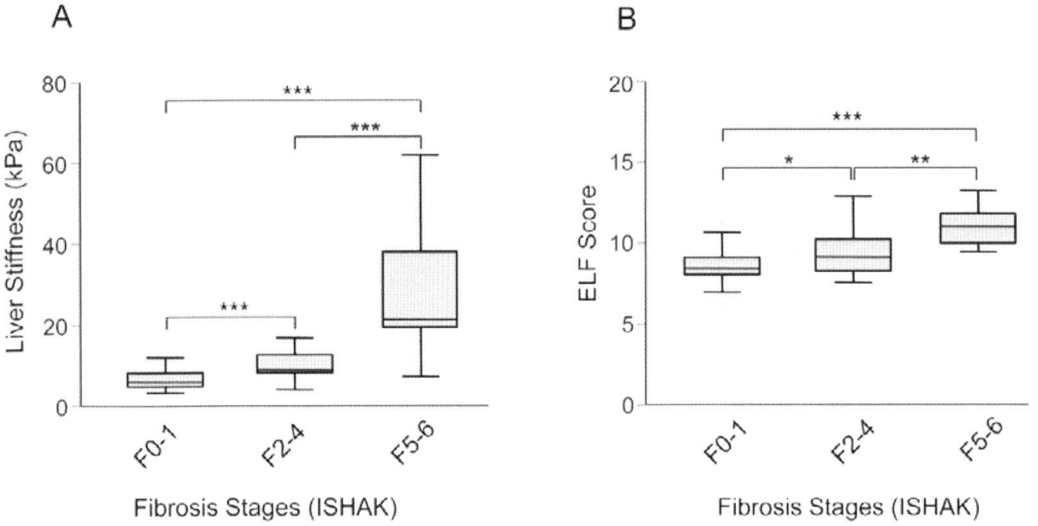

Figure 1. Measurement of liver stiffness by transient elastography and serological detection of ELF score in patients with chronic liver diseases and minimal (F0-1), moderate (F2-4) or high (F5-6) stages of fibrosis. Data are presented as box plots including medians and 25th and 75th percentiles. Both non-invasive methods can significantly discriminate between the different fibrosis stages. Transient elastography (A) allowed a better discrimination between minimal and moderate fibrosis stages ($p<0.01$) compared to ELF score (B; $p<0.05$). *$P<0.05$; **$P<0.01$; ***$P<0.001$. ELF, enhanced liver fibrosis.

Predictive Value of the ELF Score and Transient Elastography to Detect Clinically Relevant or Progressed Fibrosis Stages

We then calculated the cut-off values of the ELF Score and transient elastography to correctly predict clinically relevant stages of fibrosis (≥F2) or progressed fibrosis/cirrhosis (≥F5) with the best compromise sensitivity/specificity. To this end, we performed a ROC plot analysis including all patients (n = 102) with different fibrosis stages. The cut-off value of transient elastography of 8.5 kPa correctly predicted fibrosis stages of ≥F2 with a sensitivity of 86% and a specificity of 73% (AUC 0.92, confidence interval (CI) 95%: 0.85–0.98; **Figure 2A**). Similar results were obtained for the ELF score with a cut-off value of 8.99 that predicts clinically relevant fibrosis stages with a sensitivity of 86% and a specificity of 70% (AUC 0.87; CI95%: 0.78–0.96; **Figure 2B**). Compared to transient elastography that revealed with a cut-off value of 17.45 kPa a sensitivity of 91% and a specificity of 100% (AUC 0.95; CI95%: 0.87–1.0) for prediction of fibrosis stages of ≥F5 (**Figure 2C**), the ELF score showed a cut-off value (9.39) with higher sensitivity (100%) but lower specificity (77%; AUC 0.93; CI95%: 0.88–0.99; **Figure 2D**) for detection of progressed fibrosis/cirrhosis. However, the cut-off value of the ELF score to predict ≥F2 (8.99) was close to the cut-off value to predict ≥F5 (9.39). In contrast, the cut-off values of transient elastography for prediction of ≥F2 or ≥F5 fibrosis stages showed higher differences.

Table 2. Correlation of ELF score or liver stiffness measured by transient elastograpgy with histological fibrosis.

	ELF Score	Liver Stiffness	ISHAK F
ELF Score		r = 0.479**	r = 0.525**
Liver Stiffness	r = 0.479**		r = 0.587**
ISHAK F	r = 0.525**	r = 0.587**	

**Correlation is significant at the 0.01 level (2-tailed). ELF, enhanced liver fibrosis.

Influence of Liver Inflammation on Transient Elastography and ELF Score

To analyze a potential influence of liver inflammation on ELF score and transient elastography, we performed regression analyses comparing ALT or AST levels with ELF score and transient elastography. Both methods of fibrosis detection significantly correlated with AST and ALT levels (**Figure 3**). The ELF score showed a higher correlation with aminotransferase levels compared to transient elastography (**Table 3**). Similarly, the ELF score revealed a significantly higher correlation with inflammatory liver injury (ISHAK A-D) compared to transient elastography (**Table 3**). Thus, these data imply that the ELF score is more strongly influenced by inflammatory disease activity compared to transient elastography. In contrast to the ELF score, liver stiffness showed a weak but significant correlation with the percentage of liver steatosis (**Table 3**). To analyze the influence of inflammation or steatosis on prediction of relevant (≥F2) or progressed (≥F5) fibrosis stages, we performed a multivariate logistic regression analysis. This analysis showed that neither transient elastography nor the ELF score were significantly influenced by steatosis or inflammation (ISHAK A-D or ALT levels) in prediction of relevant or progressed fibrosis stages.

Discussion

Chronic liver diseases represent a substantial public health problem with a worldwide mortality of around 800.000 deaths per year [30]. A common pathological feature of chronic liver disease is fibrosis which is characterized by the progressive development of collagen-rich extracellular matrix and decreased matrix degradation due to an increase of inhibitors of matrix degradating enzymes, e.g. TIMPs [31]. Progression of liver fibrosis can result in liver cirrhosis with clinical complications due to loss of liver

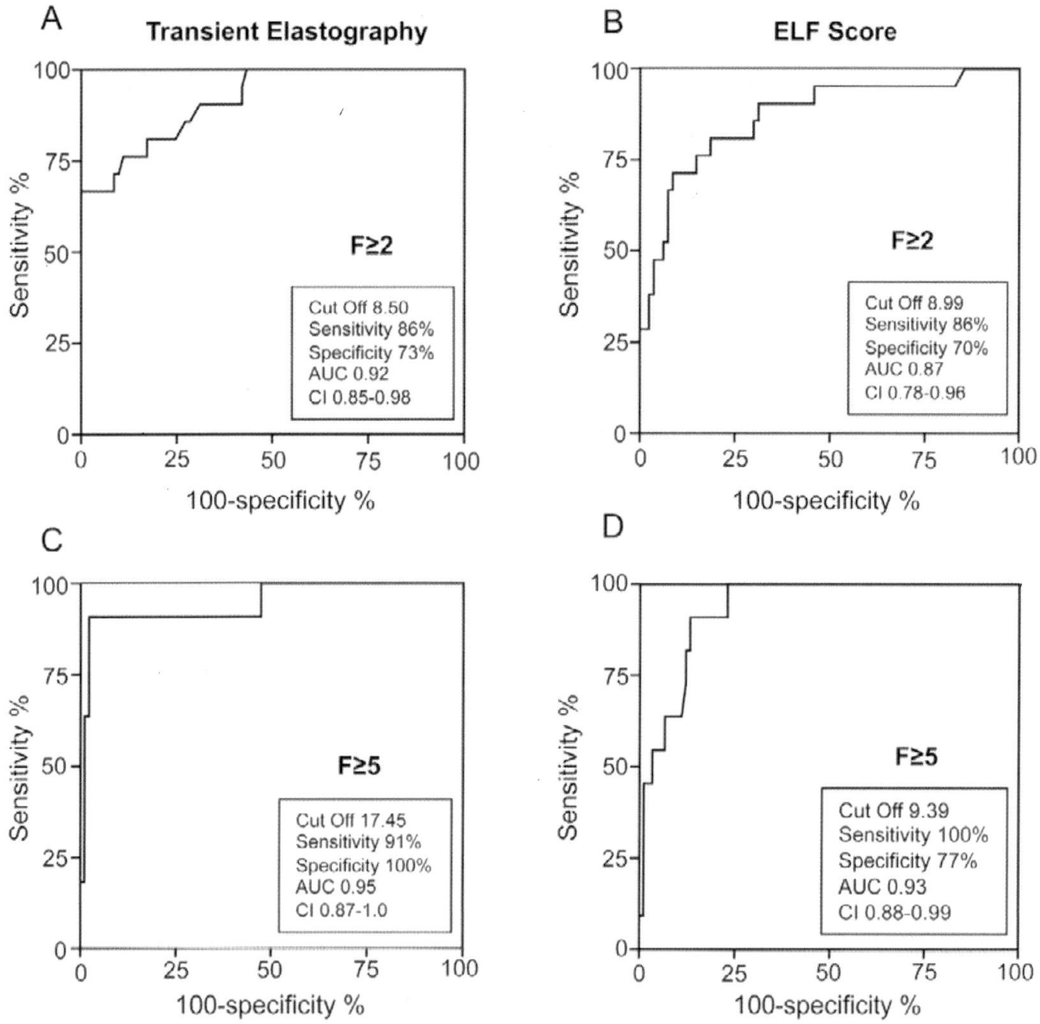

Figure 2. Prediction of relevant or advanced fibrosis stages by transient elastography and ELF score. The cut-off values of transient elastography (A, C) and ELF score (B, D) to predict fibrosis stages ≥F2 (A, B) or ≥F5 (C, D) with best compromise sensitivity/specificity were determined by ROC plot analysis. AUC, area under the curve; ELF, enhanced liver fibrosis; ROC, receiver operating characteristics.

function and portal hytertension. Advanced fibrosis/cirrhosis are also considered a pre-cancerous state that provides a microenvironment which allows for the development of hepatocellular carcinoma. Thus, screening for fibrosis progression with non-invasive methods in everyday general practice is required to identify patients with increased risk of developing liver cirrhosis and associated complications. Vice versa, there is increasing evidence indicating that successful treatment of various chronic liver diseases is associated with fibrosis regression [32]. Moreover, novel antifibrotic agents targeting different factors of fibrogenesis revealed promising results in animal models [33]. Monitoring of fibrosis regression during therapy of chronic liver diseases might be therefore also important for evaluation of treatment efficacy.

Ideally, non-invasive markers of liver fibrosis should be liver-specific and easy to perform with high diagnostic performance (compromise sensitivity/specificity) for accurate fibrosis staging. Among the most studied non-invasive detection methods of liver fibrosis is transient elastography. A prospective study in patients with chronic liver diseases demonstrated that measurement of liver stiffness by transient elastography is a reliable method to predict moderate or severe fibrosis stages, but shows less accuracay to differentiate between lower fibrosis stages according to METAVIR [7,34], which was in line with observations of other studies [35–37]. In our prospective study of patients with chronic liver diseases, transient elastography was able to significantly ($p<0.01$) discriminate not only between moderate and high but also between low and moderate fibrosis stages according to Ishak classification [29]. Differences in the applied fibrosis scores as well as interobserver variability might account for the lower overlapping range between minimal and moderate fibrosis stages observed in the present compared to the latter studies. Indeed, interobserver agreement for transient elastography was found to be significantly reduced in patients with lower degrees of hepatic fibrosis [38,39].

Compared to transient elastography, the ELF score revealed a lower significance ($p<0.05$) for discrimination between low and moderate fibrosis stages and showed a broad overlapping range for those stages. Nevertheless, AUC values for prediction of relevant fibrosis (≥F2) are high for both non-invasive methods with similar sensitivity and specificity. Both transient elastopgraphy and ELF score showed also a comparable high diagnostic accuracy to predict progressed fibrosis/cirrhosis (≥F5). The cut off-value of transient elastography for prediction of progressed fibrosis

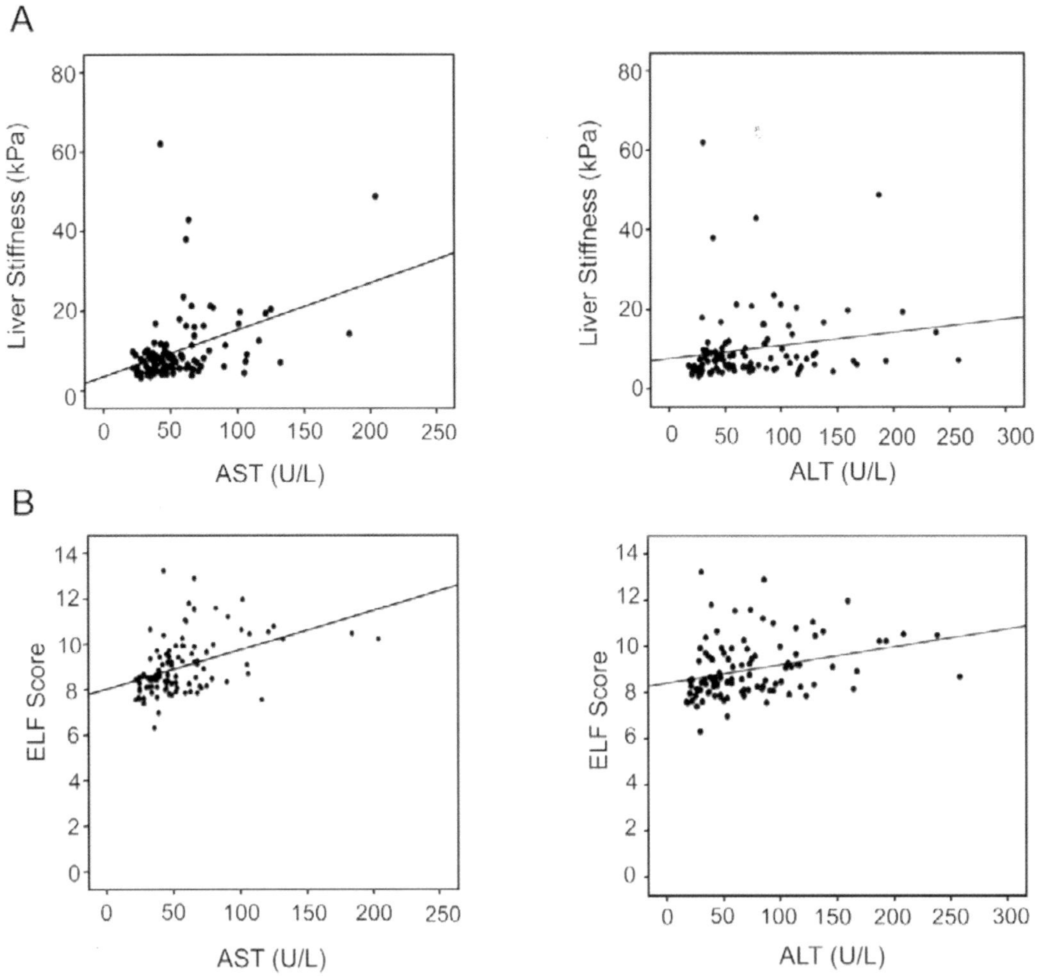

Figure 3. Regression analyses correlating liver stiffness measured by transient elastography or the ELF score with AST or ALT levels. A significant correlation (at 0.01/two tailed) was observed between liver stiffness (A) and AST or ALT levels as well as between ELF score (B) and AST or ALT levels. ALT, alanine aminotransferase; AST, aspartate aminotransferase; ELF, enhanced liver fibrosis.

evaluated in this study was nearly the same (17.5 kPa) compared to that (17.6 kPa) of a previous study [7]. However, transient elastography showed a lower sensitivity for detection of fibrosis ≥F5 compared to the ELF score.

A recent study showed lower diagnostic performance for transient elastography in detection of liver cirrhosis compared to lower fibrosis stages [40]. One explanation for this observation could be that liver stiffness measurement topographically reflects liver architecture which is characterized by fibrotic septa and regenerative nodules in cirrhosis. Moreover, the architecture of liver cirrhosis shows differences between various liver diseases which might influence the sensitivity of cirrhosis detection by transient elastography. In contrast to transient elastography, the ELF score showed a lower specificity to predict progressed fibrosis. In this context it is interesting to note that the ELF score showed a higher correlation with ALT levels and with histological inflammatory liver injury compared to transient elastography. Thus, inflammatory disease activity might account for the lower specificity to detect progressed fibrosis by the ELF score. This might also be the reason for the lower performance of the ELF score compared to transient elastography in prediction of advanced fibrosis which has been recently demonstrated in patients with chronic hepatitis B [41].

Table 3. Correlation of ELF score or liver stiffness measured by transient elastography with histological disease activity (ISHAK A-D), steatosis and aminotransferase levels.

	ELF Score	Liver Stiffness
AST	r = 0.475**	r = 0.431**
ALT	r = 0.362**	r = 0.297**
Steatosis %	r = 0.010	r = 0.257**
ISHAK A-D	r = 0.417**	r = 0.212*

Correlation is significant at the **0.01 or *0.05 level (2-tailed).
ELF, enhanced liver fibrosis.

There is also increasing evidence that liver stiffness is influenced by acute exacerbation of liver disease with ALT flares resulting in overestimation, e.g. up to three fold increase, of liver stiffness values [42–44]. Nevertheless, in acute liver failure it has been observed that liver stiffness correlates with tissue repair, e.g. markers of fibrogenesis [45]. However, we found a weaker correlation of transient elastography with ALT values and histological disease activity compared to the ELF score. This might be explained by the lack of disease flares with only moderately increased aminotransferase levels in the present study. In line with this observation, liver stiffness was not correlated with histological activity in chronic hepatitis C virus-infected patients that usually do not show ALT flares [35,36]. Instead, we found a weak but significant correlation of transient elastography with steatosis which was not observed with the ELF test.

It has been reported that liver stiffness values are higher in subjects with enhanced BMI or metabolic syndrome [39,46]. A multivariate analysis in patients with alcoholic liver disease showed a significant influence of steatosis on liver stiffness measurement [47]. In contrast, other studies did not reveal an influence of steatosis on fibrosis stage assessment by transient elastography [8,36,37]. Further studies are therefore needed to evaluate the influence of different grades of steatosis on liver stiffness measurements. A recently performed study comparing ultrasound-based methods with ELF score appeared confirming the diagnostic accuracy of those non-invasive methods for prediction of relevant fibrosis or cirrhosis [48]. However, the number of non-transplant patients with chronic liver diseases included in this study was lower (n = 59) compared to our study (n = 102), and unfortunately no information about possible variables that might influence fibrosis such as inflammation or steatosis was provided. Furthermore, the discriminative power of both methods for lower fibrosis stages, which is often relevant for clinical decision-making, remains unclear in this report.

Our present large biopsy-controlled prospective study showed that the ELF score reveals similar diagnostic accuracy to predict relevant (≥F2) or advanced (≥F5) stages of fibrosis compared with transient elastography. However, the cut-off values of the ELF score to predict relevant stages of fibrosis are close to the cut-off value for detection of progressed fibrosis whereas the respective cut-off values for transient elastography showed a higher difference. The ELF score appears less discriminative in lower fibrosis stages compared to transient elastography. Furthermore, the ELF score showed a higher correlation with inflammatory liver injury compared to transient elastography. These observations should be considered when making clinical interpretations or decisions on the base of ELF score values.

Author Contributions

Conceived and designed the experiments: HB, MJB, KSO, MPM, WR. Performed the experiments: KW, WR. Analyzed the data: HB, MJB, KSO, MPM, WR, KW, BV, MJB. Wrote the paper: HB, WR, KSO.

References

1. Bravo AA, Sheth SG, Chopra S (2001) Liver biopsy. N Engl J Med 344: 495–500.
2. Castéra L, Nègre I, Samii K, Buffet C (1999) Pain experienced during percutaneous liver biopsy. Hepatology 30: 1529–1530.
3. Bedossa P, Dargère D, Paradis V (2003) Sampling variability of liver fibrosis in chronic hepatitis C. Hepatology 38: 1449–1457.
4. Rousselet MC, Michalak S, Dupré F, Croué A, Bedossa P, et al. (2005) Sources of variability in histological scoring of chronic viral hepatitis. Hepatology 41: 257–264.
5. Afdhal NH (2003) Diagnosing fibrosis in hepatitis C: is the pendulum swinging from biopsy to blood tests? Hepatology 37: 972–974.
6. Regev A, Berho M, Jeffers LJ, Milikowski C, Molina EG, et al. (2002) Sampling error and intraobserver variation in liver biopsy in patients with chronic HCV infection. Am J Gastroenterol 97: 2614–2618.
7. Foucher J, Chanteloup E, Vergniol J, Castéra L, Le Bail B, et al. (2006) Diagnosis of cirrhosis by transient elastography (FibroScan): a prospective study. Gut 55: 403–408.
8. Sandrin L, Fourquet B, Hasquenoph JM, Yon S, Fournier C, et al. (2003) Transient elastography: a new non-invasive method for assessment of hepatic fibrosis. Ultrasound Med Biol 29: 1705–1713.
9. Castéra L, Foucher J, Bernard PH, Carvalho F, Allaix D, et al. (2010) Pitfalls of liver stiffness measurement: a 5-year prospective study of 13,369 examinations. Hepatology 51: 828–835.
10. Lichtinghagen R, Bahr MJ (2004) Noninvasive diagnosis of fibrosis in chronic liver disease. Expert Rev Mol Diagn 4: 715–726.
11. Parkes J, Guha IN, Roderick P, Rosenberg W (2006) Performance of serum marker panels for liver fibrosis in chronic hepatitis C. J Hepatol 44: 462–474.
12. Martínez SM, Crespo G, Navasa M, Forns X (2011) Noninvasive assessment of liver fibrosis. Hepatology 53: 325–335.
13. McHutchison JG, Blatt LM, de Medina M, Craig JR, Conrad A, et al. (2000) Measurement of serum hyaloronic acid in patients with chronic hepatitis C and its relationship to liver histology. Consensus Interferon Study Group. J Gastroenterol Hepatol 15: 945–951.
14. Lichtinghagen R, Huegel O, Seifert T, Haberkorn CI, Michels D, et al. (2000) Expression of matrix metalloproteinase-2 and -9 and their inhibitors in peripheral blood cells of patients with chronic hepatitis C. Clin Chem 46: 183–192.
15. Lebensztejn DM, Sobaniec-Lotowska ME, Bauer M, Kaczmarski M, Voelker M, et al. (2005) Serum fibrosis markers as predictors of an antifibrotic effect of interferon alfa in children with chronic hepatitis B. Eur J Gastroenterol Hepatol 17: 843–848.
16. Rosenberg WM, Voelker M, Thiel R, Becka M, Burt A, et al. (2004) Serum markers detect the presence of liver fibrosis: a cohort study. Gastroenterology 127: 1704–1713.
17. Sebastiani G, Alberti A (2006) Non invasive fibrosis biomarkers reduce but not substitute the need for liver biopsy. World J Gastroenterol 12: 3682–3694.
18. Nobili V, Parkes J, Bottazzo G, Marcellini M, Cross R, et al. (2009) Performance of ELF serum markers in predicting fibrosis stage in pediatric non-alcoholic fatty liver disease. Gastroenterology 136: 160–167.
19. Parkes J, Guha IN, Roderick P, Harris S, Cross R, et al. (2011) Enhanced Liver Fibrosis (ELF) test accurately identifies liver fibrosis in patients with chronic hepatitis C. J Viral Hepat 18: 23–31.
20. Friedrich-Rust M, Rosenberg W, Parkes J, Herrmann E, Zeuzem S, et al. (2010) Comparison of ELF, FibroTest and FibroScan for the non-invasive assessment of liver fibrosis. BMC Gastroenterol 10: 103.
21. Mayo MJ, Parkes J, Adams-Huet B, Combes B, Mills AS, et al. (2008) Prediction of clinical outcomes in primary biliary cirrhosis by serum enhanced liver fibrosis assay. Hepatology 48: 1549–1557.
22. Noble PW, Liang J, Jiang D (2011) Hyaluronan as an immune regulator in human diseases. Physiol Rev 91: 221–264.
23. Kong X, Horiguchi N, Mori M, Gao B (2012) Cytokines and STATs in Liver Fibrosis. Front Physiol 3: 69.
24. Cao Q, Mak KM, Ren C, Lieber CS (2004) Leptin stimulates tissue inhibitor of metalloproteinase-1 in human hepatic stellate cells: respective roles of the JAK/STAT and JAK-mediated H_2O_2-dependent MAPK pathways. J Biol Chem 279: 4292–4304.
25. Bataller R, Brenner DA (2005) Liver fibrosis. Clin Invest 115: 209–218.
26. Canbay A, Higuchi H, Bronk SF, Taniai M, Sebo TJ, et al. (2002) Fas enhances fibrogenesis in the bile duct ligated mouse: a link between apoptosis and fibrosis. Gastroenterology 123: 1323–1330.
27. Fadok VA, Bratton DL, Konowal A, Freed PW, Westcott JY, et al. (1998) Macrophages that have ingested apoptotic cells in vitro inhibit proinflammatory cytokine production through autocrine/paracrine mechanisms involving TGF-beta, PGE2, and PAF. J Clin Invest 101: 890–898.
28. Paik YH, Schwabe RF, Bataller R, Russo MP, Jobin C, et al. (2003) Toll-like receptor 4 mediates inflammatory signaling by bacterial lipopolysaccharide in human hepatic stellate cells. Hepatology 37: 1043–1055.
29. Ishak K, Baptista A, Bianchi L, Callea F, De Groote J, et al. (1995) Histological grading and staging of chronic hepatitis. J Hepatol 22: 696–699.
30. Williams R (2006) Global challenges in liver disease. Hepatology 44: 521–526.
31. Iredale JP (2007) Models of liver fibrosis: exploring the dynamic nature of inflammation and repair in a solid organ. J Clin Invest 117: 539–548.
32. Ellis EL, Mann DA (2012) Clinical evidence for the regression of fibrosis. J Hepatol 56: 1171–1180.
33. Kisseleva T, Brenner DA (2011) Anti-fibrogenic strategies and the regression of fibrosis. Best Pract Res Clin Gastroenterol 25: 305–317.
34. The French METAVIR Cooperative Study Group (1994) Intraobserver and interobserver variations in liver biopsy interpretation in patients with chronic hepatitis C. Hepatology 20: 15–20.
35. Castéra L, Vergniol J, Foucher J, Le Bail B, Chanteloup E, et al. (2005) Prospective comparison of transient elastography, Fibrotest, APRI, and liver biopsy for the assessment of fibrosis in chronic hepatitis C. Gastroenterology 128: 343–350.
36. Ziol M, Handra-Luca A, Kettaneh A, Christidis C, Mal F, et al. (2005) Noninvasive assessment of liver fibrosis by measurement of stiffness in patients with chronic hepatitis C. Hepatology 41: 48–54.
37. Wong VW, Vergniol J, Wong GL, Foucher J, Chan HL, et al. (2010) Diagnosis of fibrosis and cirrhosis using liver stiffness measurement in nonalcoholic fatty liver disease. Hepatology 51: 454–462.

38. Fraquelli M, Rigamonti C, Casazza G, Conte D, Donato MF, et al. (2007) Reproducibility of transient elastography in the evaluation of liver fibrosis in patients with chronic liver disease. Gut 56: 968–973.
39. Castéra L, Forns X, Alberti A (2008) Non-invasive evaluation of liver fibrosis using transient elastography. J Hepatol 48: 835–847.
40. Lee MH, Cheong JY, Um SH, Seo YS, Kim DJ, et al. (2010) Comparison of surrogate serum markers and transient elastography (Fibroscan) for assessing cirrhosis in patients with chronic viral hepatitis. Dig Dis Sci 55: 3552–3560.
41. Kim BK, Kim HS, Park JY, Kim do Y, Ahn SH, et al. (2012) Prospective validation of ELF test in comparison with Fibroscan and FibroTest to predict liver fibrosis in Asian subjects with chronic hepatitis B. PLoS One 7: e41964.
42. Coco B, Oliveri F, Maina AM, Ciccorossi P, Sacco R, et al. (2007) Transient elastography: a new surrogate marker of liver fibrosis influenced by major changes of transaminases. J Viral Hepat 14: 360–369.
43. Arena U, Vizzutti F, Corti G, Ambu S, Stasi C, et al. (2008) Acute viral hepatitis increases liver stiffness values measured by transient elastography. Hepatology 47: 380–384.
44. Sagir A, Erhardt A, Schmitt M, Häussinger D (2008) Transient elastography is unreliable for detection of cirrhosis in patients with acute liver damage. Hepatology 47: 592–595.
45. Dechêne A, Sowa JP, Gieseler RK, Jochum C, Bechmann LP, et al. (2010) Acute liver failure is associated with elevated liver stiffness and hepatic stellate cell activation. Hepatology 52: 1008–1016.
46. Roulot D, Czernichow S, Le Clésiau H, Costes JL, Vergnaud AC, et al. (2008) Liver stiffness values in apparently healthy subjects: influence of gender and metabolic syndrome. J Hepatol 48: 606–613.
47. Nahon P, Kettaneh A, Tengher-Barna I, Ziol M, de Lédinghen V, et al. (2008) Assessment of liver fibrosis using transient elastography in patients with alcoholic liver disease. J Hepatol 49: 1062–1068.
48. Crespo G, Fernández-Varo G, Mariño Z, Casals G, Miquel R, et al. (2012) ARFI, FibroScan®, ELF, and their combinations in the assessment of liver fibrosis: A prospective study. J Hepatol 57: 281–287.

28

The Frequency and Determinants of Liver Stiffness Measurement Failure: A Retrospective Study of "Real-Life" 38,464 Examinations

Dong Ji[1¶], Qing Shao[1¶], Ping Han[2], Fan Li[1], Bing Li[1], Hong Zang[3], Xiaoxia Niu[1], Zhongbin Li[1], Shaojie Xin[3]*, Guofeng Chen[1]*

1 Liver Fibrosis Diagnosis and Treatment Center, 302 Military Hospital of China, Beijing, China, **2** Tumor Radiotherapy Center, 302 Military Hospital of China, Beijing, China, **3** Liver Failure Diagnosis and Treatment Center, 302 Military Hospital of China, Beijing, China

Abstract

Objective: To investigate the frequency and determinants of liver stiffness measurement (LSM) failure by means of FibroScan in "real-life" Chinese patients.

Methods: A total of 38,464 "real-life" Chinese patients in 302 military hospital of China through the whole year of 2013, including asymptomatic carrier, chronic hepatitis B, chronic hepatitis C, liver cirrhosis (LC), alcoholic liver disease, autoimmune liver disease, hepatocellular carcinoma (HCC) and other, were enrolled, their clinical and biological parameters were retrospectively investigated. Liver fibrosis was evaluated by FibroScan detection. S probe (for children with height less than 1.20 m) and M probe (for adults) were used. LSM failure defined as zero valid shots (unsuccessful LSM), or the ratio of the interquartile range to the median of 10 measurements (IQR/M) greater than 0.30 plus median LSM greater or equal to 7.1 kPa (unreliable LSM).

Results: LSM failure occurred in 3.34% of all examinations (1286 patients out of 38,464), among them, there were 958 cases (2.49%) with unsuccessful LSM, and 328 patients (0.85%) with unreliable LSM. Statistical analyses showed that LSM failure was independently associated with body mass index (BMI) greater than 30 kg/m^2, female sex, age greater than 50 years, intercostal spaces (IS) less than 9 mm, decompensated liver cirrhosis and HCC patients. There were no significant differences among other diseases. By changing another skilled operator, success was achieved on 301 cases out of 1286, which reduced the failure rate to 2.56%, the decrease was significant ($P<0.0001$).

Conclusions: The principal reasons of LSM failure are ascites, obesity and narrow of IS. The failure rates of HCC, decompensated LC, elder or female patients are higher. These results emphasize the need for adequate operator training, technological improvements and optimal criteria for specific patient subpopulations.

Editor: Do Young Kim, Yonsei University College of Medicine, Republic of Korea

Funding: This work was supported by Beijing Natural Science Foundation (7122177, http://www.bjnsf.org/) and National Natural Science Foundation of China (81371799, http://www.nsfc.gov.cn/). The funders had no role in study design, data collection and analysis, decision to publish, or preparation of the manuscript.

Competing Interests: The authors have declared that no competing interests exist.

* Email: XinShaojie302@163.com (SJX); bjchen302@aliyun.com (GFC)

¶ These authors contributed equally to this work.

Introduction

Formation and accumulation of fibrosis in the liver is the common pathway of chronic liver diseases (CLD) that represent a major cause of morbidity and mortality worldwide. An accurate assessment of the extent of liver fibrosis is important for predicting the prognosis and determining the appropriate management of patients with CLD [1–4]. Until recently, liver biopsy (LB) is still considered as the best way for this purpose, and remains the gold standard in assessing liver histology. Although percutaneous LB is a safe procedure, it is an invasive one with rare but potentially life-threatening complications, resulting which can lead to treatment delay. Ultimately, its accuracy has been questioned because of sampling errors and inter- or intra-observer variability. So, noninvasive techniques have developed recently and become more popular every day due to better patient compliance. Liver stiffness measurement (LSM) using FibroScan (Echosens, Paris, France) is one of these novel noninvasive methods for assessing liver fibrosis and therefore cirrhosis, both in chronic hepatitis C and other CLD [5–9]. A LSM was considered reliable if the ratio of the interquartile range to the median of 10 measurements (IQR/M) less than 0.3, or IQR/M >0.30 with median liver stiffness <7.1 kPa. The diagnostic accuracy of FibroScan is excellent for cirrhosis and mild fibrosis. Because FibroScan is a user-friendly technique that can be performed rapidly at bedside, with immediate results and high acceptance of patients and physicians, it is likely to become an important tool in clinical practice in the near future [10–15].

However, FibroScan has its own limitation: its results may be influenced by high alanine aminotransferase (ALT) level and extrahepatic cholestasis. In addition, FibroScan is difficult in patients with obesity, narrow intercostal spaces, or ascites [16–19]. In this study, we retrospectively investigated the frequency and determinants of LSM failure in "real-life" Chinese patients, based on 38,464 examinations.

Patients and Methods

Patients

The cohort study included 38,464 "real-life" patients with CLD due to various causes, who had undergone FibroScan detection at 302 military hospital of China, Beijing, China, through a whole year of 2013. Hepatitis B (HBV) or C (HCV) virus infection was diagnosed by serological detection of HBV surface antigen and HCV antibody, and was based on 2012 Asian-Pacific consensus statement on the management of chronic hepatitis B issued by Asian Pacific Association for the study of the liver and 2011 European HCV clinical practice guidelines issued by European association for the study of the liver [20,21], respectively. Alcoholic liver disease (ALD) was diagnosed in patients with consumption of at least 40 g alcohol daily for at least 5 years. The diagnosis of hepatocellular carcinoma (HCC) was established using combination of elevated AFP and typical findings on tri-phasic CT or MRI. Other diseases were diagnosed according to the current criteria. LSMs are median values of successful acquisitions. The following clinical and biological parameters were recorded at the time of LSM: age, sex, body mass index (BMI), intercostal space (IS), and ALT.

The written informed consents were obtained from all patients for their clinical records to be used in this study, and their information was anonymized and de-identified prior to analysis. The study was approved by ethics committee of 302 military hospital of China and was conducted in accordance with the ethical standards formulated in the Helsinki Declaration.

Liver stiffness measurement

Liver stiffness was measured using FibroScan device (Echosens, Paris, France) according to the manufacturer's instructions. Measurements were performed on the right lobe of the liver through the IS with patients lying in a dorsal decubitus with the right arm in maximal abduction. S probe (for children with height less than 1.20 m) and M probe (for adults) were used. The tip of the transducer probe was covered with coupling gel and placed on the skin, between the ribs at the level of the right lobe of the liver. The operator, assisted by a time-motion ultrasound image, located a liver portion that was at least 6-cm thick and free of large vascular structures. When the target area had been located, the operator pressed the probe button to commence the measurements. Ten validated measurements were performed on each patient. The results were expressed in kilopascals (kPa), with a higher value reflecting a stiffer liver and more severe liver fibrosis. The results were considered failure when no value was obtained after at least 10 shots (unsuccessful LSM), or when the IQR/M greater than 0.30 plus median LSM greater or equal to 7.1 kPa (unreliable LSM). If a patient had a LSM failure, the second LSM examination was performed with another skilled operator at least 2 days, but no longer than 1 week after first examination.

Statistical analysis

All statistical analyses were performed using the SPSS version 19.0 (SPSS Inc., Chicago, IL, USA). In descriptive analyses, continuous variables were expressed as mean ± standard deviation and categorical variables as absolute figures and percentages. Chi-squared test was used for categorical variables and Fisher's exact test when appropriate. Continuous variables with skewed distribution were analyzed using Mann-Whitney test. Factors significantly associated with the outcome in univariate analyses were entered in a multivariate logistic model. Odd ratios were estimated from the model and are given with their 95% confidence intervals (CI). A *P*-value of <0.05 was considered significant.

Results

Patient characteristics

A total of 38,464 examinations were performed, mean age was 43.5±12.2 years (from 11 to 90 years), 13112 (34.1%) of patient was older than 50 years, 9541 (24.8%) were females, mean BMI was 24.2±3.4 kg/m^2, 3536 (9.2%) were obesity (BMI≥30 kg/m^2). The median (IQR) of LSM value and ALT were 7.6 (5.5–12.3) kPa and 39 (23–89) IU/ml. The mean examination duration was 4 min and 35 seconds.

The distribution of enrolled patients grouped by years was almost normal one, the percentage of patients with 40–49 years old was the highest (32.5%), and there were significant differences on FibroScan values according to age groups (Figure 1A).

Based on BMI, there were no differences among patients with BMI<30 kg/m^2, however, for those patients with BMI≥30 kg/m^2, LSM value raised with their BMI increasing significantly (Figure 1B).

Indications for LSM by means of FibroScan were chronic asymptomatic HBV carrier (AsC) 0.6%, chronic viral hepatitis (CH) 65.4%, compensated liver cirrhosis related to viral hepatitis (LC-1) 22.7%, decompensated LC related to viral hepatitis (LC-2) 3.1%, alcoholic liver disease (ALD) 2.5%, autoimmune liver disease (AILD) 2.8%, drug-induced liver injure (DILIN) 1.1%, hepatocellular carcinoma (HCC) 1.5%, and other diseases (including liver Transplant Recipient, hepatolenticular degeneration, and Budd-chiari syndrome) 0.3%. With the progress of chronic viral hepatitis, the LSM value increased significantly (P< 0.0001) (Figure 1C).

Frequency of LSM Failure in the total population

Overall, LSM failed in 1286 patients (3.34%), which included 958 cases (2.5%) with unsuccessful LSM, and 328 cases (0.9%) with unreliable LSM (Figure 2A). Mean age of these 1286 patients was 51.1±9.5 years, 869(67.6%) were females. LSM values were obtained in 37178 (96.66%) patients. LSM failure ranged from 1.90% in AsC patients to 12.36% in patient with decompensated LC (most of them with obvious ascites), Chi-squared test showed that LSM failure rate was statistical significant high in decompensated LC and HCC patients ($P<0.0001$) compared with the total failure rate (3.34%) (Figure 2B). On second examination (at least two days, but no longer than one week after first examination) by changing another skilled operator, the fail rate reduced to 2.56% (985 cases).

Factors associated with LSM failure

Altogether five factors showed significant association with LSM failure, the distribution of these 5 factors is presented in Figure 3A. Multivariate analysis showed that LSM failure was independently associated with the following factors: ascites (OR 13.475, 95% CI

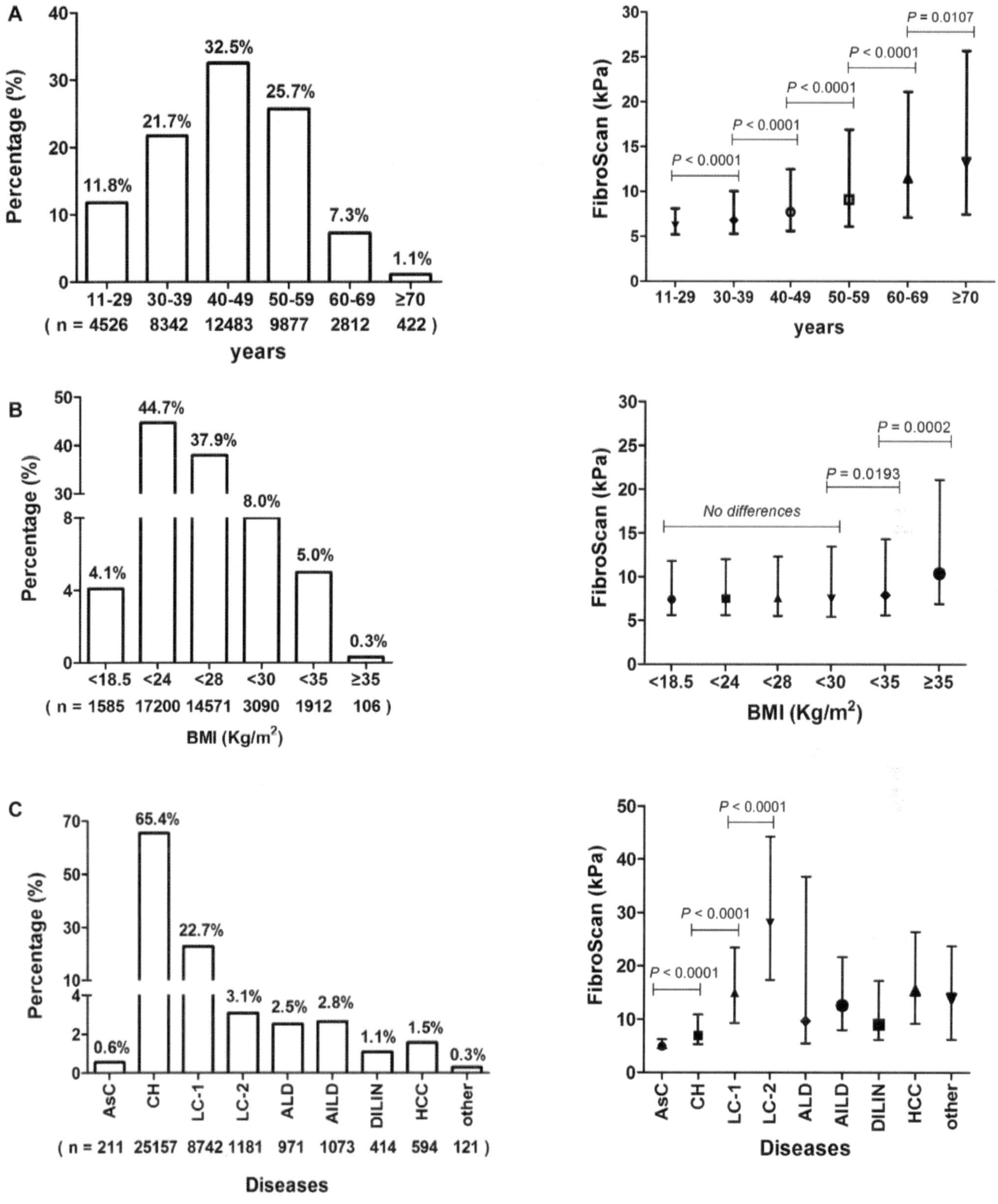

Figure 1. Summary of 38,464 LSM examinations according to age, BMI, and diseases group. LSM values are presented as median (interquartile range). Nonparametric test (Mann-Whitney test) is used to analyze the differences between each two groups. Patients' percentage and FibroScan value distribution are analyzed according to age (A), BMI (B), and diseases (C) group. AsC, chronic asymptomatic HBV carrier; CH, chronic hepatitis; LC-1, compensated liver cirrhosis; LC-2, decompensated liver cirrhosis; ALD, alcoholic liver disease; AILD, autoimmune liver disease; DILIN, drug-induced liver injure; HCC, hepatocellular carcinoma (HCC); other includes liver transplant recipient, hepatolenticular degeneration, and Budd-chiari syndrome.

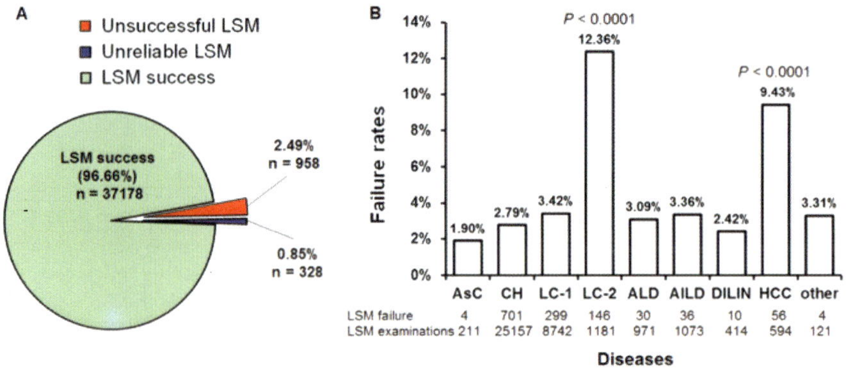

Figure 2. Frequency of LSM failure according to different diseases. LSM failure rate in 38,464 LSM examinations is overviewed (A), and Chi-square test is applied to find the unsuccessful and unreliable LSM rate differences between each disease group and the total failure rate (B). AsC, chronic asymptomatic HBV carrier; CH, chronic hepatitis; LC-1, compensated liver cirrhosis; LC-2, decompensated liver cirrhosis; ALD, alcoholic liver disease; AILD, autoimmune liver disease; DILIN, drug-induced liver injure; HCC, hepatocellular carcinoma (HCC); other includes liver transplant recipient, hepatolenticular degeneration, and Budd-chiari syndrome.

5.594–32.456), BMI greater than 30 kg/m^2 (OR 6.902, 95% CI 2.632–18.179), age older than 50 years (OR 6.571, 95% CI 2.671–16.169), IS narrower than 9 mm (OR 5.435, 95% CI 2.191–13.483), and female (OR 3.074, 95% CI 1.219–7.757). Univariate analysis had the similar results (Figure 3B).

Discussion

Hepatic fibrosis is the final result of CLD and is a wound healing process similar to those observed in other organs. So, early diagnosis of fibrosis or cirrhosis is an important clinical issue, as it is a pivotal factor in determining a treatment plan for antiviral therapy and predicting the overcome of CLD [22–24]. LSM was first studied in Western populations with chronic hepatitis C. Recently, it has been used in the assessment of other hepatic fibrosis-related non-HCV etiologies such as HBV, ALD, AILD and non-alcoholic hepatitis [25–28]. All of these studies have shown that LSM values correlate strongly with METAVIR fibrosis staging by LB. LSM is measured through a device that is called FibroScan which is composed of an ultrasound transducer probe mounted on the axis of a vibrator. Vibrations of mild amplitude and low frequency are transmitted by the transducer, inducing an elastic shear wave that propagates through the underlying tissues. Pulse echo ultrasound acquisition is used to follow the propagation of the shear wave and to measure its velocity, which is directly related to tissue stiffness: the stiffer the tissue, the faster the shear wave propagates. FibroScan measures liver stiffness in a volume that is approximately a cylinder 1 cm wide and 4 cm long, between 2.5 cm and 6.5 cm below the skin surface. This volume is at least 100 times bigger than a biopsy sample. FibroScan examination is painless, rapid (less than 5 min) method with a steep learning curve and requires the experience of only 50–100 examinations to be able to make proficient determinations, which is easy to perform at the bedside or in the outpatient clinic. In various studies, the accuracy of FibroScan results was similar to that of serum non-invasive markers for the diagnosis of significant fibrosis, sometimes with inadequate figures (<80%), and showed excellent performance for the diagnosis of cirrhosis.

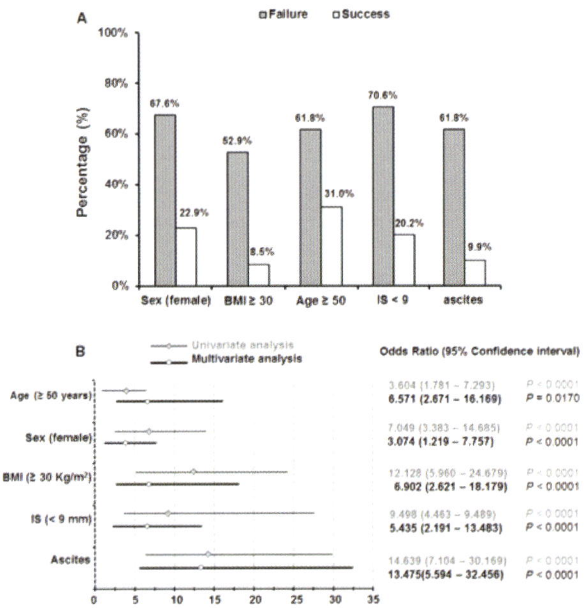

Figure 3. Distribution of factors significantly associated with LSM failure. Patients' percentage distribution according to the factors associated with LSM failure is showed (A), and the significances were determined by univariate and multivariate analyses (B). Intercostal space (IS).

Over the last few years, LSM has been increasingly used as a noninvasive measurement for the assessment of liver fibrosis and even adopted as first-line screening tool for patients with CLD. Although the usefulness of LSM has been established, there is relatively limited data on its failure. The current study is to clarify the reason of LSM failure and comprehend the factors contributed to LSM failure. LSM can be difficult in obese patients or in those with narrow IS and impossible in patients with ascites. Failure rates range between 2.4% and 9.4% in the different studies [29–32].

In the present study, we could not obtain 1286 valid measurements in 38,464 examinations, which led to a failure rate of 3.34%. Among them, there were 958 cases (2.5%) with unsuccessful LSM, and 328 cases (0.9%) with unreliable LSM. These data were similar as to the previous study which also performed in Chinese patients [33]. A significant decrease in the failure rate was observed in patients undergoing second examination (3.34% at 1st versus 2.56% at 2nd examination, $P<0.0001$). To address the reasons for a higher successful LSM on 2nd examination, we thought that the experience of operators (e.g.

probe positioning, probe pressure) might be a major factor, but patients body position, respiratory movements or even patients' psychological state also could influence the results of LSM, the impacts of these factors need more researches to be clarified.

Regarding the etiologies of CLD, we found that the failure rates in decompensated LC and HCC patients were significant higher than other diseases, which might be associated with ascites complication in decompensated LC patients and uneven distribution of liver parenchyma of HCC patients. We also found that LSM is more difficult in patients with IS narrower than 9 mm compared with those normal IS patients. These results suggest that operator experience might be important to gain the valid results, and operators should be fully trained before work in clinic.

Another important determinant of LSM failure was obesity (BMI≥30 kg/m^2). Our study showed that 52.9% of LSM failure was patient with BMI more than 30 kg/m^2, while only 8.5% in LSM success. The reason we supposed that obesity patients are large waist circumference, and the subcutaneous and prehepatic fat thickness is increased, attenuating both elastic waves and ultrasound and making LSM impossible with a regular probe that is calibrated for a given distance between the liver and the chest wall. Recently, the manufacturer of transient elastography developed a new XL probe for obese patients, it is possible to generate low-frequency ultrasound to evaluate deeper liver tissue. A study showed the success rate of measurement by XL probe can be as high as 90% even in obese patients [34]. Another study of 193 consecutive nonalcoholic fatty liver disease (NAFLD) patients (35% patients with BMI≥30 kg/m^2) showed that XL probe was more likely to achieve 10 valid measurements compared with M probe (95% vs. 81%; $P<0.001$) in these patients, and among patients with BMI≥30 kg/m^2, 93% had successful LSM using XL probe, compared with only 60% when M probe was used ($P<0.0001$). The study also emphasized that because validation data on XL probe are less extensive than those on M probe (XL probe tends to generate higher IQR/M), M probe should be used in all patients as first line. In the patients who failed M probe measurements, XL probe could be used as a salvage technique to ensure higher successful measurements in most obese patients [35]. The other important point is that LSM values obtained with XL probe were typically 1.0–2.0 kPa lower than those obtained with M probe [36,37], So in order to improve the diagnosis accuracy of XL probe for obese patients, more clinical researches should be performed to set up the optimal criteria and standard procedure of XL probe examination.

LSM failure rate is relatively high in patients with HCC and decompensated LC, IS narrower than 9 mm, BMI more than 30 kg/m^2, female sex, and age older than 50 years, these results emphasize the need for adequate operator training, technological improvements, and optimal protocol establishment in specific patient subpopulations.

In conclusion, LSM by means of FibroScan is a promising, reproducible noninvasive technique of evaluation which could be used in numerous clinical situations, and efforts should be made to avoid examination failure and set up the standard of its practice.

Acknowledgments

We thank Ya Li, Qiaomin Wang, and Huidan Cui for their excellent technical assistance.

Author Contributions

Conceived and designed the experiments: SJX GFC. Performed the experiments: DJ QS PH BL HZ XXN. Analyzed the data: DJ. Contributed reagents/materials/analysis tools: FL ZBL. Contributed to the writing of the manuscript: DJ.

References

1. Singh S, Fujii LL, Murad MH, Wang Z, Asrani SK, et al. (2013) Liver Stiffness Is Associated With Risk of Decompensation, Liver Cancer, and Death in Patients With Chronic Liver Diseases: A Systematic Review and Meta-analysis. Clin Gastroenterol Hepatol 11: 1573–1584.
2. Povero D, Busletta C, Novo E, di Bonzo LV, Cannito S, et al. (2010) Liver fibrosis: a dynamic and potentially reversible process. Histol Histopathol 25: 1075–1091.
3. Ferraioli G, Tinelli C, Dal Bello B, Zicchetti M, Lissandrin R, et al. (2013) Performance of liver stiffness measurements by transient elastography in chronic hepatitis. World J Gastroenterol 19: 49–56.
4. Castera L (2012) Noninvasive methods to assess liver disease in patients with hepatitis B or C. Gastroenterology 142: 1293–1302.
5. Duarte-Rojo A, Altamirano JT, Feld JJ (2012) Noninvasive markers of fibrosis: key concepts for improving accuracy in daily clinical practice. Ann Hepatol 11: 426–439.
6. Sanchez-Conde M, Montes-Ramirez ML, Miralles P, Alvarez JM, Bellón JM, et al. (2010) Comparison of transient elastography and liver biopsy for the assessment of liver fibrosis in HIV/hepatitis C virus-coinfected patients and correlation with noninvasive serum markers. J Viral Hepat 17: 280–286.
7. Afdhal NH (2012) Fibroscan (transient elastography) for the measurement of liver fibrosis. Gastroenterol Hepatol (NY), 8: 605–607.
8. Wong GL (2013) Transient elastography: Kill two birds with one stone? World J Hepatol 5: 264–274.
9. Kumar R, Rastogi A, Sharma MK, Bhatia V, Tyagi P, et al. (2013) Liver stiffness measurements in patients with different stages of nonalcoholic fatty liver disease: diagnostic performance and clinicopathological correlation. Dig Dis Sci 58: 265–274.
10. Kim SU, Lee JH, Kim do Y, Ahn SH, Jung KS, et al. (2012) Prediction of liver-related events using fibroscan in chronic hepatitis B patients showing advanced liver fibrosis. PLoS One 7:e36676.
11. Saad Y, Said M, Idris MO, Rabee A, Zakaria S (2013) Liver stiffness measurement by fibroscan predicts the presence and size of esophageal varices in egyptian patients with HCV related liver cirrhosis. J Clin Diagn Res 7: 2253–2257.
12. Crespo G, Fernández-Varo G, Mariño Z, Casals G, Miquel R, et al. (2012) ARFI, FibroScan, ELF, and their combinations in the assessment of liver fibrosis: a prospective study. J Hepatol 57: 281–287.
13. Sporea I, Nicolita D, Sirli R, Deleanu A, Tudora A, et al. (2011) Assessment of noninvasive liver stiffness in inactive HBsAg carriers by transient elastography: Fibroscan in inactive HBsAg carriers. Hepat Mon 11: 182–185.
14. Kim SU, Kim JK, Park YN, Han KH (2012) Discordance between liver biopsy and Fibroscan in assessing liver fibrosis in chronic hepatitis b: risk factors and influence of necroinflammation. PLoS One 7:e32233.
15. Kim SU, Kim do Y, Park JY, Lee JH, Ahn SH, et al. (2010) How can we enhance the performance of liver stiffness measurement using FibroScan in diagnosing liver cirrhosis in patients with chronic hepatitis B? J Clin Gastroenterol 44: 66–71.
16. Osaki A, Kubota T, Suda T, Igarashi M, Nagasaki K, et al. (2010) Shear wave velocity is a useful marker for managing nonalcoholic steatohepatitis. World J Gastroenterol 16: 2918–2925.
17. Buster EH, Hansen BE, Lau GK, Piratvisuth T, Zeuzem S, et al. (2009) Factors that predict response of patients with hepatitis B e antigen-positive chronic hepatitis B to peginterferon-alfa. Gastroenterology 137: 2002–2009.
18. Marcellin P, Ziol M, Bedossa P, Douvin C, Poupon R, et al. (2009) Non-invasive assessment of liver fibrosis by stiffness measurement in patients with chronic hepatitis B. Liver Int 29: 242–247.
19. Janssens E, Spahr L, Rubbia-Brandt L, Giostra E, Bihl F (2010) Hepatic amyloidosis increases liver stiffness measured by transient elastography. Acta Gastroenterol Belg 73: 52–54.
20. Liaw YF, Kao JH, Piratvisuth T, Chan HLY, Chien RN, et al. (2012) Asian-Pacific consensus statement on the management of chronic hepatitis B: a 2012 update. Hepatol Int 6: 531–561.
21. European Association of the Study of the Liver (2012) 2011 European Association of the Study of the Liver hepatitis C virus clinical practice guidelines. Liver Int 32: 2–8.
22. Fraquelli M, Rigamonti C (2007) Diagnosis of cirrhosis by transient elastography: what is hidden behind misleading results. Hepatology 46: 282.
23. Forestier J, Dumortier J, Guillaud O, Ecochard M, Roman S, et al. (2010) Noninvasive diagnosis and prognosis of liver cirrhosis: a comparison of biological scores, elastometry, and metabolic liver function tests. Eur J Gastroenterol Hepatol 22: 532–540.
24. Kim BK, Han KH, Park JY, Ahn SH, Chon CY, et al. (2010) A novel liver stiffness measurement-based prediction model for cirrhosis in hepatitis B patients. Liver Int 30: 1073–1081.

25. Millonig G, Reimann FM, Friedrich S, Fonouni H, Mehrabi A, et al. (2008) Extrahepatic cholestasis increases liver stiffness (FibroScan) irrespective of fibrosis. Hepatology 48: 1718–1723.
26. Kim SU, Ahn SH, Park JY, Kang W, Kim do Y, et al. (2009) Liver stiffness measurement in combination with noninvasive markers for the improved diagnosis of B-viral liver cirrhosis. J Clin Gastroenterol 43: 267–271.
27. Corpechot C, El Naggar A, Poujol-Robert A, Ziol M, Wendum D, et al. (2006) Assessment of biliary fibrosis by transient elastography in patients with PBC and PSC. Hepatology 43: 1118–1124.
28. Lemoine M, Katsahian S, Ziol M, Nahon P, Ganne-Carrie N, et al. (2008) Liver stiffness measurement as a predictive tool of clinically significant portal hypertension in patients with compensated hepatitis C virus or alcoholrelated cirrhosis. Aliment Pharmacol Ther 28: 1102–1110.
29. Nahon P, Kettaneh A, Tengher-Barna I, Ziol M, de Lédinghen V, et al. (2008) Assessment of liver fibrosis using transient elastography in patients with alcoholic liver disease. J Hepatol 49: 1062–1068.
30. Kirk GD, Astemborski J, Mehta SH, Spoler C, Fisher C, et al. (2009) Assessment of liver fibrosis by transient elastography in persons with hepatitis C virus infection or HIV-hepatitis C virus coinfection. Clin Infect Dis 48: 963–972.
31. Fraquelli M, Rigamonti C, Casazza G, Conte D, Donato MF, et al. (2007) Reproducibility of transient elastography in the evaluation of liver fbrosis in patients with chronic liver disease. Gut 56: 968–973.
32. Castera L, Forns X, Alberti A (2008) Non-invasive evaluation of liver fibrosis using transient elastography. J Hepatol 48: 835–847.
33. Wong GL, Wong VW, Chim AM, Yiu KK, Chu SH, et al. (2011) Factors associated with unreliable liver stiffness measurement and its failure with transient elastography in the Chinese population. J Gastroenterol Hepatol 26: 300–305.
34. Myers RP, Pomier-Layrargues G, Kirsch R, Pollett A, Duarte-Rojo A, et al. (2012) Feasibility and diagnostic performance of the FibroScan XL probe for liver stiffness measurement in overweight and obese patients. Hepatology 55: 199–208.
35. Wong VW, Vergniol J, Wong GL, Foucher J, Chan AW, et al. (2012) Liver stiffness measurement using XL probe in patients with nonalcoholic fatty liver disease. Am J Gastroenterol 107: 1862–1871.
36. de Lédinghen V, Vergniol J, Foucher J, El-Hajbi F, Merrouche W, et al. (2010) Feasibility of liver transient elastography with FibroScan using a new probe for obese patients. Liver Int 30: 1043–1048.
37. Friedrich-Rust M, Hadji-Hosseini H, Kriener S, Herrmann E, Sircar I, et al. (2010) Transient elastography with a new probe for obese patients for non-invasive staging of nonalcoholic steatohepatitis. Eur Radiol 20: 2390–2396.

29

New Susceptibility and Resistance HLA-DP Alleles to HBV-Related Diseases Identified by a Trans-Ethnic Association Study in Asia

Nao Nishida[1,2*¶], Hiromi Sawai[2¶], Koichi Kashiwase[3], Mutsuhiko Minami[3], Masaya Sugiyama[1], Wai-Kay Seto[4], Man-Fung Yuen[4], Nawarat Posuwan[5], Yong Poovorawan[5], Sang Hoon Ahn[6], Kwang-Hyub Han[6], Kentaro Matsuura[7], Yasuhito Tanaka[7], Masayuki Kurosaki[8], Yasuhiro Asahina[9,10], Namiki Izumi[8], Jong-Hon Kang[11], Shuhei Hige[12], Tatsuya Ide[13], Kazuhide Yamamoto[14], Isao Sakaida[15], Yoshikazu Murawaki[16], Yoshito Itoh[17], Akihiro Tamori[18], Etsuro Orito[19], Yoichi Hiasa[20], Masao Honda[21], Shuichi Kaneko[21], Eiji Mita[22], Kazuyuki Suzuki[23], Keisuke Hino[24], Eiji Tanaka[25], Satoshi Mochida[26], Masaaki Watanabe[27], Yuichiro Eguchi[28], Naohiko Masaki[1], Kazumoto Murata[1], Masaaki Korenaga[1], Yoriko Mawatari[1], Jun Ohashi[29], Minae Kawashima[2], Katsushi Tokunaga[2], Masashi Mizokami[1*]

1 The Research Center for Hepatitis and Immunology, National Center for Global Health and Medicine, Ichikawa, Chiba, Japan, **2** Department of Human Genetics, Graduate School of Medicine, The University of Tokyo, Bunkyo-ku, Tokyo, Japan, **3** HLA Laboratory, Japanese Red Cross Kanto-Koshinetsu Block Blood Center, Koutou-ku, Tokyo, Japan, **4** Department of Medicine, Queen Mary Hospital, Hong Kong, **5** Faculty of Medicine, Chulalongkorn University, Bangkok, Thailand, **6** Department of Internal Medicine, Yonsei University College of Medicine, Seoul, South Korea, **7** Department of Virology & Liver Unit, Nagoya City University Graduate School of Medical Sciences, Nagoya, Aichi, Japan, **8** Division of Gastroenterology and Hepatology, Musashino Red Cross Hospital, Musashino, Tokyo, Japan, **9** Department of Liver Disease Control, Tokyo Medical and Dental University, Bunkyo-ku, Tokyo, Japan, **10** Department of Gastroenterology and Hepatology, Tokyo Medical and Dental University, Bunkyo-ku, Tokyo, Japan, **11** Department of Internal Medicine, Teine Keijinkai Hospital, Sapporo, Hokkaido, Japan, **12** Department of Internal Medicine, Hokkaido University Graduate School of Medicine, Sapporo, Hokkaido, Japan, **13** Division of Gastroenterology, Department of Medicine, Kurume University School of Medicine, Kurume, Fukuoka, Japan, **14** Department of Gastroenterology and Hepatology, Okayama University Graduate School of Medicine, Dentistry, and Pharmaceutical Sciences, Okayama, Okayama, Japan, **15** Gastroenterology and Hepatology, Yamaguchi University Graduate School of Medicine, Ube, Yamaguchi, Japan, **16** Faculty of Medicine, Tottori University, Tottori, Tottori, Japan, **17** Molecular Gastroenterology and Hepatology, Kyoto Prefectural University of Medicine, Kyoto, Kyoto, Japan, **18** Department of Hepatology, Osaka City University Graduate School of Medicine, Osaka, Osaka, Japan, **19** Department of Gastroenterology, Nagoya Daini Red Cross Hospital, Nagoya, Aichi, Japan, **20** Department of Gastroenterology and Metabology, Ehime University Graduate School of Medicine, Toon, Ehime, Japan, **21** Department of Gastroenterology, Kanazawa University Graduate School of Medicine, Kanazawa, Ishikawa, Japan, **22** Department of Gastroenterology and Hepatology, National Hospital Organization Osaka National Hospital, Osaka, Osaka, Japan, **23** Division of Gastroenterology and Hepatology, Department of Internal Medcine, Iwate Medical University, Morioka, Iwate, Japan, **24** Division of Hepatology and Pancreatology, Kawasaki Medical College, Kurashiki, Okayama, Japan, **25** Department of Medicine, Shinshu University School of Medicine, Matsumoto, Nagano, Japan, **26** Division of Gastroenterology and Hepatology, Saitama Medical University, Iruma, Saitama, Japan, **27** Department of Gastroenterology, Kitasato University School of Medicine, Sagamihara, Kanagawa, Japan, **28** Department of Internal Medicine, Saga Medical School, Saga, Saga, Japan, **29** Faculty of Medicine, University of Tsukuba, Tsukuba, Ibaraki, Japan

Abstract

Previous studies have revealed the association between SNPs located on human leukocyte antigen (*HLA*) class II genes, including *HLA-DP* and *HLA-DQ*, and chronic hepatitis B virus (HBV) infection, mainly in Asian populations. *HLA-DP* alleles or haplotypes associated with chronic HBV infection or disease progression have not been fully identified in Asian populations. We performed trans-ethnic association analyses of *HLA-DPA1*, *HLA-DPB1* alleles and haplotypes with hepatitis B virus infection and disease progression among Asian populations comprising Japanese, Korean, Hong Kong, and Thai subjects. To assess the association between *HLA-DP* and chronic HBV infection and disease progression, we conducted high-resolution (4-digit) *HLA-DPA1* and *HLA-DPB1* genotyping in a total of 3,167 samples, including HBV patients, HBV-resolved individuals and healthy controls. Trans-ethnic association analyses among Asian populations identified a new risk allele *HLA-DPB1*09:01* ($P = 1.36\times10^{-6}$; OR = 1.97; 95% CI, 1.50–2.59) and a new protective allele *DPB1*02:01* ($P = 5.22\times10^{-6}$; OR = 0.68; 95% CI, 0.58–0.81) to chronic HBV infection, in addition to the previously reported alleles. Moreover, *DPB1*02:01* was also associated with a decreased risk of disease progression in chronic HBV patients among Asian populations ($P = 1.55\times10^{-7}$; OR = 0.50; 95% CI, 0.39–0.65). Trans-ethnic association analyses identified Asian-specific associations of *HLA-DP* alleles and haplotypes with HBV infection or disease progression. The present findings will serve as a base for future functional studies of HLA-DP molecules in order to understand the pathogenesis of HBV infection and the development of hepatocellular carcinoma.

Editor: Ferruccio Bonino, University of Pisa, Italy

Funding: This work was supported by a Grant-in-Aid from the Ministry of Health, Labour, and Welfare of Japan H24-Bsou-kanen-ippan-011 and H24-kanen-ippan-004 to Masashi Mizokami, H23-kanen-005 to Katsushi Tokunaga, H25-kanen-wakate-013 to Nao Nishida, and H25-kanen-wakate-012 to Hiromi Sawai. This work was also supported by The Grant for National Center for Global Health and Medicine 22-shi-302 to Masashi Mizokami and 24-shi-107 to Nao Nishida. Partial support by Grant-in-Aid from the Ministry of Education, Culture, Sports, Science of Japan [grant number 22133008] for Scientific Research on Innovative Areas to Katsushi Tokunaga, [grant number 24790728] for Young Scientists (B) to Nao Nishida, and [grant number 25870178] for Young Scientists (B) to Hiromi Sawai, is also acknowledged. The funders had no role in study design, data collection and analysis, decision to publish, or preparation of the manuscript.

Competing Interests: The authors have declared that no competing interests exist.

* E-mail: mmizokami@hospk.ncgm.go.jp (MM); nishida-75@umin.ac.jp (NN)

These authors contributed equally to this work.

Introduction

Hepatitis B virus (HBV) infection is a major global health problem, resulting in 0.5–1.0 million deaths per year [1]. The prevalence of chronic HBV infection varies. About 75% of the chronic carriers in the world live in Southeast Asia and East Pacific [2]. Due to the introduction of vaccination programs, the prevalence of HBV infection in many countries has gradually been decreasing with consequent decreases in HBV-related hepatocellular carcinoma (HCC) [3]. Although some HBV carriers spontaneously eliminate the virus, about 10–15% of carriers develop liver cirrhosis (LC), liver failure and HCC [4]. Moreover, the progression of liver disease was revealed to be associated with the presence of several distinct mutations in HBV infections [5]. Genetic variations in *STAT4* and *HLA-DQ* genes were recently identified as host genetic factors in a large-scale genome-wide association study (GWAS) for HBV-related HCC in China [6].

With regard to the genes associated with susceptibility to chronic HBV infection, *HLA-DP* and *HLA-DQ* genes were identified by GWAS in Japanese and Thai populations in 2009 [7] and 2011 [8], respectively. In addition, our previous GWAS confirmed and identified the association of SNP markers located on *HLA-DPA1* (rs3077) and *HLA-DPB1* (rs9277535) genes with susceptibility to chronic hepatitis B (CHB) and HBV clearance in Japanese and Korean subjects[9]. The significant associations of *HLA-DP* with CHB and HBV clearance have mainly been detected in Asian populations, such as Japanese [8,9], Thai [7], Chinese [10–12], and Korean [9]. In 2012, the association between *HLA-DPA1* gene SNPs and persistent HBV infection was replicated in a Germany non-Asian population for the first time; however, this showed no association with HBV infection [13]. These results seem to be explained by the fact that allele frequencies of both rs3077 (0.155, 0.587 and 0.743 for C allele, on HapMap CEU, JPT, and YRI) and rs9277535 (0.261, 0.558 and 0.103 for G allele, on HapMap CEU, JPT, and YRI) are markedly different between populations. Moreover, the previous study showed that HBsAg seropositivity rates were higher in Thailand and China (5–12%) than in North America and Europe (0.2–0.5%) [2]. These results suggest that comparative analyses of *HLA-DP* alleles and haplotypes in Asian populations would clarify key host factors of the susceptible and protective *HLA-DP* alleles and haplotypes for CHB and HBV clearance. Here, we performed trans-ethnic analyses of *HLA-DP* alleles and haplotypes in Asian populations comprising Japanese, Korean, Hong Kong and Thai individuals. The findings from this study will serve as a base for future functional studies of HLA-DP molecules.

Results

Characteristics of studied subjects

The characteristics of a total of 3,167 samples, including Japanese, Korean, Hong Kong and Thai subjects, are shown in Table 1. Each population included three groups of HBV patients, resolved individuals and healthy controls. The clinical definitions of HBV patients and resolved individuals are summarized in Materials and Methods. Some of the Japanese and all of the Korean samples overlapped with the subjects in our previous study [9,14].

We performed genotyping for *HLA-DPA1* and *HLA-DPB1* in all 3,167 samples, and a total of 2,895 samples were successfully genotyped. The characteristics of successfully genotyped samples are shown in Table S1.

Association of *HLA-DPA1* and *HLA-DPB1* alleles in Asian populations

As for a general Asian population, including 464 Japanese, 140 Korean, 156 Hong Kong, and 122 Thai subjects, five *HLA-DPA1* alleles and twenty-four *HLA-DPB1* alleles were observed (Table S2). The frequencies of *HLA-DPA1* and *HLA-DPB1* alleles were similar between Japanese and Korean subjects. On the other hand, the number of alleles with frequencies of 1–2% was larger in Hong Kong and Thai populations, despite the small sample size. Although the frequencies of *HLA-DP* alleles varied in Asian populations, *HLA-DPB1*05:01* was the most prevalent with over 30% in all populations.

The associations of *HLA-DPA1* and *HLA-DPB1* alleles with chronic HBV infection (i.e., comparison between HBV patients and healthy controls) are shown in Table S2. To avoid false positives caused by multiple testing, the significance levels were corrected based on the numbers of *HLA-DPA1* and *HLA-DPB1*

Table 1. Number of individuals in this study.

Population	Japanese	Korean	Hong Kong	Thai
Total number of samples	1,291	586	661	629
HBV patients	489	340	281	390
IC	114	-	-	-
CH	147	175	187	198
AE	21	-	-	-
LC	38	-	-	-
HCC	169	165	94	192
Mean age (y)	57.1	44.7	57.9	52.0
(min-max)	(20–84)	(18–74)	(32–86)	(21–84)
Gender (M/F)	338/151	265/75	239/42	289/101
Resolved individuals*	335	106	190	113
HCV (−)	249	106	190	113
HCV (+)	86	-	-	-
Mean age (y)	59.7	43.1	40.0	48.2
(min-max)	(18–87)	(12–66)	(18–60)	(39–66)
Gender (M/F)	173/162	61/45	113/77	83/30
Healthy controls	467	140	190	126
Mean age (y)	39.0**	33.7	26.2	46.6
(min-max)	(23–64)	(1–59)	(16–60)	(38–79)
Gender (M/F)	370/97	67/73	87/103	73/53

Abbreviation: IC, Inactive Carrier; CH, Chronic Hepatitis; AE, Acute Exacerbation; LC, Liver Cirrhosis; HCC, Hepatocellular Carcinoma.
* Resolved individuals were HBsAg negative and HBcAb positive.
** 419 of 467 healthy controls were de-identified, without information on age.

alleles in the focal population. Briefly, the significance level was set at 0.05/(# of observed alleles at each locus) in each population (see Materials and Methods). With regard to high-risk alleles of *HLA-DPA1*, the most prevalent allele *HLA-DPA1*02:02* was significantly associated with susceptibility to HBV infection in Japanese ($P = 3.45 \times 10^{-4}$; OR = 1.39; 95% CI, 1.16–1.68) and Korean subjects ($P = 2.66 \times 10^{-5}$; OR = 1.89; 95% CI, 1.39–2.58), whereas this association was not observed in Hong Kong or Thai subjects. The association of *HLA-DPA1*02:01* with susceptibility to HBV infection was significant only in Japanese ($P = 2.61 \times 10^{-7}$; OR = 1.88; 95% CI, 1.46–2.41). The significant association of *HLA-DPA1*01:03* with protection against HBV infection was commonly observed among four Asian populations (Table S2). The pooled OR and 95% CI were 0.51 and 0.41–0.63, respectively in a meta-analysis ($P = 3.15 \times 10^{-10}$) (Fig. S1A).

As shown in Table S2, *HLA-DPB1* shows higher degree of polymorphism than *HLA-DPA1*. The most common allele in Asian populations, *HLA-DPB1*05:01*, was significantly associated with HBV susceptibility in both Japanese and Korean subjects. Although *HLA-DPB1*05:01* showed no significant association in the Hong Kong and Thai populations, the same direction of association (i.e., HBV susceptibility) was observed. Meta-analysis of the four populations revealed a significant association between *HLA-DPB1*05:01* and susceptibility to HBV infection ($P = 1.51 \times 10^{-4}$; OR = 1.45; 95% CI, 1.19–1.75) (Fig. S1B). The frequency of *HLA-DPB1*09:01* was significantly elevated in Japanese HBV patients (15.7%) as compared with healthy controls (8.7%) ($P = 3.70 \times 10^{-6}$; OR = 1.94; 95% CI, 1.45–2.62), and this association was most significant (i.e., the smallest P value) in the Japanese population. Because of lower allele frequencies of *HLA-DPB1*09:01* or lack of statistical power in the other populations, no significant associations were observed. A common allele in Thai subjects, *HLA-DPB1*13:01*, was significantly associated with susceptibility to HBV infection ($P = 2.49 \times 10^{-4}$; OR = 2.17; 95% CI, 1.40–3.47) with the same direction of associations in Japanese and Hong Kong (OR = 1.52 and 1.40, respectively).

*HLA-DPB1*04:02* was identified as the most protective allele for HBV infection in Japanese ($P = 1.59 \times 10^{-7}$; OR = 0.37; 95% CI, 0.24–0.55) and Korean subjects ($P = 1.27 \times 10^{-7}$; OR = 0.19; 95% CI, 0.10–0.38). Both *HLA-DPB1*02:01* and *HLA-DPB1*04:01* were also significantly associated with protection in the Japanese population, and the former was significantly associated with protection in Hong Kong subjects ($P = 9.17 \times 10^{-4}$; OR = 0.49; 95% CI, 0.32–0.76). This common allele among four Asian populations, *HLA-DPB1*02:01*, showed a significant association with protection against HBV infection ($P = 5.22 \times 10^{-6}$; OR = 0.68; 95% CI, 0.58–0.81) in a meta-analysis (Fig. S1B).

The frequencies of associated *HLA-DP* alleles in a comparison of HBV patients with healthy controls (Table S2) or with HBV-resolved individuals (Table S3) were similar in all four Asian populations. In the Japanese population, the associations of susceptible and protective *HLA-DPB1* alleles to chronic HBV infection seem weaker in the comparison of HBV patients with HBV-resolved individuals than in the comparison of HBV patients with healthy controls. Moreover, the results of association analyses showed no difference in the comparison of HBV patients with HBV-resolved individuals, including or excluding HCV positive individuals (Table S3). In contrast, the association became stronger in the comparison of HBV patients with HBV-resolved individuals among the Korean subjects. The protective allele *HLA-DPB1*04:01* was also identified to have a strong association with HBV clearance in Hong Kong subjects (Table S3). Moreover, in Hong Kong subjects, the *HLA-DPB1*05:01* associated with the risk for HBV infection showed lower frequency in HBV-resolved individuals (42.9%) than in the healthy controls (48.1%), which accounts for a strong association in the comparison of HBV patients with HBV-resolved individuals ($P = 6.24 \times 10^{-3}$; OR = 1.64; 95% CI, 1.14–2.36). Although the number of samples was insufficient, *HLA-DP*100:01* showed a significant association with protection against HBV infection in the Hong Kong population ($P = 3.05 \times 10^{-6}$; OR = 0.03; 95% CI, 0.0007–0.20).

Table 2. Association of number of *DPB1*02:01* alleles (i.e., 0, 1 or 2) with disease progression in CHB patients assessed by multivariate logistic regression analysis adjusted for age and sex.

Population	P value	OR (95% CI)
Japanese	0.000177	0.47 (0.32–0.70)
Korean	0.025358	0.55 (0.33–0.93)
Hong Kong	0.040842	0.46 (0.22–0.97)
Thai	0.087782	0.58 (0.31–1.08)
All*	1.55×10^{-7}	0.50 (0.39–0.65)

*Population was adjusted using dummy variables.

As for disease progression in CHB patients among Asian populations, a protective effect of *HLA-DPB1*02:01* on disease progression was observed in the Japanese ($P = 4.26 \times 10^{-5}$; OR = 0.45; 95% CI, 0.30–0.67) and Korean populations ($P = 8.74 \times 10^{-4}$; OR = 0.47; 95% CI, 0.29–0.75) (Table S4). Multivariate logistic regression analysis adjusted for age and sex revealed that the number of *DPB1*02:01* alleles (i.e., 0, 1, or 2) was significantly associated with disease progression in CHB patients in Japanese ($P = 1.77 \times 10^{-4}$; OR = 0.47; 95% CI, 0.32–0.70) (Table 2). Moreover, protective effects of *DPB1*02:01* on disease progression in Asian populations ($P = 1.55 \times 10^{-7}$; OR = 0.50; 95% CI, 0.39–0.65) were detected in a multivariate logistic regression analysis adjusted for age, gender, and population (Table 2).

Associations of *DPA1-DPB1* haplotypes in Asian populations

The estimated frequencies of *HLA DPA1-DPB1* haplotypes are shown in Table S5. The most frequent haplotype among the four Asian populations was *DPA1*02:02-DPB1*05:01*. The number of haplotypes with low frequencies of 1–2% was 10 in both Japanese and Korean subjects, whereas more haplotypes appeared with frequencies of 1–2% in Hong Kong and Thai subjects. The associations of *DPA1-DPB1* haplotypes with HBV infection are shown in Table S5. In the Japanese population, *DPA1*02:01-DPB1*09:01* showed the most significant association with susceptibility to HBV infection ($P = 3.38 \times 10^{-6}$; OR = 1.95; 95% CI, 1.46–2.64). The most common haplotype in the four Asian populations, *DPA1*02:02-DPB1*05:01*, was found to be significantly associated with susceptibility to HBV infection in the Japanese and Korean subjects ($P = 7.40 \times 10^{-4}$; OR = 1.37; 95% CI, 1.14–1.66 for Japanese, and $P = 4.50 \times 10^{-6}$; OR = 2.02; 95% CI, 1.48–2.78 for Korean). In the Thai subjects, *HLA-DPB1*13:01* was the most significant risk allele for HBV infection (Table S2); however, no significant associations were found for the three different haplotypes bearing *HLA-DPB1*13:01*: *DPA1*02:01-DPB1*13:01*, *DPA1*02:02-DPB1*13:01*, and *DPA1*04:01-DPB1*13:01*,indicating that the association of *HLA-DPB1*13:01* with susceptibility to HBV infection did not result from a specific *DPA1-DPB1* haplotype or combination with a specific *DPA1* allele.

In the Japanese population, both haplotypes *DPA1*01:03-DPB1*04:01* and *DPA1*01:03-DPB1*04:02* showed significant associations with protection against HBV infection ($P = 1.17 \times 10^{-5}$; OR = 0.32; 95% CI, 0.18–0.56 for *DPA1*01:03-DPB1*04:01* and $P = 1.95 \times 10^{-7}$; OR = 0.37; 95% CI, 0.24–0.55 for *DPA1*01:03-DPB1*04:02*). In the Korean subjects, a significant association of *DPA1*01:03-DPB1*04:02* was also demonstrated; however, no association was observed for *DPA1*01:03-DPB1*04:01*. Because the observed number of each haplotype was small, none of the other haplotypes showed a significant association with protection against HBV infection.

In order to identify trans-ethnic DPA1-DPB1 haplotypes associated with HBV infection, a meta-analysis was performed. A meta-analysis further revealed that the *DPA1*01:03-DPB1*02:01* haplotype was significantly associated with protection against HBV infection ($P = 1.45 \times 10^{-5}$; OR = 0.69; 95% CI, 0.58–0.82) (Fig. S1C).

Discussion

Among 2.2 billion individuals worldwide who are infected with HBV, 15% of these are chronic carriers. Of chronic carriers, 10–15% develops LC, liver failure and HCC, and the remaining individuals eventually achieve a state of nonreplicative infection, resulting in HBsAg negative and anti-HBc positive, i.e. HBV-resolved individuals. To identify host genetic factors associated with HBV-related disease progression may lead HBV patients to discriminate individuals who need treatment.

The *HLA-DPA1* and *HLA-DPB1* genes were identified as host genetic factors significantly associated with CHB infection, mainly in Asian populations [7–12], and not in European populations [13]. In the previous association analyses of *HLA-DPB1* alleles with HBV infection, one risk allele *HLA-DPB1*05:01* (OR = 1.52; 95% CI, 1.31–1.76), and two protective alleles, *HLA-DPB1*04:01* (OR = 0.53; 95% CI, 0.34–0.80) and *HLA-DPB1*04:02* (OR = 0.47; 95% CI, 0.34–.64), were identified in the Japanese population [7]. In this study, we further identified a new risk allele *HLA-DPB1*09:01* (OR = 1.94; 95% CI, 1.45–2.62) for HBV infection and a new protective allele *HLA-DPB1*02:01* (OR = 0.71; 95% CI, 0.56–0.89) in the Japanese population, in addition to the previously reported alleles (Table S2) [7]. The discrepancy in the association of *HLA-DPB1*09:01* allele with risk for HBV infection in a previous study [7] results from the elevated frequency of *HLA-DPB1*09:01* in the controls (12.2%), which is higher than our controls (8.7%). In this study, healthy subjects were recruited as controls. In contrast, individuals that were registered in BioBank Japan as subjects with diseases other than CHB were recruited as controls in the previous study [7], which may have included patients with diseases with which *HLA-DPB1*09:01* is associated. Although no significant association of *HLA-DPB1*09:01* with risk for HBV infection was observed in the Korean subjects, *HLA-DPB1*09:01* appears to have a susceptible effect on HBV infection, as it showed the same direction of association. When the association analyses in Japanese and Korean subjects were combined in meta-analysis, the association was statistically significant ($P = 1.36 \times 10^{-6}$; OR = 1.97; 95% CI, 1.50–2.59). Thus, *HLA-DPB1*09:01* may be a Northeast Asian-specific allele associated with risk for HBV infection.

Moreover, a significant association of *HLA-DPB1*13:01* with risk of HBV infection (OR = 2.17; 95% CI, 1.40–3.47) was identified in the Thai subjects. However, the frequency of *HLA-DPB1*13:01* in Thai healthy controls (11.5% in the present study) reportedly varies, ranging from 15.4% to 29.5%, due to the population diversity [15–17]. Therefore, a replication analysis is required to confirm the association of *HLA-DPB1*13:01* with HBV infection in the Thai subjects. There were four other marginally associated *HLA-DPB1* alleles with low allele frequencies below 5% in HBV patients and healthy controls, including *HLA-DPB1*28:01*, *-DPB1*31:01*, *-DPB1*100:01*, and *-DPB1*105:01*, in the Hong Kong and Thai subjects. Because these infrequent alleles may have resulted from false positive associations, the association needs to be validated in a large number of subjects.

*HLA-DPB1*02:01* showed a significant association with protection against HBV infection in both Japanese and Hong Kong populations (Table S2); however, the *HLA-DPB1*02:01* allele was not associated with HBV infection in the previous study [7]. Although *HLA-DPB1*02:01* showed no association in either Korean or Thai populations, a significant association of *HLA-DPB1*02:01* with protection against HBV infection among four Asian populations was detected in meta-analysis ($P = 5.22 \times 10^{-6}$; OR = 0.68; 95% CI, 0.58–0.81) (Fig. S1B). We therefore conclude that the present finding is not a false positive.

A recent report showed that *HLA-DPB1*02:01:02*, **02:02*, **03:01:01*, **04:01:01*, **05:01*, **09:01*, and **14:01* were significantly associated with response to booster HB vaccination in Taiwan neonatally vaccinated adolescents [18]. The *HLA-DPB1*02:01:02*, **02:02*, **03:01:01*, **04:01:01*, and **14:01* were significantly more frequent in recipients whose post-booster titers of antibodies against HBV surface antigen (anti-HBs) were detectable, on the other hand, *HLA-DPB1*05:01* and **09:01* were significantly more frequent in recipients who were undetectable. Moreover, the *HLA-DPB1*05:01* and **09:01* significantly increase the likelihoods of undetectable pre-booster anti-HBs titers. These results seem consistent with our findings, in which *HLA-DPB1*05:01* and **09:01* are associated with susceptibility to chronic hepatitis B infection.

We also identified a protective effect of *HLA-DPB1*02:01* allele on disease progression in Asian populations. Previous studies identified the association of HLA class II genes including *HLA-DQ* and *HLA-DR* with development of HBV related hepatocellular carcinoma in the Chinese population [6,19,20]. In this study using Japanese and Korean samples, we identified significant associations between *HLA-DPB1*02:01* and disease progression in CHB patients ($P = 4.26 \times 10^{-5}$; OR = 0.45; 95% CI, 0.30–0.67, for Japanese and $P = 8.74 \times 10^{-4}$; OR = 0.47; 95% CI, 0.29–0.75 for Korean) (Table S4). Although the association of *HLA-DPB1*02:01* with disease progression was weaker after adjustment for age and gender in Korean subjects ($P = 2.54 \times 10^{-2}$; OR = 0.55; 95% CI, 0.33–0.93), the same direction of association was observed (i.e. protective effect on disease progression) (Table 2). The protective effects of *HLA-DPB1*02:01* on disease progression showed a significant association after adjustment for age and gender in the Japanese population ($P = 1.77 \times 10^{-4}$; OR = 0.47; 95% CI, 0.32–0.70); moreover, a significant association between *HLA-DPB1*02:01* was observed among four Asian populations, under which population was adjusted by using dummy variables in a multivariate logistic regression analysis ($P = 1.55 \times 10^{-7}$; OR = 0.50; 95% CI, 0.39–0.65) (Table 2).

The *HLA-DPA1* and *HLA-DPB1* belong to the HLA class II alpha and beta chain paralogues, which make a heterodimer consisting of an alpha and a beta chain on the surface of antigen presenting cells. This HLA class II molecule plays a central role in the immune system by presenting peptides derived from extracellular proteins. We identified two susceptible haplotypes (*DPA1*02:02-DPB1*05:01* and *DPA1*02:01-DPB1*09:01*) and three protective haplotypes (*DPA1*01:03-DPB1*04:01*, *DPA1*01:03-DPB1*04:02*, and *HLA-DPA1*01:03-DPB1*02:01*) to chronic hepatitis B infection, which may result in different binding affinities between HLA-DP subtypes and extracellular antigens. Although functional analyses of HLA-DP subtypes to identify HBV-related peptides are not fully completed, identification of susceptible and protective haplotypes as host genetic factors would lead us to understand the pathogenesis of HBV infection including viral factors.

In summary, we identified a new risk allele *HLA-DPB1*09:01*, which was specifically observed in Northeast Asian populations, Japanese and Korean. Moreover, a new protective allele *HLA-DPB1*02:01* was identified among four Asian populations: Japanese, Korean, Hong Kong and Thai. The protective allele *HLA-DPB1*02:01* was associated with both chronic HBV infection and disease progression in chronic HBV patients. Identification of a total of five alleles, including two risk alleles (*DPB1*09:01* and *DPB1*05:01*) and three protective alleles (*DPB1*04:01*, *DPB1*04:02* and *DPB1*02:01*), would enable HBV-infected individuals to be classified into groups according to the treatment requirements. Moreover, the risk and protective alleles for HBV infection and disease progression, identified in this study by means of trans-ethnic association analyses, would be key host factors to recognize HBV-derived antigen peptides. The present results may lead to subsequent functional studies into HLA-DP molecules and viral factors in order to understand the pathogenesis of HBV infection and development of hepatocellular carcinoma.

Materials and Methods

Ethics Statement

All study protocols conform to the relevant ethical guidelines, as reflected in the *a priori* approval by the ethics committee of National Center for Global Health and Medicine, and by the ethics committees of all participating universities and hospitals, including The University of Tokyo, Japanese Red Cross Kanto-Koshinetsu Block Blood Center, The University of Hong Kong, Chulalongkorn University, Yonsei University College of Medicine, Nagoya City University Graduate School of Medical Sciences, Musashino Red Cross Hospital, Tokyo Medical and Dental University, Teine Keijinkai Hospital, Hokkaido University Graduate School of Medicine, Kurume University School of Medicine, Okayama University Graduate School of Medicine, Yamaguchi University Graduate School of Medicine, Tottori University, Kyoto Prefectural University of Medicine, Osaka City University Graduate School of Medicine, Nagoya Daini Red Cross Hospital, Ehime University Graduate School of Medicine, Kanazawa University Graduate School of Medicine, National Hospital Organization Osaka National Hospital, Iwate Medical University, Kawasaki Medical College, Shinshu University School of Medicine, Saitama Medical University, Kitasato University School of Medicine, Saga Medical School, and University of Tsukuba.

Written informed consent was obtained from each patient who participated in this study and all samples were anonymized. For Japanese healthy controls, 419 individuals were de-identified with information about gender, and all were recruited after obtaining verbal informed consent in Tokyo prior to 1990. For the 419 Japanese healthy individuals, written informed consent was not obtained because the blood sampling was conducted before the "Ethical Guidelines for Human Genome and Genetic Sequencing Research" were established in Japan. Under the condition that DNA sample is permanently de-linked from the individual, this study was approved by the Research Ethics Committee of National Center for Global Health and Medicine.

Characteristics of studied subjects

All of the 3,167 genomic DNA samples were collected from individuals with HBV, HBV-resolved individuals (HBsAg-negative and anti-HBc-positive) and healthy controls at 26 multi-center hospitals throughout Japan, Korea, Hong Kong, and Thailand (Table 1). In a total of 1,291 Japanese and 586 Korean samples, 1,191 Japanese individuals and all 586 Korean individuals were included in our previous study [9]. With regard to additional Japanese individuals, we collected samples from 48 healthy controls at Kohnodai Hospital, and 52 HBV patients at Okayama University Hospital and Ehime University Hospital, including 26 individuals with LC and 26 individuals with HCC. A total of 661 Hong Kong samples and 629 Thai samples were collected at Queen Mary Hospital and Chulalongkorn University, respectively.

HBV status was measured based on serological results for HBsAg and anti-HBc with a fully automated chemiluminescent enzyme immunoassay system (Abbott ARCHITECT; Abbott Japan, Tokyo, Japan, or LUMIPULSE f or G1200; Fujirebio, Inc., Tokyo, Japan). For clinical staging, inactive carrier (IC) state was defined by the presence of HBsAg with normal ALT levels over 1 year (examined at least four times at 3-month intervals) and without evidence of liver cirrhosis. Chronic hepatitis (CH) was defined by elevated ALT levels (>1.5 times the upper limit of normal [35 IU/L]) persisting over 6 months (by at least 3 bimonthly tests). Acute exacerbation (AE) of chronic hepatitis B was defined as an elevation of ALT to more than 10 times the upper limit of normal (ULN, 58 IU/L) and bilirubin to at least three times ULN (15 μmol/L). LC was diagnosed principally by ultrasonography (coarse liver architecture, nodular liver surface, blunt liver edges and hypersplenism), platelet counts<100,000/cm^3, or a combination thereof. Histological confirmation by fine-needle biopsy of the liver was performed as required. HCC was diagnosed by ultrasonography, computerized tomography, magnetic resonance imaging, angiography, tumor biopsy or a combination thereof.

The Japanese control samples from HBV-resolved subjects (HBsAg-negative and anti-HBc-positive) at Nagoya City University-affiliated healthcare center were used by comprehensive agreement (anonymization in a de-identified manner) in this study. Some of the unrelated and anonymized Japanese healthy controls were purchased from the Japan Health Science Research Resources Bank (Osaka, Japan). One microgram of purified genomic DNA was dissolved in 100 μl of TE buffer (pH 8.0) (Wako, Osaka, Japan), followed by storage at −20°C until use.

Genotyping of *HLA-DPA1* and *HLA-DPB1* alleles

High resolution (4-digit) genotyping of *HLA-DPA1* and *-DPB1* alleles was performed for HBV patients, resolved individuals, and healthy controls in Japan, Korea, Hong Kong, and Thailand. LABType SSO HLA DPA1/DPB1 kit (One Lambda, CA) and a Luminex Multi-Analyte Profiling system (xMAP; Luminex, Austin, TX) were used for genotyping, in according with the manufacturer's protocol. Because of the small quantity of genomic DNA in some Korean samples, we performed whole genome amplification for a total of 486 samples using GenomiPhi v2 DNA Amplification kit (GE Healthcare Life Sciences, UK), in accordance with the manufacturer's instruction.

A total of 2,895 samples were successfully genotyped and characteristics of these samples are summarized in Table S1.

Statistical analysis

Fisher's exact test in two-by-two cross tables was used to examine the associations between *HLA-DP* allele and chronic HBV infection or disease progression in chronic HBV patients, using statistical software R2.9. To avoid false-positive results due to multiple testing, significance levels were adjusted based on the number of observed alleles at each locus in each population. For *HLA-DPA1* alleles, the number of observed alleles was 3 in Japanese, 4 in Korean, 5 in Hong Kong, and 5 in Thai subjects. Therefore, the significant levels for α were set at $\alpha = 0.05/3$ in Japanese, $\alpha = 0.05/4$ in Korean, $\alpha = 0.05/5$ in Hong Kong, and $\alpha = 0.05/5$ in Thai subjects. In the same way, significant levels for *HLA-DPB1* alleles were $\alpha = 0.05/10$, 0.05/11, 0.05/12, and 0.05/16, respectively. Multivariate logistic regression analysis adjusted for age and sex (used as independent variables) was applied to assess associations between the number of *DPB1*02:01* alleles (i.e., 0, 1, or 2) and disease progression in CHB patients. To examine the effect of *DPB1*02:01* allele on disease progression in all populations, population was further adjusted by using three dummy variables (i.e., (c1, c2, c3) = (0, 0, 0) for Japanese, (1, 0, 0) for Korean, (0, 1, 0) for Hong Kong, and (0, 0, 1) for Thai) in a multivariate logistic regression analysis. We obtained the following regression equation: logit(p) = −3.905+0.083*age+(−0.929)*sex+(−0.684)**DPB1*02:01*+1.814*c1+(−0.478)*c2+0.782*c3. Significance levels in the analysis of disease progression in CHB patients were set as $\alpha = 0.05/10$ in Japanese, $\alpha = 0.05/11$ in Korean, $\alpha = 0.05/15$ in Hong Kong, and $\alpha = 0.05/15$ in Thai subjects. The phase of each individual (i.e., a combination of two *DPA1-DPB1* haplotypes) was estimated using PHASE software [21], assuming samples are selected randomly from a general population. In comparison of the estimated *DPA1-DPB1* haplotype frequencies, significant levels were set as $\alpha = 0.05/14$ in Japanese, $\alpha = 0.05/17$ in Korean, $\alpha = 0.05/17$ in Hong Kong, and $\alpha = 0.05/18$ in Thai subjects. Meta-analysis was performed using the DerSimonian-Laird method (random-effects model) in order to calculate pooled OR and its 95% confidence interval (95% CI). We applied meta-analysis for alleles with frequency>1% in all four Asian populations. The significance levels in meta-analysis were adjusted by the total number of statistical tests; $\alpha = 0.05/20$ for *DPA1* alleles, $\alpha = 0.05/57$ for *DPB1* alleles, and $\alpha = 0.05/74$ for *DPA1-DPB1* haplotypes.

Supporting Information

Figure S1 Comparison of odds ratios in association analyses for *HLA-DP* with chronic HBV infection among four Asian populations: (A) *HLA-DPA1* alleles; (B) *HLA-DPB1* alleles; and (C) *HLA DPA1-DPB1* haplotypes. Meta-analysis was performed using the DerSimonian-Laird method (random-effects model) to calculate pooled OR and its 95% confidence interval (95% CI). Bold depicts a statistically significant association after correction of significance level.

Table S1 Individuals with successfully genotyped for *HLA-DPA1* and *HLA-DPB1*.

Table S2 Frequencies of HLA-DP alleles in HBV patients and healthy controls among Asian populations.

Table S3 Frequencies of HLA-DP alleles in HBV patients and resolved individuals among Asian populations.

Table S4 Associations of HLA-DPB1 alleles with disease progression in CHB patients among Asian populations.

Table S5 Estimated frequencies of HLA DPA1-DPB1 haplotypes in HBV patients and healthy controls among Asian populations.

Acknowledgments

We would like to thank all the patients and families who contributed to the study. We are also grateful to Ms. Mayumi Ishii (National Center for Global Health and Medicine), Ms. Megumi Sageshima, Yuko Hirano, Natsumi Baba, Rieko Shirahashi, Ayumi Nakayama (University of Tokyo), and Yuko Ohara (Japanese Red Cross Kanto-Koshinetsu Block Blood Center) for technical assistance.

Author Contributions

Conceived and designed the experiments: NN HS MS KT M. Mizokami. Performed the experiments: NN HS KK Y. Mawatari M. Kawashima M. Minami. Analyzed the data: NN HS M. Kawashima JO. Contributed reagents/materials/analysis tools: W-KS M-FY NP YP SHA K-HH K. Matsuura YT M. Kurosaki YA NI J-HK SH TI KY IS Y. Murawaki YI AT EO YH MH SK EM KS KH ET SM MW YE NM K. Murata M. Korenaga KT M. Mizokami. Wrote the paper: NN HS JO KT M. Mizokami.

References

1. Chen DS (1993) From hepatitis to hepatoma: lessons from type B viral hepatitis. Science 262: 369–370.
2. Custer B, Sullivan SD, Hazlet TK, Iloeje U, Veenstra DL, et al. (2004) Global epidemiology of hepatitis B virus. J Clin Gastroenterol 38: S158–168.
3. Zidan A, Scheuerlein H, Schule S, Settmacher U, Rauchfuss F (2012) Epidemiological pattern of hepatitis B and hepatitis C as etiological agents for hepatocellular carcinoma in iran and worldwide. Hepat Mon 12: e6894.
4. Pungpapong S, Kim WR, Poterucha JJ (2007) Natural history of hepatitis B virus infection: an update for clinicians. Mayo Clin Proc 82: 967–975.
5. Kim DW, Lee SA, Hwang ES, Kook YH, Kim BJ (2012) Naturally occurring precore/core region mutations of hepatitis B virus genotype C related to hepatocellular carcinoma. PLoS One 7: e47372.
6. Jiang DK, Sun J, Cao G, Liu Y, Lin D, et al. (2013) Genetic variants in STAT4 and HLA-DQ genes confer risk of hepatitis B virus-related hepatocellular carcinoma. Nat Genet 45: 72–75.
7. Kamatani Y, Wattanapokayakit S, Ochi H, Kawaguchi T, Takahashi A, et al. (2009) A genome-wide association study identifies variants in the HLA-DP locus associated with chronic hepatitis B in Asians. Nat Genet 41: 591–595.
8. Mbarek H, Ochi H, Urabe Y, Kumar V, Kubo M, et al. (2011) A genome-wide association study of chronic hepatitis B identified novel risk locus in a Japanese population. Hum Mol Genet 20: 3884–3892.
9. Nishida N, Sawai H, Matsuura K, Sugiyama M, Ahn SH, et al. (2012) Genome-wide association study confirming association of HLA-DP with protection against chronic hepatitis B and viral clearance in Japanese and Korean. PLoS One 7: e39175.
10. Guo X, Zhang Y, Li J, Ma J, Wei Z, et al. (2011) Strong influence of human leukocyte antigen (HLA)-DP gene variants on development of persistent chronic hepatitis B virus carriers in the Han Chinese population. Hepatology 53: 422–428.
11. An P, Winkler C, Guan L, O'Brien SJ, Zeng Z (2011) A common HLA-DPA1 variant is a major determinant of hepatitis B virus clearance in Han Chinese. J Infect Dis 203: 943–947.
12. Li J, Yang D, He Y, Wang M, Wen Z, et al. (2011) Associations of HLA-DP variants with hepatitis B virus infection in southern and northern Han Chinese populations: a multicenter case-control study. PLoS One 6: e24221.
13. Vermehren J, Lotsch J, Susser S, Wicker S, Berger A, et al. (2012) A common HLA-DPA1 variant is associated with hepatitis B virus infection but fails to distinguish active from inactive Caucasian carriers. PLoS One 7: e32605.
14. Sawai H, Nishida N, Mbarek H, Matsuda K, Mawatari Y, et al. (2012) No association for Chinese HBV-related hepatocellular carcinoma susceptibility SNP in other East Asian populations. BMC Med Genet 13: 47.
15. Chandanayingyong D, Stephens HA, Fan L, Sirikong M, Longta P, et al. (1994) HLA-DPB1 polymorphism in the Thais of Southeast Asia. Hum Immunol 40: 20–24.

16. Chandanayingyong D, Stephens HA, Klaythong R, Sirikong M, Udee S, et al. (1997) HLA-A, -B, -DRB1, -DQA1, and -DQB1 polymorphism in Thais. Hum Immunol 53: 174–182.
17. Maneemaroj R, Stephens HA, Chandanayingyong D, Longta K, Bejrachandra S (1997) HLA class II allele frequencies in northern Thais (Kamphaeng Phet). J Med Assoc Thai 80 Suppl 1: S20–24.
18. Wu TW, Chu CC, Ho TY, Chang Liao HW, Lin SK, et al. (2013) Responses to booster hepatitis B vaccination are significantly correlated with genotypes of human leukocyte antigen (HLA)-DPB1 in neonatally vaccinated adolescents. Hum Genet.
19. Hu L, Zhai X, Liu J, Chu M, Pan S, et al. (2012) Genetic variants in human leukocyte antigen/DP-DQ influence both hepatitis B virus clearance and hepatocellular carcinoma development. Hepatology 55: 1426–1431.
20. Li S, Qian J, Yang Y, Zhao W, Dai J, et al. (2012) GWAS identifies novel susceptibility loci on 6p21.32 and 21q21.3 for hepatocellular carcinoma in chronic hepatitis B virus carriers. PLoS Genet 8: e1002791.
21. Stephens M, Smith NJ, Donnelly P (2001) A new statistical method for haplotype reconstruction from population data. Am J Hum Genet 68: 978–989.

52-Week Efficacy and Safety of Telbivudine with Conditional Tenofovir Intensification at Week 24 in HBeAg-Positive Chronic Hepatitis B

Teerha Piratvisuth[1]*, Piyawat Komolmit[2], Tawesak Tanwandee[3], Wattana Sukeepaisarnjaroen[4], Henry L. Y. Chan[5], Mário G. Pessôa[6], Eduardo Fassio[7], Suzane K. Ono[8], Fernando Bessone[9], Jorge Daruich[10], Stefan Zeuzem[11], Hugo Cheinquer[12], Rashidkhan Pathan[13], Yuhong Dong[14], Aldo Trylesinski[14]

1 NKC Institute of Gastroenterology and Hepatology, Prince of Songkla University, Songklanagarind Hospital, Hat-Yai, Songkhla, Thailand, **2** Division of Gastroenterology, Department of Medicine, Chulalongkorn University, Bangkok, Thailand, **3** Siriraj Hospital, Bangkok, Thailand, **4** Department of Medicine, Srinagarind Hospital, Khon Kaen University, Khon Kaen, Thailand, **5** Department of Medicine and Therapeutics, The Chinese University of Hong Kong, Hong Kong, Hong Kong S.A.R, **6** Hospital das Clinicas da Faculdade de Medicina da Universidade de São Paulo, São Paulo, Brazil, **7** Hospital Nacional Prof. Alejandro Posadas, Buenos Aires, Argentina, **8** Departamento de Gastroenterologia da Faculdade de Medicina da Universidade de São Paulo, São Paulo, Brazil, **9** Catedra de Clınica Medica, Universidad Nacional de Rosario, Rosario, Antigua and Barbuda, **10** Hospital de Clínicas San Martín, University of Buenos Aires, Buenos Aires, Argentina, **11** Klinikum der Johann Wolfgang Goethe-Universitaet, Frankfurt am Main, Germany, **12** Gastroenterology Division, Hospital de Clínicas de Porto Alegre, Universidade Federal do Rio Grande do Sul (UFRGS), Porto Alegre, Brazil, **13** Novartis Pharmaceuticals, East Hanover, New Jersey, United States of America, **14** Novartis Pharma AG, Basel, Switzerland

Abstract

Background and Aims: The Roadmap concept is a therapeutic framework in chronic hepatitis B for the intensification of nucleoside analogue monotherapy based on early virologic response. The efficacy and safety of this approach applied to telbivudine treatment has not been investigated.

Methods: A multinational, phase IV, single-arm open-label study (ClinicalTrials.gov ID NCT00651209) was undertaken in HBeAg-positive, nucleoside-naive adult patients with chronic hepatitis B. Patients received telbivudine (600 mg once-daily) for 24 weeks, after which those with undetectable serum HBV DNA (<300 copies/mL) continued to receive telbivudine alone while those with detectable DNA received telbivudine plus tenofovir (300 mg once-daily). Outcomes were assessed at Week 52.

Results: 105 patients commenced telbivudine monotherapy, of whom 100 were included in the efficacy analysis. Fifty-five (55%) had undetectable HBV DNA at Week 24 and continued telbivudine monotherapy; 45 (45%) received tenofovir intensification. At Week 52, the overall proportion of undetectable HBV DNA was 93% (93/100) by last-observation-carried-forward analysis (100% monotherapy group, 84% intensification group) and no virologic breakthroughs had occurred. ALT normalization occurred in 77% (87% monotherapy, 64% intensification), HBeAg clearance in 43% (65% monotherapy, 16% intensification), and HBeAg seroconversion in 39% (62% monotherapy, 11% intensification). Six patients had HBsAg clearance. Myalgia was more common in the monotherapy group (19% versus 7%). No decrease in the mean glomerular filtration rate occurred in either treatment group at Week 52.

Conclusions: Telbivudine therapy with tenofovir intensification at Week 24, where indicated by the Roadmap strategy, appears effective and well tolerated for the treatment of chronic hepatitis B.

Editor: Javier R. Lama, Asociacion Civil Impacta Salud y Educacion, Peru

Funding: These authors have no support or funding to report.

Competing Interests: The authors have read the journal's policy and have the following conflicts: RP, YD, and AT are all employees of Novartis, the funder of this study. The following employees of Novartis Pharma played key roles in the design, execution and analysis of the study and in the drafting of this manuscript: Efsevia Albanis, Patricia Lopez, Claudio Avila, and George Harb (study design and data analysis); Weibin Bao (data analysis); Michele Gysen, Joe Mostillo, Kevin Poirier (study operations); Mechthild Jung (study operations and manuscript preparation); Charles Koehne (manuscript preparation). Editorial assistance with the drafting of the manuscript in association with the authors was provided by a professional medical writer (Nicholas Fitch) with funding from Novartis Pharma AG. There are no patents, products in development, or marketed products to declare.

* E-mail: teerha.p@psu.ac.th

Introduction

There are approximately 400 million people worldwide who are chronically infected with hepatitis B virus (HBV), of whom 75% live in the Asia-Pacific region. Chronic hepatitis B results in liver disease progressing to cirrhosis and hepatocellular carcinoma (HCC) and is responsible for approximately one million liver-related deaths per annum [1].

Treatment of HBV involves finite administration of pegylated or unpegylated interferon alfa, or indefinite administration of anti-HBV nucleoside/nucleotide analogues. Five such analogues are currently available. Lamivudine, a deoxycytidine analogue, was the first nucleoside approved for use in HBV and lamivudine monotherapy remains common despite high rates of treatment-emergent drug resistance [2]. Entecavir is a deoxyguanosine analogue with a high genetic barrier to resistance in treatment-naive patients [3]. However, lamivudine resistance predisposes HBV to subsequent entecavir resistance [4]. Telbivudine is an L-deoxythymidine analogue with superior efficacy to lamivudine [5] but a similar resistance profile [6]. Finally, the nucleotides adefovir and tenofovir are both acyclic mimetics of deoxyadenosine monophosphate which retain activity against lamivudine- and telbivudine-resistant HBV [6]. However, adefovir is associated with dose-dependent nephrotoxicity which restricts its dosing to 10 mg daily [7], at which dose it demonstrates inferior virologic efficacy to the other agents [8–10]. There are also concerns about the long-term safety of tenofovir, which is associated with significant loss of renal function in HIV treatment [11].

HBV viral replication is a key driver for disease progression and is associated with the development of cirrhosis and HCC [12]. The initial goal of treatment is to suppress viral replication; thereafter, sustained (on-treatment) or maintained (off-treatment) suppression of circulating HBV DNA is associated with improved serological responses and long-term outcomes [13,14]. The emergence of drug-resistant HBV results in breakthrough viremia leading to hepatitis and liver disease progression. To ensure good long-term outcomes, the conservation of HBV DNA suppression is essential.

Early virologic response, particularly at Week 24, is associated with better long-term outcomes in chronic HBV, while detectable HBV DNA at Week 24 is associated with a higher incidence of on-therapy drug resistance [14,15]. This predictive association has lead an international group of experts to propose the so-called "Roadmap" concept – a therapeutic algorithm for the conditional intensification of nucleoside monotherapy based on early virologic response [16]. In the Roadmap, monotherapy is continued if plasma virus is undetectable (HBV DNA <300 copies/mL) at Week 24; while for those with detectable HBV DNA defined options exist for either intensification or continued monotherapy. The Roadmap principle is widely accepted in clinical practice [17], but has yet to be prospectively evaluated. In this study, we sought to confirm prospectively the clinical utility of the Roadmap by investigating whether the conditional intensification of telbivudine monotherapy with tenofovir, when indicated by the algorithm, results in effective virologic suppression in nucleoside-naive, HBeAg-positive patients with chronic hepatitis B. We present 52-week primary efficacy and safety data.

Materials and Methods

The protocol for this trial and supporting CONSORT checklist are available as supporting information; see Checklist S1 and Protocol S1.

Ethics Statement

Written informed consent was obtained and eligibility assessed at a screening visit up to 6 weeks before the first dose of telbivudine. The study was approved by the institutional review boards/independent ethics committees of each study center and was conducted in compliance with the principles of the Declaration of Helsinki and in compliance with all International Conference on Harmonization Good Clinical Practice Guidelines and local regulatory requirements.

Patients

This study (ClinicalTrials.gov ID NCT00651209) had a multinational, single-arm, open-label design. Male and female adults ($\geq$18 years) were recruited between April 2008 and September 2009 from 17 clinical centers in Argentina (n = 3), Brazil (4), China [Hong Kong] (2), Germany (4) and Thailand (4). Major inclusion criteria were: documented chronic hepatitis B with detectable HBsAg at screening and for at least 6 months prior; HBeAg-positive (HBeAg+) and HBeAb-negative at screening; serum HBV DNA $\geq$5 $\log_{10}$ copies/mL by COBAS Amplicor HBV Monitor® assay (Roche Molecular Systems Inc., Pleasanton, California); screening alanine aminotransferase (ALT) between 1.3× and 10× the upper limit of normal (ULN) with evidence of chronic liver inflammation ($\geq$2 elevated ALT or aspartate aminotransferase values over at least 6 months). Exclusion criteria included: co-infection with hepatitis C virus, hepatitis D virus or HIV; hepatic decompensation; any prior nucleoside treatment or interferon/immunomodulator treatment in the 6 months before screening, or chronic renal insufficiency or serum creatinine clearance below 50 mL/min.

Study Design

Patient disposition is shown in Figure 1 and the study design in Figure 2. Total treatment period is 104 weeks with the primary analysis at 52 weeks. Planned study visits occurred at Weeks 2, 4, 8, 12, 16, 24, 26, 30, 40, 48, and 52. All patients received oral telbivudine (600 mg once daily) for the first 24 weeks. At Week 26, patients with detectable HBV DNA at Week 24 ($\geq$300 copies/mL by COBAS Amplicor) received tenofovir disoproxil fumarate (300 mg once daily) in addition to telbivudine throughout the remaining time on study. Patients with undetectable HBV DNA (<300 copies/mL) at Week 24 continued to receive telbivudine monotherapy.

Efficacy and Safety Analyses

The primary efficacy endpoint was the proportion of patients with undetectable HBV DNA at Week 52. Secondary endpoints included the rate of virological breakthrough; HBV DNA reductions from baseline and proportions with undetectable HBV DNA at each study visit; ALT normalization rates at Weeks 24 and 52, and rates of HBeAg and HBsAg loss and seroconversion at Week 52.

Clinical and laboratory adverse events were graded according to pre-specified criteria and reported relationship to study drug was at investigator discretion. ALT flares were defined according to AASLD criteria [18]. Glomerular filtration rates (GFR) at each visit were estimated using both the Cockcroft-Gault [19] and the Modification Of Diet In Renal Disease Study (MDRD) equations [20,21].

Statistical Analysis

The primary efficacy endpoint was analyzed as a binary variable using last-observation-carried-forward (LOCF) imputa-

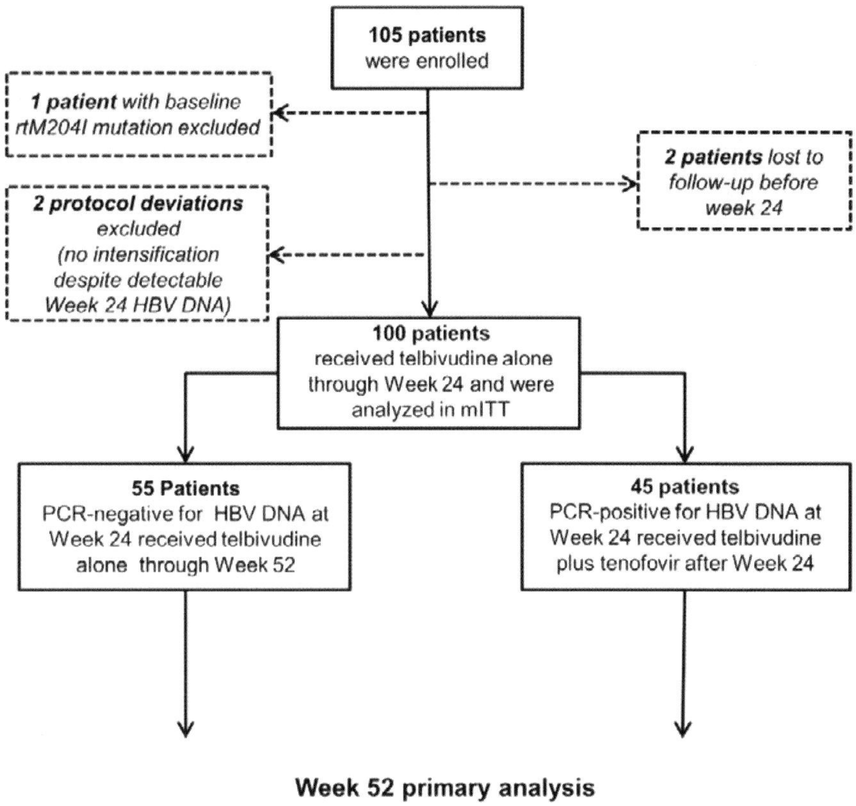

Figure 1. Patient disposition.

tion. The primary endpoint and all binary secondary endpoints were summarized at each visit, with the 95% confidence interval calculated using the normal approximation method for binomial proportion. Differences in baseline demographics and disease characteristics between patients who remained on telbivudine monotherapy through Week 52 and those who added tenofovir after Week 24 were assessed for significance using Fisher's exact test for categorical variables and two-sided t-tests for continuous variables. Changes from baseline in GFR at Week 52 were assessed for significance using two-sided, paired t-tests. Statistical analyses were carried out using SAS ver 1.3 (SAS Institute, Inc. Carey, NC, USA).

The full intention-to-treat (ITT) population comprised all patients who received at least one dose of telbivudine. As this was a study of a specific therapeutic algorithm, a per-protocol population was derived for efficacy assessments – i.e. the efficacy population – which excluded one patient with a confirmed baseline rtM204I resistance mutation to telbivudine/lamivudine, 2 patients lost to follow-up before Week 24, and 2 protocol violators who did not receive tenofovir despite detectable Week 24 HBV DNA. The safety population for adverse event monitoring comprised the full ITT population as defined.

This was a single-arm study, hence the sample size was not based on power for statistical comparison between treatment groups. The primary objective was to demonstrate antiviral efficacy by estimating the proportion of patients with HBV DNA <300 copies/mL at Week 52.

Based on the pivotal phase III GLOBE study (NCT00057265) [15], approximately 44% of patients treated with telbivudine were anticipated to have HBV DNA <300 copies/mL at Week 24, of whom 95% would still be <300 copies/mL at Week 52. By contrast, it was assumed from GLOBE data that only 34% of patients with HBV DNA of 300 copies/mL or above at Week 24 would fall to below 300 copies/mL by Week 52 on telbivudine monotherapy, giving an overall proportion of 60% with <300 copies/mL at Week 52. It was assumed that adding tenofovir at Week 24 for those with ≥300 HBV DNA copies/mL would increase the proportion who subsequently fell to <300 copies/mL at Week 52 to at least 50%. With 100 patients, and under these assumptions, the estimated 95% confidence interval was 70% ±9%, which gave over 95% chance to show a higher rate of HBV DNA <300 copies/mL over telbivudine mono therapy in GLOBE and also provided a reasonably accurate estimate. However, it remains important to note that the two groups after Week 24– telbivudine and telbivudine plus tenofovir – were not randomized and hence statistical comparisons are limited. In particular, the lack of randomization, and confounding by Week 24 response to telbivudine, precludes efficacy comparison between the telbivudine and telbivudine plus tenofovir groups.

Results

Patient Disposition

The efficacy population comprised 100 patients and the safety population 105 patients (Figure 2).

Patient demographics and baseline characteristics are shown in Table 1, stratified according to treatment after Week 24. Compared with those who remained on telbivudine monotherapy, a higher proportion of intensification patients had baseline HBV DNA ≥9 $\log_{10}$ copies/mL (73.3% versus 36.4% of those remaining on monotherapy; P<0.001). Mean baseline ALT was also higher in those who remained on monotherapy (167.2 U/L

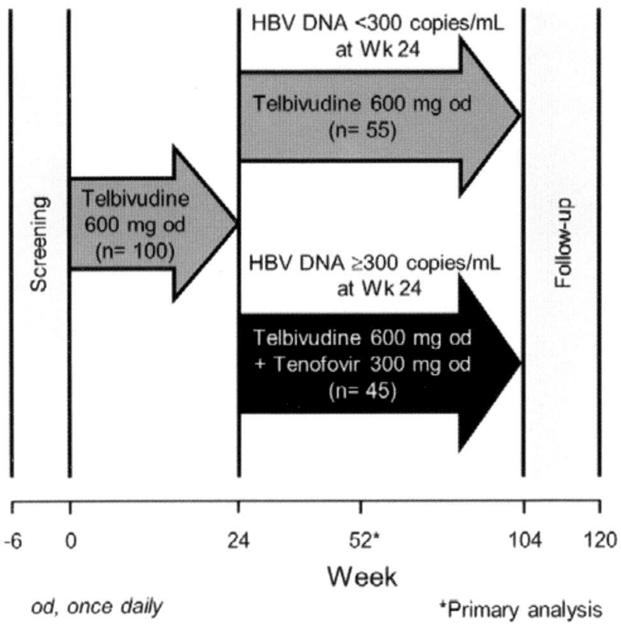

Figure 2. Study design.

versus 93.2 U/L; P = 0.0045). Other characteristics were broadly similar between those who did and did not receive intensification.

A total of 99/100 patients in the efficacy population (99%) completed Week 52. There was one discontinuation in the telbivudine plus tenofovir group for loss to follow-up after Week 30.

Efficacy

At Week 24, 55 of 100 patients (55%) in the efficacy population had undetectable HBV DNA and continued to receive monotherapy. All of these 55 patients remained undetectable at Week 52 on telbivudine monotherapy. The remaining 45 patients (45%) received telbivudine plus tenofovir after Week 24, of whom 38 (84.4%) had undetectable DNA at Week 52. Of these 45 patients, 12 had baseline HBV DNA <9 $\log_{10}$ copies/mL (of whom 3 also had baseline ALT ≥2×ULN) and 33 had ≥9 $\log_{10}$ copies/mL. All (12/12) of the patients with baseline HBV DNA <9 $\log_{10}$ copies/mL, and 78.8% (26/33) of those with ≥9 $\log_{10}$ copies/mL, achieved undetectable DNA at week 52.

The overall rate of undetectable HBV DNA at Week 52 (primary endpoint) was therefore 93% (93/100) by LOCF analysis. This value was the same by a strict ITT missing = failure analysis, as one patient lost to follow-up after Week 30 had detectable HBV DNA (2.67 log) at last visit.

Primary and secondary efficacy endpoints are shown in Table 2. Figure 3 shows mean changes from baseline in HBV DNA by visit for the two treatment groups. By LOCF analysis, mean reduction from baseline in HBV DNA at Week 24 was −6.2 $\log_{10}$ copies/mL in patients who continued to receive telbivudine alone, versus −6.0 $\log_{10}$ copies/mL in those who subsequently received tenofovir. The Week 24 mean reduction remained stable at −6.2 $\log_{10}$ through Week 52 in those who continued telbivudine monotherapy, while the addition of tenofovir resulted in an additional 1.4 $\log_{10}$ reduction at Week 52 in the intensification group.

Table 1. Demographics and baseline characteristics (efficacy population) according to post-Week 24 treatment.

Characteristic		Telbivudine	Telbivudine+tenofovir	*P value*	Overall
N		55	45		100
Age, mean (SD) y		37 (10.4)	40 (15.0)	0.2394	38 (12.7)
Male, n (%)		37 (67)	30 (67)	1.0000	67 (67)
Weight, mean (SD) kg		69.7 (15.0)	65.5 (13.5)	0.1419	67.8 (14.4)
Race, n (%)	Caucasian	11 (20)	16 (36)	0.0550	27 (27)
	Black	0	1 (2)		1 (1)
	Asian	41 (75)	28 (62)		69 (69)
	Other	3 (6)	0		3 (3)
HBV genotype, n (%)	A	6 (11)	8 (18)	0.2192	14 (14)
	B	5 (9)	6 (13)		11 (11)
	C	35 (64)	22 (49)		57 (57)
	D	1 (2)	5 (11)		6 (6)
	F	7 (13)	3 (7)		10 (10)
	Intermediate	1 (2)	1 (2)		2 (2)
Serum ALT, mean (SD) U/L		167.2 (162.2)	93.2 (57.8)	**0.0045**	133.9 (131.2)
Serum HBV DNA (copies/mL), n (%)	5– <6 $\log_{10}$	4 (7)	1 (2)		5 (5)
	6– <7 $\log_{10}$	7 (13)	1 (2)		8 (8)
	7– <8 $\log_{10}$	11 (20)	4 (9)		15 (15)
	8– <9 $\log_{10}$	13 (24)	6 (13)		19 (19)
	≥9 $\log_{10}$	20 (36)	33 (73)	**<0.001**	53 (53)
GFR, mean (SD) mL/min/1.73 m^2 by MDRD		93.4 (15.1)	92.1 (18.5)	0.6873	92.8 (16.6)

Table 2. Results of efficacy endpoints up to Week 52 (efficacy population, LOCF).

n (%)	Efficacy endpoint	Telbivudine monotherapy (n = 55)	Telbivudine+Tenofovir (n = 45)	Overall (N = 100)
Week 24	HBV DNA <300 copies/mL	55/55 (100)	0/45	55/100 (55.0)
Week 52	HBV DNA <300 copies/mL	55/55 (100)	38/45 (84.4)	93/100 (93.0)
	Virologic breakthrough	0/55 (0)	0/45 (0)	0/100 (0)
	HBeAg loss*	36/55 (65.5)	7/44 (15.9)	43/99 (43.4)
	HBeAg seroconversion*	34/55 (61.8)	5/44 (11.4)	39/99 (39.4)
	HBsAg loss*	1/55 (1.8)	5/44 (11.4)	6/99 (6.1)
	HBsAg seroconversion*	0/55 (0)	3/44 (6.8)	3/99 (3.0)
	ALT normalization	48/55 (87.3)	29/45 (64.4)	77/100 (77.0)

*HBeAg/HBsAg loss and seroconversion were evaluated at Week 52 only without LOCF imputation. HBeAg/HBsAg data were unavailable for 1/45 patients receiving telbivudine + tenofovir.

Overall, 43.4% of patients (43/99) with available data at Week 52 lost HBeAg and 39.4% (39/99) achieved HBeAg seroconversion. Rates of HBeAg loss and seroconversion among those who remained on monotherapy (65.5% and 61.8%, respectively) were approximately fourfold higher than among those who received intensification (15.9% and 11.4%, respectively). HBsAg clearance at Week 52 occurred in 6.1% (6/99) and HBsAg seroconversion in 3.0% (3/99). Of the six patients with HBsAg loss, one (Genotype B) was in the monotherapy group and five (3 Genotype A, 1 F;1 B) in the intensification group; four were Hispanic Caucasians and two were other races, and all had baseline HBV DNA >9 log_{10} copies/mL.

Overall, 77% of patients achieved ALT normalization at Week 52: 48/55 (87%) in the monotherapy group and 29/45 (64%) in the intensification group.

No virologic breakthrough and no genotypic resistance over 52 weeks was observed.

Safety

Adverse events through Week 52 in the safety population are shown in Table 3. Adverse events were similar to the GLOBE study and balanced between treatment groups.

There were no deaths. Five serious adverse events occurred, comprising one case each of atrial septal defect, gallbladder polyp, vascular injury and spontaneous abortion on telbivudine alone; and one foot fracture on telbivudine plus tenofovir. No event was considered treatment related.

There were no reports of myopathy, myositis, rhabdomyolysis, lactic acidosis, pancreatitis or peripheral neuropathy. One patient reported mild muscle weakness. The study treatment was interrupted and patient followed up in-study. This patient (highest creatine kinase 1866 IU/mL) did not have objective evidence of decreased muscle strength or abnormal EMG or muscle biopsy results. Myalgia occurred in 13 patients. Twelve were mild and one was moderate. Twelve resolved and one was followed up in-study. Twelve patients continued the study treatment without

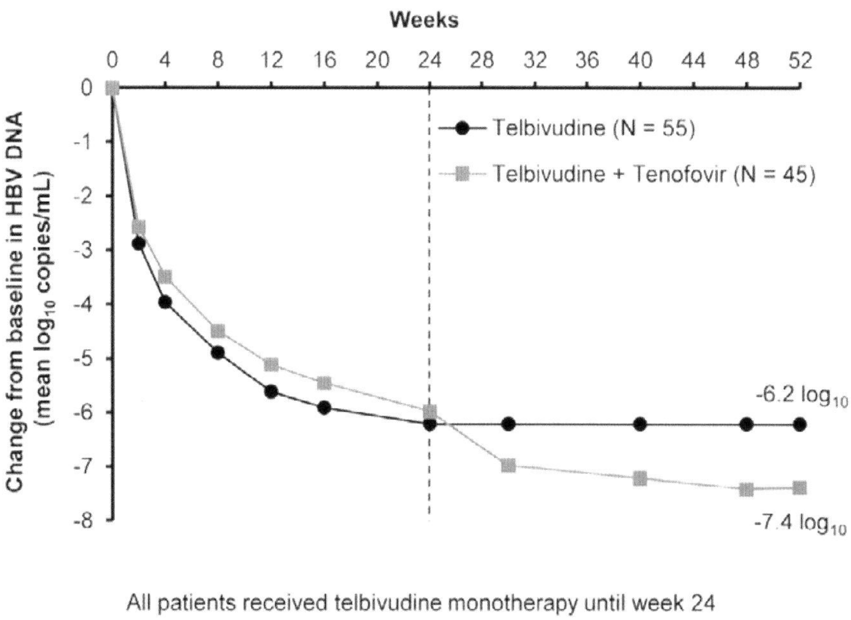

Figure 3. Changes from baseline in HBV DNA by post-Week 24 treatment (efficacy population).

Table 3. Most common (≥5%) all-cause adverse events through Week 52 (safety population).

		Tenofovir intensification (n = 46)		
n (%)	**Telbivudine monotherapy (n = 59)**	**Telbivudine only period**	**Tenofovir add on period**	**Overall*(N = 105)**
Total patients with any event	**42 (71.2)**	**23 (50.0)**	**20 (43.5)**	**73 (69.5)**
Myalgia	10 (16.9)	3 (6.5)	1 (2.2)	13 (12.4)
Headache	6 (10.2)	5 (10.9)	1 (2.2)	12 (11.4)
Upper respiratory tract infection	4 (6.8)	4 (8.7)	1 (2.2)	9 (8.6)
Dyspepsia	4 (6.8)	0 (0.0)	3 (6.5)	7 (6.7)
Arthralgia	1 (1.7)	2 (4.3)	3 (6.5)	5 (4.8)
Diarrhoea	3 (5.1)	1 (2.2)	1 (2.2)	5 (4.8)
Nausea	2 (3.4)	0 (0.0)	3 (6.5)	5 (4.8)
Dizziness	3 (5.1)	1 (2.2)	0 (0.0)	4 (3.8)
Fatigue	3 (5.1)	1 (2.2)	0 (0.0)	4 (3.8)
Pain in extremity	3 (5.1)	1 (2.2)	0 (0.0)	4 (3.8)
Pyrexia	3 (5.1)	1 (2.2)	0 (0.0)	4 (3.8)
Vomiting	1 (1.7)	0 (0.0)	3 (6.5)	4 (3.8)
Nasopharyngitis	3 (5.1)	0 (0.0)	1 (2.2)	4 (3.8)
Upper abdominal pain	0 (0.0)	3 (6.5)	0 (0.0)	3 (2.9)
Cough	0 (0.0)	2 (4.3)	1 (2.2)	3 (2.9)

*Intensification patients may have had an event during both the telbivudine only and intensification periods. Overall numbers with an indicated event may therefore be less than the row total.

interruption and one discontinued. Six myalgia cases were not suspected to be related to study treatment.

Grade 3 or grade 4 creatine kinase elevations occurred in two patients in the monotherapy group (one grade 3 at Week 48 and one grade 4 at Week 49) and two intensification group patients (one grade 3 at Week 16 on telbivudine alone and another at Week 52 on telbivudine plus tenofovir).

Two patients experienced an ALT flare. Both occurred under initial telbivudine monotherapy (Weeks 4 and 8) in patients who later received intensification. Both flare patients had undetectable HBV DNA at Week 52.

There were no renal events other than one treatment-unrelated case of moderate renal colic. No patient reported with creatinine increase. Mean Week 52 GFR was significantly higher than baseline in both treatment groups. Overall mean GFR change to week 52 by the MDRD and the Cockcroft-Gault formulae was 6.9 mL/min and 8.3 mL/min, respectively, in the monotherapy group; and 7.4 mL/min and 6.2 mL/min, respectively, in the intensification group ($P<0.01$ for all comparisons). Figure 4 shows week 52 GFR changes (MDRD) stratified by baseline GFR. No significant GFR decline was noted in patients with low baseline GFR, although numbers were small.

Discussion

In providing a framework for the conditional intensification of monotherapy, the Roadmap [16] provides a rational approach to improve long-term outcomes, while minimizing the risk of drug resistance due to continued sub-optimal monotherapy or adverse events associated with unnecessary combination treatment. Under the Roadmap, nucleosides with a low genetic barrier to resistance (e.g. lamivudine) are intensified with a non-cross-resistant second agent if any HBV replication is still measurable at Week 24. Although telbivudine is more potent than lamivudine with less on-treatment resistance [5,15], it is closest to lamivudine in terms of the features informing Roadmap decisions; and intensification was applied to any patient with detectable Week 24 viremia. The requirement for a non-cross-resistant second agent predicates the use of adefovir or tenofovir [6], with tenofovir the better choice due to greater potency [10].

Over half the patients achieved undetectable Week 24 viremia on telbivudine alone, and, following tenofovir intensification of the remaining 45%, the overall proportion of undetectable HBV DNA was greater than 90% at Week 52. The additional reduction in HBV DNA seen following tenofovir intensification of viremic patients is presumably due to additive antiviral activity. There was no in-study comparator to estimate the treatment effect of tenofovir intensification over continued telbivudine monotherapy in viremic patients. Nor was tenofovir monotherapy investigated, or the effect of switching viremic patients to tenofovir as opposed to adding it to telbivudine. However, historical data suggest that intensification would have significantly improved Week 52 outcomes over what would have been seen had telbivudine monotherapy been continued. In GLOBE [15] a broadly similar rate of undetectable viremia at Week 24 (45%) was seen in HBeAg+ telbivudine patients to that seen here (55%), but with a substantially lower rate of undetectable DNA at Week 52 (60%). GLOBE also showed lower rates of undetectable HBV DNA, ALT normalization and HBeAg seroconversion at Week 52, and higher rates of drug resistance at Week 48, for patients with detectable Week 24 viremia [15], although the design of these analyses precludes cross-study comparison. Similar results were observed in a study of telbivudine versus lamivudine in over 300 Chinese patients [22]. Finally, in the two-year GLOBE analyses, 82% (166/203) of HBeAg+ patients with undetectable Week 24 HBV remained undetectable through two years, but only 36% (89/247) of those with detectable Week 24 DNA were undetectable at the end of Year 2 [23].

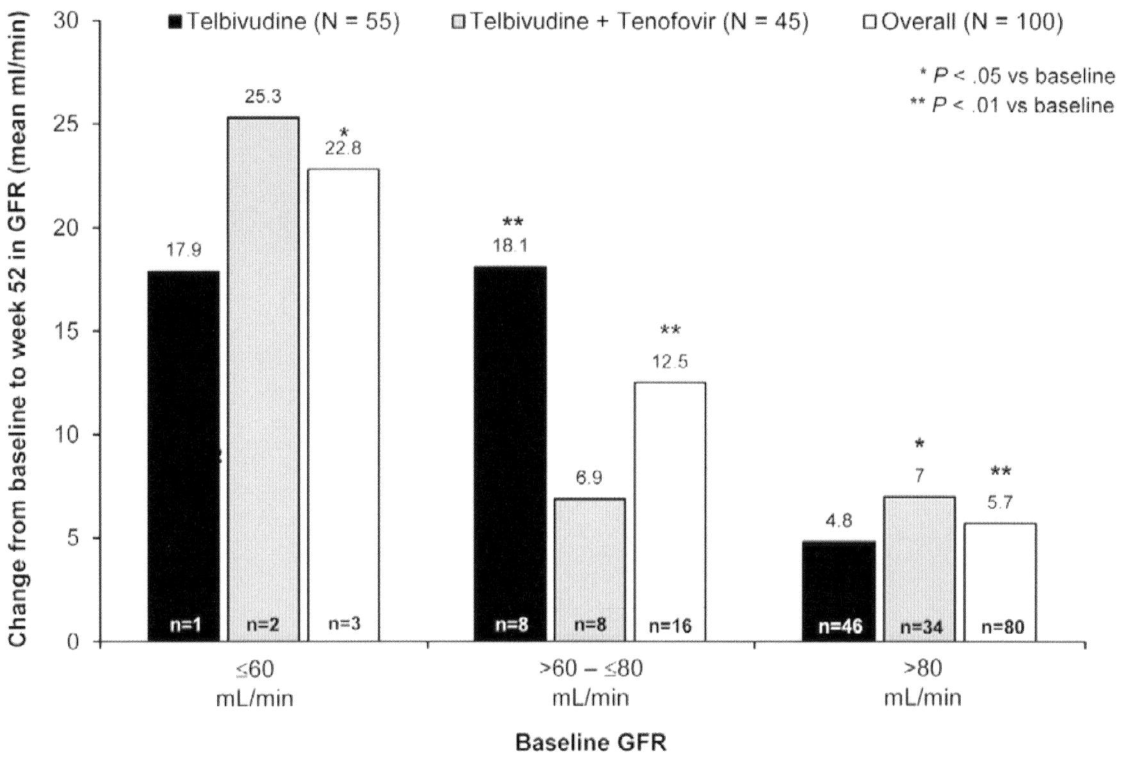

Figure 4. Week 52 glomerular filtration rate (MDRD) changes, by baseline rate and treatment (efficacy population).

HBeAg clearance and seroconversion rates were very high (Table 2), with most (approximately 85% of cases) occurring in those with undetectable Week 24 viremia who remained on telbivudine monotherapy. Effective clearance and seroconversion of HBeAg therefore appears to be a function of early and complete virologic suppression. The 6% rate of HBsAg loss at 1 year of treatment was also substantially higher than the typically reported per-annum rates of <1% on nucleosides and approximately 3% on interferon treatment [24,25]. The association of HBsAg response with intensification (5/6 cases of loss and all three cases of seroconversion) suggests a potential synergistic effect between tenofovir and telbivudine that merits longer-term investigation in a larger dataset.

Safety and tolerability were consistent with GLOBE, and, other than myalgia, muscle-related events were rare. Of 13 patients with myalgia, most (12/13) experienced mild events and most (12/13) resolved sponataneously.

No renal toxicity was observed after 24 weeks of tenofovir plus telbivudine. Mean GFR at week 52 was significantly higher than baseline in both the monotherapy and intensification groups. These findings are consistent with both 2-year clinical data from a study of telbivudine versus lamivudine in decompensated HBV disease [26]. Furthermore, retrospective analyses of seven studies (2500 patients) in both compensated and decompensated disease showed consistent GFR improvements on telbivudine treatment for up to 6 years compared with GFR declines on lamivudine therapy. Improvement was greatest in patients more than 50 years old and those with abnormal baseline GFR; and was not associated with baseline ascites, virologic response or reduction in Child-Pugh score [27]. GFR improvement on telbivudine stands in contrast to the declines over time observed in studies of tenofovir [28] and entecavir [29]. Interestingly, GFR modeling data from Mauss *et al.* predict a year-on-year GFR reduction of approximately 2 mL/min in untreated HBV monoinfection which is halved, but not abolished, by monotherapy with lamivudine, adefovir, entecavir or tenofovir [30]. Telbivudine was not studied in the Mauss model, and more research is needed to confirm and provide a mechanism for the apparent dissimilarity of telbivudine to the other nucleosides with respect to GFR preservation.

The Roadmap algorithm does not consider baseline HBV DNA in treatment decisions [16]. However, in this study, high baseline DNA was predictive of detectable Week 24 viremia requiring intensification. Almost three-quarters of patients who received tenofovir had baseline HBV DNA ≥9 $\log_{10}$ copies/mL. In future, baseline viremia may need to be considered in any treatment algorithm where decisions are made on the presence of detectable viremia early on therapy.

In conclusion, telbivudine with conditional tenofovir intensification according to the Roadmap algorithm was well tolerated and, over 52 weeks, resulted in very high rates of undetectable HBV DNA, ALT normalization, and HBeAg/HBsAg clearance and seroconversion in nucleoside-naive HBeAg+ patients with chronic HBV infection, along with an improvement in GFR. The Roadmap appears to be a highly effective approach to HBV treatment and 104-week data from this study are awaited.

Supporting Information

Table S1 List of ethics committees/institutional review boards.

Checklist S1 CONSORT checklist.

Protocol S1 Study protocol.

Author Contributions

Critical manuscript review and amendment: TP PK TT WS HLYC MGP EF SKO FB JD SZ HC RP YD AT. Conceived and designed the experiments: TP RP YD AT. Performed the experiments: TP PK TT WS HLYC MGP EF SKO FB JD SZ HC. Analyzed the data: TP RP YD AT. Wrote the paper: YD.

References

1. McMahon BJ (2005) Epidemiology and natural history of hepatitis B. Semin Liver Dis 25 (Suppl 1): 3–8.
2. Yuen MF, Seto WK, Chow DH, Tsui K, Wong DK, et al. (2007) Long-term lamivudine therapy reduces the risk of long-term complications of chronic hepatitis B infection even in patients without advanced disease. Antivir Ther 12: 1295–1303.
3. Tenney DJ, Rose RE, Baldick CJ, Pokornowski KA, Eggers BJ, et al. (2009) Long-term monitoring shows hepatitis B virus resistance to entecavir in nucleoside-naive patients is rare through 5 years of therapy. Hepatology 49: 1503–1514.
4. Tenney DJ, Levine SM, Rose RE, Walsh AW, Weinheimer SP, et al. (2004) Clinical emergence of entecavir-resistant hepatitis B virus requires additional substitutions in virus already resistant to Lamivudine. Antimicrob Agents Chemother 48: 3498–3507.
5. Liaw YF, Gane E, Leung N, Zeuzem S, Wang Y, et al. (2009) 2-Year GLOBE trial results: telbivudine Is superior to lamivudine in patients with chronic hepatitis B. Gastroenterology 136: 486–495.
6. Yang H, Qi X, Sabogal A, Miller M, Xiong S, et al. (2005) Cross-resistance testing of next-generation nucleoside and nucleotide analogues against lamivudine-resistant HBV. Antivir Ther 10: 625–633.
7. Izzedine H, Hulot JS, Launay-Vacher V, Marcellini P, Hadziyannis SJ, et al. (2004) Renal safety of adefovir dipivoxil in patients with chronic hepatitis B: two double-blind, randomized, placebo-controlled studies. Kidney Int 66: 1153–1158.
8. Chan HL, Heathcote EJ, Marcellin P, Lai CL, Cho M, et al. (2007) Treatment of hepatitis B e antigen positive chronic hepatitis with telbivudine or adefovir: a randomized trial. Ann Intern Med 147: 745–754.
9. Leung N, Peng CY, Hann HW, Sollano J, Lao-Tan J, et al. (2009) Early hepatitis B virus DNA reduction in hepatitis B e antigen-positive patients with chronic hepatitis B: A randomized international study of entecavir versus adefovir. Hepatology 49: 72–79.
10. Marcellin P, Heathcote EJ, Buti M, Gane E, de Man RA, et al. (2008) Tenofovir disoproxil fumarate versus adefovir dipivoxil for chronic hepatitis B. N Engl J Med 359: 2442–2455.
11. Cooper RD, Wiebe N, Smith N, Keiser P, Naicker S, et al. (2010) Systematic review and meta-analysis: renal safety of tenofovir disoproxil fumarate in HIV-infected patients. Clin Infect Dis 51: 496–505.
12. Chen CJ, Yang HI, Iloeje UH (2009) Hepatitis B virus DNA levels and outcomes in chronic hepatitis B. Hepatology 49: S72–S84.
13. Mommeja-Marin H, Mondou E, Blum MR, Rousseau F (2003) Serum HBV DNA as a marker of efficacy during therapy for chronic HBV infection: analysis and review of the literature. Hepatology 37: 1309–1319.
14. Yuen MF, Sablon E, Hui CK, Yuan HJ, Decraemer H, et al. (2001) Factors associated with hepatitis B virus DNA breakthrough in patients receiving prolonged lamivudine therapy. Hepatology 34: 785–791.
15. Lai CL, Gane E, Liaw YF, Hsu CW, Thongsawat S, et al. (2007) Telbivudine versus lamivudine in patients with chronic hepatitis B. N Engl J Med 357: 2576–2588.
16. Keeffe EB, Zeuzem S, Koff RS, Dieterich DT, Esteban-Mur R, et al. (2007) Report of an international workshop: Roadmap for management of patients receiving oral therapy for chronic hepatitis B. Clin Gastroenterol Hepatol 5: 890–897.
17. European Association For The Study Of The Liver (2009) EASL Clinical Practice Guidelines: management of chronic hepatitis B. J Hepatol 50: 227–242.
18. Lok AS, McMahon BJ (2007) Chronic hepatitis B. Hepatology 45: 507–539.
19. Cockcroft DW, Gault MH (1976) Prediction of creatinine clearance from serum creatinine. Nephron 16: 31–41.
20. National Kidney Foundation (2002) K/DOQI clinical practice guidelines for chronic kidney disease: evaluation, classification, and stratification. Part 5. Evaluation of laboratory measurements for clinical assessment of kidney disease. Am J Kidney Dis 39: S76–S110.
21. Levey AS, Bosch JP, Lewis JB, Greene T, Rogers N, et al. (1999) A more accurate method to estimate glomerular filtration rate from serum creatinine: a new prediction equation. Modification of Diet in Renal Disease Study Group. Ann Intern Med 130: 461–470.
22. Jia JD, Hou JL, Yin YK, Xu DZ, Tan DM, et al. (2007) [The degree of HBV suppression with 24 week telbivudine- or lamivudine-treatment in hepatitis B patients predicts the efficacy of the treatment at week 52]. Zhonghua Gan Zang Bing Za Zhi 15: 342–345.
23. Zeuzem S, Gane E, Liaw YF, Lim SG, DiBisceglie A, et al. (2009) Baseline characteristics and early on-treatment response predict the outcomes of 2 years of telbivudine treatment of chronic hepatitis B. J Hepatol 51: 11–20.
24. Andersson KL, Chung RT (2009) Monitoring during and after antiviral therapy for hepatitis B. Hepatology 49: S166–S173.
25. Liaw YF, Chu CM (2009) Hepatitis B virus infection. Lancet 373: 582–592.
26. Gane EJ, Chan HL, Choudhuri G, Suh DJ, Chutaputti A, et al. (2010) Treatment of decompensated HBV-cirrhosis: results from 2-years randomized trial with telbivudine or lamivudine [Abstract]. J Hepatol (Suppl. 1): S4.
27. Gane EJ, Deray G, Piratvisuth T, Chan HL, Zeuzem S, et al. (2011) Renal function is improved for Chronic Hepatitis B (CHB) patients treated with telbivudine [Abstract]. Hepatol (Suppl. 1): 1044A-1045A.
28. van Bömmel F, de Man R, Ferenci P, Bronowiki JP, Fülöp B, et al. (2009) Long-term follow-up evaluation of the efficacy and safety of tenofovir disoproxil fumarate (TDF) in a European multicenter (nucleos(t)ide experienced) hepatitis B virus HBV-infected cohort. 60th Annual Meeting of the American Association for the Study of Liver Diseases, Boston, MA, USA; Oct 30 - Nov 3, 2009 [Abstract 221]. Available: http://www.hivandhepatitis.com/2009icr/aasld/posters/vanBommel.ppt. Accessed 2012 Jul 31.
29. Gish RG, Mangahas MF, Baqai SF, Shaw RE, Clark MD, et al. (2010) Risk of renal toxicity with tenofovir DF (TFD) for chronic hepatitis B (CHB) [Abstract]. Hepatol 52 (Suppl. 1): 529A.
30. Mauss S, Berger F, Filmann N, Hueppe D, Henke J, et al. (2011) Effect of HBV polymerase inhibitors on renal function in patients with chronic hepatitis B. J Hepatol 55: 1235–1240.

Analysis of Hepatitis B Virus Intrahepatic Covalently Closed Circular DNA and Serum Viral Markers in Treatment-Naive Patients with Acute and Chronic HBV Infection

Weijie Li[1,2]⁹, Jingmin Zhao[3]⁹, Zhengsheng Zou[2], Yan Liu[2], Baosen Li[2], Ying Sun[2], Xiaodong Li[2], Shuhong Liu[3], Shaoping Cai[2], Weimin Yao[2], Shaojie Xin[2], Fengmin Lu[1]*, Dongping Xu[1,2]*

1 Department of Microbiology, Peking University Health Science Center, Beijing, China, **2** Institute of Infectious Diseases and Medical Center for Liver Failure, Beijing 302 Hospital, Beijing, China, **3** Department of Pathology, Beijing 302 Hospital, Beijing, China

Abstract

Background: This study aimed to investigate the relationships of intrahepatic cccDNA with serum HBsAg and with HBV DNA in treatment-naive patients throughout acute and chronic HBV infection.

Methods: A total of 120 patients who had a liver biopsy were enrolled, including 19 with acute hepatitis B (AHB), and 101 patients with chronic HBV infection (CHB) of whom were 10 in immune-tolerant (IT) phase, 59 in immune-clearance (IC) phase, 8 in low-replicative (LR) phase, and 24 in HBeAg-negative hepatitis (ENH) phase. Intrahepatic cccDNA, serum HBsAg and serum HBV DNA levels were comparatively analyzed.

Results: The median intrahepatic cccDNA levels were 0.18 4.80, 3.81, 0.22 and 0.97 copies/cell for patients with AHB, CHB-IT, CHB-IC, CHB-LR, and CHB-ENH, respectively. In AHB patients, intrahepatic cccDNA was positively correlated with serum HBsAg ($r = 0.665$, $P = 0.003$), as well as serum HBV DNA ($r = 0.536$, $P = 0.022$). In CHB patients, intrahepatic cccDNA was positively correlated with serum HBsAg in the IC phase ($r = 0.392$, $P = 0.005$), and with serum HBV DNA in the IC phase ($r = 0.301$, $P = 0.036$) and ENH phase ($r = 0.588$, $P = 0.013$). HBV replicative efficiency, defined as the ratio of serum HBV DNA to intrahepatic cccDNA, was obviously lower in AHB and CHB-LR patients than in CHB-IT, CHB-IC and CHB-ENH patients (0.70 and 0.53 vs. 1.12, 1.09 and 0.99, $P < 0.001$, values were logarithmic transformed for analysis). In CHB-IC patients, HBV replicative efficiency was positively correlated with histological activity index of liver inflammation ($r = 0.308$, $P = 0.009$).

Conclusion: Serum HBsAg and HBV DNA levels may reflect the amount of active intrahepatic cccDNA in treatment-naive AHB and CHB-IC patients. Reduced intrahepatic cccDNA and HBV replicative efficiency may imply effective immune control of HBV infection.

Editor: Haitao Guo, Drexel University College of Medicine, United States of America

Funding: This work was supported by the National Natural Science Foundation of China (81171617), and 12th Five-Year High-Tech Grand (2010gxjs009), and 12th Five-Year Special Grand project for Infectious Diseases (2012ZX10004503). The funders had no role in study design, data collection and analysis, decision to publish, or preparation of the manuscript. The funders had no role in study design, data collection and analysis, decision to publish, or preparation of the manuscript.

Competing Interests: The authors have declared that no competing interests exist.

* E-mail: xudongping302@sina.com (DX); lu.fengmin@hsc.pku.edu.cn (FL)

⁹ These authors contributed equally to this work.

Introduction

Chronic hepatitis B virus (HBV) infection remains a serious health problem. Around 350–400 million people worldwide and 93 million in China are chronic HBV surface antigen (HBsAg) carriers [1,2]. Chronic HBV infection is associated with high risk of developing liver cirrhosis and hepatocellular carcinoma [3]. One crucial step in HBV life cycle is the formation of covalently closed circular DNA (cccDNA), which serves as original template for viral replication and plays an important role in the persistence of HBV infection [4,5,6]. Quantitation of intrahepatic HBV cccDNA is suggested to be valuable in evaluating anti-HBV therapeutic efficacy and estimating treatment endpoint [7,8,9,10,11,12]. In addition, HBV cccDNA level is considered to be a valuable marker for HBV recurrence after liver transplantation and extrahepatic HBV infection [13,14].

The major obstacle for quantitation of cccDNA in clinic is the requirement for invasive liver biopsy. Therefore, finding serum surrogate maker of intrahepatic cccDNA is clinically meaningful. Recently, correlation between serum HBsAg and HBV DNA levels with intrahepatic cccDNA level has been actively investigated for patients with chronic hepatitis B infection (CHB) [15,16,17]. Serum HBsAg and HBV DNA levels were suggested

Table 1. Definitions of phases of persistent HBV infection.

Phase	HBeAg status	HBV DNA (IU/ml)	ALT* (U/L)
immune tolerance (IT)	(+)	>107	<ULN
immune clearance (IC)	(+)	>2000	>2× ULN
low-replicative (LR)	(−)	<2000	<ULN
HBeAg(-) hepatitis (ENH)	(−)	>2000	>2× ULN

*In IT and LR groups patients with ALT activity of <1.5 ULN were accepted if no inflammation in liver biopsy was observed. In IC and ENH groups patients with ALT activity of >ULN were accepted if significant inflammation.

to serve as a surrogate markers of intrahepatic cccDNA for evaluating effectiveness and endpoint of anti-HBV treatment for patients with chronic hepatitis B, particularly for HBeAg-positive patients. However, controversial conclusion existed. For examples, patients on treatment with nucleos(t)ide analogs with greater reductions in levels of cccDNA had greater reductions in HBsAg, but these reductions were not statistically significant [11]; serum HBV DNA, but not HBsAg, reflected the amount of cccDNA and the replicatvive efficiency of HBV in patients with HBeAg-negative hepatitis B [12]. Similarly, inconsistent results were documented on the relationship between intrahepatic cccDNA and serum HBV DNA among HBeAg-positive patients prior to antiviral treatment [7,16].

The dynamic processes of intrahepatic and serum HBV replication markers and histopathological damage are suggested to be complex in CHB patients [18,19]. The production of HBsAg by the cccDNA can be independent of the replication of the virus [16], and study results could be influenced by disease stages, antiviral treatments, sample resource and size, and cccDNA quantitative assays. There is still a paucity of data presenting the correlation of intrahepatic cccDNA with serum viral markers in patients with acute hepatitis B (AHB) and treatment-naive CHB patients at different natural phases. This study aimed to investigate the relationship between intrahepatic cccDNA and serum viral markers including HBsAg and HBV DNA throughout natural phases of acute and chronic HBV infection.

Materials and Methods

Study Subjects

The study population consisted of 19 AHB and 101 CHB Chinese patients who were admitted to Beijing 302 Hospital from January 2008 to December 2012. CHB patients comprised of 10 in immune-tolerant (IT) phase, 59 in immune-clearance (IC) phase, 8 in low-replicative (LR) phase, and 24 in HBeAg-negative (ENH) phase. The diagnosis criteria for acute and chronic hepatitis B were according to the 2000 Xi'an Viral Hepatitis Management Scheme issued by the Chinese Society of Infectious Diseases and Parasitology and the Chinese Society of Hepatology, of the Chinese Medical Association [20], and had been described in details in our previous studies [21,22]. The definitions of phases of persistent HBV-infection were shown in Table 1 according to previous definitions [23]. The clinical backgrounds of patients were summarized in Table 2. In the 32 HBeAg-negative patients, 27 harbored G1896A and (or) A1762T+G1764A mutations (19 with G1896A, 18 with A1762T+G1764A, and 10 with the both). HBeAb was positive for 29 of the 32 HBeAg-negative patients. Patients co-infected with hepatitis A, C, D, E, and F virus, or patients with autoimmune or metabolic liver disease were excluded. The study was approved by ethics committee of Beijing 302 Hospital and the written informed consents were obtained from all patients.

Sample Collection, Quantitation of Serum HBsAg and HBV DNA

Liver biopsy was obtained from all patients. Sera were collected on the same day of liver biopsy for biochemical, virological and serological analyses. The titer of serum HBsAg was quantitated by a chemiluminescence assay using the Architect i2000SR platform and Abbott Architect HBsAg reagents (Abbott Laboratories, Chicago, IL), according to the manufacture's instruction. The lower limit of detection was 0.05 IU/mL. If the initial test value was higher than the upper limit of detection (250 IU/mL), the samples were diluted (1:500) and reassessed. Serum HBV DNA was quantitated by Taqman real-time polymerase chain reaction using commercially available HBV-DNA real-time quantitative PCR kit (Fosun Pharmaceutical Co., Ltd., Shanghai, China) with a lower detection limit of 100 IU/mL, or COBAS AmpliPrep/COBAS TaqMan (Roche Diagnostics, Mannheim, Germany) with a lower detection limit of 12 IU/mL if needed.

Table 2. Clinical details of the studied patients.

	AHB (n = 19)	CHB-IT (n = 10)	CHB-IC (n = 59)	CHB-LR (n = 8)	CHB-ENG (n = 24)	*P* value
Gender (M/F)	15/4	7/3	49/10	4/4	17/7	0.257
Age (years)	32 (24–41)	18 (10–34)	30 (14–43)	30 (15–42)	35 (23–41)	0.332
TBil (μmol/L)	122 (33.9–171.5)	8.4 (5.7–13.1)	12.2 (8.6–24.6)	10.7 (7.8–12.8)	15.0 (8.8–20.4)	<0.001
Albumin (g/L)	39 (36–41)	40 (38–41)	40 (37–43)	39 (38–42.3)	41 (38–46)	0.330
Albumin/globulin	1.4 (1.2–1.8)	1.7 (1.4–1.9)	1.6 (1.3–1.9)	1.5 (1.4–1.8)	1.6 (1.3–1.9)	0.871
Cholinesterase (IU/L)	5661(4270–7225)	7662 (6091–8634)	5899 (4827–7364)	7920 (5788–9544)	6332 (5127–7851)	0.210
ALT (IU/L)	1571(1014–2142)	33 (17–39)	132 (62–398)	20 (17–32)	138 (63–346)	<0.001
HBV DNA (log_{10} IU/mL)	3.88 (2.87–4.80)	7.95 (7.35–8.32)	6.43 (4.86–7.84)	3.08 (2.44–3.14)	6.1 (5.21–8.01)	<0.001
HBeAg	Positive	Positive	Positive	Negative	Negative	
HBV genotype (B/C)	7/12	2/8	11/48	1/7	4/20	

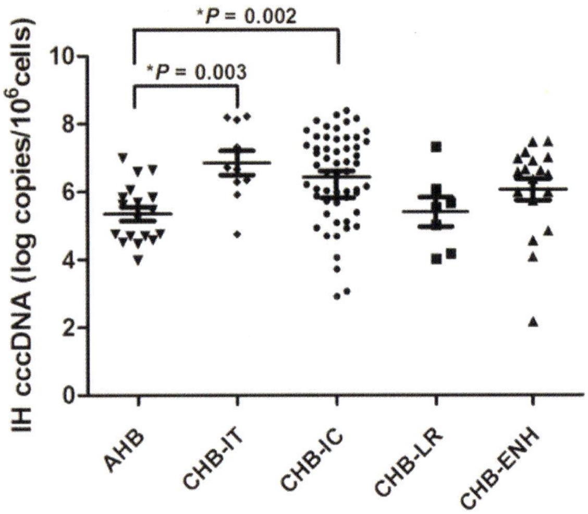

Figure 1. Comparison of intrahepatic (IH) HBV cccDNA levels among patients with different clinical presentations. The horizontal lines illustrate the 25th, 50th, and 75th percentiles of the cccDNA levels. Symbols * and ** represent *P* value less than 0.01 and 0.05, respectively. AHB, acute hepatitis B; CHB, chronic HBV infection; IT, immune-tolerant; IC, immune-clearance; LR, low-replicative; ENH, HBeAg-negative hepatitis.

HBV Genotype Classification

HBV genotype assignment as based on phylogenetic analysis of the 1,225-bp-long S/Pol gene sequence (nucleotides 54 to 1278) as we described previously [24]. Phylogenetic and molecular evolutionary analyses were performed in MEGA version 4. Phylogenetic trees were constructed using neighbor-joining (NJ) analysis with bootstrap test confirmation performed on 1,000 resampling standard reference sequences acquired from the online Hepatitis Virus Database (http://www.ncbi.nlm.nih.gov/projects/genotyping/formpage.cgi).

Histological Examination of Liver Tissues

Histological sections of liver biopsy specimens were stained with hematoxylin-eosin. Histologic grading of necroinflammation and staging of fibrosis were performed using Knodell histological activity index (HAI) (range 0 to 18) and the Ishak fibrosis score (range 0 to 6) respectively, as previously described [18,25,26]. The degree of necroinflammation was classified into score 0–3, 4–8, 9–12, and >score 12 groups. The stage of fibrosis was classified into 4 groups based on the Ishak fibrosis scores.

Quantitation of Intrahepatic HBV cccDNA

Intrahepatic HBV cccDNA was extracted and quantitated by the assay as we described previously [27]. Briefly, about 30 µm formalin fixed paraffin-embedded (FFPE) liver biopsy tissue was sectioned to 6 µm each for DNA extraction. To prevent contamination, disposable tweezers, brush and interleaver were used and sectioning blades were carefully cleaned with 70% ethanol after every sampling. The DNA was extracted using QIAamp FFPE DNA Mini Kit (QIAGEN, GmbH, Hilden, Germany) according to the instructions of the manufacturer. PSAD (Epicentre, Madison, WI, USA) was used to digest HBV rcDNA, replicative dsDNA and ssDNA. Afterwards, rolling Circle Amplification (RCA) was conducted to selectively amplify circle DNA. Using the RCA products as template, HBV cccDNA was further amplified and quantified with TaqMan real-time PCR mediated by a pair of cccDNA-selective primers and a probe that targets the gap region between the two direct repeat regions (DR1 and DR2) of the viral genome. To quantitate cell numbers, a set of primers and a probe for reference control DNA segment of human beta-actin were used in the real-time PCR process. Cell numbers were calculated based on an estimation of 6.667 pg/hgDNA per cell.

Statistical Analysis

Data were presented as median and inter-quartile range. Differences between variables was tested by Student's *t*-test or one-way ANOVA test where it is appropriate. Regression and

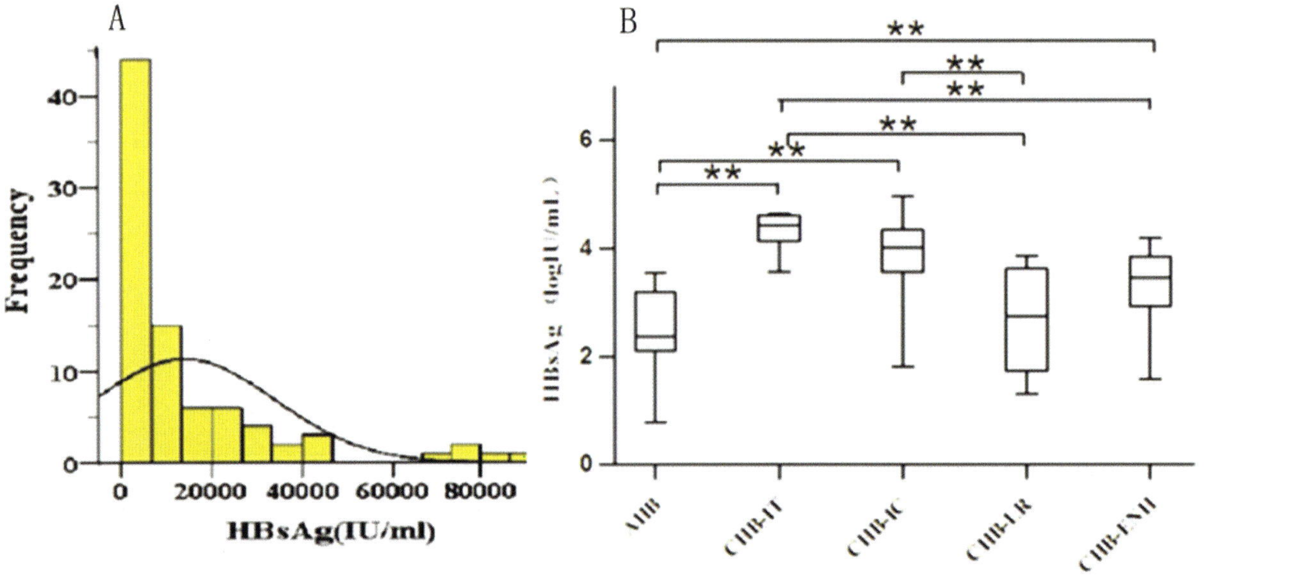

Figure 2. Quantitation of serum HBsAg for 120 HBV-infected patients with different clinical presentations. The distribution of serum HBsAg level across the study population (A). Comparison of serum HBsAg levels among patients with different clinical presentations (B). Symbol ** represent *P* value less than 0.01.

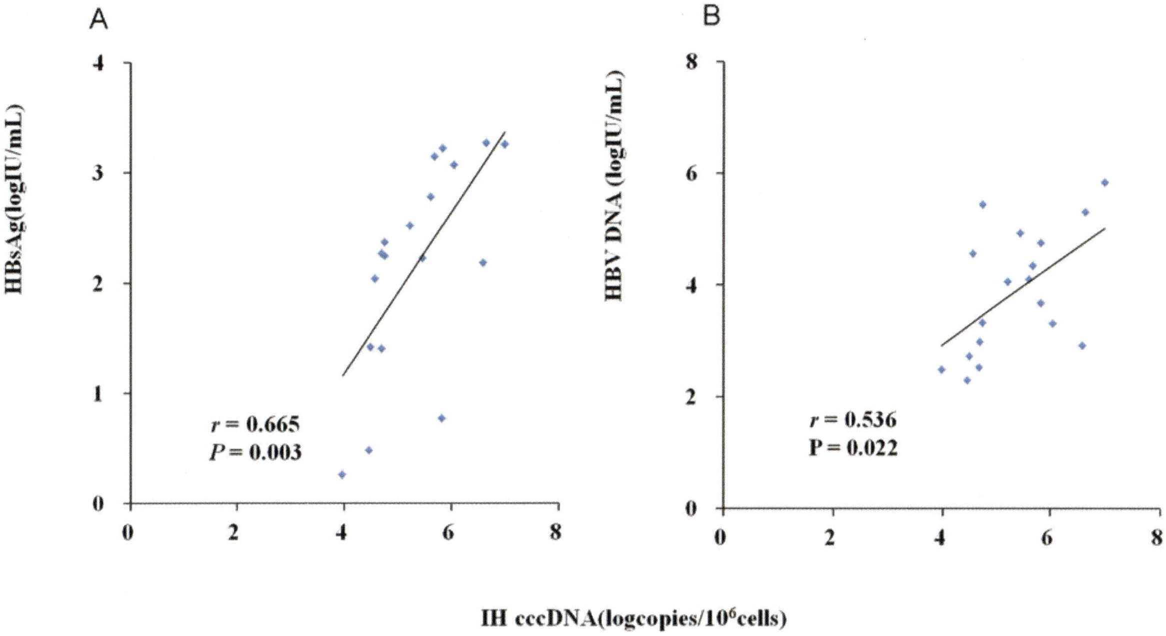

Figure 3. Analysis of correlation between intrahepatic (IH) HBV cccDNA and serum HBV markers for 19 patients with acute hepatitis B. Correlation between intrahepatic HBV cccDNA level and serum HBsAg level (A). Correlation between intrahepatic HBV cccDNA level and serum HBV DNA level (B).

Pearson's correlation analysis were applied to compare the data obtained by real-time PCR methods. A *P*-value (2-tailed) of <0.05 was considered statistically significant. All statistical analyses were carried out in Statistical Program for Social Sciences (SPSS 18.0 for Windows; SPSS Inc., Chicago, IL).

Results

Intrahepatic HBV cccDNA Levels in Different Groups of Patients

The median (25th–75th centile) intrahepatic cccDNA levels were 0.17 (0.04–0.68), 4.80 (4.66–136.97), 3.81 (0.23–29.43), 0.22 (0.11–1.02) and 0.97 (0–7.09) copies/cell in patients with AHB, CHB-IT, CHB-IC, CHB-LR, and CHB-ENH, respectively. HBV cccDNA level was significantly lower in patient with AHB than in

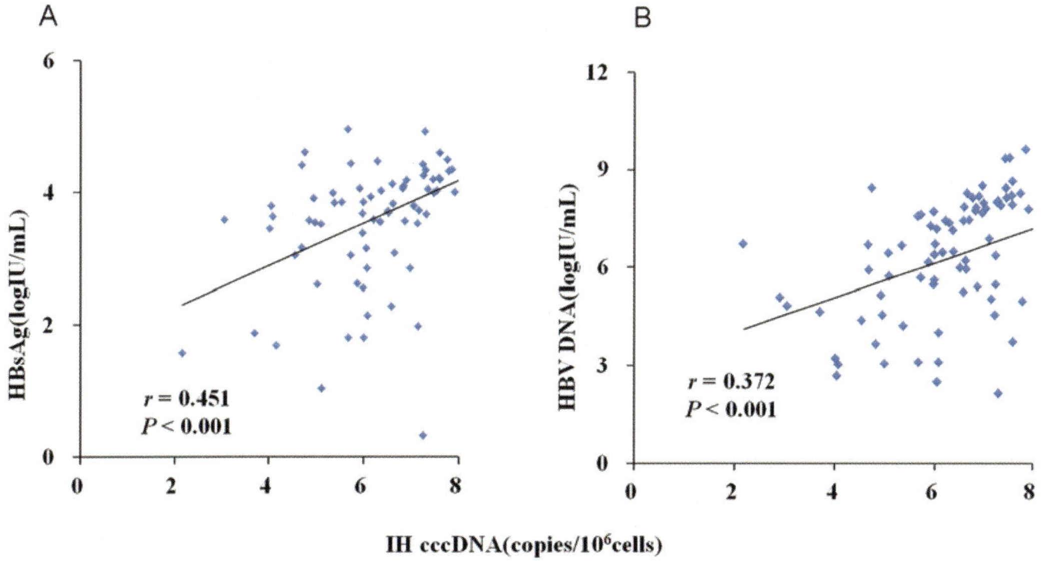

Figure 4. Overall analysis of correlation between intrahepatic (IH) HBV cccDNA and serum HBV markers across 101 patients with chronic HBV infection. Correlation between IH cccDNA level and serum HBsAg level (A). Correlation between IH cccDNA level and serum HBV DNA level (B).

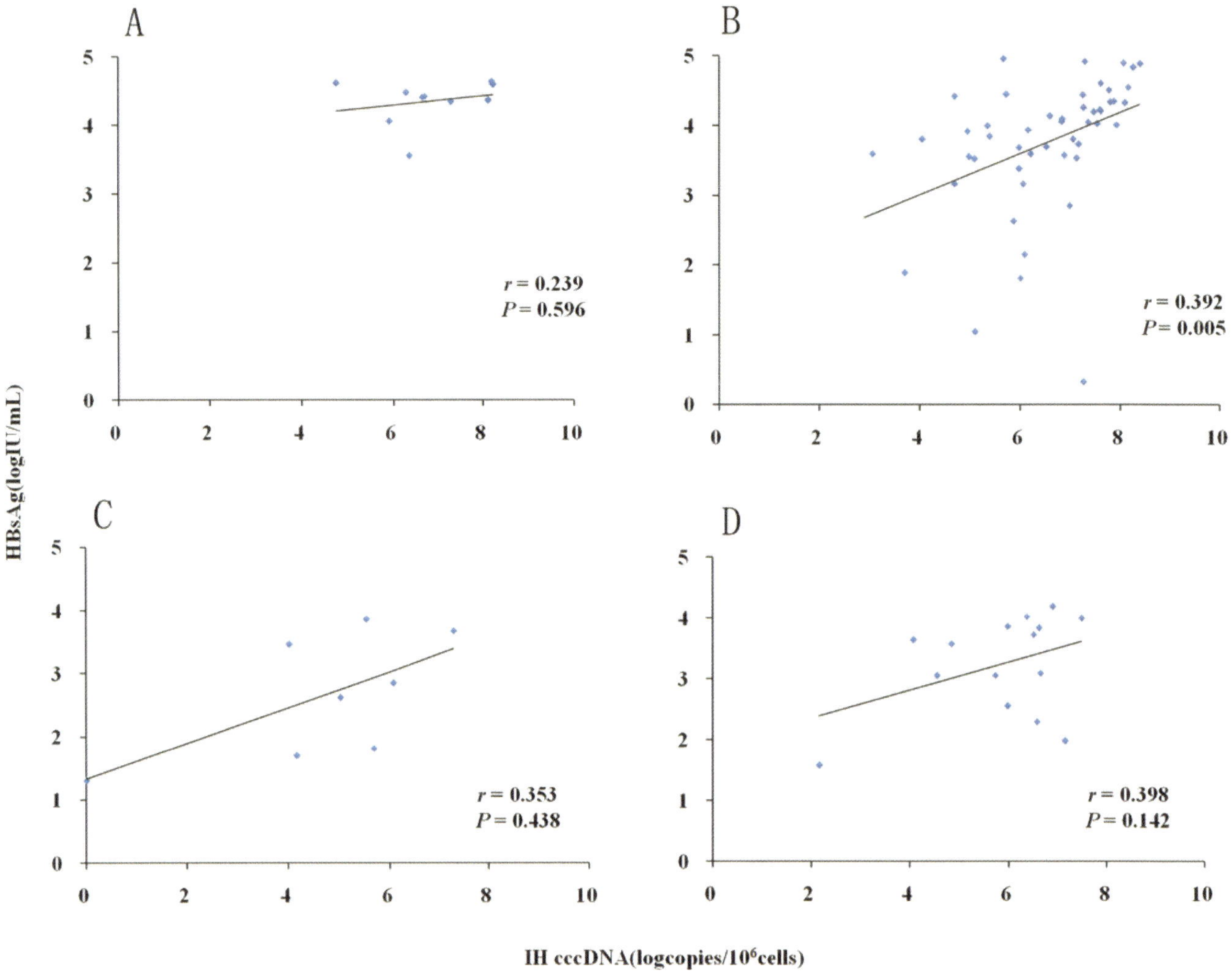

Figure 5. Phase-categorized analysis of correlation between intrahepatic (IH) HBV cccDNA level and serum HBsAg level for patients with chronic HBV infection. Analysis for 10 patients in immune-tolerant phase (A). Analysis for 59 patients in immune-clearance phase (B). Analysis for 8 patients in low-replicative phase (C). Analysis for 24 patients in HBeAg-negative hepatitis phase (D).

patients with CHB-IT and CHB-IC patients; CHB-IT and CHB-IC patients had a significantly higher cccDNA level than CHB-LR patients (Figure 1).

Serum HBsAg Levels in Different Groups of Patients

As shown in Figure 2A, the distribution of serum HBsAg level across the study population was skewed (median 3850, range 1.9–91 000 IU/ml in studied population). AHB patients had a significantly lower median serum HBsAg level than CHB patients (186 IU/ml vs. 6,330 IU/ml, $P<0.001$). Specifically, HBsAg level was different between AHB patients and CHB-IT/CHB-IC/CHB-ENH but not CHB-LR patients. The median serum HBsAg levels for CHB patients in different phases were 22 550 IU/ml (range 3 610–43 900 IU/ml) in CHB-IT patients, 8 680 IU/ml (range 2.1–91 000 IU/ml) in CHB-IC, 563 IU/ml (range 2.1–7 210 IU/ml) in CHB-LR patients, and 2 895 IU/ml (range 38–15 400 IU/ml) in ENH patients, respectively. CHB-IT patients had a significantly higher HBsAg level than CHB-LR and CHB-ENH patients. CHB-IC patients had a significantly higher HBsAg level than CHB-LR patients (Figure 2B).

Correlation of Intrahepatic cccDNA with Serum HBsAg and Serum HBV DNA

In AHB patients, positive correlation was observed between intrahepatic cccDNA and serum HBV DNA ($r=0.536$, $P=0.022$), as well as HBsAg level ($r=0.665$, $P=0.003$) (Figure 3).

In the entire cohort of CHB patients, positive correlation was observed between intrahepatic cccDNA level and serum HBsAg level ($r=0.451$, $P<0.001$), as well as serum HBV DNA level ($r=0.372$, $P<0.001$) (Figure 4). When analyzing the different phases of patients separately, the significant correlation between intrahepatic cccDNA level and serum HBsAg level was only observed in the IC phase rather than in other three phases (Figure 5); and significant correlation between intrahepatic cccDNA level and serum HBV DNA level was observed in the IC and ENH phases rather than in the IT and LR phases (Figure 6).

Dynamics of Serum HBsAg and HBV DNA Levels

In AHB patients, a progressive reduction of serum HBsAg level was observed, which was closely associated with a rapid decline of serum HBV DNA level (Figure 7). The reduction medians (25th–

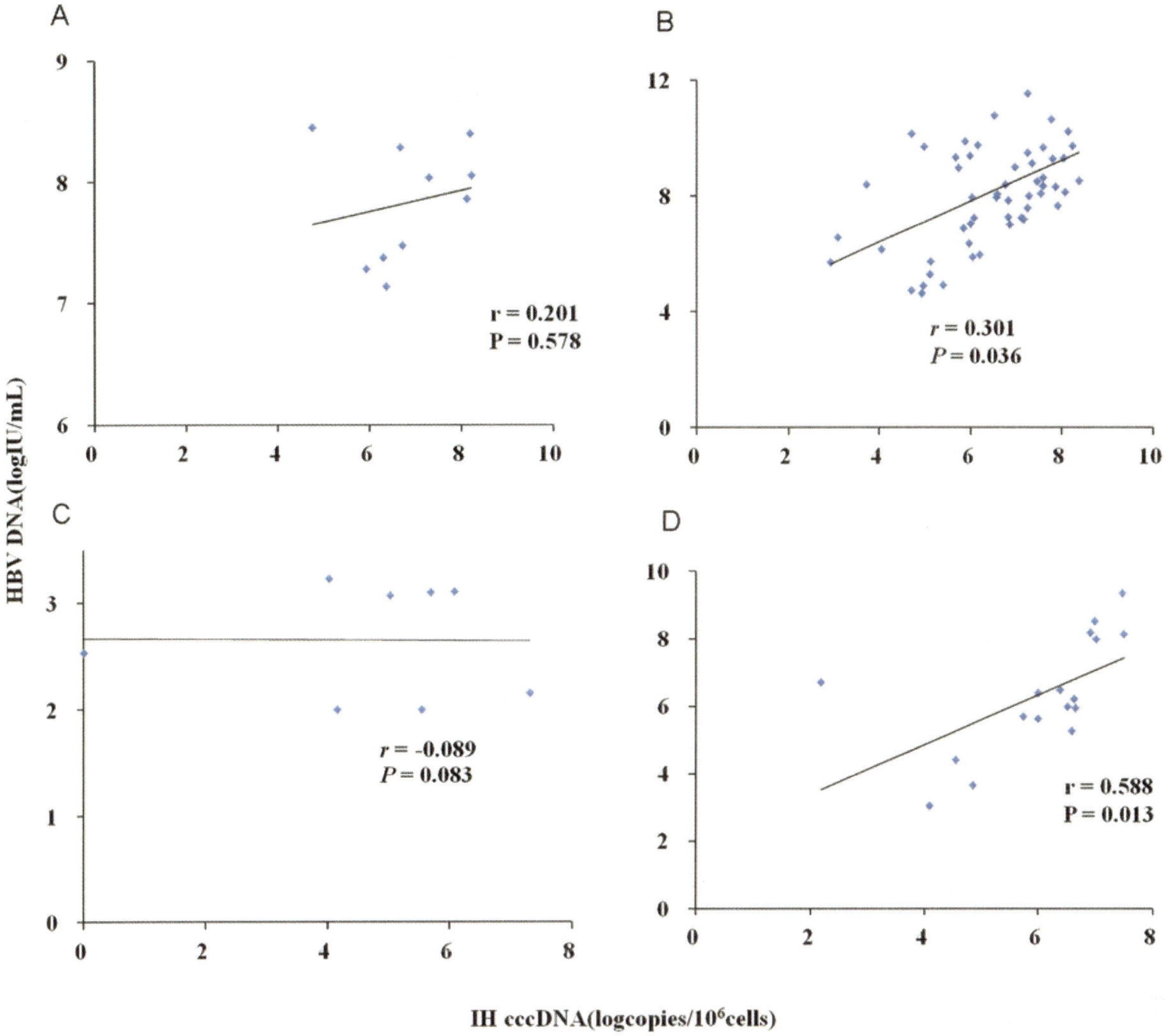

Figure 6. Phase-categorized analysis of correlation between intrahepatic (IH) HBV cccDNA level and serum HBV DNA level for patients with chronic HBV infection in different phases. Analysis for 10 patients in immune-tolerant phase (A). Analysis for 59 patients in immune-clearance phase (B). Analysis for 8 patients in low-replicative phase (C). Analysis for 24 patients in HBeAg-negative hepatitis phase (D).

75th centile) were 0.62 (0.20–2.07) and 2.54 (2.30–2.99) $\log_{10}$ IU/mL for serum HBsAg and HBV DNA 14 days post patient admission, respectively. By contrast, in CHB patients. serum HBsAg level changed much slower and its associations with HBV DNA level was weak or missing.

Comparison of HBV Replicative Efficiency among Different Groups of Patients

HBV replicative efficiency, defined as the ratio of serum HBV DNA to intrahepatic cccDNA ($\log_{10}$ serum HBV DNA/$\log_{10}$ cccDNA (copies/10^6 cells) [12], was analyzed. The replicative efficiency medians (25th–75th centile) were 0.70 (0.55–0.81) in AHB patients, 1.12 (1.01–1.24) in CHB-IT patients, 1.09 (0.78–1.20) in CHB-IC patients, 0.53 (0.22–0.66) in CHB-LR patients, and 0.99 (0.91–1.06) CHB-ENH patients. AHB and CHB-LR patients had significantly lower replicative efficiency than CHB-IT, CHB-IC and CHB-ENH patients ($P<0.001$). The values of HBV replicative efficiency were not statistically different among CHB-IT, CHB-IC, and CHB-ENH patients.

In CHB patients, HBV replicative efficiency was positively associated with alanine aminotransferase (ALT) level ($r=0.390$, $P<0.001$). Further analysis showed that replicative efficiency was correlated with ALT level only in CHB-IC patients ($r=0.515$, $P<0.001$), but not in CHB-IT patients ($r=0.333$, $P=0.347$), CHB-LR patients ($r=0.653$, $P=0.180$), or CHB-ENH patients ($r=0.221$, $P=0.393$).

In CHB-IC patients, HBV replicative efficiency had a correlation with the histological grade of active inflammation ($r=0.348$, $P=0.030$). The replicative efficiency medians (25th–75th centile) were 0.97 (0.64–1.14), 1.07 (0.91–1.23), and 1.13 (1.05–1.20) in score 0–3, 4–8 and 9–12 groups, exhibiting a stepwise elevation with the increase of the inflammation grade. By contrast, HBV replicative efficiency was not correlated with stage of fibrosis (r = 0.189, P = 0.248) (Figure 8). In the other 3 phases of CHB patients, no significant correlation was observed between HBV replicative efficiency and the liver histological activities (data not shown).

Discussion

This study for the first time revealed the comprehensive relationship of intrahepatic cccDNA with serum HBsAg and

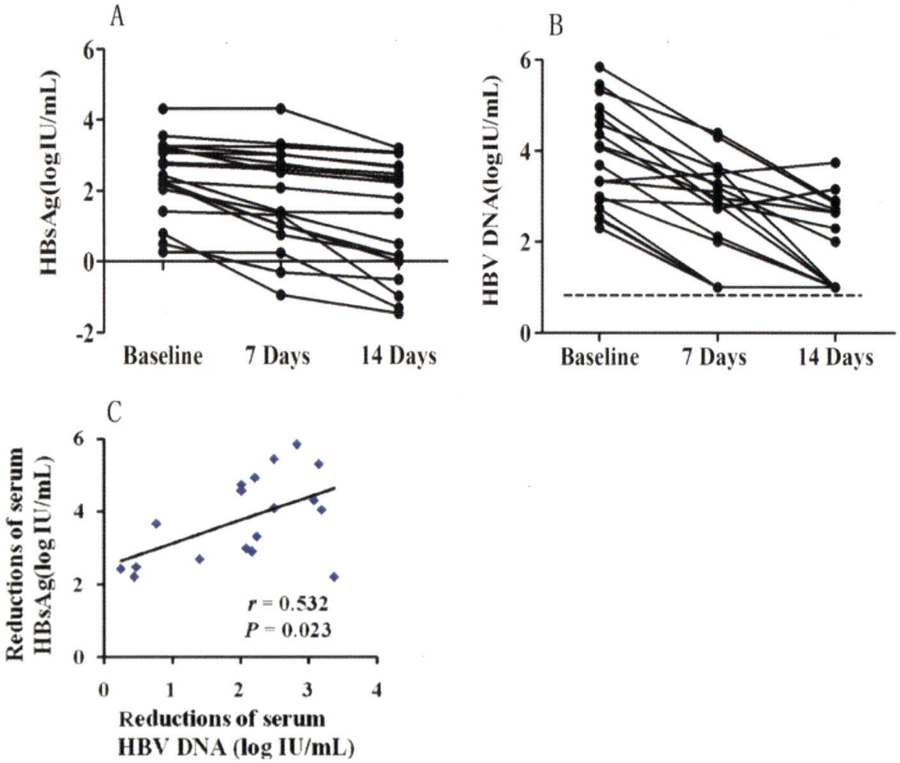

Figure 7. Monitoring of serum HBsAg and HBV DNA levels in patients with acute hepatitis B. Dynamical change of serum HBsAg level (A). Dynamical change of serum HBV DNA level (B). Association of reductions between serum HBsAg level and HBV DNA level 14 days post patient admission (C).

HBV DNA throughout the natural phases of both acute and chronic HBV infections. Previous studies have not described intrahepatic cccDNA with serum markers in AHB patients, nor CHB patients in the LR phase, owing to the particular difficulty in obtaining liver biopsy from these patients in clinical practice. The current study made a great effort to fill up the knowledge gap.

Intrahepatic cccDNA level was significantly lower in AHB patients than that in CHB patients in this study. Dynamical observation showed that both serum HBsAg and HBV DNA levels

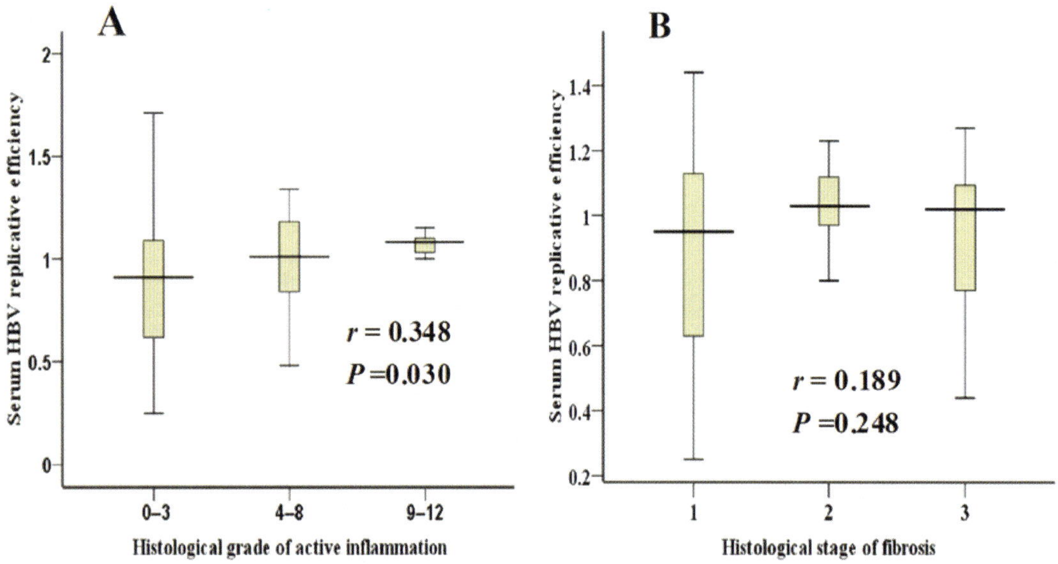

Figure 8. Relationship of HBV replicative efficiency with histological activitiesin CHB-IC patients. Correlation between HBV replicative efficiency and histological grade of active inflammation (A). Correlation between HBV replicative efficiency and histological stage of fibrosis(B).

progressively declined in a short period of time with a good correlation to each other. These evidence suggested that active anti-HBV immune response in AHB patients could effectively eliminate intrahepatic cccDNA and the effect was reflected well in peripheral. Thus, serum HBsAg and HBV DNA levels could serve as surrogate markers for intrahepatic cccDNA level in AHB patients.

In this study, HBV replicative efficiency was significantly lower in AHB patients than in CHB patients in overall, but CHB-LR patients had a low HBV replicative efficiency value similarly as in AHB patients. Consistently, patients with inactive HBeAg-negative chronic hepatitis B was observed to have a lower cccDNA level and a lower viral replicative efficiency than patients with active HBeAg-negative chronic hepatitis B [12]. This suggested that rate of active cccDNA loss was faster than the rate of total cccDNA loss when HBV activity is well checked by host immunity, such that reduced replicative efficiency may imply effective immune control of HBV infection.

Discrepancy in the relationship between intrahepatic HBV cccDNA level and histological activities has been described from previous studies [12,18,28,29]. In this study, intrahepatic cccDNA level was not correlated with histological activities of liver inflammation or fibrosis. Our results are consistent with that by Lin et al [12] and by Guner et al [18]. The reason for the lack of correlation may be that histopathological damage was developed over time or that damage was mainly caused by differences in immune response [18]. Interestingly, we found that HBV replicative efficiency (ratio of $\log_{10}$ serum HBV DNA to $\log_{10}$ intrahepatic cccDNA) was correlated with the histological index of inflammation activity and ALT level in CHB-IC patients, suggesting that HBV replicative efficiency was a valuable indicator associated with liver damage in the IC phase.

One limitation of the study is the relatively small sample size for CHB-LR and CHB-IT groups. In addition, HBV cccDNA activity could be influenced by epigenetic regulation, including DNA methylation, histoneacetylation, and microRNAs [30,31]. Whether these factors influence the association between intrahepatic cccDNA and serum viral markers needs further clarification.

In summary, the major findings of this study are that (i) Intrahepatic cccDNA levels were significantly lower in patients with AHB and CHB-LR than patients with CHB-IT, CHB-IC, and CHB-ENH. (ii) intrahepatic cccDNA level is positively correlated with serum HBsAg level in untreated AHB and CHB-IC patients, and with serum HBV DNA level in the AHB, CHB-IC, and CHB-ENH patients. (iii) Reduced HBV replicative efficiency may imply effective immune control of HBV infection. (iv) In CHB-IC patients, HBV replicative efficiency is positively correlated with inflammation in the liver. These findings provided new insights on the clinical implications of intrahepatic cccDNA and the serum viral markers in different stages of HBV infection.

Author Contributions

Conceived and designed the experiments: DX FL JZ. Performed the experiments: WL XL SL SC WY. Analyzed the data: WL YL YS. Contributed reagents/materials/analysis tools: JZ ZZ BL SX. Wrote the paper: WL DX.

References

1. European Association For The Study Of The Liver (2012) EASL clinical practice guidelines: Management of chronic hepatitis B virus infection. J Hepatol, 57: 167–185. doi: 10.1016/j.jhep.2012.02. 010.
2. Chinese Society of Hepatology and Chinese Society of Infectious Diseases (2011) Chinese Medical Association, The guideline of prevention and treatment for chronic hepatitis B (2010 version). Zhonghua Gan Zang Bing Za Zhi (Chinese J Hepatol) 19: 13–24. doi:10.3760/cma.j.issn.1007-3418.2011.01.007.
3. Papatheodoridis GV, Manolakopoulos S, Dusheiko G, Archimandritis AJ (2008) Therapeutic strategies in the management of patients with chronic hepatitis B virus infection. Lancet Infect Dis 8: 167–178. doi:10.1016/S1473-3099(07)70264-5.
4. Zoulim F (2005) New insight on hepatitis B virus persistence from the study of intrahepatic viral cccDNA. J Hepatol 42: 302–308. doi:10.1016/j.jhep.2004.12.015.
5. Laras A, Koskinas J, Dimou E, Kostamena A, Hadziyannis SJ (2006) Intrahepatic levels and replicative activity of covalently closed circular hepatitis B virus DNA in chronically infected patients. Hepatology 44: 694–702. doi:10.1002/hep.21299.
6. Levrero M, Pollicino T, Petersen J, Belloni L, Raimondo G, et al. (2009) Control of cccDNA function in hepatitis B virus infection. J Hepatol 51: 581–592. doi:10.1016/j.jhep.2009.05.022.
7. Werle-Lapostolle B, Bowden S, Locarnini S, Wursthorn K, Petersen J, et al. (2004) Persistence of cccDNA during the natural history of chronic hepatitis B and decline during adefovir dipivoxil therapy. Gastroenterology 126: 1750–1758. doi:10.1053/j.gastro.2004.03.018.
8. Sung JJ, Wong ML, Bowden S, Liew CT, Hui AY, et al. (2005) Intrahepatic hepatitis B virus covalently closed circular DNA can be a predictor of sustained response to therapy. Gastroenterology 128: 1890–1897. doi:10.1053/j.gastro.2005.03.009.
9. Bourne EJ, Dienstag JL, Lopez VA, Kostamena A, Hadziyannis SJ (2007) Quantitative analysis of HBV cccDNA from clinical specimens: correlation with clinical and virological response during antiviral therapy. J Viral Hepat 14: 55–63. doi:10.1111/j.1365-2893.2006.00775.x.
10. Takkenberg B, Terpstra V, Zaaijer H, Weegink C, Dijkgraaf M, et al. (2011) Intrahepatic response markers in chronic hepatitis B patients treated with peginterferon alpha-2a and adefovir. J Gastroenterol Hepatol 26: 1527–1535. doi: 10.1111/j.1440-1746.2011.06766.x.
11. Wong DK, Seto WK, Fung J, Ip P, Huang FY, et al. (2013) Reduction of hepatitis B surface antigen and covalently closed circular DNA by nucleos(t)ide analogues of different potency. Clin Gastroenterol Hepatol 11: 1004–10.e1. doi: 10.1016/j.cgh.2013.01.026.
12. Lin LY, Wong VW, Zhou HJ, Chan HY, Gui HL, et al. (2010) Relationship between serum hepatitis B virus DNA and surface antigen with covalently closed circular DNA in HBeAg-negative patients. J Med Virol, 82: 1494–1500. doi:10.1002/jmv.21863.
13. Lenci I, Marcuccilli F, Tisone G, Di Paolo D, Tariciotti L, et al. (2010) Total and covalently closed circular DNA detection in liver tissue of long-term survivors transplanted for HBV-related cirrhosis. Dig Liver Dis 42: 578–584. doi:10.1016/j.dld.2009.12.003.
14. Lu L, Zhang HY, Yueng YH, Cheung KF, Luk JM, et al. (2009) Intracellular levels of hepatitis B virus DNA and pregenomic RNA in peripheral blood mononuclear cells of chronically infected patients. J Viral Hepat 16: 104–112.doi: 10.1111/j.1365-2893.
15. Wursthorn K, Lutgehetmann M, Dandri M, Volz T, Buggisch P, et al. (2006) Peginterferon alpha-2b plus adefovir induce strong cccDNA decline and HBsAg reduction in patients with chronic hepatitis B. Hepatology 44: 675–684. doi:10.1002/hep.21282.
16. Chan HL, Wong VW, Tse AM, Tse CH, Chim AM, et al. (2007) Serum hepatitis B surface antigen quantitation can reflect hepatitis B virus in the liver and predict treatment response. Clin Gastroenterol Hepatol 5: 1462–1468. doi:10.1016/j.cgh.2007.09.005.
17. Wang M, Qiu N, Lu S, Xiu D, Yu J, et al. (2013) Serum hepatitis B surface antigen is correlated with intrahepatic total HBV DNA and cccDNA in treatment-naïve patients with chronic hepatitis B but not in patients with HBV related hepatocellular carcinoma. J Med Virol 85: 219–227. doi: 10.1002/jmv.23461.
18. Guner R, Karahocagil M, Buyukberber M, Kandemir O, Ural O, et al. (2011) Correlation between intrahepatic hepatitis B virus cccDNA levels and other activity markers in patients with HBeAg-negative chronic hepatitis B infection. Eur J Gastroenterol Hepatol 23: 1185–1191. doi:10.1097/MEG.0b013e32834-ba13a.
19. Chan HL, Wong VW, Wong GL, Tse CH, Chan HY, et al. (2010) A longitudinal study on the natural history of serum hepatitis B surface antigen changes in chronic hepatitis B. Hepatology 52: 1232–1241. doi:10.1002/hep.23803.
20. Chinese Society of Infectious Diseases and Parasitology, Chinese Society of Hepatology. (2000) Management scheme of diagnostic and therapy criteria of viral hepatitis. Zhonghua Gan Zang Bing Za Zhi (Chinese J Hepatol) 6: 324–329.
21. Liu Y, Zhong Y, Zou Z, Xu Z, Li B, et al. (2010) Features and clinical implications of hepatitis B virus genotypes and mutations in basal core promoter/precore region in 507 Chinese patients with acute and chronic hepatitis B. J Clin Virol 47: 243–247. doi:10.1016/j.jcv.2009.12.013.

22. Xu Z, Liu Y, Liu L, Li X, Bai S, et al. (2013) Association of Interferon-gamma induced protein 10 promoter polymorphisms with the disease progression of hepatitis B virus infection in Chinese Han population. PLOS ONE 8: e72799. doi:10.1371/journal.pone.0072799.
23. Jaroszewicz J, Serrano BC, Wursthorn K, Deterding K, Schlue J, et al. (2010) Hepatitis B surface antigen (HBsAg) levels in the natural history of hepatitis B virus (HBV) infection: A European perspective. J Hepatol 52: 514–522. doi:10.1016/j.jhep.2010.01.014.
24. Li X, Wang L, Zhong Y, Wong VW, Xu Z, et al. (2010) Hepatitis B virus (HBV) subgenotypes C2 and B2 differ in lamivudine- and adefovir-resistance-associated mutational patterns in HBV-infected Chinese patients. J Clin Microbiol 48: 4363–4369. doi: 10.1128/JCM.01518-10.
25. Seto WK, Wong DK, Fung J, Ip PP, Yuen JC, et al. (2012) High hepatitis B surface antigen levels predict insignificant fibrosis in hepatitis B e antigen positive chronic hepatitis B. PLoS One 7: e43087. doi:10.1371/journal.pone.0043087.
26. Wong DK, Yuen MF, Yuan H, Sum SS, Hui CK, et al. (2004) Quantitation of covalently closed circular hepatitis B virus DNA in chronic hepatitis B patients. Hepatology 40: 727–737. doi: 10.1002/hep.20353.
27. Zhong Y, Han J, Zou Z, Liu S, Ren X, et al. (2011) Quantitation of HBV covalently closed circular DNA in micro formalin fixed paraffin-embedded liver tissue using rolling circle amplification in combination with real-time PCR. Clin Chim Acta 412: 1905–1911. doi:10.1016/j.cca.2011.06.031.
28. Takkenberg RB, Zaaijer HL, Menting S, Kandemir O, Ural O, et al. (2010) Detection of hepatitis B virus covalently closed circular DNA in paraffin-embedded and cryo-preserved liver biopsies of chronic hepatitis B patients. Eur J Gastroenterol Hepatol 22: 952–960. doi:10.1097/MEG.0b013e32834-ba13a.
29. Larsson SB, Eilard A, Malmström S, Hannoun C, Dhillon AP, et al. (2013) HBsAg quantification for identification of liver disease in chronic hepatitis B virus carriers. Liver Int doi: 10.1111/liv.12345. [Epub ahead of print].
30. Kim JW, Lee SH, Park YS, Hwang JH, Jeong SH, et al. (2011) Replicative activity of hepatitis B virus is negatively associated with methylation of covalently closed circular DNA in advanced hepatitis B virus infection. Inter virology 54, 316–325. doi:10.1159/000321450.
31. Zhang X, Hou J, Lu M (2013) Regulation of hepatitis B virus replication by epigenetic mechanisms and micro RNAs. Front Genet 14: 202. doi:10.3389/fgene.2013.00202.

Discordance between Liver Biopsy and FibroTest in Assessing Liver Fibrosis in Chronic Hepatitis B

Mi Sung Park[1], Beom Kyung Kim[1,2,3], Jae Yoeun Cheong[4], Dong Joon Kim[5], Jun Yong Park[1,2,3], Do Young Kim[1,2,3], Sang Hoon Ahn[1,2,3,6], Kwang-Hyub Han[1,2,3,6], Chae Yoon Chon[1,2,3], Seung Up Kim[1,2,3]*

1 Department of Internal Medicine, Yonsei University College of Medicine, Seoul, Korea, **2** Institute of Gastroenterology, Yonsei University College of Medicine, Seoul, Korea, **3** Liver Cirrhosis Clinical Research Center, Seoul, Korea, **4** Department of Gastroenterology, Ajou University School of Medicine, Suwon, Korea, **5** Department of Internal Medicine, Hallym University College of Medicine, Chuncheon, Korea, **6** Brain Korea 21 Project for Medical Science, Seoul, Korea

Abstract

Background and Aims: The FibroTest (FT) demonstrated excellent diagnostic performance in the prediction of liver fibrosis in patients with chronic hepatitis B (CHB). Here, we aimed to identify predictors of discordance between FT and liver biopsy (LB) in Asian patients with CHB.

Methods: Consecutive patients with CHB who underwent both LB and FT on the same day between 2007 and 2010 were recruited from three medical institutes. Laboratory evaluations including specific parameters for calculating FT score, such as α2-macroglobulin, apolipoprotein A1, haptoglobin, γ-glutamyl transpeptidase, and total bilirubin levels, were obtained. The Batts and Ludwig scoring system was used for histological analysis.

Results: A total of 330 patients (200 male and 130 female) were analyzed. Discordances of at least two fibrosis stages between FT and LB were observed in 30 (9.1%) patients; using FT, fibrosis was underestimated in 25 patients and overestimated in 5 patients with reference to LB. Patients with discordance had a higher proportion of F3–4 ($P<0.001$) and F4 ($P=0.012$) compared with those with nondiscordance. The discordance rate was significantly higher in those with F3–4 than those with F1–2 (15.4% vs. 3.0%, $P<0.001$). Multivariate analysis demonstrated F3–4 at LB as the only independent factor for discordance ($P<0.001$; odds ratio 5.95). After adjusting fibrosis stages, neither necroinflammatory activity on histology nor serum ALT level influenced FT values independently.

Conclusion: Advanced fibrosis stage (F3–4) is the sole factor of discordance between FT and LB in Asian patients with CHB.

Editor: James Fung, The University of Hong Kong, Hong Kong

Funding: This study was supported by the Liver Cirrhosis Clinical Research Center, in part by a grant from the Korea Healthcare Technology R & D Project, Ministry of Health and Welfare, Republic of Korea (no.A102065), and by the Yonsei Liver Blood Bank (YLBB), in part by a grant from Sanofi-Aventis Korea. BioPredictive kindly provided the complimentary service for calculation of FT score. The funders had no role in study design, data collection and analysis, decision to publish, or preparation of the manuscript.

Competing Interests: The authors received funding from commercial sources, Sanofi-Aventis Korea and BioPredictive; this study was supported by the Yonsei Liver Blood Bank (YLBB) in part by a grant from Sanofi-Aventis Korea and BioPredictive kindly provided the complimentary service for calculation of FT score.

* E-mail: ksukorea@yuhs.ac

These authors contributed equally to this work.

Introduction

Accurate assessment of the severity of liver fibrosis in patients with chronic hepatitis B (CHB) is necessary not only to predict the long-term clinical course, but also to determine whether and when to begin antiviral therapy. To-date, liver biopsy (LB) has been the gold standard for assessing liver fibrosis. However, it is often limited because of its invasiveness, cost, risk of complications, poor acceptance, lack of availability of expert practitioners, and intra/inter-observer variability [1,2]. These factors make sequential LBs unfeasible, especially when repeated examinations are required to monitor the response to antiviral or anti-fibrotic treatment. Consequently, these limitations have stimulated research into noninvasive approaches. So far, two kinds of noninvasive surrogates have been identified: (1) ultrasound-based methods such as transient elastography [3,4] or acoustic radiation force impulse (ARFI) [5], and (2) biochemical marker-based methods such as the aspartate aminotransferase (AST)-to-platelet ratio index (APRI) [6], AST-to-alanine aminotransferase (ALT) ratio [7], and FibroTest (FT) (BioPredictive, Paris, France) [8], all of which combine several biochemical parameters [9].

Of these, the FT was first proposed by Poynard *et al.* [8] in 2001. It is a scoring algorithm that uses a panel of five biochemical markers, including α2-macroglobulin, apolipoprotein A1, haptoglobin, γ-glutamyl-transpeptidase (GGT), and total bilirubin to assess liver fibrosis adjusted by age and gender. Since FT was initially investigated in Caucasian populations with chronic hepatitis C (CHC), its performance as a surrogate marker for LB has been studied extensively and has shown a good correlation with histological liver fibrosis stage [10–12]. In addition, a recent study reported that FT can also predict liver fibrosis with comparable accuracy to transient elastography in Asian patients with CHB [13].

However, such indirect methods as noninvasive surrogates for LB, including the FT, are always subject to discordance compared with fibrosis staging by LB. Thus, identification of factors associated with the discordance between noninvasive surrogates and LB may enable us to determine the optimal method among several noninvasive tests. Furthermore, if the effects of other clinical variables (*i.e.*, necroinflammatory activity) on FT values other than the fibrosis stage itself are elucidated, the optimal timing for evaluation of the intrahepatic fibrotic burden could be better determined, ultimately avoiding underestimation or overestimation of the real fibrotic burden.

However, to our knowledge, investigations of these issues are scarce so far, especially for the FT. In this study, we aimed to identify predictors of discordance between LB and the FT and to investigate the potential effects of necroinflammation on FT values in Asian patients with CHB.

Patients and Methods

Patients

Consecutive patients with CHB who underwent both LB and the FT on the same day at Severance Hospital, Yonsei University College of Medicine, Seoul, Korea, Ajou University School of Medicine, Suwon, Korea, and Hallym University College of Medicine, Chuncheon, Korea between January 2007 and December 2010 were considered eligible for this study. LB was performed to assess the severity of fibrosis and inflammation prior to treatment.

The exclusion criteria were as follows: previous history of antiviral therapy; history of hepatocellular carcinoma treatment at the time of LB; LB specimen shorter than 20 mm; coinfection with human immunodeficiency virus or hepatitis C or D virus; alcohol ingestion in excess of 40 g/day for more than 3 years; and Child-Pugh classification of B or C.

The study was performed in accordance with the ethical guidelines of the 1975 Declaration of Helsinki. Written informed consent was obtained from each participant or responsible family member after possible complications of the diagnostic procedures had been fully explained.

Serum Biochemical Markers and FT Score Calculation

All laboratory data including specific parameters for calculating the FT score, such as α2-macroglobulin level, apolipoprotein A1 level, haptoglobin level, γ-GGT level, and total bilirubin level, were obtained on the same day as the FT and LB. BioPredictive kindly provided the complimentary service for calculation of FT score. The discriminant cutoff values for fibrosis stage as estimated by the FT were based on a previous study (F1, FT <0.32; F2, $0.32\leq$ FT <0.52; F3, $0.52\leq$ FT <0.68; F4, FT ≥ 0.68) [13].

Liver Biopsy Examination

Percutaneous LB was performed using a 16G disposable needle. The LB specimens were fixed in formalin and embedded in paraffin. Sections 4 mm thick were then stained with hematoxylin and eosin and Masson's trichrome. All liver tissue samples were evaluated by an experienced hepatopathologist in each institute blinded to the patients' clinical histories. Specimens that were shorter than 17 mm and considered by the pathologists to be unsuitable for fibrosis assessment were excluded from the analysis. Liver histology was evaluated semiquantitatively according to the Batts and Ludwig scoring system [14]. Fibrosis was staged on a 0–4 scale: F0, no fibrosis; F1, portal fibrosis; F2, periportal fibrosis; F3, septal fibrosis; and F4, cirrhosis. Significant fibrosis was defined as F2 or more, advanced fibrosis as F3 or more, and cirrhosis as F4.

Statistical Analysis

Continuous variables of patients with discordance and those without were compared with independent *t*-tests or Mann-Whitney U tests, as appropriate. The chi-squared or Fisher's exact tests were used for categorical variables. Based on previous studies [15–17], discordance was defined as a discordance of at least two stages between fibrosis stages determined by the FT and LB. Subsequent multivariate analysis using binary logistic regression analyses was performed to identify independent factors related to discordance between fibrosis stage of the FT and LB. Odds ratios (ORs) and corresponding 95% confidence intervals (CIs) were also indicated.

Statistical analyses were performed using the SPSS software (ver. 18.0; SPSS Inc., Chicago, IL, USA). In all analyses, a value of $P<0.05$ was taken to indicate statistical significance.

Results

Baseline Characteristics of the Study Population

A total of 628 consecutive patients were screened for possible inclusion in the study. Based on the above exclusion criteria, a total of 330 patients (200 male and 130 female) were finally analyzed (Figure 1).

Baseline characteristics of study cohort are summarized in Table 1. The median age was 44 years, and male gender predominated (n = 200, 60.6%). The median AST and ALT levels were 42 IU/L (range, 12–385) and 51 IU/L (range, 5–551), respectively. All patients had well-preserved liver functions with Child-Pugh class A.

Liver Histology and Corresponding FT Values

The median length of LB samples was 22 mm (range, 20–25). The distribution of FT values according to maximal inflammatory activity in each fibrosis stage is shown in Table 2. The mean FT values increased significantly as fibrosis stage increased (0.23±0.17 for F1, 0.35±0.18 for F2, 0.59±0.21 for F3, and 0.71±0.21 for F4; all $P<0.001$ between each fibrosis stage) (Table 2 and Figure 2).

Using discriminant cutoff values to predict each fibrosis state (F1, F2, F3, and F4) by the FT (values were suggested in a previous study [13]), a discordance of at least two stages (gray) between the

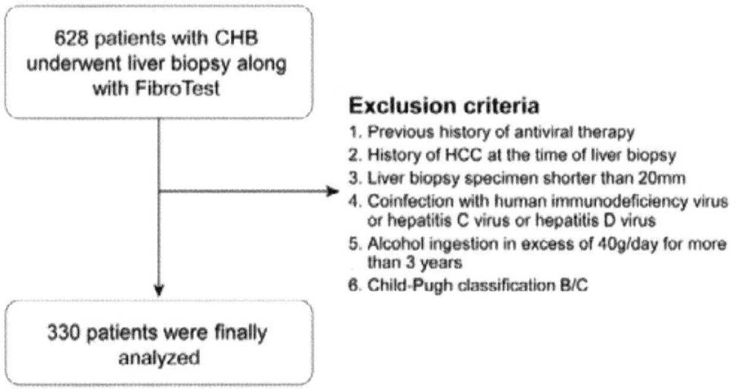

Figure 1. Flow chart describing the selection of the study population. CHB; Chronic hepatitis B, HCC; hepatocellular carcinoma.

Table 1. Baseline characteristics (n = 330).

Variables	Value
Demographic data	
Age (years)	44 (20–83)
Male gender	200 (60.6)
Body mass index (kg/m^2)	23.4 (15.1–35.8)
Obesity (≥30 kg/m^2)	9 (2.7)
Laboratory data	
Serum albumin (g/dL)	4.3 (2.9–5.4)
Total bilirubin (mg/dL)	0.7 (0.2–2.0)
Aspartate aminotransferase (IU/L)	42 (12–385)
Alanine aminotransferase (IU/L)	51 (5–551)
Prothrombin time (INR)	1.1 (0.91–1.25)
Platelet count (10^9/L)	186 (80–489)

Values are expressed as median (range) or no. (%).
INR, international normalized ratio.

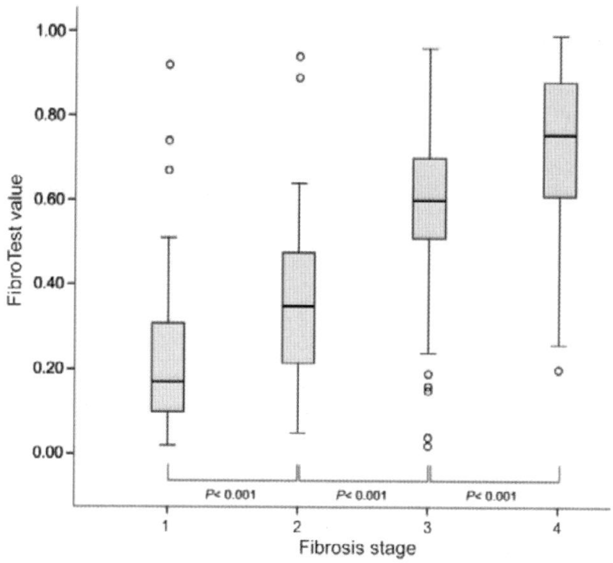

Figure 2. Box plots of FT values according to fibrosis stage. Mean FT values increase significantly as fibrosis stage increase (0.17 for F1 (range, 0.02–0.92), 0.35 for F2 (range, 0.05–0.94), 0.6 for F3 (range, 0.02–0.96), and 0.76 for F4 (range, 0.2–0.99), all $P<0.001$ among fibrosis stages).

FT and LB was observed in 30 (9.1%) patients (Table 3). On the whole, using the FT, fibrosis stage was underestimated in 25 patients and overestimated in 5 patients with reference to LB (Table 3).

Factors Affecting the Discordance between Histology and FT Values

When we compared baseline characteristics of patients with nondiscordance and those with discordance, patients with discordance had a higher proportion of F3–4 ($P<0.001$) and F4 ($P=0.012$) than those with nondiscordance, with statistical significance (Table 4). The discordance rate was significantly higher in patients with F3–4 than in those with F1–2 (15.4% vs. 3.0%, respectively; $P<0.001$) (Figure 3).

Subsequent multivariate analysis demonstrated that F3–4 at the time of LB was selected as the only independent factor for discordance between the two tests showing a positive correlation ($P<0.001$; adjusted OR, 5.95; 95% CI 2.22–15.96) (Table 5).

Influence of Histological Necroinflammation and ALT Level on FT Values

Although significant differences in necroinflammatory activity and serum ALT level between patients with discordance and those with nondiscordance were not detected (Table 4), previous studies of ultrasound-based tests such as transient elastography and ARFI [5,16,18] reported overestimation of fibrosis due to secondary effects of high ALT levels and/or necroinflammation. Thus, we further analyzed the influence of histological necroinflammation and ALT level in our cohort.

FT values between patients with maximal activity of grades 1–2 and 3–4 were statistically equivalent in each fibrosis stage (all $P>0.05$, Figure 4). In addition, there was no significant difference in FibroTest value between patients with normal ALT and those with high ALT in each fibrosis stage (all $P>0.05$, Figure 5).

Factors Affecting Discordance Based on External Cutoff Values

When we used the external cutoff values from BioPredictive (0.49, 0.59, and 0.75 for F ≥2, F ≥3, and F >4, respectively), discordances between the FT and LB were found in 41 (12.4%) patients; 36 patients were underestimated using the FT, whereas 5 patients were overestimated. Similarly, a higher proportion of patients with an advanced fibrosis stage (F3–4) were identified in patients with discordance ($P<0.001$). On multivariate analysis, advanced fibrosis stage (F3–4) was the only predictor positively

Table 2. Liver histology and corresponding FT values (n = 330).

Fibrosis		FT value*	Maximal activity^a		FT value*
Stage	**no. (%)**	**Mean ± SD**	**Grade**	**no.**	**Mean ± SD**
1	65 (19.7)	0.23±0.17	1	32	0.22±0.18
			2	26	0.24±0.18
			3	6	0.21±0.11
			4	1	0.07
2	103 (31.2)	0.35±0.18	1	11	0.35±0.15
			2	51	0.32±0.18
			3	27	0.38±0.19
			4	14	0.40±0.14
3	84 (25.5)	0.59±0.21	1	6	0.49±0.16
			2	28	0.58±0.21
			3	39	0.61±0.20
			4	11	0.58±0.24
4	78 (23.6)	0.71±0.21	1	7	0.75±0.24
			2	53	0.72±0.21
			3	16	0.68±0.21
			4	2	0.76±0.11

FT values* are described as mean ± standard deviation.
Maximal activity^a grade was defined as the higher one between lobular and periportal activity.

Table 3. Distribution of fibrosis stages according to histology and FT.

Fibrosis stage estimated by histology	Fibrosis stage estimated by FT			
	F1	F2	F3	F4
	FT<0.32	0.32≤FT<0.52	0.52≤FT<0.68	FT≥0.68
F1 (n = 65)	50	12	**1**	**2**
F2 (n = 103)	46	40	45	**2**
F3 (n = 84)	**11**	12	36	25
F4 (n = 78)	**8**	**6**	10	54
Total (n = 330)	115	70	92	83

affecting discordance between the FT and LB ($P<0.001$; adjusted OR 9.31, 95% CI 3.55–24.42) (Table S1).

Discussion

The FT is known to show good diagnostic performance with reference to fibrosis stages of LB in not only the Caucasian population with CHC, but also Asian patients with CHB [10–13]. However, noninvasive surrogates for LB including the FT, no matter how they achieve their excellent diagnostic performance, are inherently subject to discordance compared with the fibrosis staging by LB primarily because noninvasive surrogates indirectly assess the total fibrotic burden instead of the architectural changes in liver parenchyma, which is the major factor in histological evaluation [19]. Nevertheless, because LB is the current gold standard, identification of factors associated with the discordance between noninvasive surrogates and LB is an important prerequisite for accurate assessment of the intrahepatic fibrotic burden. However, investigations on this issue are scarce so far, especially for the FT. In addition, data on the influence of necroinflammation on the FT value are lacking, which can be an important issue for two reasons: first, patients in whom LB is required usually have evidence of necroinflammation along with fibrotic burden; and second, probable effects (*i.e.*, overestimation of fibrosis stage) of necroinflammation have been reported for several surrogate tests [5]. Therefore, our findings will assist formulation of guidelines for optimal evaluation of the intrahepatic fibrotic burden, ultimately avoiding underestimation or overestimation of the real fibrotic burden.

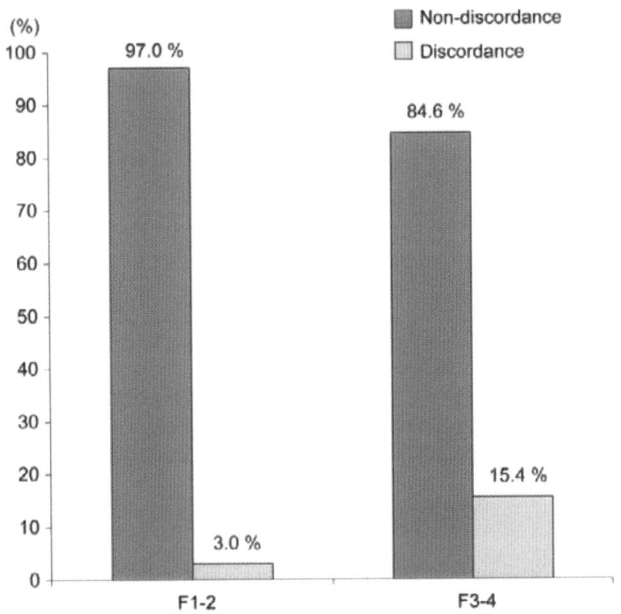

Figure 3. Percentage of patients with non-discordance and those with discordance in fibrosis stage 1–2 (F1–2) vs. fibrosis stage 3–4 (F3–4). Patients with F3–4 had the significantly higher proportion of discordance than those with F1–2 (15.4% vs. 3.0%, $P<0.001$).

To our knowledge, this is the first study to investigate the prevalence of the discordance between LB and the FT and its predictors in Asian patients with CHB in a relative large cohort from three medical institutes. Advanced fibrosis (F3–4) at LB is a sole factor attributed to discordance between fibrosis stages by LB and the FT, indicating a greater chance of agreement between LB and the FT when patients with CHB show F0–2 at the time of LB. Indeed, most discordance in this study was caused by underestimation of liver fibrosis by the FT in patients with F3–4 (11 cases of F3 and 14 of F4 of 30 discordant cases). Furthermore, we analyzed the additional influence of histological necroinflammatory activity and serum ALT level on FT values in each fibrosis stage; neither affected either the likelihood of discordance or FT value itself. Interestingly, when we used the external cutoff values from BioPredictive, an advanced fibrosis stage of F3–4 was selected again as the only predictor of discordance.

In contrast to the FT, for transient elastography, a fibrosis stage of F0–2 is the only factor that predicts significant discordance with reference to LB in Asian patients with CHB, and necroinflammation (*i.e.*, serum ALT level more than twice the upper normal limit) has been identified as a significant confounder, which non-specifically increases liver stiffness values and thus leads to overestimation of the fibrosis stage [15–18,20]. Therefore, with active necroinflammation or ALT flares, measuring liver stiffness using transient elastography should be delayed after stabilization of necroinflammation and normalization of serum ALT to exclude such undesirable overestimating effects [21]. Such contradictory results of the FT and transient elastography are noteworthy in that they might be mutually complementary in assessing liver fibrosis in terms of combining the FT with transient elastography to enhance the diagnostic accuracy.

However, paradoxically, a histological stage of F0–2 favoring the use of the FT or F3–4 favoring the use of transient elastography cannot be revealed without LB. Therefore, the optimal diagnostic algorithm for use of these two noninvasive surrogates remains unresolved. The French guideline for

Table 4. Comparison of patients with non-discordance and those with discordance.

Variables	Patients with non-discordance (n = 300, 90.9%)	Patients with discordance (n = 30, 9.1%)	*P* value
Clinical variables			
Age (years)	44 (20–83)	43 (24–65)	NS
Male gender	186 (62.0)	14 (46.7)	NS
Body mass index (kg/m^2)	23.5 (15.1–35.8)	23.1 (18.7–31.3)	NS
Obesity (≥30 kg/m^2)	7 (2.3)	2 (6.7)	NS
Aspartate aminotransferase (IU/L)	42 (16–385)	38 (12–70)	NS
Alanine aminotransferase (IU/L)	49 (7–551)	55 (5–157)	NS
Platelet count (10^9/L)	186 (80–489)	175 (100–283)	NS
Fibrosis stage			
F2–4	238 (79.3)	27 (90.0)	NS
F3–4	137 (45.7)	25 (83.3)	<0.001
F4	63 (21.0)	14 (46.7)	0.012
Maximal activity[a]			
A2–4	249 (83.0)	26 (86.7)	NS
A3–4	107 (35.7)	9 (30.0)	NS
A4	27 (9.0)	4 (13.3)	NS

Maximal activity[a] grade was defined as the higher one between lobular and periportal activity.
Values are expressed as median (range) or no. (%).

diagnosis of uncomplicated cirrhosis [22] is an example in which the FT and transient elastography are recommended as the first-line noninvasive diagnostic tools for liver fibrosis. In these guidelines, the fibrosis stage can be confirmed without LB for a given patient if the respective fibrosis stage based on the FT and transient elastography coincides, whereas LB is recommended when there is a discordant result in fibrosis staging between the FT and transient elastography. However, although this diagnostic strategy is based mostly on accumulated data from studies on CHC, it seems reasonable to combine the FT with transient elastography for enhanced diagnostic accuracy in assessing liver fibrosis in patients with CHB when we

Table 5. Factors affecting discordance between FT and histology.

	Univariate	Multivariate	
	P value	*P* value	Adjusted odds ratio (95% confidence interval)
Clinical data			
Age (years)	NS		
Male gender	NS		
Body mass index (kg/m^2)	NS		
Aspartate aminotransferase (IU/L)	NS		
Alanine aminotransferase (IU/L)	NS		
Platelet count (10^9/L)	NS		
Fibrosis stage			
F4 (vs. F1–3)	0.003		
F3–4 (vs. F1–2)	<0.001	<0.001	5.95 (2.22–15.96)
F2–4 (vs. F1)	NS		
Maximal activity[a]			
A4 (vs. A1–3)	NS		
A3–4 (vs. A1–2)	NS		
A2–4 (vs. A1)	NS		

Maximal activity[a] grade was defined as the higher one between lobular and periportal activity.
NS, not significant.

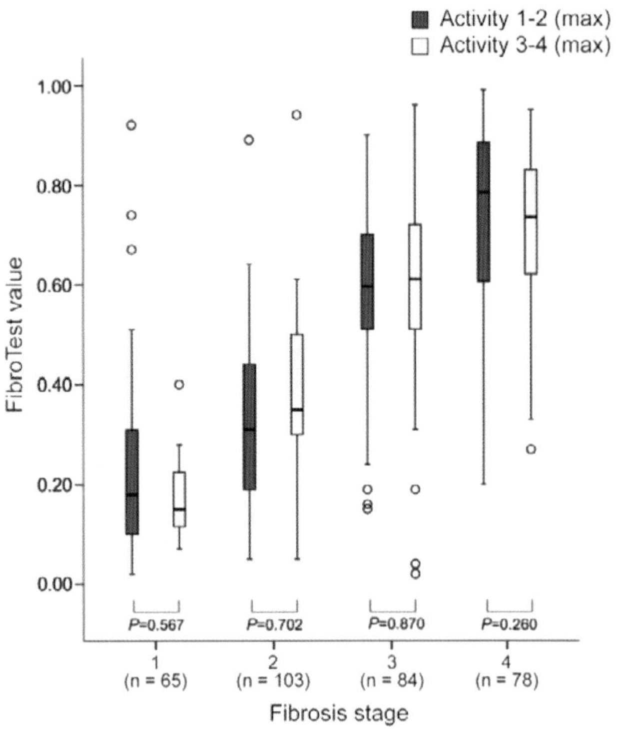

Figure 4. Distribution of FT values according to fibrosis stage and maximal activity grade 1–2 vs. 3–4. FT values were statistically equivalent between maximal activity grade 1–2 and 3–4 when stratified by each fibrosis stage (all $P>0.05$).

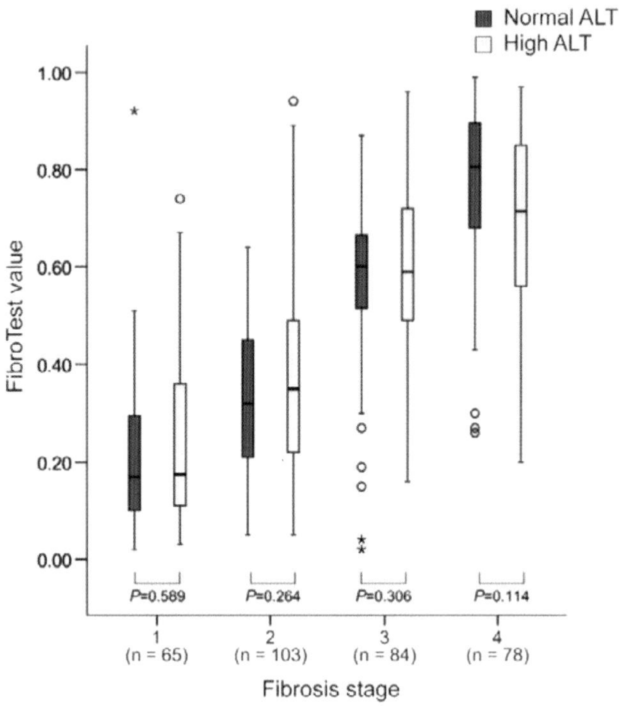

Figure 5. FT values between patients with normal ALT and those with high ALT in each fibrosis stage. FT values were statistically equivalent between two groups (all $P>0.05$).

consider the relatively lower performance of transient elastography in patients with CHB than in those with CHC [4]. The paucity of data regarding FT in patients with CHB and the increase in cost of addition of the FT should also be addressed in future studies.

This study has several strengths. First, a relatively large number of subjects from three medical institutes were consecutively enrolled, and the study population was homogenous and representative of patients with CHB generally seen in clinical practice. Second, because we recruited only patients who underwent baseline blood tests on the same day as LB, potential bias due to the gap between the two tests might have been prevented. Third, by demonstrating predictors of discordance between the FT and LB and proposing a rationale for combining several noninvasive surrogates to enhance the diagnostic accuracy, our findings will facilitate future studies that aim to propose a new noninvasive diagnostic algorithm for liver fibrosis in Asian patients with CHB.

However, we are also aware of several limitations of our study. First, there were no subjects with F0 fibrosis. Because three medical centers in this study are tertiary referral hospitals and one of the largest medical centers in Korea, patients with relatively more advanced disease are likely to be referred for close follow-up. This might have resulted in a selection bias and eventually a spectrum bias because the diagnostic performance of a given noninvasive test tends to increase in general in a cohort with high disease prevalence. Thus the diagnostic performances of FT might have been overestimated in our cohort. Therefore, another independent external validation study in a population with minimal fibrotic burden should be performed to provide more generalizable results in patients with CHB-related chronic liver disease. Second, we could not investigate the clinical role of the FT as a noninvasive monitoring tool to predict dynamic changes in liver fibrosis because a follow-up FT was not available. Third, although we identified predictors of discordance, it is unclear whether the long-term prognosis of patients with discordance differs from that of patients with nondiscordance. In addition, whether we should follow the results of the FT or LB to start treatment intervention and predict the prognosis of a given patient is unclear. Clarification of these issues requires longitudinal studies using solid end-points such as hepatocellular carcinoma or liver-related death.

In conclusion, advanced fibrosis stage (F3–4) showed a positive correlation with discordance between LB and the FT in patients with CHB. Furthermore, necroinflammation and ALT levels were not factors predictive of accuracy. Future studies should focus on methods of enhancing the diagnostic accuracy of the FT in clinical practice.

This manuscript was checked by a professional editing service (www.textcheck.com, certificate link: http://www.textcheck.com/certificate/jNAqDE).

Acknowledgments

The authors are grateful to Dong-Su Jang, (Medical Illustrator, Medical Research Support Section, Yonsei University College of Medicine, Seoul, Korea) for his help with the figures.

Author Contributions

Patient management: JYP DYK SHA KHH CYC. Conceived and designed the experiments: MSP BKK SUK. Performed the experiments: MSP BKK SUK. Analyzed the data: MSP BKK JYC DJK SUK. Contributed reagents/materials/analysis tools: MSP BKK SUK. Wrote the paper: MSP BKK SUK.

References

1. Bravo AA, Sheth SG, Chopra S (2001) Liver biopsy. N Engl J Med 344: 495–500.
2. Poynard T, Halfon P, Castera L, Charlotte F, Le Bail B, et al. (2007) Variability of the area under the receiver operating characteristic curves in the diagnostic evaluation of liver fibrosis markers: impact of biopsy length and fragmentation. Aliment Pharmacol Ther 25: 733–739.
3. Sandrin L, Fourquet B, Hasquenoph JM, Yon S, Fournier C, et al. (2003) Transient elastography: a new noninvasive method for assessment of hepatic fibrosis. Ultrasound Med Biol 29: 1705–1713.
4. Kim SU, Han KH, Ahn SH (2010) Transient elastography in chronic hepatitis B: an Asian perspective. World J Gastroenterol 16: 5173–5180.
5. Yoon KT, Lim SM, Park JY, Kim do Y, Ahn SH, et al. (2012) Liver stiffness measurement using acoustic radiation force impulse (ARFI) elastography and effect of necroinflammation. Dig Dis Sci 57: 1682–1691.
6. Wai CT, Greenson JK, Fontana RJ, Kalbfleisch JD, Marrero JA, et al. (2003) A simple noninvasive index can predict both significant fibrosis and cirrhosis in patients with chronic hepatitis C. Hepatology 38: 518–526.
7. Sheth SG, Flamm SL, Gordon FD, Chopra S (1998) AST/ALT ratio predicts cirrhosis in patients with chronic hepatitis C virus infection. Am J Gastroenterol 93: 44–48.
8. Imbert-Bismut F, Ratziu V, Pieroni L, Charlotte F, Benhamou Y, et al. (2001) Biochemical markers of liver fibrosis in patients with hepatitis C virus infection: a prospective study. Lancet 357: 1069–1075.
9. Han KH, Yoon KT (2008) New diagnostic method for liver fibrosis and cirrhosis. Intervirology 51 Suppl 1: 11–16.
10. Shaheen AA, Wan AF, Myers RP (2007) FibroTest and FibroScan for the prediction of hepatitis C-related fibrosis: a systematic review of diagnostic test accuracy. Am J Gastroenterol 102: 2589–2600.
11. Poynard T, Morra R, Halfon P, Castera L, Ratziu V, et al. (2007) Meta-analyses of FibroTest diagnostic value in chronic liver disease. BMC Gastroenterol 7: 40.
12. Halfon P, Munteanu M, Poynard T (2008) FibroTest-ActiTest as a non-invasive marker of liver fibrosis. Gastroenterol Clin Biol 32: 22–39.
13. Kim BK, Kim SU, Kim HS, Park JY, Ahn SH, et al. (2012) Prospective validation of FibroTest in comparison with liver stiffness for predicting liver fibrosis in Asian subjects with chronic hepatitis B. PLoS One 7: e35825.
14. Batts KP, Ludwig J (1995) Chronic hepatitis. An update on terminology and reporting. Am J Surg Pathol 19: 1409–1417.
15. Lucidarme D, Foucher J, Le Bail B, Vergniol J, Castera L, et al. (2009) Factors of accuracy of transient elastography (fibroscan) for the diagnosis of liver fibrosis in chronic hepatitis C. Hepatology 49: 1083–1089.
16. Kim SU, Kim JK, Park YN, Han KH (2012) Discordance between liver biopsy and Fibroscan(R) in assessing liver fibrosis in chronic hepatitis b: risk factors and influence of necroinflammation. PLoS One 7: e32233.
17. Kim SU, Seo YS, Cheong JY, Kim MY, Kim JK, et al. (2010) Factors that affect the diagnostic accuracy of liver fibrosis measurement by Fibroscan in patients with chronic hepatitis B. Aliment Pharmacol Ther 32: 498–505.
18. Coco B, Oliveri F, Maina AM, Ciccorossi P, Sacco R, et al. (2007) Transient elastography: a new surrogate marker of liver fibrosis influenced by major changes of transaminases. J Viral Hepat 14: 360–369.
19. Kim SU, Han KH, Ahn SH (2011) Non-invasive assessment of liver fibrosis: the gap between ideal and real. J Gastroenterol Hepatol 26: 937–939.
20. Arena U, Vizzutti F, Corti G, Ambu S, Stasi C, et al. (2008) Acute viral hepatitis increases liver stiffness values measured by transient elastography. Hepatology 47: 380–384.
21. Park H, Kim SU, Kim D, Kim do Y, Ahn SH, et al. (2012) Optimal time for restoring the reliability of liver stiffness measurement in patients with chronic hepatitis B experiencing acute exacerbation. J Clin Gastroenterol 46: 602–607.
22. Fontaine H, Petitprez K, Roudot-Thoraval F, Trinchet JC, Association francaise pour l'etude du f, et al. (2007) Guidelines for the diagnosis of uncomplicated cirrhosis. Gastroenterol Clin Biol 31: 504–509.

Permissions

All chapters in this book were first published in PLOS ONE, by The Public Library of Science; hereby published with permission under the Creative Commons Attribution License or equivalent. Every chapter published in this book has been scrutinized by our experts. Their significance has been extensively debated. The topics covered herein carry significant findings which will fuel the growth of the discipline. They may even be implemented as practical applications or may be referred to as a beginning point for another development.

The contributors of this book come from diverse backgrounds, making this book a truly international effort. This book will bring forth new frontiers with its revolutionizing research information and detailed analysis of the nascent developments around the world.

We would like to thank all the contributing authors for lending their expertise to make the book truly unique. They have played a crucial role in the development of this book. Without their invaluable contributions this book wouldn't have been possible. They have made vital efforts to compile up to date information on the varied aspects of this subject to make this book a valuable addition to the collection of many professionals and students.

This book was conceptualized with the vision of imparting up-to-date information and advanced data in this field. To ensure the same, a matchless editorial board was set up. Every individual on the board went through rigorous rounds of assessment to prove their worth. After which they invested a large part of their time researching and compiling the most relevant data for our readers.

The editorial board has been involved in producing this book since its inception. They have spent rigorous hours researching and exploring the diverse topics which have resulted in the successful publishing of this book. They have passed on their knowledge of decades through this book. To expedite this challenging task, the publisher supported the team at every step. A small team of assistant editors was also appointed to further simplify the editing procedure and attain best results for the readers.

Apart from the editorial board, the designing team has also invested a significant amount of their time in understanding the subject and creating the most relevant covers. They scrutinized every image to scout for the most suitable representation of the subject and create an appropriate cover for the book.

The publishing team has been an ardent support to the editorial, designing and production team. Their endless efforts to recruit the best for this project, has resulted in the accomplishment of this book. They are a veteran in the field of academics and their pool of knowledge is as vast as their experience in printing. Their expertise and guidance has proved useful at every step. Their uncompromising quality standards have made this book an exceptional effort. Their encouragement from time to time has been an inspiration for everyone.

The publisher and the editorial board hope that this book will prove to be a valuable piece of knowledge for researchers, students, practitioners and scholars across the globe.

Contributors

Yun-Hsuan Lee, Chia-Yang Hsu, Chen-Wei Chu, Po-Hong Liu, Cheng-Yuan Hsia, Chien-Wei Su, Yi-You Chiou, Han-Chieh Lin and Teh-Ia Huo
Faculty of Medicine, National Yang-Ming University School of Medicine, Taipei, Taiwan

Yi-Hsiang Huang
Institute of Clinical Medicine, National Yang-Ming University School of Medicine, Taipei, Taiwan

Teh-Ia Huo
Institute of Pharmacology, National Yang-Ming University School of Medicine, Taipei, Taiwan

Chia-Yang Hsu, Po-Hong Liu, Yi-Hsiang Huang, Chien-Wei Su, Han-Chieh Li and Teh-Ia Huo
Department of Medicine, Taipei Veterans General Hospital, Taipei, Taiwan

Cheng-Yuan Hsia
Department of Medicine, Taipei Veterans General Hospital, Taipei, Taiwan

Yi-You Chiou
Department of Radiology, Taipei Veterans General Hospital,Taipei, Taiwan

Chen-Wei Chu and Yun-Hsuan Lee
Department of Medicine, Yuanshan Branch of Taipei Veterans General Hospital, Taipei, Taiwan

Chia-Yang Hsu
Department of Biostatistics, University of California Los Angeles, Los Angeles, California, United States of America

Julia Starmann, Maria Fälth and Holger Sültmann
Unit Cancer Genome Research, German Cancer Research Center and National Center for Tumor Diseases, Heidelberg, Germany

Maria Fälth
Cellzome/GlaxoSmithKline, Heidelberg, Germany

Walter Spindelböck, Katja-Lauren Lanz and Michael Trauner
Laboratory of Experimental and Molecular Hepatology, Division of Gastroenterology and Hepatology, Department of Internal Medicine, Medical University of Graz, Austria

Carolin Lackner
Institute of Pathology, Medical University of Graz, Austria

Michael Trauner
Division of Gastroenterology and Hepatology, Department of Internal Medicine III, Medical University of Vienna, Vienna, Austria

Seung Up Kim, Ji Hoon Lee, Do Young Kim, Sang Hoon Ahn, Kyu Sik Jung, Kwang-Hyub Han, Chae Yoon Chon and Jun Yong Park
Department of Internal Medicine, Yonsei University College of Medicine, Seoul, Korea

Seung Up Kim, Do Young Kim, Sang Hoon Ahn, Kwang-Hyub Han, Chae Yoon Chon and Jun Yong Park
Institute of Gastroenterology, Yonsei University College of Medicine, Seoul, Korea

Eun Hee Choi
Department of Biostatistics, Yonsei University College of Medicine, Seoul, Korea

Young Nyun Park
Department of Pathology, Yonsei University College of Medicine, Seoul, Korea

Seung Up Kim, Do Young Kim, Sang Hoon Ahn, Kwang-Hyub Han, Chae Yoon Chon and Jun Yong Park
Liver Cirrhosis Clinical Research Center, Seoul, Korea

Sang Hoon Ahn,Young Nyun Park and Kwang-Hyub Han
Brain Korea 21 Project of Medical Science, Seoul, Korea

Susan Costantini, Francesca Capone, Eliana Guerriero, Angela Sorice and Giuseppe Castello
INT "G. Pascale" - Oncology Research Centre of Mercogliano, Mercogliano, Italy

Raffaele Marfella and Giuseppe Paolisso
Department of Geriatrics and Metabolic Diseases, Second University of Naples, Naples,
Italy

Patrizia Maio
Unità Operativa Malattie Infettive, Azienda Ospedaliera di Rilievo Nazionale "San Giuseppe Mosçati", Avellino, Italy

Michele Di Stasio
Institute of Food Science - CNR, Avellino, Italy

Giovanni Colonna
Department of Biochemistry and Biophysics and Interdepartmental Research Center for Computational and Biotechnological Sciences, Second University of Naples,Naples, Italy

Robert P. Favier, Bart Spee, Baukje A. Schotanus, Hille Fieten, Bas Brinkhof, Cornelia S. Viebahn, Louis C. Penning and Jan Rothuizen
Department of Clinical Sciences of Companion Animals, Faculty of Veterinary Medicine, Utrecht University, Utrecht, The Netherlands

Ted S. G. A. M. van den Ingh
TCCI Consultancy BV, Utrecht,The Netherlands

Martin-Walter Welker, David Reichert, Simone Susser, Christoph Sarrazin, Yolanda Martinez, Stefan Zeuzem, Albrecht Piiper and Bernd Kronenberger
Medizinische Klinik 1, Klinikum der Johann Wolfgang Goethe-Universita¨t, Theodor-Stern-Kai 7, Frankfurt am Main, Germany

Eva Herrmann
Fachbereich Medizin, Institut für Biostatistik und mathematische Modellierung, Johann Wolfang Goethe-Universität, Frankfurt am Main, Germany

Roberto Muga, Arantza Sanvisens, Daniel Fuster, Jordi Tor and Elisenda Martínez
Department of Internal Medicine, Hospital Universitari Germans Trias i Pujol, Universitat Autònoma Barcelona, Barcelona, Spain

Daniel Fuster
Section of General Internal Medicine,Boston Medical Center, Boston University School of Medicine, Boston, Massachusetts, United States of America

Santiago Pérez-Hoyos
Department of Public Health, Institut de Recerca Hospital Vall d'Hebrón, Universitat Auto`noma Barcelona, Barcelona, Spain

Alvaro Muñoz
Department of Epidemiology, Johns Hopkins University, Bloomberg School of Public Health, Baltimore,Maryland, United States of America

Bettina Langhans, Hans Dieter Nischalke, Simone Arndt, Ingrid Braunschweiger, Jacob Nattermann, Tilman Sauerbruch and Ulrich Spengler
Department of Internal Medicine I, University of Bonn, Bonn, Germany

Fu-Hsiung Su, Hung-Yi Chiou, Chien-Tien Su and Chih-Ching Yeh
School of Public Health, College of Public Health and Nutrition, Taipei Medical University, Taipei, Taiwan

Fu-Hsiung Su and Chien-Tien Su
Department of Family Medicine, Taipei Medical University Hospital, Taipei, Taiwan

Shih-Ni Chang
The Ph.D. Program for Cancer Biology and Drug Discovery, China Medical University, Taichung, Taiwan

Shih-Ni Chang
Institute of Biomedical Sciences,Academia Sinica, Taipei, Taiwan

Shih-Ni Chang, Pei-Chun Chen and Fung-Chang Sung
Management Office for Health Data, China Medical University Hospital, Taichung, Taiwan

Pei-Chun Chen
Graduate Institute of Epidemiology and Preventive Medicine, National Taiwan University College of Public Health, Taipei, Taiwan

Fung-Chang Sung and Chih-Ching Yeh
Department of Public Health, China Medical University, Taichung, Taiwan

Shiang-Fu Huang
Department of Otolaryngology, Head and Neck Surgery, Chang Gung Memorial Hospital, Chang Gung University, Tao-Yuan, Taiwan

Hung-Yi Chiou
Center of Excellence for Cancer Research, Taipei Medical University, Taipei, Taiwan

Cheng-Chieh Lin
Department of Family Medicine, China Medical University Hospital, Taichung, Taiwan
School of Medicine,College of Medicine, China Medical University, Taichung, Taiwan
Department of Healthcare Administration, College of Health Science, Asia University, Taichung, Taiwan

Stephanie Villar, Sandra Ortiz-Cuaran, Behnoush Abedi-Ardekani, Doriane Gouas, Andre Nogueira da Costa and Pierre Hainaut
International Agency for Research on Cancer, Lyon, France

Amelie Plymoth
Karolinska Institute, Stockholm, Sweden

Thiravud Khuhaprema, Anant Kalalak and Suleeporn Sangrajrang
National Cancer Institute, Bangkok, Thailand

Marlin D. Friesen and John D. Groopman
Bloomberg School of Public Health, Johns Hopkins University, Baltimore, Maryland, United States of America

Pierre Hainaut
International Prevention Research Institute, Lyon, France

Jian Han, Yaxin Lei, Lin Liu, Peng Liu, Junke Xia, Yulin Zhang, Hang Zeng, Lin Wang, Ling Wang and Hui Zhuang
Department of Microbiology, School of Basic Medical Sciences, Peking University Health Science Center, Beijing, China

Wen-Juei Jeng, Chun-Yen Lin,Chang-Wen Huang, Chien-Hao Huang and I-Shyan Sheen
Division of Hepatology, Department of Gastroenterology and Hepatology, Linkou Medical Center, Chang Gung Memorial Hospital, Taoyuan, Taiwan

Chun-Yen Lin, Ji-Yih Chen and I-Shyan Sheen
College of Medicine, Chang Gung University, Taoyuan, Taiwan

Ji-Yih Chen
Department of Rheumatology, Allergy and Immunology, Linkou Medical Center, Chang Gung Memorial Hospital,Taoyuan, Taiwan

Wen-Juei Jeng
Institute of Clinical Medicine, National Yang-Ming University, Taipei, Taiwan

José A. Agúndez and Carmen Mart ínez
Department of Pharmacology, University of Extremadura, Cáceres, Spain

Elena García-Martin
Department of Biochemistry and Molecular Biology, University of Extremadura, Cáceres, Spain

María L. Maestro and Marta Vidaurreta
Genomics Unit, Service of Clinical Biochemistry, Hospital Clínico San Carlos, Instituto de Investigación Sanitaria del Hospital Clínico San Carlos (IdISSC), Madrid, Spain

Francisca Cuenca and Marta Agreda
Liver Unit, Service of Gastroenterology, Hospital Clínico San Carlos, Instituto de Investigación Sanitaria del Hospital Clínico San Carlos (IdISSC), Madrid, Spain

Luis Ortega and Gabriela Díaz-Zelaya
Service of Pathology, Hospital Clínico San Carlos, Instituto de Investigacio´n Sanitaria del Hospital Clínico San Carlos (IdISSC), Madrid, Spain

Miguel Carballo
Laboratory of Molecular Genetics,Hospital de Terrassa, Terrassa (Barcelona), Spain

Avelina Suárez
Service of Clinical Microbiology, Hospital Clínico San Carlos (IdISCC), Madrid, Spain

Manuel Díaz-Rubio and José M. Ladero
Liver Unit, Service of Gastroenterology, Hospital Clínico San Carlos, Department of Medicine, Medical School, Universidad Complutense, Instituto de Investigación Sanitaria del Hospital Clínico San Carlos (IdISSC), Madrid, Spain

Christoph Roderburg, Tobias Mollnow, Cardenas, Katharina Berger, Henning Zimmermann, Alexander Koch, Mihael Vucur, Christian Trautwein, Frank Tacke and Tom Luedde
Department of Medicine III, University Hospital RWTH Aachen, Aachen, Germany

Brenda Bongaerts
Department of Pathology, Maastricht University Medical Center, Maastricht, The Netherlands

Natalia Elfimova and Margarete Odenthal
Institute for Pathology, University Hospital Cologne, Cologne, Germany

Mark Luedde
Department of Cardiology and Angiology, University of Kiel, Kiel, Germany

Claus Hellerbrand
Department of Internal Medicine I, University of Regensburg, Regensburg, Germany

Carmine Rossi, Ian Shrier, Lee Marshall, Sonya Cnossen and Chris Greenaway
Centre for Clinical Epidemiology and Community Studies of the Lady Davis Institute for Medical Research, Jewish General Hospital, Montreal, Canada

Carmine Rossi, Ian Shrier, Kevin Schwartzman, Marina B. Klein and Chris Greenaway
Department of Epidemiology, Biostatistics and Occupational Health, McGill University, Montreal, Canada

Kevin Schwartzman
Respiratory Epidemiology and Clinical Research Unit, Montreal Chest Institute, McGill University, Montreal, Canada

Marina B. Klein
Division of Infectious Diseases, McGill University Health Centre, McGill University, Montreal, Canada

Guido Schwarzer
Institute of Medical Biometry and Medical Informatics, University of Freiburg, Freiburg, Germany

Chris Greenaway
Division of Infectious Diseases, Jewish General Hospital, McGill University, Montreal, Canada

Beom Kyung Kim, Seung Up Kim, Jun Yong Park, Sang Hoon Ahn,Chae Yoon Chon, In Rae Cho, Dong-Hoo Joh, Kwang-Hyub Han and Do Young Kim
Department of Internal Medicine, Yonsei University College of Medicine, Seoul, Korea

Beom Kyung Kim, Seung Up Kim, Jun Yong Park, Sang Hoon Ahn, Chae Yoon Chon, Kwang-Hyub Han and Do Young Kim
Yonsei Institute of Gastroenterology, Yonsei University College of Medicine, Seoul, Korea

Hyon Suk Kim
Department of Laboratory Medicine, Yonsei University College of Medicine, Seoul, Korea

Young Nyun Park
Department of Pathology, Yonsei University College of Medicine, Seoul, Korea

Beom Kyung Kim, Seung Up Kim, Jun Yong Park, Sang Hoon Ahn, Chae Yoon Chon, Kwang-Hyub Han and Do Young Kim
Liver Cirrhosis Clinical Research Center, Yonsei University College of Medicine, Seoul, Korea

Sang Hoon Ahn, Kwang-Hyub Han and Do Young Kim
Brain Korea 21 Project for Medical Science, Yonsei University College of Medicine, Seoul, Korea

Salvatore Petta, Fabio Salvatore Macaluso, Maria Rosa Barcellona, Calogero Cammà, Vito Di Marco and Antonio Craxı
Sezione di Gastroenterologia, DiBiMIS, University of Palermo, Palermo, Italy

Daniela Cabibi
Cattedra di Anatomia Patologica, University of Palermo, Palermo, Italy

Chia-Yang Hsu, Yun-Hsuan Lee, Po-Hong Liu, Cheng-Yuan Hsia, Chieh Lin, Yi-You Chiou and Fa-Yauh Lee
Faculty of Medicine, National Yang-Ming University School of Medicine, Taipei, Taiwan

Yi-Hsiang Huang
Institute of Clinical Medicine, National Yang-Ming University School of Medicine, Taipei, Taiwan

Teh-Ia Huo
Institute of Pharmacology, National Yang-Ming University School of Medicine, Taipei, Taiwan

Chia-Yang Hsu, Yun-Hsuan Lee, Po-Hong Liu, Fa-Yauh Lee and Teh-Ia Huo
Department of Medicine, Taipei Veterans General Hospital, Taipei, Taiwan

Cheng-Yuan Hsia
Department of Surgery, Taipei Veterans General Hospital, Taipei, Taiwan

Yi-You Chiou
Department of Radiology, Taipei Veterans General Hospital,Taipei, Taiwan.

Chia-Yang Hsu
Department of Biostatistics, UCLA, Los Angeles, California, United States of America

Tung-Hung Su, Chun-Jen Liu, Tai-Chung Tseng, Chen-Hua Liu, Hung-Chih Yang, Pei-Jer Chen, Jia-Horng Kao and Ding-Shinn Chen
Department of Internal Medicine, National Taiwan University Hospital, Taipei, Taiwan

Tung-Hung Su, Chun-Jen Liu, Tai-Chung Tseng, Chen-Hua Liu, Chi-Ling Chen, Pei-Jer Chen, Jia-Horng Kao and Ding-Shinn Chen
Graduate Institute of Clinical Medicine, National Taiwan University College of Medicine, Taipei, Taiwan

Tung-Hung Su, Chun-Jen Liu, Chen-Hua Liu, Pei-Jer Chen, Jia-Horng Kao and Ding-Shinn Chen
Hepatitis Research Center, National Taiwan University Hospital, Taipei, Taiwan

Tai-Chung Tseng
Division of Gastroenterology, Department of Internal Medicine, Buddhist Tzu Chi General Hospital Taipei Branch, Taipei, Taiwan

Hung-Chih Yang
Department of Microbiology, National Taiwan University College of Medicine, Taipei, Taiwan

Mei-Zhu Hong, Wen-Qi Huang, Feng Min and Jin-Chao Xu
Department of Infectious Diseases, Chenggong Hospital affiliated to Xiamen University (The 174th Hospital of PLA), Xiamen, China

Zhen Lin
Department of Pathology,Chenggong Hospital affiliated with Xiamen University (The 174th Hospital of PLA), Xiamen, China

Kuang-Nan Fang
Department of Statistics, School of Economics, Xiamen University,Xiamen, China

Jin-Shui Pan
Department of Gastroenterology, Zhongshan Hospital affiliated with Xiamen University, Xiamen, China

Anonh Xeuatvongsa
National Immunization Program, Ministry of Health, Lao PDR, Simeuang Road, Vientiane, Lao PDR

Kenichi Komada, Tomomi Kitamura and Masahiko Hachiya
Bureau of International Cooperation, National Center for Global Health and Medicine, Shinjuku, Tokyo, Japan

Thongchanh Sisouk, Darouny Phonekeo,Bounthanom Sengkeopa-seuth and Vilasak Som-Oulay
National Center for Laboratory and Epidemiology, Ministry of Health, Lao PDR, Simeuang Road, Vientiane, Lao PDR

Koji Ishii and Takaji Wakita
Department of Virology II, National Institute of Infectious Diseases, Musashi-murayama, Tokyo, Japan

Masaya Sugiyama
Hepatology Research Center, National Center for Global Health and Medicine, Ichikawa, Chiba, Japan

Yuan Kong, Xiaoping Wang, Yushu Shang, Wenhua Liang, Xiaoting Ling,Zhiyong Guo and Xiaoshun He
Organ Transplant Center, The First Affiliated Hospital, Sun Yat-sen University, Guangzhou, China

Paul M. Schroder
Department of Medical Microbiology and Immunology, University of Toledo College of Medicine, Toledo, Ohio, United States of America

Antoaneta A. Markova, Verena Schlaphoff, Sebastian Lunemann, Birgit Bremer,, Michael P. Manns1,Markus Cornberg and Heiner Wedemeyer
Department of Gastroenterology, Hepatology and Endocrinology, Hannover Medical School, Hannover, Germany

Ulrike Mihm
Department of Medicine 1, JW Goethe-University Hospital, Frankfurt am Main, Germany

Natalie Filmann and Eva Herrmann
Institute of Biostatistics and Mathematical Modelling, Faculty of Medicine, JW Goethe-University, Frankfurt am Main, Germany

Thomas Berg
Department of Internal Medicine, Division of Gastroenterology and Rheumatology, University of Leipzig, Leipzig, Germany

Qintao Lai, Shiwu Ma, Jun Ge, Zuxiong Huang, Xuan Huang, Xiaotao Jiang, Yongyin Li,Mingxia Zhang, Xiaoyong Zhang, Jian Sun, William G. H. Abbott and Jinlin Hou
Hepatology Unit and Key Lab for Organ Failure Research, Department of Infectious Diseases, Nanfang Hospital, Southern Medical University, No. 1838, North Guangzhou
Avenue, Guangzhou, China

Shiwu Ma
Department of Infectious Diseases, Kunming General Hospital of PLA, Kunming, China

Xiaotao Jiang
Department of immunology, Basic Medicine School, Southern Medical University, Auckland City Hospital, Auckland, New Zealand

William G. H. Abbott
The New Zealand Liver Transplant Unit, Auckland City Hospital, Auckland, New Zealand

Shantel Olivares, Richard M. Green and Anne S. Henkel
Division of Gastroenterology and Hepatology, Northwestern University Feinberg School of Medicine, Chicago, Illinois, United States of America

I-Cheng Lee, Chen-Hao Lin, Yi-Hsiang Huang, Teh-Ia Huo, Chien-Wei Su, Ming-Chih Hou,Hui-Chun Huang, Kuei-Chuan Lee, Che-Chang Chan and Han-Chieh Lin
Division of Gastroenterology, Department of Medicine, Taipei Veterans General Hospital, Taipei, Taiwan

Ming-Chih Hou
Endoscopy Center for Diagnosis and Treatment, Taipei Veterans General Hospital, Taipei, Taiwan

I-Cheng Lee, Chen-Hao Lin, Yi-Hsiang Huang, Chien-Wei Su, Kuei-Chuan Lee and Che-Chang Chan
Institute of Clinical Medicine, National Yang-Ming University School of Medicine, Taipei, Taiwan

Teh-Ia Huo
Institute of Pharmacology,National Yang-Ming University School of Medicine, Taipei, Taiwan

Ming-Wei Lin
Institute of Public Health, National Yang-Ming University School of Medicine, Taipei, Taiwan

I-Cheng Lee
Department of Medicine, National Yang-Ming University Hospital, I-Lan, Taiwan

Shou-Dong Lee
Cheng Hsin General Hospital, Taipei, Taiwan

Kristin Wahl, Michael P. Manns and Heike Bantel
Department of Gastroenterology, Hepatology and Endocrinology, Hannover Medical School, Hannover, Germany

William Rosenberg
Centre for Hepatology, University College London Institute of Liver and Digestive Health, Division of Medicine, University College London, London, United Kingdom

Bernhard Vaske
Institute of Biometry, Hannover Medical School,Hannover, Germany

Klaus Schulze-Osthoff
Interfaculty Institute of Biochemistry, University of Tübingen, Tübingen, Germany

Matthias J. Bahr
Sana Kliniken, Lübeck, Germany

Dong Ji, Qing Shao, Fan Li, Bing Li, Xiaoxia Niu, Zhongbin Li and Guofeng Chen
Liver Fibrosis Diagnosis and Treatment Center, 302 Military Hospital of China, Beijing, China

Ping Han
Tumor Radiotherapy Center, 302 Military Hospital of China, Beijing, China

Hong Zang and Shaojie Xin
Liver Failure Diagnosis and Treatment Center, 302 Military Hospital of China, Beijing, China

Nao Nishida and Masaya Sugiyama, Naohiko Masaki, Kazumoto Murata, Masaaki Korenaga and Yoriko Mawatari
The Research Center for Hepatitis and Immunology, National Center for Global Health and Medicine, Ichikawa, Chiba, Japan

Hiromi Sawai, Minae Kawashima and Katsushi Tokunaga
Department of Human Genetics, Graduate School of Medicine, The University of Tokyo, Bunkyo-ku, Tokyo, Japan

Koichi Kashiwase and Mutsuhiko Minami
HLA Laboratory, Japanese Red Cross Kanto-Koshinetsu Block Blood Center, Koutou-ku, Tokyo, Japan

Kay Seto and Man-Fung Yuen
Department of Medicine, Queen Mary Hospital, Hong Kong

Nawarat Posuwan and Yong Poovorawan
Faculty of Medicine, Chulalongkorn University, Bangkok, Thailand

Sang Hoon Ahn and Kwang-Hyub Han
Department of Internal Medicine, Yonsei University College of Medicine, Seoul, South Korea

Kentaro Matsuura and Yasuhito Tanaka
Department of Virology and Liver Unit, Nagoya City University Graduate School of Medical Sciences, Nagoya, Aichi, Japan

Masayuki Kurosaki and Namiki Izumi
Division of Gastroenterology and Hepatology, Musashino Red Cross Hospital, Musashino, Tokyo, Japan

Yasuhiro Asahina
Department of Gastroenterology and Hepatology, Tokyo Medical and Dental University, Bunkyo-ku, Tokyo, Japan

Jong-Hon Kang
Department of Internal Medicine, Teine Keijinkai Hospital, Sapporo, Hokkaido, Japan

Shuhei Hige
Department of Internal Medicine, Hokkaido University Graduate School ofMedicine, Sapporo, Hokkaido,Japan

Tatsuya Ide
Division of Gastroenterology, Department of Medicine, Kurume University School of Medicine, Kurume, Fukuoka, Japan

Kazuhide Yamamoto
Department of Gastroenterology and Hepatology, Okayama University Graduate School of Medicine, Dentistry, and Pharmaceutical Sciences, Okayama, Okayama, Japan

Isao Sakaida
Gastroenterology and Hepatology,Yamaguchi University Graduate School ofMedicine, Ube, Yamaguchi, Japan

Yoshikazu Murawaki
Faculty of Medicine, Tottori University, Tottori, Tottori, Japan

Yoshito Itoh
Molecular Gastroenterology and Hepatology, Kyoto Prefectural University of Medicine, Kyoto, Kyoto, Japan

Akihiro Tamori
Department of Hepatology, Osaka City University Graduate School of Medicine, Osaka, Osaka

Etsuro Orito
Department of Gastroenterology, Nagoya Daini Red Cross Hospital, Nagoya, Aichi, Japan

Yoichi Hiasa
Department of Gastroenterology and Metabology, Ehime University Graduate School of Medicine, Toon, Ehime, Japan

Masao Honda and Shuichi Kaneko
Department of Gastroenterology, Kanazawa University Graduate School of Medicine, Kanazawa, Ishikawa, Japan

Eiji Mita
Department of Gastroenterology and Hepatology, National Hospital Organization Osaka National Hospital, Osaka, Osaka, Japan

Kazuyuki Suzuki
Division of Gastroenterology and Hepatology, Department of InternalMedcine, Iwate Medical University, Morioka, Iwate, Japan

Keisuke Hino
Division of Hepatology and Pancreatology, Kawasaki Medical College, Kurashiki, Okayama, Japan

Eiji Tanaka
Department of Medicine, Shinshu University School of Medicine, Matsumoto, Nagano, Japan

Satoshi Mochida
Division of Gastroenterology and Hepatology, Saitama Medical University, Iruma, Saitama, Japan

Masaaki Watanabe
Department of Gastroenterology, Kitasato University School ofMedicine, Sagamihara, Kanagawa, Japan

Yuichiro Eguchi
Department of Internal Medicine, Saga Medical School, Saga, Saga, Japan

Jun Ohashi
Faculty of Medicine, University of Tsukuba, Tsukuba, Ibaraki, Japan

Teerha Piratvisuth
NKC Institute of Gastroenterology and Hepatology, Prince of Songkla University, Songklanagarind Hospital, Hat-Yai, Songkhla, Thailand

Piyawat Komolmit
Division of Gastroenterology,Department of Medicine, Chulalongkorn University, Bangkok, Thailand

Tawesak Tanwandee
Siriraj Hospital, Bangkok, Thailand

Wattana Sukeepaisarnjaroen
Department of Medicine, Srinagarind Hospital, Khon Kaen University, Khon Kaen, Thailand

Henry L. Y. Chan
Department of Medicine and Therapeutics, The Chinese University of Hong Kong, Hong Kong, Hong Kong S.A.R

Mário G. Pessôa
Hospital das Clinicas da Faculdade de Medicina da Universidade de São Paulo, São Paulo, Brazil

Eduardo Fassio
Hospital Nacional Prof. Alejandro Posadas, Buenos Aires, Argentina, 8 Departamento de Gastroenterologia da Faculdade de Medicina da Universidade de São Paulo, São Paulo, Brazil

Suzane K. Ono
Departamento de Gastroenterologia da Faculdade de Medicina da Universidade de São Paulo, São Paulo, Brazil

Fernando Bessone
Catedra de Clınica Medica, Universidad Nacional de Rosario, Rosario,Antigua and Barbuda

Jorge Daruich
Hospital de Clínicas San Martín, University of Buenos Aires, Buenos Aires, Argentina

Stefan Zeuzem
Klinikum der Johann Wolfgang Goethe-Universitaet,Frankfurt am Main, Germany

Hugo Cheinquer
Gastroenterology Division, Hospital de Clínicas de Porto Alegre, Universidade Federal do Rio Grande do Sul (UFRGS), Porto Alegre, Brazil

Rashidkhan Pathan
Novartis Pharmaceuticals, East Hanover, New Jersey, United States of America

Yuhong Dong and Aldo Trylesinski
Novartis Pharma AG, Basel, Switzerland

Weijie Li and Fengmin Lu
Department of Microbiology, Peking University Health Science Center, Beijing, China

Weijie Li, Zhengsheng Zou, Yan Liu, Baosen Li, Ying Sun, Xiaodong Li, Shaoping Cai, Weimin Yao, Shaojie Xin and Dongping Xu
Institute of Infectious Diseases and Medical Center for Liver Failure, Beijing 302 Hospital, Beijing, China

Jingmin Zhao
Department of Pathology, Beijing 302 Hospital, Beijing, China

Mi Sung Park, Beom Kyung Kim, JaeJun Yong Park, Do Young Kim, Sang Hoon Ahn, Kwang-Hyub Han, Chae Yoon Chon, Seung Up Kim
Department of Internal Medicine, Yonsei University College of Medicine, Seoul, Korea

Beom Kyung Kim, Jun Yong Park, Young Kim, Sang Hoon Ahn, Kwang-Hyub Han, Chae Yoon Chon and Seung Up Kim
Institute of Gastroenterology, Yonsei University College of Medicine, Seoul,Korea

Beom Kyung Kim, Jun Yong Park, Young Kim, Sang Hoon Ahn, Kwang-Hyub Han, Chae Yoon Chon and Seung Up Kim
Liver Cirrhosis Clinical Research Center, Seoul, Korea

Jae Yoeun Cheong
Department of Gastroenterology, Ajou University School of Medicine, Suwon, Korea

Dong Joon Kim
Department of Internal Medicine, Hallym University College of Medicine, Chuncheon, Korea

Sang Hoon Ahn and Kwang-Hyub Han
Brain Korea 21 Project for Medical Science, Seoul, Korea

Index